MEASUREMENT OF NURSING OUTCOMES

VOLUME ONE

Carolyn F. Waltz, Ph.D., R.N., F.A.A.N., is a professor and coordinator of evaluation at the University of Maryland School of Nursing and is Program Director of the "Measurement of Clinical and Educational Nursing Outcomes" grant funded by the Division of Nursing and Program Director of the "Accreditation Outcomes Project," National League for Nursing, which is funded by the Helene Fuld Health Trust Fund. She received her B.S. and M.S. degrees from the University of Maryland and her Ph.D. from the University of Delaware. She has published numerous books, chapters, journals, and articles on measurement, nursing outcomes, and evaluation. To date, she has served as consultant to more than 100 universities and institutions nationally and internationally regarding topics such as measurement, program evaluation, and nursing outcomes.

Ora L. Strickland, Ph.D., R.N., F.A.A.N., is a professor in the School of Nursing of the University of Maryland at Baltimore where she is also the Project Director of the Measurement of Clinical and Educational Nursing Outcomes Project. Dr. Strickland earned a doctoral degree in child development and family relations from the University of North Carolina, Greensboro. She took a master's degree in maternal and child health nursing from Boston University, Massachusetts, and received a bachelor's degree in nursing from North Carolina Agricultural and Technical State University. As a nationally known specialist in nursing research, measurement, evaluation, maternal and child health and parenting, Dr. Strickland is frequently called upon as a consultant by universities, health care agencies, community organizations, and governmental agencies. She has presented over 100 public lectures, speeches, and workshops and her research has been featured in newspapers and on radio and television. Dr. Strickland is on the editorial boards of several professional journals.

MEASUREMENT OF NURSING OUTCOMES

Volume One
Measuring Client Outcomes

Carolyn F. Waltz
R.N., Ph.D., F.A.A.N.
Ora L. Strickland
R.N., Ph.D., F.A.A.N.
Editors

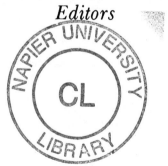

SPRINGER PUBLISHING COMPANY
New York

CA   QA 610.73 WAL

Copyright © 1988 by Springer Publishing Company, Inc.

Springer Publishing Company, Inc.
536 Broadway
New York, NY 10012

93 94 95 96 97 / 5 4 3

LIBRARY OF CONGRESS
Library of Congress Cataloging-in-Publication Data

Measurement of nursing outcomes/Carolyn F. Waltz, Ora L. Strickland,
    editors.
        p.   cm.
    Includes bibliographies and indexes.
    Contents: v. 1. Measuring client outcomes – v. 2. Measuring
nursing performance.
    ISBN 0-8261-5271-6 (v. 1). ISBN 0-8261-5272-4 (v. 2)
    ISBN 0-8261-5270-8 (2 vol. set)
    1. Nursing audit. 2. Nursing – Standards. I. Waltz, Carolyn
Feher. II. Strickland, Ora.
    [DNLM: 1. Nursing – methods. 2. Nursing – standards.
3. Personnel Management. WY 16 M484]
    RT85.5.M434   1988
    362.1'73'068 – dc19
    DNLM/DLC   88-19961
    for Library of Congress   CIP

Printed in the United States of America

CONTENTS

Preface   *ix*

Contributors   *xiii*

Part I   ILLNESS-ORIENTED MEASURES

1   Measuring the Stressful Experience of Hospital   3
    Discharge Following Acute Myocardial
    Infarction
    Jean C. Toth

2   Revision and Testing of the Haussman and   24
    Hegyvary Outcome Measure for Myocardial
    Infarction
    Sandra R. Edwardson

3   Denial and Anxiety in Second-Day Myocardial   48
    Infarction Patients
    Karen R. Robinson

4   Information Preferences and   62
    Information-Seeking in Hospitalized Surgery
    Patients
    Sarah S. Strauss

5   The Measurement of Compliance as a Nursing   81
    Outcome
    Gail Hilbert

6   Measuring Health Goal Attainment in Patients   109
    Imogene M. King

7   The Self-Administered ADL Scale for Persons   129
    with Multiple Sclerosis
    Elsie E. Gulick

8   Measuring the Clinical Outcomes of the Patient   161
    with Chronic Pain
    Gail C. Davis

9   Assessing Client Risk for Pressure Sores   186
    Davina J. Gosnell

10 Measuring Children's Fears of Medical   202
    Experiences
    *Marion E. Broome, Astrid Hellier, Thayer
    Wilson, Sandra Dale, Cathryn Glanville*

11 Reliability and Validity of Selected Measures of   216
    Chemotherapy - Induced Nausea and Vomiting
    *Susan C. McMillan, Linda H. Johnston,
    Kathy Tedford and Candace Harley*

12 Evaluation of Measures Assessing Family   231
    Responses to Chronic Illness
    Martha J. Foxall and Patrice Watson

Part II   ASSESSING THE WHOLE PERSON – MEASURING WELLNESS

13 Confirmatory Factor Analysis of the Jalowiec   287
    Coping Scale
    Anne Jalowiec

14 Measuring Social Support: Revision and   309
    Further Development of the Personal
    Resource Questionnaire
    Clarann Weinert

15 Functional Assessment of the Elderly: The   328
    Iowa Self-Assessment Inventory
    Woodrow W. Morris, Kathleen C. Buckwalter

16 Reliability and Validity of the Lifestyle   352
    Assessment Questionnaire
    Judith M. Richter

17 Validity and Reliability of a Measure of   377
    Women's Health Beliefs
    Carol Ann Gramse

18 Measuring Family Well-Being: Conceptual   396
    Model, Reliability, Validity, and Use
    Shirley M. Caldwell

19   Identifying Social and Intellectual Stimulation   423
      Available to Young Children in the Home
      Helen Lerner

      **Part III   MEASURING FACTORS IN COMMUNITY
                   BASED CARE**

20   Specific Outcomes of Nurse-Directed   443
      Colorectal Cancer Screening
      Roberta L. Messner, Sylvia S. Gardner

21   The Measurement of Client Outcomes in   457
      Home Health Care Agencies
      Sarah B. Keating

22   The Measurement of Nursing Outcomes for   475
      Home Health Care
      Janet I. Felman, Robert J. Richard

      Part IV   MEASURING QUALITY OF CARE

23   The Individualized Care Index   499
      Gwen van Servellen

24   Measuring Patient Satisfaction with Nursing   523
      Care: A Magnitude Estimation Approach
      Lillian Eriksen

      Part V   FUTURE DIRECTIONS

25   Measurement of Clinical Outcomes for the   541
      Improvement of Nursing Care: Issues,
      Dilemmas and Future Directions
      Marianne K. Zalar

Appendix   Measurement of Clinical and Educational   549
             Nursing Outcomes Project: Project
             Participants and Topic Areas

Index   557

PREFACE

The major purpose of this publication and its companion volume is to disseminate information about the measurement of clinical and educational nursing outcomes. More specifically, these volumes include nursing measurement tools, comprehensive measurement protocols for the tools, presentation of results in testing the tools (including reliability and validity assessment), discussion of results, and conclusions (including the utility of the instruments for measuring outcomes of nursing education and practice).

The tools and other methods resulted from the efforts of selected participants in the Measurement of Clinical and Educational Nursing Outcomes Project, a two-and-one-half year continuing education project administered by Drs. Carolyn F. Waltz and Ora L. Strickland at the University of Maryland School of Nursing and funded by the Division of Nursing, Special Projects Branch. Nurse researchers, clinicians, and educators from across the nation were provided the opportunity to refine their skills in nursing measurement through a series of three intensive workshops and individualized consultations. The project focused on the development and testing of clinical and educational outcome measurement tools in nursing. Enrollment was limited to nurses actively involved in research or education and selection for participation was on a competitive basis.

The objectives of the project were to:

1. Introduce participants to new and expanded measurement theories and practices that are germane to the measurement of clinical and educational outcomes in nursing.
2. Provide opportunities for participants to scrutinize measurement tools and devices currently utilized in nursing to measure outcomes in terms of new advances in measurement theory and practices.
3. Provide opportunities for participants to apply new and expanded measurement principles and practices to the development and testing of sound tools for the measurement of clinical and educational outcomes in nursing.
4. Provide for the dissemination of information about measurement of clinical and educational outcomes in nursing through the publication of workshop proceedings and outcome measures developed and/or tested by participants.

The workshops were led and facilitated by experts in measurement, nursing education, and nursing research. Each participant developed and/

or modified and tested a tool to measure a nursing outcome variable. In addition to Drs. Waltz and Strickland, the consultants involved in the workshops and in providing consultation to participants were:

Ada Sue Hinshaw, R.N., Ph.D., F.A.A.N.	Director, National Center for Nursing Research National Institutes of Health
Wealtha C. McGurn, R.N., Ph.D., C.P.N.P.	Director, Nursing Research School of Nursing The University of Texas Health Science Center at San Antonio
Marylin T. Oberst, R.N., Ed.D., F.A.A.N.	Associate Professor, School of Nursing University of Wisconsin-Madison

One hundred and four participants were selected by a committee composed of nursing leaders located throughout the United States. Of these, ninety-three of the participants continued with the project for the whole two-and-one-half year period. A listing of the participants, their degrees, afflilations, and project titles is included in the Appendix.

The papers published here were selected from those developed through the project, and include tools developed, modified, and/or tested by project participants, as well as presentations by other nurses who have developed tools to measure nursing outcome variables. These were presented at a conference open to the profession at large, and attended by approximately 250 individuals.

In essence, Volume 1 is a compendium of tools applicable to clinical settings – clusters of topic areas that address client outcomes related to illness, and those related to wellness, community-based care, and quality of care. Some of the major topic areas include, but are not limited to, coping, anxiety, stress, cadiac care, pediatric care, nursing of clients with long-term health problems, and patient-related outcome variables. Volume 2 presents tools that focus on provider-centered outcomes also resulting from the project. For example, some of the major topic areas for education include, but are not limitied to, socialization to the professional role, continuing education, clinical competencies, and student assessment.

The measurement protocol for each tool includes the following:

1. A critical review and analysis of the literature related to the outcome variable/concept selected.
2. A review and analysis of existing tools and procedures for measuring the selected outcome variable.
3. The conceptual basis of the measure.
4. Purpose and/or objectives of the measure.
5. Procedures for construction, revision, or further development of the measure.

6. Procedure for administration and scoring.
7. Methodology for testing the reliability and validity of the measure including approach to data collection, procedure for protection of human subjects where appropriate and statistical analysis procedures.

The reader will find in these volumes a collection of tools for the measurement of clinical and educational outcome variables that represents some of the finest work to date.

A variety of substantive topic areas are addressed, and in addition protoypes of methodologies for the measurement of outcome variables whose utility extends well beyond a given topic area are provided. Other benefits to the reader result from the following: all tools are conceptually based; extensive reviews of the literature and bibliographies provide state-of-the-art information regarding measurement of nursing outcomes; all tools and methods are well grounded in sound measurement theory and practices; both norm-referenced and criterion-referenced measurement frameworks are used and varied types of instrumentation, including but not limited to clinical simulations and magnitude estimation scaling, are represented; newly developed measures as well as modifications of existing methods are included; reliability and validity data are provided for all tools, often in cases where such information was not available before; and varied methods for determining reliability and validity with unrealized potential in nursing measurement such as confirmatory factor analysis and the multitrait multimethod approach are applied in an easily understood and replicable manner.

CAROLYN F. WALTZ, R.N., PH.D., F.A.A.N.
Program Director
Measurement of Clinical and Educational
    Nursing Outcomes Project and Professor
    and Coordinator for Evaluation
University of Maryland, School of Nursing

ORA L. STRICKLAND, R.N., PH.D., F.A.A.N.
Project Director
Measurement of Clinical and Educational
    Nursing Outcomes Project and Professor
University of Maryland, School of Nursing

CONTRIBUTORS

Marion E. Broome, R.N. Ph.D.
Assistant Professor
School of Nursing
Medical College of Georgia
Augusta, Georgia

Kathleen C. Buckwalter, R.N., Ph.D.
Associate Professor
College of Nursing
The University of Iowa
Iowa City, Iowa

Shirley M. Caldwell, R.N.C., Ed.D.
Assistant Professor of Nursing
Vanderbilt University
School of Nursing
Nashville, Tennessee

Sandra Dale, M.S., M.E.d.
Assistant Professor
School of Nursing
Medical College of Georgia
Augusta, Georgia

Gail C. Davis, B.S.N., M.E.d., Ed.D.
Associate Professor
Texas Christian University
Harris College of Nursing
Fort Worth, Texas

Sandra R. Edwardson, R.N., Ph.D.
Assistant Professor
University of Minnesota
School of Nursing
Minneapolis, Minnesota

Lillian Eriksen, R.N., D.S.N.
Assistant Professor
The University of Texas
Health Science Center-Houston
Houston, Texas

Janet I. Feldman, R.N., Ph.D.
Assistant Professor
Area Coordinator, Nursing Management
Center for Nursing
Northwestern University
Chicago, Illinois

Sylvia S. Gardner, R.N., M.S., C.A.N.P.
Nurse Practitioner, Ambulatory Care
VA Medical Center
Huntington, West Virginia

Cathryn Glanville, R.N., M.A.
Associate Professor
School of Nursing
Medical College of Georgia
Augusta, Georgia

Davina J. Gosnell, R.N., Ph.D.
Associate Professor, Nursing
Kent State University
Kent, Ohio

Carol Ann Gramse, R.N., Ph.D., C.N.A.
Clinical Associate Professor of Nursing
State University of New York at Stony Brook
School of Nursing
Stony Brook, New York

Elsie E. Gulick, R.N., Ph.D.
Assistant Professor and Acting Director
Office of Research
Rutgers, The State University of New Jersey
College of Nursing
Newark, New Jersey

Candace Harley
Staff Assistant/Data Coordinator
J. A. Haley Veterans Hospital
Tampa, Florida

Astrid Hellier, R.N., M.N.
Instructor
School of Nursing
Medical College of Georgia
Augusta, Georgia

Gail Hilbert, R.N., D.N.Sc.
Assistant Dean Undergraduate Studies
Widener University
School of Nursing
Chester, Pennsylvania

Anne Jalowiec, R.N., Ph.D.
Assistant Professor of Community
Health Nursing
Loyola University of Chicago
Chicago, Illinois

Linda H. Johnston, M.S., A.R.N.P.
Oncology Nurse Practitioner
J. A. Haley Veterans Hospital
Tampa, Florida

Sarah B. Keating, R.N., C-PNP, Ed.D.
Chair and Professor
Department of Nursing
San Francisco State University
San Francisco, California

Imogene M. King, R.N., Ed.D.
Professor
University of South Florida
College of Nursing
Tampa, Florida

Helen Lerner, R.N., Ph.D.
Assistant Professor of Nursing
Herbert H. Lehman College
Bronx, New York

Susan C. McMillan, R.N., Ph.D.
Associate Professor
University of South Florida
College of Nursing
Tampa, Florida

Roberta L. Messner, M.S.N., R.N.C., C.I.C.
Infection Control Nurse
VA Medical Center
Huntington, West Virginia

Woodrow W. Morris, Ph.D.
Professor Emeritus and Consultant
to the Dean
College of Medicine
The University of Iowa
Iowa City, Iowa

Robert J. Richard, M.A.
Research Associate
Division of General Internal Medicine
University of California–San Francisco
San Francisco, California

Judith M. Richter, R.N., Ph.D.
Associate Professor
University of Northern Colorado
School of Nursing
Greely, Colorado

Karen R. Robinson, R.N., M.S.
Day Supervisor, Nursing Service
Medical Center
Fargo, North Dakota

Sarah S. Strauss. R.N., Ph.D.
Nursing Service Research Nurse
Virginia Commonwealth University
Medical College of Virginia Hospitals
and School of Nursing
Richmond, Virginia

Kathy Tedford, R.N.
Oncology Nurse Clinician
University of South Florida
Medical Clinics
Tampa, Florida

Jean C. Toth, R.N., CCRN, D.N.Sc.
Associate Professor of Cardiovascular
Nursing
The Catholic University of America
Washington, DC

Gwen van Servellen, R.N., Ph.D.
Associate Professor
School of Nursing
University of California–Los Angeles
Los Angeles, California

Clarann Weinert, S.C., R.N., Ph.D.
Education Director/Associate
Professor
College of Nursing
Montana State University
Bozeman, Montana

Thayer Wilson, R.N., M.N.
Assistant Professor
School of Nursing
Medical College of Georgia
Augusta, Georgia

Marianne K. Zalar, R.N., Ed.D.
President
ZBS Research Associates
San Mateo, California

PART I
Illness-Oriented Measures

1

Measuring the Stressful Experience of Hospital Discharge Following Acute Myocardial Infarction

Jean C. Toth

This chapter discusses the Stress of Discharge Assessment Tool, a measure of stress experienced at hospital discharge following acute myocardial infarction.

PURPOSE OF MEASURE

The purposes of this research were to develop an instrument to measure the stress that patients with acute myocardial infarction (AMI) experience at the time of hospital discharge and to identify variables that may be predictors of this stress. The instrument developed is the Stress of Discharge Assessment Tool (SDAT).

REVIEW OF THE LITERATURE

Although mortality rates from cardiovascular disease have been declining since the early 1970s, this group of diseases claims more American lives each year than all other causes combined (American Heart Association [AHA], 1984; McIntosh, Stamler, & Jackson, 1978; McMillan, 1979; Schettler, 1975). AMI accounts for 56.5% of these deaths (AHA, 1984).

Since the advent of the coronary care unit (CCU), mortality from AMI

This research was supported in part by The American Heart Association, Nation's Capital Affiliate's Clinical Nursing Research Fellowship program, and by The Computer Center, The Catholic University of America, Washington, DC.

Requests for permission to use and photocopy the Stress of Discharge Assessment Tool (SDAT) may be obtained by writing to Jean C. Toth, R.N., CCRN, D.N.Sc., School of Nursing, The Catholic University of America, Washington, DC 20064.

during hospitalization has been reduced from approximately 30% of patients admitted to CCUs to 15% (Garrity, 1975; Grace, 1975; McGurn, 1981). The incidence and degree of morbidity and the incidence of mortality, however, have reciprocally increased. For example, 50% of post-AMI patients experience angina pectoris, 15% die within one year following hospital discharge, and 3% to 5% die each subsequent year from their heart disease (AHA, 1984; Goldberg, Szkol, Tonascia, & Kennedy, 1981; Segev & Schlesinger, 1981; Weinberg, Col, & Madhaven, 1982). Morbidity is also evidenced through the grief of family members and through the personal, psychological, and economic hardships of sick persons that accompany and follow illness (Volicer, 1974).

One of the roles of nursing is to initiate in-hospital interventions designed to reduce morbidity and mortality following hospital discharge. These interventions include teaching aimed toward increasing patients' knowledge of the effects of AMI and the recommendation of changes in their life-styles. Studies that have measured patient knowledge before and after such teaching programs, however, reveal that the patients did not remember the content presented to them (Rahe, Scalzi, & Shine, 1975; Scalzi, Burke, & Greenland, 1980). Explanations of these findings by the researchers included the fact that during hospitalization patients are preoccupied with survival and with family and work crises, and are not able to retain information.

These explanations were supported by Guzzetta (1979), who found a significant inverse relationship between anxiety of hospitalized AMI patients and learning, and they are in agreement with educational literature which indicates that high levels of stress interfere with learning (Conley, 1973; Redman, 1980; Sawry & Telford, 1964). A major source of stress for AMI patients at the time customarily targeted for teaching is the anticipation of hospital discharge.

The Stress of Hospital Discharge

Discharge from the hospital following AMI occurs when daily assessment of the patient's condition is no longer necessary (Toth, 1980; Weinberg et al., 1982). Although hospital discharge is generally viewed by the patient as tangible evidence of progress, increased stress is not unusual (Cassem & Hackett, 1973; Dellipiani et al., 1976; Guzzetta, 1979; Wishnie, Hackett, & Cassem, 1971).

Of special concern to nursing, then, are interventions aimed at reducing the stress that AMI patients experience near hospital discharge prior to engaging in activities designed to increase patient knowledge. Barriers to the assessment of the magnitude of stress, and therefore stress reduction, include the absence of reported personality instruments that measure the effect of stressors specific to AMI patients and limited research on variables that may be predictors of stress at hospital discharge.

Review of the literature does reveal, however, that multiple situational factors may be implicated in the degree of stress that patients experience following AMI. These variables include the presence of persistent cardiac symptoms, lower socioeconomic status, younger age, previous history of AMI, not being married, and having a more severe AMI (Andreoli, Fowkes, Zipes, & Wallace, 1979; Cassem & Hackett, 1973; Coleman, 1969; Dellipiani et al., 1976; Goldberg et al., 1981; Wishnie et al., 1971). Research findings on these variables, however, have not included information related to the combined and independent contribution of the variables, nor has their effect been reported measured at the time of hospital discharge.

DEFINITIONS OF TERMS

Stress

Theoretical Definition

Stress was theoretically defined as a generalized stimulation of the autonomic nervous system, which results in alerting the individual to the presence of a stressor(s) and mobilizes resources for coping with the changes in feelings that result (Selye, 1977).

Operational Definition

Stress was operationally defined as scores on the SDAT, which was developed during the study.

Acute Myocardial Infarction

Theoretical Definition

AMI was theoretically defined as an acute obstruction in coronary artery blood flow to an area of cardiac muscle, which results in myocardial cellular death (Andreoli et al., 1979; Guyton, 1981).

Operational Definition

AMI was operationally defined as the death of cardiac tissue as documented by cardiac history, electrocardiographic changes, and/or above normal elevations in the blood serum level of creatine phosphokinase-MB (CPK-MB).

Variables influencing stress that were studied included persistent cardiac symptoms, socioeconomic status, age, previous history of AMI, marital status, and the severity of the AMI.

Persistent Cardiac Symptoms

Persistent cardiac symptoms were operationally defined to include one or more of the following conditions that occurred at any time during hospitalization: (a) cardiac arrest, (b) cardiac rhythms that required electrical cardioversion and/or temporary or permanent cardiac pacing, (c) a new AMI or an extension of the AMI, (d) pulmonary edema, (e) presence of a cardiac condition(s) requiring aortic balloon pumping, (f) pericarditis, and (g) the return of angina pectoris; plus one or more of the following conditions after transfer from the CCU: congestive heart failure and/or cardiac rhythm disturbances preceding readmission of the patient to the CCU.

Socioeconomic Status

Socioeconomic status (SES) was operationally defined as the number of (whole) years of formal education the patients stated they had completed.

Age

Age was operationally defined as the age of the patient in whole years at the time of discharge from the hospital.

Previous History of AMI

Previous history of AMI was operationally defined as one or more AMIs prior to the present hospitalization as documented by the patient's medical records and/or by the statement of the patient.

Marital Status

Marital status was operationally defined as being married or not being married (to include those patients who were divorced, separated, or widowed) at the time of hospital discharge.

Severity of the AMI

Theoretical Definition

Severity of the AMI was theoretically defined as the amount of damage to the myocardium, as measured by the degree of elevation in the blood serum isoenzyme CPK-MB (Cohen, Pantaleo, & Shell, 1982; Guyton, 1981; Johnston & Bolton, 1982; Roberts, 1981; Roberts & Sobel, 1976).

Operational Definition

The severity of the AMI was operationally defined as the highest blood level of CPK-MB recorded on the patient's medical record, provided the isoenzyme was measured within 12 hr of cardiac symptoms and in the absence of myocardial electrical stimulation (defibrillation or cardioversion), cardiopulmonary resuscitation, and pericarditis.

CONCEPTUAL FRAMEWORK: THE PSYCHOPHYSIOLOGIC STRESS MODEL

The Psychophysiologic Stress Model (Toth, 1984) (see Figure 1.1) was used to guide the study. Based on the work of Selye (1956, 1976, 1977, 1980) and the physiologic consequences of stress (Chidsey, 1971; Folkow & Neil, 1971; Guyton, 1981), it illustrates the interplay of multiple stressors on affective and physiologic behavior that can increase the likelihood of a relapse of the AMI patient, the problem under investigation. The model also incorporates information from the following sources: review of the literature related to stressors specific to AMI patients, interviews with post-AMI patients and their families, and clinical experience with AMI patients.

The General Adaptation Syndrome

Selye (1980) defined stress as "the nonspecific response of the body to any demand made upon it" (p. 125). Selye (1980) labeled these demands stressors and emphasized that they can be physical and/or psychological in nature. Changes that occur in the body when exposed to stressors form

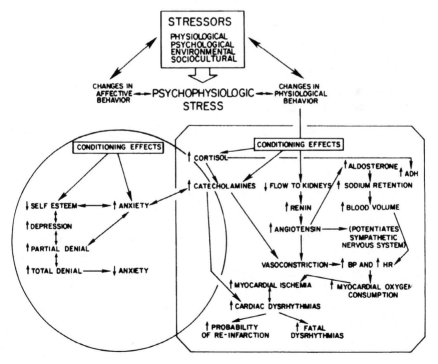

FIGURE 1.1 Psychophysiologic stress model.

what Selye (1956) defined as the general adaptation syndrome or GAS. The GAS includes the alarm reaction and the stages of resistance and exhaustion.

Alarm Reaction

The alarm reaction consists of two phases. The first, the shock phase, is characterized by a generalized stimulation of the autonomic nervous system, which results in alerting the individual to the presence of a stressor(s). The mobilization of resources for coping with the felt stress response represents what Selye (1980) defined as the countershock phase. Mechanisms of adaptation that occur during the alarm reaction include an increase in adrenocorticotropic hormone (ACTH) and cortisol, and the liberation of catecholamines, which increase the heart rate and blood pressure (Folkow & Neil, 1971; Selye, 1980).

Stage of resistance

Selye (1956) stated that this stage of the GAS occurs in response to successful adaptation to stress. Selye (1980) noted that during this stage the physical symptoms of stress almost disappear. In the event, however, that the demand (the presence or reappearance of stressors) is severe or prolonged, the alarm reaction reappears (Selye, 1980).

Stage of Exhaustion

The stage of exhaustion occurs when adaptive mechanisms are no longer able to restore equilibrium. In this stage the signs of the alarm reaction occur in an irreversible form and lead to the death of the individual (Selye, 1980).

Psychophysiologic Stress

The psychophysiologic stress response is manifested by changes in affective and physiologic behavior. These changes occur in response to moments of manifest threat, in response to any increase in alertness, and in response to an increase in the number or magnitude of psychological, physiologic, situational, and/or sociocultural stressors (Guzzetta & Forsyth, 1979; Toth, 1984). Examples of these stressors include the meaning the AMI has for the patients' short- and long-term plans, physical effects from the AMI, interference with customary ways of meeting daily needs, and changes in role. The response of the AMI patient to these multiple stressors, or psychophysiologic stress, translates into specific physiologic consequences, analogous to Selye's (1980) stage of alarm.

Changes in Affective Behavior

Although the affective response of AMI patients to stressors is modified by what Selye (1980) described as conditioning effects (individual differences), a pattern of behavior has been identified in the literature. This pattern includes a decrease in self-esteem, increases in anxiety and depression, and either partial or total denial (Cassem & Hackett, 1971, 1973; Dellipiani et al., 1976; Garrity & Klein, 1975; Gentry & Haney, 1975; Hackett, Cassem, & Wishnie, 1968, 1969; Pranulis, 1975; Speedling, 1982, Wishnie et al., 1971). With the exception of total denial, which may temporarily increase feelings of well-being (Garrity & Klein, 1975; Hackett et al., 1968), changes in affective behavior generally result in increased stress for AMI patients. Changes in affective behavior may result from or lead to changes in physiologic behavior.

Changes in Physiologic Behavior

The physiologic response to stressors was also described by Selye (1980) as being modified by conditioning effects. The response, however, is predictable and occurs in the same manner regardless of the type of stressor or demand made on the body (Selye, 1980).

The physiologic response of AMI patients to stressors includes the response of the heart muscle to the catecholamines of epinephrine and norepinephrine (Chidsey, 1971, Lefkowitz, 1976). The net effect of this response in areas of myocardial ischemia is further ischemia and an increased likelihood of dysrhythmias (Folkow & Neil, 1971). Persistent dysrhythmias, which decrease cardiac output and also increase cardiac ischemia, can precipitate congestive heart failure, an extension of the infarction, and/or ventricular fibrillation. The overall response of the noncoronary vasculature to catecholamines is vasoconstriction with a concommitant rise in heart rate and blood pressure (Folkow & Neil, 1971).

The stress response also leads to the retention of sodium through the mechanism of increased antidiuretic hormone (ADH) production (Raab, 1971). Other changes in physiologic behavior, illustrated in Figure 1.1, include the release of renin and angiotensin in response to a decreased blood flow through the kidney and potentiation of the sympathetic nervous system.

Summary

The Psychophysiologic Stress Model, which incorporates concepts from the GAS, physiology, and psychology, explains both the disease process that may result in AMI and the undesirable effects of multiple stressors for the patient recovering from AMI. This framework was also used to guide the development of items for the SDAT and to support the activities of nurses to reduce morbidity and mortality of AMI patients following hospital discharge by reducing their psychophysiologic stress response.

STRESS OF DISCHARGE ASSESSMENT TOOL

The SDAT (see pp. 21) is a 60-item, norm-referenced, paper-and-pencil test that measures the impact of stressors specific to AMI patients at the time of hospital discharge. It takes the patient approximately 20 min to answer it.

Scoring the SDAT

Scores on each item in the SDAT range from one to five points depending on the patient's degree of agreement with the item. A high score indicates high stress for that item, and a low score indicates low stress. The total possible score ranges from 60 to 300 points.

The SDAT has two parts. Part A contains 46 items that measure stressors common to most AMI patients; for example, "I am sure that I had a heart attack" (item 4). There are five possible responses to each of the items: strongly agree, agree, uncertain, disagree, strongly disagree.

Part B contains 14 items that measure the effect of stressors that may not be common to all AMI patients; for example, "My illness means that I might have to change my job" (item 55). Because of this, the additional response choice – "does not apply to me" – is provided. Items in each part measure how the AMI patient feels at the time the SDAT is answered and are not intended to measure knowledge.

METHODOLOGY FOR DEVELOPING THE SDAT

Content for the SDAT was determined through a review of the literature, interviews with former AMI patients and their families, clinical experi-

TABLE 1.1 Content Areas of the SDAT

Content area[a]	Number of items[b]
Feelings toward self	
Anxiety	4
Control	5
Denial	3
Depression	4
Perceived knowledge	5
Readiness for discharge	3
Self-esteem	1
Severity of illness	1
Social comparison	1
Spirituality	1
Total	28
Feelings toward others	
Communication	5
Responsibility to others	1
Social support	7
Total	13
Anticipation of problems	
Home-related problems	13
Work (financial)–related problems	6
Total	19

[a]Listed in alphabetical order.
[b]$N = 60$.

ence, and the expertise of an eight-member panel. The panel included two cardiovascular clinical nurse specialists, a cardiovascular nurse educator from a university setting, a cardiovascular nurse educator from a clinical setting, one cardiovascular rehabilitation nurse specialist, two staff nurses with more than 5 years, experience in CCUs and/or post-CCUs, and an educational psychologist.

Modifications to the SDAT were made in response to the panel's judgment on the clarity of the directions and items, the appropriateness of the content, the sequence of the items, and the scoring and recoding of items. Table 1.1 contains the content areas of items on the SDAT. Twenty-eight items measure the effect of stressors related to the individual reaction of the patient to the AMI, 13 items measure the effect of stressors related to others, and the remaining 19 items measure the anticipation of problems that may occur following hospital discharge.

METHODOLOGY FOR TESTING

The SDAT was evaluated on a sample of 104 AMI patients from three hospitals in the Washington DC metropolitan area, who answered it from 1 to 48 hr prior to hospital discharge. Their ages ranged from 38 to 86 years with a mean (M) of 63.6 years and a standard deviation (SD) of 10.5 years. Three-fourths were males and one-fourth females. The years of formal education ranged from 1 to 22 years (M = 12.0 years, SD = 4.3 years). Eighty percent were Caucasian and the remainder were black.

Data related to the nominal-level independent variables of the study included the following: 60% of the subjects had persistent cardiac symptoms during hospitalization, 35% were married, and 30% had a previous history of AMI. SES, age, and severity of the AMI were measured using interval data.

Scores on the SDAT ranged from 86 to 168 points (M = 132.2 points, SD = 18.0 points). Seventy-two percent of the scores fell between +1 SD and −1 SD.

Reliability and validity

The internal consistency of the SDAT was evaluated using Cronbach's (1960) coefficient alpha during the pilot and main study. Subjects in the pilot study (N = 25) were from two hospitals in the Washington DC metropolitan area; the reliability was 0.84. During the main study a third setting, also in the Washington DC area, was included. The reliability of the SDAT for the 104 subjects in the main study was 0.85.

Content validity was supported by the panel of experts. Each member of the panel reviewed the SDAT twice. During the initial review, panel members were asked to evaluate the clarity of directions and items and the appropriateness of the content, specify what topics (stressors) were missing, evaluate whether changing the sequence of the items might decrease the likelihood of biasing the responses of subjects, and validate the recoding of items. All eight members made comments and suggestions. As a result of the reviews, the wording of specific items was clarified, new items were added to measure stressors that had not been included, items that addressed more than one stressor were expanded into two or more items, and the sequence of the items was modified. Agreement on the recoding of items was reached during this review, and no changes were made. During the second review, agreement was reached relating to clarity, content, and sequencing of items. Suggestions from this review also resulted in changing the name of the instrument from Patient Questionnaire to Patient Survey. No item was deleted.

Concurrent validation of content within the SDAT related to the measurement of anxiety and depression, and their clinical manifestations were evaluated through the concurrent administration of a second instrument, the Anxiety-Depression (A-D) Scale for Medically Ill Patients (Sgroi, Holland, & Solkoff, 1970).

The A-D Scale is a participant-observer instrument that contains Anxiety (15 items) and Depression (13 items) subscales. Validity of the A-D Scale was established by its authors. Interrater reliability of the A-D Scale was evaluated on the first 10 subjects in the pilot study.

Mean percent agreement between the researcher and a second rater was 95% on both the Anxiety and Depression subscales. The Pearson product-moment correlation between raters for the anxiety subscale was $r(10) = 0.84$ and $r(10) = 0.77$ for the depression subscale. Internal consistency was measured using Cronbach's (1960) coefficient alpha on all study subjects ($N = 104$) and was 0.79 for the Anxiety subscale and 0.76 for the Depression subscale.

Pearson product-moment correlations between scores on the SDAT and scores on the Anxiety subscale [$r(104) = 0.18$, $p = 0.03$] and on the Depression subscale [$r(104) = 0.34$, $p < .001$] were statistically significant but low to moderately low in magnitude. These findings provide some support for the concurrent validity of the SDAT and validity related to the constructs of anxiety and depression within the SDAT. In addition, since the A-D Scale measures solely anxiety and depression and their effects, some support exists for the discriminate validity of the SDAT.

Validity of the major construct of stress was supported by the homogeneity of items in the SDAT. Item analysis revealed that 81.7% of the item-to-total correlations were greater than 0.20. Of the 60 items, 57 were found to have item-to-total correlations ranging from 0.08 to 0.54. The remaining three had item-to-total correlations close to zero.

Most Stressful Concerns at Hospital Discharge

Item analysis was also used to evaluate the contribution of individual items to the total score of the SDAT. The items with low item-to-total correlations (i.e., those representing the situations most troublesome to the subjects) were item 10 (I feel disappointed that I got sick), item 48 (My partner (important person) worries too much about me), item 16 (I find it hard to believe that this illness has happened to me), and item 45 (Sometimes I worry about having another heart attack). The range of score means for these items was 3.22 to 3.98, and the SDs ranged from 1.03 to 1.32. Interestingly, three of these four items measured stressors related to the self. The SD was similar in the four items.

REVISIONS TO THE SDAT

Item analysis was used again to guide revision of the SDAT for a subsequent study to measure stress over time. Revisions were minor and included the rewording of items to improve clarity of those with low item-to-total correlations and to reflect the magnitude of stress AMI patients experience whether answering the instrument at hospital discharge or during recovery at home. For example, one item was reworded from "I know what to do if I get any heart pain (angina) after I go home" to "I know what to do if I get any heart pain (angina)." No item was added or deleted. The revisions were reviewed by panel members and resulted in the second version of the SDAT.

Hypothesis Testing

Six research hypotheses, based on theory and/or research related to variables that may affect the magnitude of stress following AMI, were tested using regression analysis with scores on the SDAT as the dependent variable. The hypotheses were

H1: AMI patients who have persistent cardiac symptoms during hospitalization will experience more stress at hospital discharge than those who do not have persistent cardiac symptoms.

H2: AMI patients of lower SES will experience more stress at hospital discharge than those of higher SES.

H3: AMI patients who are younger will experience more stress at hospital discharge than those who are older.

H4: AMI patients who have a previous history of AMI will experience more stress at hospital discharge than those who do not have a previous history of AMI.

H5: AMI patients who are not married will experience more stress at hospital discharge than those who are married.

H6: Patients who have a more serious AMI will experience more stress at hospital discharge than those who have a less serious AMI.

TABLE 1.2 Summary of Regression Analysis with SDAT Scores as the Dependent Variable[a]

Step	Variable	df	R^2 Change	F^b
Blocking variables				
1	Hospital type	2,101	0.047	2.50
2	Hours before discharge	1,100	0.028	3.07
Independent variables				
3	Persistent symptoms	1,99	0.008	0.90
4	SES	1,98	0.007	0.77
5	Age	1,97	0.002	0.17
6	Previous history of AMI	1,96	0.005	0.51
7	Marital status	1,95	0.001	0.06
8	Severity of AMI	1,94	0.038	4,13*

[a] $N = 104$.
[b] Value of F for R^2 changes when variable enters into the equation.
*$p < 0.05$.

Analysis of Data Related to the Hypotheses

A hierarchical model was used to test the hypotheses (Kerlinger & Pedhazur, 1973). A summary of the regression analysis is presented in table 1.2. Two blocking variables were entered into the regression model to control for variance associated with the type of hospital in which the AMI patients were treated and the number of hours prior to hospital discharge that they completed the SDAT. The independent variables were then entered into the regression equation in the order illustrated in Table 1.2. Table 1.2 shows that only one of the independent variables, the severity of the AMI, reached statistical significance (set at alpha = 0.05). However, the variable explained only 3.8% of the variance in scores. Hypothesis 6, patients who have a more serious AMI will experience more stress at hospital discharge than those who have a less serious AMI, was supported ($F(1,94) = 4.13$, $p < 0.05$). The remaining five hypotheses were not supported.

CONCLUSIONS

Conclusions from the research included the following:

1. The reliability and validity of the SDAT was supported.
2. The severity of the AMI may be a predictor of stress at hospital discharge.
3. The following variables, previously reported to increase stress following AMI, may not affect stress at hospital discharge: persistent cardiac symptoms, SES, age, previous history of AMI, and marital status.

4. The behavior of the partner (important person) was found to be a major source of stress for AMI patients at the time of their discharge from the hospital.

Implications for Nursing

The major implication for nursing is that an instrument about which preliminary statements can be made regarding reliability and validity is available to nurses as an additional means to measure the stress AMI patients experience at hospital discharge. Assessment information is needed so that nurses can initiate interventions designed to reduce the stress these patients may experience prior to engaging them in cardiac rehabilitation teaching programs. In addition, the SDAT can be used by nurses as an independent variable to measure the effect of different types of stress reduction programs with AMI patients prior to their discharge from the hospital.

That the severity of the AMI as measured by CPK-MB blood values may be a predictor of which patients may experience high stress at hospital discharge is especially useful to nurses because CPK-MB values are generally known within 12 to 24 hr after the admission of the patient to the hospital. CPK-MB values are also routinely obtained on all AMI patients and are not an additional expense for the patient.

Another implication for nursing is that variables that have been reported to be associated with stress following AMI may not be predictors of which patients may experience increases in stress specifically at hospital discharge. Therefore, nurses need to use other methods to assess the stress that AMI patients may have surrounding discharge from the hospital. Some of these methods, in addition to the SDAT, are assessment of increases in heart rate, blood pressure, and cardiac dysrhythmias during situations stressful for this group of patients.

Nurses are keenly aware that the partner or important person can be a source of stress to the AMI patient. The finding that the item "My partner (important person) worries too much about me" was the second most stressful situation measured, lends empirical support to this awareness. One way to reduce this source of stress might be to include the partner or important person in the cardiac rehabilitation teaching program.

Recommendations

Based on the results of this study, the following recommendations are made:

1. That the SDAT be used with other samples of AMI patients for the purpose of replicating the results.
2. That the SDAT be used as a dependent variable to measure the

effectiveness of different types of stress reduction programs for AMI patients.
3. That development of the SDAT continue.

REFERENCES

American Heart Association. (1984). *Heart facts; 1984.* Dallas, TX; Author.

Andreoli, K. G., Fowkes, V. H., Zipes, D. P., & Wallace, A. G. (1979). *Comprehensive cardiac care* (2nd ed.). St. Louis: C. V. Mosby.

Cassem, N. H., & Hackett, T. P. (1971). Psychiatric consultation in a coronary care unit. *Annals of Internal Medicine, 75,* 9-14.

Cassem, N. H., & Hackett, T. P. (1973). Psychological rehabilitation of myocardial infarction patients in the acute phase. *Heart and Lung, 2,* 382-388.

Chidsey, C. A., III. (1971). Neural and hormonal control of the circulation. In H.L. Conn & O. Horwitz (Eds.), *Cardiac and vascular diseases* (vol. 1, pp. 41-53). Philadelphia: Lea & Febiger.

Cohen, J. A., Pantaleo, N., & Shell, W. E. (1982). A message from the heart: What isoenzymes can tell you about your cardiac patient. *Nursing, 12,* 47-49.

Coleman, J. C. (1969). *Psychology and effective behavior.* Glenview, IL: Scott, Foresman.

Conley, V. C. (1973). *Curriculum and instruction in nursing.* Boston: Little, Brown.

Cronbach, L. J. (1960). *Essentials of psychological testing* (2nd ed.). New York: Harper & Row.

Dellipiani, A. W., Cay, E. L., Philip, A. E., Vetter, N. J., Colling, W. A., Donaldson, R. J., & McCormack, P. (1976). Anxiety after a heart attack. *British Heart Journal, 38,* 752-757.

Folkow, B., & Neil, E. (1971). *Circulation.* New York: Oxford University Press.

Garrity, T. F. (1975). Morbidity, mortality, and rehabilitation. In W. D. Gentry & R. B. Williams, Jr. (Eds.), *Psychological aspects of myocardial infarction and coronary care* (pp. 124-133). St. Louis: C. V. Mosby.

Garrity, T. F., & Klein, R. F. (1975). Emotional response and clinical severity as early determinants of six-month mortality after myocardial infarction. *Heart and Lung, 4,* 730-737.

Gentry, W. D., & Haney, T. (1975).. Emotional and behavioral reaction to acute myocardial infarction. *Heart and Lung, 4,* 738-745.

Goldberg, R., Szkol, M., Tonascia, J., & Kennedy, H. (1981). A population-based study of factors associated with the prognosis of acute myocardial infarction. *Heart and Lung, 10,* 833-840.

Grace, W. J. (1975). Intermediate coronary care units revisited (Editorial). *Chest, 67,* 510.

Guyton, A. C. (1981). *Textbook of medical physiology* (6th ed.). Philadelphia: W.B. Saunders.

Guzzetta, C. E. (1979). Relationship between stress and learning. *Advances in Nursing Science, 1,* 35-49.

Guzzetta, C. E., & Forsyth, G. L. (1979). Nursing diagnostic pilot study: Psychophysiologic stress. *Advances in Nursing Science, 2,* 27-44.

Hackett, T. P., Cassem, N. H., & Wishnie, H. A. (1968). The coronary care unit: An appraisal of its psychological hazards. *New England Journal of Medicine, 279,* 1365-1370.

Hackett, T. P., Cassem, N. H., & Wishnie, H. A. (1969). Detection and treatment of anxiety in the coronary care unit. *American Heart Journal, 78*, 727-730.

Johnston, C. C., & Bolton, E. C. (1982). Cardiac enzymes. *Annals of Emergency Medicine, 11*, 27-35.

Kerlinger, F. W., & Pedhazur, E. J. (1973). *Multiple regression in behavioral research.* New York: Holt, Rinehart & Winston.

Lefkowitz, R. J. (1976). Beta adrenergic receptors: Recognition and regulation. *New England Journal of Medicine, 295*, 323-328.

McGurn, W. C. (1981). Cultural and psychosocial factors related to cardiac health, illness, and nursing care. In W. C. McGurn (Ed.), *People with cardiac problems: Nursing concepts* (pp. 1-14). Philadelphia: J. B. Lippincott.

McIntosh, H. D., Stamler, J., & Jackson, D. (1978). Introduction to risk factors in coronary artery disease. *Heart and Lung, 7*, 126-131.

McMillan, G. C. (1979). Part I. Cardiovascular diseases: Atherosclerotic disease and the vessel wall. *Experimental and Molecular Pathology, 31*, 163-168.

Pranulis, M. R. (1975). Coping with an acute myocardial infarction. In W. D. Gentry & R. B. Williams, Jr. (Eds.). *Psychological aspects of myocardial infarction and coronary care* (pp. 65-75). St. Louis: C. V. Mosby.

Raab, W. (1971). Cardiotoxic biochemical effects of emotional-environmental mental stresses: Fundamentals of psychocardiology. In L. Levi (Ed.), *Society, stress and disease* (pp. 331-336). New York: Oxford University Press.

Rahe, R. H., Scalzi, C., & Shine, K. (1975). A teaching evaluation questionnaire for postmyocardial infarction patients. *Heart and Lung, 4*, 759-766.

Redman, B. K. (1980). *The process of patient teaching in nursing* (2nd ed.). St. Louis: C.V. Mosby.

Roberts, R. (1981). Diagnostic assessment of myocardial infarction based on lactate dehydrogenase and creatine kinase isoenzyme. *Heart and Lung, 10*, 486-506.

Roberts, R., & Sobel, B. E. (1976). CPK isoenzymes in evaluation of myocardial ischemic injury. *Hospital Practice*, 55-62.

Sawrey, J. M., & Telford, C. W. (1964). *Educational psychology: Psychological foundations of education* (2nd ed.). Boston: Allyn & Bacon.

Scalzi, C. C., Burke, L. E., & Greenland, S. (1980). Evaluation of an inpatient educational program for coronary patients and families. *Heart and Lung, 9*, 846-853.

Schettler, G. (1977). Highlights of current research in atherosclerosis. In G.W. Haust (Eds.), *Advances in experimental medicine and biology* (pp. 9-14). New York: Plenum Press.

Segev, W., & Schlesinger, Z. (1981). Rehabilitation of patients after acute myocardial infarction – an interdisciplinary, family-oriented program. *Heart and Lung, 10*, 84-847.

Selye, H. (1956). *The stress of life.* New York: McGraw-Hill.

Selye, H. (1976). *The stress of life* (2nd ed.). New York: McGraw-Hill.

Selye, H. (1977). Selections from *The stress of life.* In A. Monat & R. S. Lazarus (Eds.), *Stress and coping: An anthology* (pp. 17-35). New York: Columbia University Press.

Selye, H. (1980). Stress and a holistic view of health for the nursing profession. In K. E. Claus & J. T. Bailey (Eds.), *Living with stress and promoting well-being* (pp. 125-136). St. Louis: C. V. Mosby.

Sgroi, S. M., Holland, J. C. B., & Solkoff, N. (1970). *Development of an Anxiety-Depression Scale for use with medically ill patients* (Mimeograph). New York: State University of New York at Buffalo, School of Medicine, Department of Psychiatry.

Speedling, E. J. (1982). *Heart attack: The family response at home and in the hospital.* New York: Tavistock.

Toth, J. C. (1980). Effect of structurded preparation for transfer on patient anxiety on leaving coronary care unit. *Nursing Research, 29*, 28-34.

Toth, J. C. (1984). Variables associated with the stressful experience of hospital discharge following acute myocardial infarction (Doctoral dissertation, The Catholic University of America, 1984). *Dissertation Abstracts International,* A82857.

Volicer, B. J. (1974). Patients' perceptions of stressful events associated with hospitalization. *Nursing Research, 23*, 235-238.

Weinberg, S. L., Col, J. J., & Madhaven, V. (1982). Prognosis after myocardial infarction – ten years of change. *Heart and Lung, 11*, 9-11.

Wishnie, H. A., Hackett, T. P., & Cassem, N. H. (1971). Psychologic hazards of convalescence following myocardial infarction. *Journal of the American Medical Association, 215*, 1292-1296.

Stress of Discharge Assessment Tool*

Part A

Directions: All of the statements in this Part (1 through 46) refer to how you are feeling now. There are *five* possible responses to each of the statements. They are:

SA = Strongly Agree

A = Agree

U = Uncertain

D = Disagree

SD = Strongly disagree

For each statement, circle the letter(s) that best describes your feeling.

1. I am glad that I will be going home from the hospital.   SA A U D SD   (6)

2. I feel more nervous today than I usually do.   SA A U D SD   (7)

3. Going home from the hospital means that my health is getting better.   SA A U D SD   (8)

4. I am sure that I had a heart attack.   SA A U D SD   (9)

5. Compared to the last 2 or 3 days, I slept better last night.   SA A U D SD   (10)

6. I have not been very sick during my stay in the hospital.   SA A U D SD   (11)

7. Since I have been in the hospital, my spiritual thinking (the meaning of life or religious background) has helped me to feel better.   SA A U D SD   (12)

8. I feel a little worried about leaving the hospital.   SA A U D SD   (13)

9. Compared to the last 2 or 3 days, my appetite is better today.   SA A U D SD   (14)

10. I feel disappointed that I got sick.   SA A U D SD   (15)

11. I feel that I was ready to go home from the hospital a couple of days ago.   SA A U D SD   (16)

12. I have at least one person that I feel   SA A U D SD   (17)
    I can talk to about myself or my
    problems.

13. I feel it is all right to ask the doctors or SA A U D SD   (18)
    the nurses questions I have about my
    illness.

14. When I go home, I feel I will be able to   SA A U D SD   (19)
    tell the difference between heart pain
    (angina) and ordinary aches and pains.

15. Since I have been in the hospital I have   SA A U D SD   (20)
    asked my doctor or nurse questions
    about my illness.

16. I find it hard to believe that this illness   SA A U D SD   (21)
    has happened to me.

17. I was having financial problems before   SA A U D SD   (22)
    I got sick.

18. I understand what physical activities   SA A U D SD   (23)
    I can do when I go home.

19. I feel depressed today.   SA A U D SD   (24)

20. When I ask questions about my illness,   SA A U D SD   (25)
    I understand the answers the doctors
    give me.

21. After my doctor says it is all right, I   SA A U D SD   (26)
    believe that my illness will not make
    much difference in my sexual activities.

22. After I go home, I know what specific   SA A U D SD   (27)
    conditions I should report to my doctor
    or nurse if they happen to me.

23. I understand what physical activities   SA A U D SD   (28)
    I should not do when I go home.

24. When I ask questions about my illness,   SA A U D SD   (29)
    I understand the answers that the
    nurses give me.

25. Compared to the last 2 or 3 days,   SA A U D SD   (30)
    I feel tired today.

26. When I go home, I will do things differ-   SA A U D SD   (31)
    ently than before I got sick.

27. Being in the hospital has resulted in a   SA A U D SD   (32)
    financial problem for me.

28. After I go home, I think it is all right to   SA A U D SD   (33)
    call my doctor or nurse if I have ques-
    tions about my care.

29. Sometimes I worry if I will be able to   SA A U D SD   (34)
    stay calm when I go home.

30. I have one or more people who depend   SA   A   U   D   SD   (35)
on me to take care of them.

31. Sometimes I do not know what ques-   SA   A   U   D   SD   (36)
tions to ask my doctor or nurse about
my illness.

32. Getting extremely upset about things is   SA   A   U   D   SD   (37)
not good for me now.

33. I understand why I got sick.   SA   A   U   D   SD   (38)

34. I sometimes worry that I will not be   SA   A   U   D   SD   (39)
able to take care of myself when I go
home.

35. When I compare myself to other people   SA   A   U   D   SD   (40)
with my kind of illness, I think that my
progress in getting well has been as
good as theirs.

36. I will be able to make the changes in   SA   A   U   D   SD   (41)
my everyday living that my doctor or
nurse has suggested.

37. I feel the same or better about myself   SA   A   U   D   SD   (42)
now than before I got sick.

38. I understand what foods I should not   SA   A   U   D   SD   (43)
eat after I go home.

39. Feeling weak is a normal reaction for   SA   A   U   D   SD   (44)
people with my illness.

40. I know what to do if I get any heart   SA   A   U   D   SD   (45)
pain (angina) after I go home.

41. I know how to get in touch with my   SA   A   U   D   SD   (46)
doctor or nurse after I leave the
hospital.

42. In the future I will be able to do most   SA   A   U   D   SD   (47)
of the same things I did before I got
sick.

43. After I go home I may have trouble   SA   A   U   D   SD   (48)
asking other people to do things for me
(for example, buying groceries).

44. I understand what kinds of food I can   SA   A   U   D   SD   (49)
eat after I go home.

45. Sometimes I worry about having   SA   A   U   D   SD   (50)
another heart attack.

46. Making some changes in the things I do   SA   A   U   D   SD   (51)
after I go home may help prevent me
from having this kind of illness again.

Part B

Directions: All of the statements in this Part (47 through 60) also refer to how you are feeling now but there are *six* possible responses to each of the statements. They are

SA = Strongly Agree
A = Agree
U = Uncertain
D = Disagree
SD = Strongly Disagree
NA = Does Not Apply to me

For each statement, circle the letter(s) which best describes your feelng.

47. My partner (important person) has helped me to feel better about myself while I have been in the hospital.   SA A U D SD NA (52)

48. My partner (important person) worries too much about me.   SA A U D SD NA (53)

49. My partner (important person) understands how I am feeling right now.   SA A U D SD NA (54)

50. My partner (important person) will help me to make the changes in my everyday living that my doctor or nurse has suggested.   SA A U D SD NA (55)

51. After my doctor says it is all right for me to resume sexual activities, my partner will be worried about that.   SA A U D SD NA (56)

52. My partner (important person) does not worry enough about me.   SA A U D SD NA (57)

53. When my doctor says it is all right, I believe I will be able to go back to work.   SA A U D SD NA (58)

54. I sometimes worry that I will not have enough money to take care of my expenses until I go back to work.   SA A U D SD NA (59)

55. My illness means that I might have to change my job.   SA A U D SD NA (60)

56. My illness means that I might lose my job.   SA A U D SD NA (61)

57. I understand why I will take medicines when I go home.   SA A U D SD NA (62)

58. I understand what the unwanted side effects are of the medicines I will take when I go home.   SA A U D SD NA (63)

59. I believe that if I am feeling all right   SA A U D SD NA (64)
after I go home, that I can stop taking
my medicines without asking my doctor
or nurse.

60. I understand that if unwanted side   SA A U D SD NA (65)
effects of my medicines happen I
should report this to my doctor or
nurse right away.

2
Revision and Testing of the Haussmann and Hegyvary Outcome Measure for Myocardial Infarction

Sandra R. Edwardson

This chapter discusses the Haussmann and Hegyvary Outcome Measure for Myocardial Infraction, a measure of patient outcome in cases of myocardial infarction.

The nature of care received by hospitalized patients has changed significantly in the past few years and continues to change. Nursing administrators faced with demands to do more with less frequently lack the information needed to explain and justify the nursing care consequences of reductions in lengths of stay and services. Policymakers and hospital administrators are demanding evidence about the impact of changes in the organization and delivery of nursing care services on patient outcomes.

This project was designed to help meet this need by evaluating and revising an instrument measuring the outcome of nursing care for myocardial infarction patients. The chapter begins with the conceptual base for the measurement. This is followed by a description of the procedure and the results of the instrument development project.

CONCEPTUAL BASIS AND REVIEW OF THE LITERATURE

Patient outcome is a widely accepted measure of the effectiveness of health care services. Numerous studies have used mortality (e.g., Detsky, Stricker, Mulley, & Thibault, 1981) or severity-adjusted death rates (Roemer, Moustafa, & Hopkins, 1968) as measures of overall quality of

Work on this study was partially supported by the Irene G. Ramey Research Fund and the Minnesota Affiliate, American Heart Association.

care and treatment in an institution. Brook and Appel (1973) were among the first to consider variables in addition to mortality, defining outcomes as the "results of care; i.e., patient response in terms of mortality, symptoms, ability to work or perform daily activities, and physiologic measurements" (p. 1323). Recent studies are including these more refined measures of outcome in an attempt to account for gradations of quality.

There is some debate in the nursing literature about the usefulness of outcomes in assessing nursing care. Phaneuf (1972), for example, favors process measures because she believes outcomes are irrelevant in some situations (such as when death is expected) and because present health care services are delivered within a medical frame of reference that is disease-oriented and hospital-oriented. Bloch (1975) spoke of the difficulty of finding outcomes that are solely attributable to nursing care. She also pointed to the difficulty in tracing the outcomes of interventions to treat the subtle psychosocial problems with which nurses work.

One other difficulty in assessing the quality of nursing care is the intervening influence of organizational factors. As Cantor (1978) pointed out, many of the functions facilitating delivery of nursing care are far removed from the bedside. Examples include personnel policies, management practices, and stability of the nursing staff. Furthermore, nursing content is sometimes insufficiently distinguished from the system's content in activities such as vital signs and other routines.

Zimmer (1974) offered a compromise position when she asserted that outcome determination should be only the first of a two-step process; once desired patient outcomes are identified, the next step is to find the most powerful and cost-effective activities that cause these outcomes.

Despite the debate as to their usefulness, outcome evaluation has been widely accepted in nursing research and practice. The Joint Commission on the Accreditation of Hospitals strongly influenced hospitals to adopt outcome evaluation by publishing the Performance Evaluation Procedure in 1974. Based on retrospective review of patient records, it measures recorded data against pre-established standards. The American Nurses' Association (ANA) (1976) has developed outcome criteria for a number of diagnoses (including myocardial infarction) that can be used in such retrospective chart audits.

Outcome measures are commonly used in studies of coronary care. Although mortality rates remain an important outcome criterion for myocardial infarction patients, researchers are increasingly concentrating on symptom relief and ability to return to work and other regular social roles. One group of investigators, for example, used the following measures in addition to death: frequency of return to work, anxiety, depression, development of angina or congestive heart failure, aneurysm formation, acute coronary insufficiency, and recurrent infarction (Hutter, Sidel, Shine, & DeSanctis, 1973). Others have investigated psychosocial adjustment as correlates of ability to remain at work, function sexually, and avoid readmission to the hospital (Fuchs & Scheidt, 1981). All of these variables have been found to be negatively affected by myocardial infarction in one study or another, although the strength of the relationships vary considerably. Despite the growing consensus about the criteria to be used in evaluating the outcome of coronary care, little effort has been devoted to developing tools to measure that outcome. Many studies have assessed the patient's health status after a myocardial infarction using well-known functional status scales (e.g., Chassin, 1982; Grant & Cohen, 1973; Zheutlin & Goldstein, 1977) or psychological assessment instruments (e.g., Gentry, Foster, & Haney, 1972; Wilson-Barnett, 1981). Among those studies that have assessed outcome criteria unique to the myocardial infarction patient, most have used investigator-developed questionnaires or interview schedules with unknown measurement properties (e.g., McPhee, Frank, Lewis, Bush, & Smith, 1983; Rahe, Scalzi, & Shine, 1975; Stern, Pascale, & Ackerman, 1977; Wilson-Barnett, 1981).

One exception to this is the work of Haussman and Hegyvary (1977), who proposed a quality assessment system similar to Zimmer's (1974) two-step approach. Their plan was to identify patients with especially poor and especially good outcomes and then systematically monitor the nursing practice believed to affect the key outcomes. Building on the outcome criteria proposed by the ANA, they developed outcome screens and process measures for several diagnostic groups, including myocardial infarction. They attempted to evaluate primarily those outcomes attributable to nursing care and measurable at the time of hospital discharge.

The Haussman and Hegyvary Outcome Criteria for Myocardial Infarction (to be referred to as the outcome measure) (Haussman & Hegyvary, 1977) is the instrument evaluated in this project. It was selected because it provides a comprehensive measure of all of the dimensions identified as relevant for the evaluation of coronary care at the time of discharge, namely, the physical and emotional status of patients, their knowledge of their illness, and prescriptions for their continued care and treatment.

The outcome measure was chosen in preference to another possible instrument, the Coronary Heart Disease Teaching Evaluation Form (Rahe, et al., 1975). Developed to test the effectiveness of a specific inpatient teaching program, the Teaching Evaluation Form tends to focus on knowledge of heart disease in general without making direct application to the patient's own health status or care and treatment plan.

DEVELOPMENT OF THE ORIGINAL MEASURE

The outcome measure described in this chapter was first developed as part of a major study by Rush-Presbyterian-St. Luke's Medical Center and the Medicus Corporation, investigating the relationship between nursing process and patient outcome. The instrument was developed by using and expanding on the ANA criteria discussed above (ANA, 1976). These criteria were divided into three categories: physical, psychological, and level of knowledge. Because of the nature of cardiac rehabilitation programs the measure was designed to be applied at the time of discharge rather than at other times in the hospitalization. After the criteria were written and defined as clearly as possible, they were reviewed by clinical specialists in cardiovascular nursing to clarify terms, descriptions, and acceptable answers. Hence, a measure of face validity was established.

PURPOSE OF REVISING THE MEASURES

The pilot phase of this investigator's research revealed some problems with the Haussman and Hegyvary (1977) instrument. This project was intended to refine the tool and reassess its reliability and validity. Specific objectives were as follows:

1. To replicate the correlation analysis and validity checks done by Haussman and Hegyvary using the data gathered on the 32 subjects in the author's pilot study; reassess the items in light of this analysis.
2. To complete an analysis of the literature since 1976 to assess whether any of the criteria originally developed on the basis of documented evidence should be revised in light of current knowledge.
3. To implement changes in the criteria and/or acceptable answers as necessary.
4. To complete an evaluation of the revised instrument's reliability and validity.

Background of the Measurement Project

The instrument development reported here is part of a larger research project with an overall goal to assess the effects of cost control measures on the content, organization, cost, and outcome of hospital services from admission through the immediate posthospitalization period for patients who have sufferred myocardial infarctions. In this research, patient outcome is conceptualized as a function of the patient's physical and emotional status, as well as a family, social, and vocational adjustment. It is assessed by using a combination of indicators including physical, social, and vocational status; the presence or absence of depression and anxiety; knowledge and skill in follow-up care; whether or not the patient was readmitted to a hospital; and the patient's location 3 to 4 months after discharge. The outcome measure evaluated here is only one of several instruments being used to achieve a comprehensive assessment of outcome.

PROCEDURE FOR REVISING MEASURE

Based on the review of the literature since 1976, analysis of data from the pilot phase of the research described, and the advice of four cardiovascular experts who served as content validators or project assistants, several modifications were made in the outcome measure. Four items were dropped. One item, which evaluated skin color as an indicator of general health status, was eliminated because there was no variance in responses to the item in either the Haussman and Hegyvary trial or this investigator's use of the item in the pilot study. Similarly, the three items comprising the psychological subscales were eliminated. One item having to do with body activation had failed to correlate with the other two items in the subscale in the Haussman and Hegyvary trial; all three items failed to produce much variance in the pilot study.

Part of an anxiety scale, developed and tested by Hargreaves (1968) for the observation of hospitalized psychiatric patients, was substituted. The response categories for each of the items in the Hargreaves scale made finer distinctions between levels of anxiety, improving the potential discriminating power of the items. Of the scale's three items, the one dealing with pacing or wandering was eliminated as not applicable to cardiac patients. The first of the two selected items had to do with verbal evidence of anxiety and the second with body activation suggesting anxiety. Nurses caring for the subjects were asked to rate the subjects' behavior during the previous eight-hr period by selecting one of four descriptions of verbal and body activity.

Other changes were made in the instrument to increase the number and specificity of acceptable answers to many of the items in the knowledge subscales. These more specific descriptors were intended to improve the reliability and validity of ratings made.

The revised instrument contains 38 items divided into eight subscales. These subscales, along with a brief description of their contents, are presented in Table 2.1.

ADMINISTRATION AND SCORING

The instrument is administered no more than 48 hr and preferably less than twelve hr before discharge. This timing is based on the fact that much discharge preparation assessed by the instrument is not completed until shortly before discharge. The tool is administered and scored by a trained nurse who observes and questions the patient and the patient's nurse. Some responses are gathered from the patient's chart.

All but three of the responses are scored on a three-point scale. Using the developer's approach, scores are weighted so that each subscale sums to 100. Total scores can range from 0 to 800.

An implicit assumption made in using total scores based on this weighting system is that each subscale is of equal importance. Because it is difficult to accept this assumption and because there is no empirical or self-evident rationale for weighting the subscales, this step in the instrument evaluation process should be interpreted as assessing the reliability and validity of a set of subscales composed of items assumed to be of equal

TABLE 2.1 Subscales and the Indicators Assessed by Each

Subscale	Indicators assessed
General Health Status	Pulse rate at rest
	Systolic blood pressure
	Diastolic blood pressure
	Respiratory rate at rest
	Quality of respirations
	Cardiac rhythm
Rest and Sleep	Freedom from chest pain
	Uninterrupted sleep (>6 hr)
	Relaxed body musculature
Activities of Daily Living	Feeding
	Dressing
	Bathing
	Personal care
	Toileting
	Walking
General Health Knowledge	Own health status
	Symptoms of fluid retention
	Ability to take own pulse
	Dates for follow-up care
Medication Knowledge	Names of prescribed drugs
	Dosage
	Schedule
	Action
	Side effects
	Action in event of side effects
	Drug interactions
Activity Knowledge	Activity limits prescribed
	Identifying own limit
	Risk factors
Nutrition Knowledge	Type of diet prescribed
	Foods to avoid
	Prescribed fluid consumption
	Reason for fluid prescription
Anxiety	Content of conversation
	Manner

importance. The measurement properties of the total instrument are also reported, acknowledging the lack of empirical support for the weighting system.

METHODOLOGY FOR TESTING

Data for the first 79 subjects enrolled in the research study were used to evaluate the instrument's validity and reliability. These subjects were patients in the first three hospitals studied: a public teaching hospital, a large tertiary private hospital, and a small suburban community hospital. All patients who were expected to fall into two Diagnostic Related Groups

(DRGs 121 and 122, myocardial infarctions with and without complications, respectively) and who were able to communicate in English were asked to participate. All but six of the 85 patients approached agreed to participate. The instrument was administered within 24 hr of hospital discharge by one of two graduate assistants, each with extensive experience in coronary care.

Reliability

The outcome instrument was evaluated for two forms of reliability, internal consistency and interrater agreement.

Internal Consistency

Internal consistency was assessed for the entire instrument and each of its subscales using the alpha statistic (Waltz, Strickland, & Lenz, 1984). The internal consistency for the subscales measuring physical status was expected to be relatively low because little variability was anticipated. But internal consistency seemed to be the most appropriate measure for the four knowledge subscales for which variability was expected to be greater.

Results of the analysis of internal consistency of the instrument are presented in Table 2.2. Alpha statistics range from 0.19 to 0.90. The overall alpha statistic for the instrument was 0.79, indicating moderately high internal consistency.

It was expected that the alphas would be low for the first three physical status subscales (General Health Status, Rest and Sleep, and Activities of Daily Living). Because the items use indicators considered to be minimum and near minimum criteria for discharge and because the measurement was made within 24 hr of discharge, little variability in scores was expected.

As is apparent from the coefficients of variation, this expectation held

TABLE 2.2 Descriptive Summary and Alpha Coefficients for the Instrument and Its Subscales

Scale	Number of items	Mean	Standard deviation	C.V.[a]	Range	Alpha
General Health Status	6	88.7	11.7	13.2	42	.41
Rest and Sleep	3	87.1	13.3	15.3	50	.19
Activities of Daily Living	6	94.4	13.2	14.0	67	.87
General Health Knowledge	7	62.2	18.1	29.2	72	.60
Medication Knowledge	7	34.6	31.2	90.2	100	.90
Activity Knowledge	3	54.9	26.5	48.4	100	.52
Nutrition Knowledge	4	52.7	30.5	58.0	100	.70
Anxiety	2	85.2	20.5	24.1	100	.86
Total Instrument	38	543.0	87.4	16.1	421	.79

[a]Coefficient of variation.

true. In several of the subscales, one item seemed to produce problems. For the General Health Status subscale, for example, elimination of the item having to do with systolic blood pressure would have improved the alpha slightly (from 0.41 to 0.46). But the alpha value for the Activities of Daily Living (ADL) subscale was unexpectedly high. Elimination of one item, ability to eat without distress, would have raised the alpha coefficient even more (from 0.87 to 0.91). The explanation for the higher alpha for the ADL subscale appears to lie in the much higher item-to-item correlations in the ADL scale. The alpha level for the Rest and Sleep subscale appears to have been attenuated by its short length (three items) and by the fact that one item, relaxation during rest periods, was negatively correlated with the other two. Removing this item would have nearly doubled the alpha value (to 0.35), although it would still be low. When the three subscales were combined into one physical status subscale, coefficient alpha was 0.58, indicating a very modest level of internal consistency.

The internal consistency values for the four knowledge subscales (General Health Knowledge, Medication Knowledge, Activity Knowledge, and Nutrition Knowledge) were higher, ranging from 0.52 to 0.90 (see Table 2.2). The alpha value of 0.52 for the Activity Knowledge subscale is not surprising in that the scale contained only three items. One item, knowledge of risk factors and their relationship to the disease, had a relatively low correlation with the other two items, and its elimination would have improved alpha for the Activity Knowledge subscale to 0.60.

The internal consistency of the other three knowledge subscales suggests that each is a moderately good to good measure of just one attribute. When the four knowledge subscales were combined into one knowledge subscale, the overall alpha was 0.84.

Because the Anxiety subscale had only two items, the value of alpha was also expected to be low. Alpha was 0.59, suggesting that this subscale has moderate internal consistency.

Interrater Reliability

The second reliability method used was interrater agreement. It was chosen in preference to test-retest methods because of the fluid nature of the constructs being measured and because it places fewer demands on seriously ill patients. The design called for two interviewers to administer the instrument jointly on three occasions. Their ratings converged quickly, going from 71% agreement on the first trial to 95% agreement on the third. Overall, the agreement was 88% in the three trials.

A goodness of fit chi square test was applied to test the reliability of the ratings. If the raters were in complete agreement, all ratings would fall along the descending diagonal of the contingency table. Since a 90% agreement standard was established, the ratings would fit the preestablished standard if 90% of them (79.2 ratings) fell along the diagonal.

The probability for the 0.61 chi-square value obtained was 0.52, indicating that the observed ratings do not differ significantly from the established model. It is concluded that the interrater reliability met the preestablished standard.

Validity

Several validation methods were used. First, two nursing experts assessed the content validity of the instrument. Then the concurrent and discriminant validity of the psychological status items were evaluated. Finally, the predictive validity of the entire instrument was estimated.

Content Validity

Two nationally recognized cardiovascular nursing experts were asked to judge the relevance of each item and its responses as indicators of the outcome variable being assessed by the subscales. There judgments were made on a four-point scale: not relevant, somewhat relevant, quite relevant, and very relevant. They agreed in 97% of their judgments. The proportion of chance agreements (Pc) was 91%, resulting in a 65% rate of nonchange agreement (K). The index of content validity (CVI), a measure of the proportion of items rated as quite or very relevant by both judges, was 0.95. Based on these findings, it is concluded that the instrument has content validity.

Concurrent Validity

The second validation method was to estimate concurrent validity of the psychological status subscale. As noted earlier, these items had been problematic in two previous applications. The subscale was reconstructed using two new items believed to measure anxiety. To assess concurrent validity, subscores on this new subscale were correlated with an established measure of psychological status, the State-Trait Anxiety Inventory-State. (Spielberger, Gorsuch, & Lushene, 1970).

The State-Trait Anxiety Inventory (STAI) provides a means for distinguishing between dispositional (trait) and transitory (state) types of anxiety. Since a cardiac episode is a threatening but relatively transitory state, the STAI-State half of the inventory was used in this study. Split-half reliability of the instrument is reported as 0.89 (Spielberger et al., 1970). Test-retest reliability over a relatively long period was reported as 0.52, a plausible value given the transient nature of the construct being measured (Newmark, 1972). In the current application, internal consistency reliability was 0.86. Concurrent validity studies based on correlation between hospital adjustment and STAI-State scores have been reported at −0.43 (Auerbach, 1973). STAI-State scores were negatively correlated with denial in a study of coronary patients, lending support to the tool's construct validity (Gentry et al., 1972).

The correlation between the new Anxiety subscale and the STAI-State was −0.28 (p = 0.006). The negative coefficient is explained by the fact that the two scales are scored in opposite directions. But the low value of the coefficients suggests the two new items may not be good measures of anxiety.

At least part of the explanation of the low coefficient appears to be related to the distribution of scores. Whereas the STAI-State produces scores that approximate a normal distribution, the Anxiety subscale produces a very skewed distribution, showing an absence of anxiety.

Comparing the STAI-State scores of the subjects in this study with norms published by its authors (Spielberger et al., 1970) also shows that the subjects were indistinguishable from normal, nonhospitalized adults. Thus, despite the low correlation between the Anxiety subscale and the STAI-State, the conclusion drawn from both instruments is the same – namely, these subjects were not experiencing anxiety. For this reason, the Anxiety subscale deserves further evaluation to assess whether advantages of the greater precision of the STAI-State instrument or other standardized tests are worth the greater respondent burden they entail.

Discriminant Validity

A second approach to estimating the validity of the Anxiety subscale was to assess the extent to which it correlates with a different construct. Since depression is another commonly observed psychological response to a myocardial infarction, scores on the Anxiety subscale were correlated with the Beck Depression Inventory (BDI) (Beck, Ward, Mendelson, Mock, & Erbaugh, 1961) also being used in the research project.

The BDI is used in both clinical practice and research. Beck et al., (1961) reported a split-half reliability of 0.93. Although Weckowicz, Muir, and Cropley (1967) report a relatively low internal consistency coefficient of 0.53, they acknowledged restricting their sample to high scorers, thereby restricting the range and lowering the coefficient. In an estimate of test-retest reliability, repeated BDI measures at one-month intervals were compared with simultaneous clinical ratings. The month-to-month changes in the parallel measures were in the same direction and in similar amounts (Little & McPhail, 1973). Concurrent validity has been established to range between 0.61 and 0.66 (Metcalfe & Goldman, 1965; Nussbaum, Witting, Hanlon, & Kurland, 1963).

The correlation between the Anxiety subscale and the BDI, using the Spearman rank correlation method, was −0.08. The fact that this correlation with a different construct is so much lower than the correlation with a similar construct (STAI-State) lends a measure of support to the validity of the Anxiety items.

Predictive Validity

One final validation procedure employed was to evaluate the predictive power of the entire outcome instrument. Although patient status was expected to change after hospitalization as the healing and recovery process progressed, it can be reasoned that the patient's status at the time of discharge should be a more or less accurate predictor of long-term adjustment. To assess predictive validity, the outcome measure was correlated with the Sickness Impact Profile (SIP) (Bergner, Bobbitt, Pollard, Martin, & Gilson, 1976) and a second STAI-State (Spielberger et al., 1970), which were administered three to four months after hospital discharge.

The SIP is a behaviorally based measure of illness-related dysfunction, assessing performance in relation to activities of daily living, mobility, social interaction, work, and emotional behavior. Its test-retest reliability has been reported as 0.88 and 0.92 (Bergner, Bobbitt, Carter, & Gilson, 1981; Pollard, Bobbitt, Bergner, Martin, & Gilson, 1976). Internal consistency estimates range between 0.94 and 0.97 (Bergner et al., 1981). Estimates of concurrent validity range from 0.27 to 0.69 (Bergner et al., 1976, 1981).

As shown in Table 2.3, the correlation between the outcome measure and SIP was −0.27, indicating that the outcome measure is not a good predictor of adjustment three to four months after discharge. (The negative sign of the coefficient is due to the fact the two instruments are scored in opposite directions.) It appears that the overall score on the outcome measure is a better predictor of the home management, physical dimension, and recreation and pastimes subscale scores of the SIP than of the overall score. All coefficients were in the expected direction except for the work subscale; those with the highest outcome scores were slightly less likely to be fully employed.

Correlations between the psychological dimension of SIP and the Anxiety subscale of the outcome measure was -0.0001, indicating the Anxiety score to be of no value in predicting psychological function as measured by the SIP. Interestingly, the correlation between the SIP psychological dimension and the STAI-State was also -0.0001. These identical coefficients suggest that both scales may be measuring the same construct.

TABLE 2.3 Correlations between Outcome Score and Sickness Impact Profile (SIP)

SIP component	Correlation with outcome score	P
Physical dimension	−.39	.01
Psychological dimension	−.17	.15
Sleep and rest	−.17	.16
Eating	−.07	.34
Work	.15	.18
Home management	−.42	.01
Recreation and pastimes	−.36	.02
Overall SIP score	−.27	.05

SUMMARY AND CONCLUSIONS

The revision of the Haussman and Hegyvary outcome screen has resulted in a set of items demonstrating high content validity and interrater reliability. The internal consistency of the subscales ranged from a low of 0.19 to a high of 0.90. At least some of the low values can be attributed to low variability within the scales and/or the limited number of items within the subscales.

Investigation of the predictive validity of the instrument showed it to be relatively weak. The outcome measure appears to be a better predictor of physical status and ability to function in home management and recreational activities three to four months after hospital discharge than it is in the areas of sleep and rest, eating, return to work, and psychological status.

Estimates of the concurrent validity of the Anxiety subscale showed it to be quite low. But this finding is tempered by the fact that the two-item scale led to the same conclusion as the more established, but also more burdensome STAI-State.

While the revised outcome measure was found to have high content validity and interrater reliability in this application, the results suggest that it would benefit from additional modifications and testings. Several points should be considered in this regard. First, the physical status indicators assess patients at rest. Results might be quite different if subjects were evaluated after simple ward activity. The addition of items to assess physical status after mild exertion may improve the instrument's predictive ability.

Second, knowledge of illness characteristics and care and treatment plans does not guarantee that the patient can or will use that knowledge. For this purpose, a patient demonstration of appropriate uses of the knowledge under conditions that simulate post-hospitalization living arrangements could be developed as part of the evaluation at the time of discharge.

A next step in the evaluation of this instrument should be to establish an empirical base for the weighting of items and subscales. For example, cardiovascular clinicians and/or patients might assign priority ratings to each of the subscales based on their judgments of the importance of the construct as a contributor to successful outcome. Alternatively, the ability of items and/or subscales in predicting specific and highly valued medium-range outcomes, such as adherence to an exercise program, recurrence of cardiac symptoms, or return to work, could be estimated.

Finally, it should be remembered that the tool provides an assessment of outcome at one point in time. In terms of evaluating the effects directly attributable to nursing care, assessing outcome at the time of discharge seems appropriate. But because of the possible effects of intervening events, it is recommended that this instrument be used in conjunction with other outcome measures if a comprehensive picture of patient recovery from myocardial infarction is needed.

REFERENCES

American Nurses' Association. (1976). *Guidelines for review of nursing care at the local level.* Kansas City, MO: Author.

Auerbach, S. M. (1973). Trait-state anxiety and adjustment to surgery. *Journal of Consulting and Clinical Psychology, 40,* 264-271.

Beck, A. T., Ward, C. H., Mendelson, M., Mock, J., & Erbaugh, J. (1961). An inventory for measuring depression. *Archives of General Psychiatry, 4,* 561-571.

Bergner, M., Bobbitt, R. A., Carter, W. B., & Gilson, B. S. (1981). The sickness impact profile: Development and final revision of a health status measure. *Medical Care, 19,* 787-805.

Bergner, M., Bobbitt, R. A., Pollard, W. E., Martin, D. P., & Gilson, B. S. (1976). The sickness impact profile: Validation of a health status measure. *Medical Care, 14,* 57-67.

Bloch, D. (1975). Evaluation of nursing care in terms of process and outcome. *Nursing Research, 24,* 256-263.

Brook, R. H., & Appel, A. A. (1973). Quality of care assessment: Choosing a method for peer review. *New England Journal of Medicine, 288,* 1323-1328.

Cantor, M.M. (1978). *Achieving nursing care standards: Internal and external.* Wakefield, MA: Nursing Resources.

Chassin, M. R. (1982). Costs and outcomes of medical intensive care. *Medical Care, 20,* 165-179.

Detsky, A. S., Stricker, S. C., Mulley, A. G., & Thibault, G. E. (1981). Prognosis, survival and the expenditure of hospital resources for patients in an intensive care unit. *New England Journal of Medicine, 305,* 667-672.

Fuchs, R., & Scheidt, S. (1981). Improved criteria for admission to cardiac care units. *Journal of the American Medical Association, 246,* 2037-2041.

Gentry, W. D., Foster, S., & Haney, T. (1972). Denial as a determinant of anxiety and perceived health status in the coronary care unit. *Psychosomatic Medicine, 34,* 39-44.

Grant, A., & Cohen, B. S. (1973). Acute myocardial infarction: Effect of a rehabilitation program on length of hospitalization and functional status at discharge. *Archives of Physiological Medicine and Rehabilitation, 54,* 201-207.

Hargreaves, W. A. (1968). A systematic nursing observation of psychopathology. *Archives of General Psychiatry, 18,* 518-531.

Haussman, R. K. D., & Hegyvary, S. T. (1977). *Monitoring quality of nursing care: Part III. Professional review for nursing: An empirical investigation.* (DHEW Publication No. HRA 77-70). Hyattsville, MD: U.S. Department of Health, Education and Welfare.

Hutter, A. M., Sidel, V. W., Shine, K. I., & DeSanctis, R. W. (1973). Early hospital discharge after myocardial infarction. *New England Journal of Medicine, 22,* 1141-1144.

Little, J. C., & McPhail, N. I. (1973). Measures of depressive mood at monthly intervals. *British Journal of Psychiatry, 122,* 447-452.

McPhee, S. J., Frank, D. H., Lewis, C., Bush, D. E., & Smith, C. R. (1983). Influence of a "discharge interview" on patient knowledge, compliance, and functional status after hospitalization. *Medical Care, 21,* 755-767.

Metcalfe, M., & Goldman, E. (1965). Validation of an inventory for measuring depression. *British Journal of Psychiatry, 111*, 240-242.

Newmark, C. S. (1972). Stability of state and trait anxiety. *Psychological Reports, 30*, 196-198.

Nussbaum, K., Wittig, B. A., Hanlon, T. E., & Kurland, A. A. (1963). Intravenous nialamide in the treatment of depressed female patients. *Comprehensive Psychiatry, 4*, 105-116.

Phaneuf, M. (1972). *The nursing audit: Profile for excellence.* New York: Appleton-Century-Crofts.

Pollard, W. E., Bobbitt, R. A., Bergner, M., Martin, D. P., & Gilson, B. S. (1976). The Sickness Impact Profile: Reliability of a health status measure. *Medical Care, 14*, 146-155.

Rahe, R. H., Scalzi, C., & Shine, K. (1975). A teaching evaluation questionnaire for postmyocardial infarction patients. *Heart and Lung, 4*, 759-766.

Roemer, M. I., Moustafa, A. T., & Hopkins, C. E. (1968). A proposed hospital quality index: Hospital death rates adjusted for case severity. *Health Services Research, 3*, 96-118.

Spielberger, C. D., Gorsuch, R. L., & Lushene, R. E. (1970). *STAI manual for the state-trait anxiety inventory.* Palo Alto, CA: Consulting Psychologist Press.

Stern, M. J., Pascale, L., & Ackerman, A. (1977). Life adjustment postmyocardial infarction. *Archives of Internal Medicine, 137*, 1680-1685.

Waltz, C., Strickland, O., & Lenz, E. (1984). *Measurement in nursing research.* Philadelphia: F. A. Davis.

Weckowicz, T. E., Muir, W., & Cropley, A. J. (1967). A factor analysis of the Beck Inventory of Depression. *Journal of Consulting Psychiatry, 31*, 23-28.

Wilson-Barnett, J. (1981). Assessment of recovery: With special reference to a study with post-operative cardiac patients. *Journal of Advanced Nursing, 6*, 435-445.

Zheutlin, S., & Goldstein, S. G. (1977). The prediction of psychosocial adjustment subsequent to cardiac insult. *Journal of Clinical Psychologg, 33*, 706-710.

Zimmer, M. (1974). Symposium on quality assurance. *Nursing Clinics of North America, 9*, 303-305.

Outcome Measure for Myocardial Infarction

GENERAL HEALTH STATUS

1. Patient maintains optimum cardiac
   output. (Check patient chart for
   record of vital signs. Scores for
   1.1-1.4 should be based on most
   recent three measures taken within
   48 hr prior to discharge. If data
   not recorded, should take vital
   signs or observe patient.)

		Scores
1.1 Pulse rate at rest	All three within 60-90/min	3
	One or two outside range 60-90/min	2
	All three outside range 60-90/min	1
1.2 Systolic blood pressure	All three within range 100-160 mm	3
	One or two outside range 100-160 mm	2
	All three outside range 100-160 mm	1
1.3 Diastolic blood pressure	All three within range 60-90 mm	3
	One or two outside range 60-90 mm	2
	All three outside range 60-90 mm	1
1.4 Respiratory rate at rest	All three within range 12-20/min	3
	One or two outside range 12-20/min	2
	All three outside range 12-20 min	1
1.5 Quality of respiration at rest (quality of respiration refers to gradations in difficulty in breathing)	Normal	3
	Shortness of breath	2
	Dyspneic	1

1.6 Cardiac rhythm is stable 48 hr prior to discharge. (Check patient chart for record of cardiac rhythm: EKG prints, M. D. notes, record of regularity of pulse. Observer judgment regarding presence or absence of arrhythmia and necessity for treatment. If data not recorded, observer should interview nurse primarily responsible for patient's care.)

Stable	3
Arrhythmias present and treated if needed	2
Arrhythmias present and not treated if needed	1

Ask nurse: Has Mr./Mrs. —— displayed any cardiac arrhythmias in the two days prior to his/her discharge?

Ask nurse: Was Mr./Mrs. —— given any treatment for his/her arrhythmias or wasn't it necessary?

REST AND SLEEP

2.1 Patient is free from chest pain 72 hr prior to discharge. (Check patient chart for indication of chest pain. Observer judgment regarding distinction between controlled and intractable angina. If data not recorded, observer should interview nurse primarily responsible for patient's care.)

Yes	3
Angina controlled by medications or rest	2
Intractable angina	1

Nurse interview: Has Mr./Mrs. —— had any chest pain in the past 3 days?

If yes: Was this generally controlled by his/her medication or by rest?

2.2 Patient has uninterrupted sleep periods 48 hr prior to discharge. (Check patient chart for sleep patterns. Interruptions include those by the nurse for medication, noise, etc., regardless of cause. If data not recorded, observer should interview nurse primarily responsible for patient's care.)

At least 6 hr in each 24 hr period with no interruption	2
Less than 6 hr in one or both 24-hr periods before discharge	1

Nurse interview: How many hours in the last two 24-hr periods would

you say Mr./Ms. -- slept without
interruption?

2.3 Body musculature is relaxed. (Check patient chart. If data not recorded, observer should interview nurse primarily responsible for patient's care.)	Relaxed during rest periods most of the time	3
	Relaxed during rest periods only sometimes	2
To nurse: Would you say Mr./Ms. -- is relaxed during rest periods most of the time, some of the time, or hardly ever?	Hardly ever relaxed during rest periods	1

ADL PERFORMANCE

3. Patient performs ADL. (Check
    patient record of performance of
    ADL. The term distress indicates
    fatigue, pain, dyspnea, etc.
    Observer judgment necessary
    regarding degree to which distress
    present. If data not recorded, inter-
    view nurse primarily responsible for
    patient's care. If nurse not avail-
    able or does not have information,
    observe patient's routine perfor-
    mance of ADL.)

    To nurse: We are trying to assess
    how easily Mr. -- performs certain
    activities of daily living. To help me
    do that, as I name an activity, can
    you tell me how Mr./Ms. -- per-
    forms it? Please indicate the cate-
    gory that best describes Mr./Ms.
    -- 's performance.

3.1 Feeding	Performs without distress	3
	Performs with some distress	2
	Will not perform	1
	Exception (note)	7
3.2 Dressing	Performs without distress	3
	Performs with some distress	2
	Will not perform	1
	Exception (note)	7
3.3 Bathing	Performs without distress	3
	Performs with some distress	2

Will not perform	1
Exception (note)	7

3.4 Personal care (mouth care, hair, shaving, makeup)

Performs without distress	3
Performs with some distress	2
Will not perform	1
Exception (note)	7

3.5 Toileting

Performs without distress	3
Performs with some distress	2
Will not perform	1
Exception (note)	7

3.6 Walking

Performs without distress	3
Performs with some distress	2
Will not perform	1
Exception (note)	7

GENERAL HEALTH KNOWLEDGE

4.1 Patient has knowledge of health status.

Source of information: Patient interview

A. What is your medical diagnosis? (correct diagnosis, medical or nonmedical terminology, myocardial infarction, heart attack, etc.)

Correct	3
Partially correct	2
Incorrect or does not know	1

B. Exactly what is an infarct/heart attack? (accurate physiological description, medical or non-medical terminology)

Correct	3
Partially correct	2
Incorrect or does not know	1

C. What kinds of activities would increase the work of your heart? (at least four activities such as walking, stair climbing, lifting, driving a car, isometrics, straining during defecation)

Correct	3
Partially correct	2
Incorrect or does not know	1

D. When would you seek medical attention? (all signs and symptoms that require a doctor's attention such as chest pain and/or dyspnea unrelieved by rest and/or medication, drug side effects, palpitations.)

Correct	3
Partially correct	2
Incorrect or does not know	1

4.2 Patient has circulatory knowledge.

C. How would you know if you are retaining a certain amount of fluid? (symptoms of fluid retention such as weight gain, shoes tight or ankles swollen in evening and disappearing by morning, pitting, coughing and rales, feeling of fullness in chest.)	Correct	3
	Partially correct	2
	Incorrect or does not know	1

4.3 Patient demonstrated ability to take own pulse. *Source of information:* Patient interview (Patient uses correct placement of fingers, optimal pressure, 30 sec., correct count within 5-10 beats.)	Correct	3
	Partially correct	2
	Incorrect or does not know	1

4.4 Patient states a date for followup care. *Source of Information:* Patient interview (Ask patient when he is scheduled to see physician for follow-up care. Compare response with recorded instruction.)	Knows	2
	Does not know	1

MEDICATION KNOWLEDGE

5. Patient has medication knowledge about all medication to be taken after discharge.

   Source of information: Patient interview
   (Compare responses with discharge orders. If patient wishes to use printed instructions, allow patient to read and then interpret instructions in own words.)

A. What are the names of the medications you will be taking at home? (Name can be generic or trade)	Correct	3
	Partially correct	2
	Incorrect or does not know	1

B. How much medication will you be taking of each type? (Dose	Correct	3
	Partially correct	2

	is correct if given in mg, partially correct if in tablets only. Observer must ask for correct dosage if answer given in tablets initially.)	Incorrect or does not know	1
C.	When will you be taking these medications? (includes both frequency and time of day)	Correct Partially correct Incorrect or does not know	3 2 1
D.	What do these drugs do for you, how do they help you? (medically intended effects of medication)	Correct Partially correct Incorrect or does not know	3 2 1
E.	What side effects should you be watching for? (potentially harmful and unintended effects)	Correct Partially incorrect Incorrect or does not know	3 2 1
F.	If you should have any side effects after taking the medication what should you do for yourself? (complete, accurate statement of self-care activities for medication side effects)	Correct Partially correct Incorrect or does not know	3 2 1
G.	What drugs should you not take along with these medications? (example: Coumadin – avoid aspirin or aspirin compounds)	Correct Partially correct Incorrect or does not know	3 2 1

ACTIVITY KNOWLEDGE

6.1 Patient has knowledge of activity limits and requirements.

Source of information: Patient interview

A.	What are your activity limits (or requirements) (Describe plan for resumption of self-care, vocation, activities to avoid such as exercise after meals, environmental considerations.)	Correct Partially correct Incorrect or does not know	3 2 1
B.	How will you know if you have done too much? (includes two of following symptoms):	Correct Partially correct Incorrect or does not know	3 2 1

Prolonged fatigue
Pain
Dyspnea, SOB lasting more
than 10 min after exercise
Tachycardia, persisting after
exercise
Dizziness
Lightheadedness
Confusion
Cold sweat
Piloerection
Cyanosis, pallor

6.2 Patient has knowledge of risk factors and relationship to disease
process.

Source of information: Patient
interview

What activities or characteristics,	Correct	3
sometimes called risk factors, may	Partially correct	2
increase the chances of having a	Incorrect or does not know	1

heart attack? (Must include smoking and obesity. Other acceptable
responses include hypertension,
hypercholesterolemia, diabetes,
lack of exercise, family history of
heart disease, oral contraception.)

NUTRITION KNOWLEDGE

7.1 Patient has knowledge of diet and
dietary instructions.

Source of information: Patient
interview

A. What type of diet are you on?	Correct	3
(Specific statement, e.g.,	Partially correct	2
500mg sodium restricted,	Incorrect or does not know	1
1500 cal, diabetic, etc.)		

B. What types of foods should you	Correct	3
avoid in order to stay on this	Partially correct	2
diet? (includes seasonings,	Incorrect or does not know	1
additives if should be avoided.)		

7.2 Patient has circulatory knowledge

Source of Information: Patient interview

A. How much fluid are you supposed to drink in a day? (specific amounts in quarts, pints, cc, etc.)	Correct Partially correct Incorrect or does not know	3 2 1
B. Why is it important for you to restrict/have a certain amount of fluid? (indicates relationship between restrictions or requirements and disease process.)	Correct Partially correct Incorrect or does not know	3 2 1

PSYCHOLOGICAL STATUS

8. By 24 hr prior to discharge patient demonstrates freedom from anxiety.
To nurse: We are trying to assess Mr./Mrs. −−'s level of anxiety. Based on your knowledge of Mr./Mrs. −−'s last 8 hr, which of the following categories best describes his/her behavior?

   A. Content of conversation

No verbal evidence of anxiety; uses nonanxiety words in conversations	No anxiety	4
Mentions being anxious once or twice during shift or only on direct questioning − does not volunteer anxious talk; patient need not refer to fear or anxiety by name.	Low anxiety	3
Occasionally talks about these feelings; worries about little difficulties; fearfully asks for reassurance; volunteers anxious talk.	Moderate anxiety	2
A large proportion of talk is about being anxious, fearful or worried; persists in anxious talk.	High anxiety	1

B. Manner

No body activation suggesting anxiety; gestures regarded as purposeful and appropriate to conversation.	No anxiety	4
Somewhat tense; occasionally appears anxious or fearful; shy; anxious quaver in voice.	Low anxiety	3
Tortured expression or mild tremor; distinct muscular tension; occasional startled or fearful expression.	Moderate anxiety	2
Continuously agitated, hand-wringing, fearfully hiding, startling, gross tremor.	High anxiety	1

Adapted from Haussman & Hegyvary. (1977). Monitoring quality of nursing care. Part III. Professional review for nursing: An empirical investigation.

3

Denial and Anxiety in Second-Day Myocardial Infarction Patients

Karen R. Robinson

This chapter discusses the Self-Appraisal Inventory, a measure of denial in post-myocardial infarction patients.

Each day many individuals are faced with stressful situations. Perhaps one of the most stressful life-threatening situations is having a myocardial infarction. How does the average individual cope with such a stress-producing event and to what degree? The literature suggests that certain defense mechanisms are employed to cope with the stressful event. It also suggests that the behavioral pattern of the patient in the coronary care unit can affect his/her morbidity and mortality. Nurses are in a strategic position to assess and intervene to promote optimal psychological as well as physical recovery.

REVIEW OF LITERATURE

It is probable that denial is one of the first adaptive behaviors or mechanisms that a patient employs during the stress-producing event of having a myocardial infarction. As reported by Freud (1946), denial is one of the earliest ego defense mechanisms used by children. As an individual matures, denial is used less frequently. Since most individuals have employed the denial mechanism at one time or another, one could reason that a coronary patient would rely on this mechanism again as a means of defense.

According to Hackett and Cassem (1969), a patient's first response to the onset of chest pain is denial. Through this defense mechanism, the individual attempts to minimize or ignore the significance of the symptoms. The patient may delay seeking medical attention for several hours, displacing the discomfort to other organ systems. When it is no longer possible to ignore the pain, and the individual either realizes or is told that he/she is having a heart attack, Cassem and Hackett (1971) contend that the individual enters the second psychologic response phase of anxiety. The individual finds himself/herself uprooted from a familiar environment and thrust into the strange surroundings of the coronary care unit. At this point the patient is preoccupied with death or its possibility. The individual is acutely aware of the disturbing symptoms of chest pain, shortness of breath, and weakness. He/she may have a sense of imminent danger or doom, or fear the unknown. As the individual starts to feel better, feelings of denial are mobilized. He/she may find it hard to believe that a heart attack has really occurred. This usually happens on the second day. Cassem and Hackett (1971) pointed out that in the next few days anxiety and denial interact, with denial protecting the individual from excessive anxiety.

Hackett, Cassem, and Wishnie (1968) suggested that a relationship may exist between the successful use of denial and morbidity/mortality in acute myocardial infarction patients. The ability to deny stress and anxiety successfully may be one of the factors that enhance the survival rate of myocardial infarction patients. Therefore, one must conclude that it is an important mechanism to investigate and measure.

For the acute myocardial infarction patient, it is not difficult to use denial as a form of coping because once the pain has been alleviated and the patient is comfortable in bed, there are no other symptoms. The patient may rationalize that nothing significant has happened.

Denial can be either healthy or unhealthy. Denial of the fact that the heart attack occurred can be adaptive behavior during the first few weeks of recovery, enabling the individual to cope with the shock and confusion. However, denial can be maladaptive if the individual ignores necessary activity restrictions or fails to take prescribed medications.

Health professionals are familiar with anxiety and denial as common responses observed in coronary patients. However, Scalzi (1973) reported that there has been a lack of emphasis, both in the literature and in practice, on identifying patterns of responses and identifying specific interventions for these behaviors.

Nurses are the health professionals who have the closest and most frequent contact with the patients. Nurses are in a position to assist the coronary patients in managing their denial; therefore, it is important for nurses to explore further the aspects of denial. How individuals use denial while in the coronary care unit or any other hospital setting to protect themselves from stress-producing events should be common knowledge for nurses. Clues that patients are using denial, whether therapeutic or nontherapeutic, may not be recognized.

It is most important that nurses recognize the manifestations of denial and then assess the degree to which denial accelerates or impedes the patient's progress toward regained health. A portion of the assessment could be accomplished by having the patient complete a denial inventory. Results of such an inventory could provide the nurse with objective data concerning the presence and degree of denial. With this information, specific nursing interventions for denial behavior can be identified for each individual patient.

REVIEW OF EXISTING MEASUREMENTS

A review of the literature was unsuccessful in locating a concise self-administered denial assessment tool. Several researchers who investigate denial were contacted by this investigator to determine their particular method of measuring denial. This investigator found that researchers measure denial primarily by two methods. One method is to ask the patient if he/she felt afraid, frightened, or apprehensive at any time during his/her hospitalization. If the patient responds negatively, he/she is classified as a denier. A positive response classifies the patient as a nondenier. However, this method does not provide the nurse with objective data concerning the degree of denial.

Another method is the use of a 31-item rating scale designed to rate behavioral characteristics associated with various degrees of denial. It contains two groups of variables: questions about the patient's typical way of tackling life's difficulties and questions about the patient's way of reacting to the present situation. It is scored by the investigator, based on a clinical interview. Each item is graded according to fixed alternatives, generally on a scale of 0 to 3. Then a total denial score is calculated for each patient (Hackett & Cassem, 1974). Several researchers have modified this particular denial scale but have continued to base scoring on the clinical interview. The problem with this type of measurement, as Hackett and Cassem cautioned, is that cross-contamination of scores by prior clinical judgment is inevitable when the same researchers do both the clinical interview and the scoring. In addition, the nature of several questions in the denial scale requires the interviewer to make inferences when rating denial behavioral characteristics of the subject.

CONCEPTUAL BASIS

The theoretical framework for the denial aspect of this study was based on Freud's (1946) theory of the mechanisms of defense. This study considered denial in the general rather than the psychoanalytic sense. Freud regarded denial as a unifying concept for various defenses but did not suggest that denial is a unitary mechanism that serves only to disclaim reality. In fact, Freud felt that denial is expressed in words, acts, and fantasies – what people do in order to counter, neutralize, and reorient themselves in the presence of danger. Denial helps us to do away with the anxiety-provoking or threatening portion of reality but only because we may then participate more fully in contending with problems (Freud, 1946).

The theoretical framework for the anxiety aspect of the study was Spielberger's (1972) trait-state anxiety theory. This theory differentiates between anxiety states and the stimulus conditions that evoke these states. Spielberger proposed two different anxiety constructs, state anxiety and trait anxiety. He conceptualized state anxiety as a transitory emotional state or condition that varies in intensity and fluctuates over time. State anxiety levels should be high in situations that the person perceives to be threatening. Spielberger, Gorsuch, Lushene, Vagg, & Jacobs (1983) stated that trait anxiety refers to "relatively stable individual differences in anxiety proneness, that is, to differences between people in the tendency to perceive stressful situations as dangerous or threatening and to respond to such situations with elevations in the intensity of their state anxiety (S-Anxiety) reactions" (p. 1). Trait anxiety levels are high in individuals who tend to perceive a larger number of situations as dangerous.

Denial has been reported as the principal way in which acute coronary patients manage the psychological stress of their illness. More often than not, denial is effective in reducing anxiety. Thus, one would reason that an individual who scores high on a denial scale would concurrently score low on an anxiety scale. If this relationship does not occur, one would question the validity of the denial scale.

PURPOSE OF THE MEASURE

Since a review of the literature demonstrated the need for an inventory that would provide objective data, the focus of this study was on the further development, refinement, and validation of an instrument to measure denial. Polit and Hungler (1978) emphasized that validating an instrument in terms of construct validity is a difficult task. Construct validity is more concerned with the underlying attribute than with the scores the instrument produces. In validating the measure of denial, the main concern was with the extent to which the measure related to situational (state) anxiety as predicted from prior research. Construct validity would be supported if one finds a denier experiencing less state anxiety than a nondenier.

An inventory such as the Self-Appraisal Inventory could provide the nurse with objective data in regard to the presence and degree of denial in the post-myocardial infarction patient. This could also enable the nurse to infer the patient's level of acceptance and understanding of his/her condition. With this information, specific nursing interventions for denial behavior could be identified for each patient.

PROCEDURE FOR FURTHER DEVELOPMENT
OF THE MEASURE

A review of the literature was unsuccessful in locating a self-administered denial measurement. Hackett and Cassem (1974) developed the Hackett-Cassem Denial Scale, a 31-item rating scale that is designed to rate behavioral characteristics associated with various degrees of denial. It is scored by the investigator, based on a clinical interview. Each item is rated on a scale of 0 to 3, and then a total score is calculated for the patient. However, a weakness of this measurement is that the nature of several questions in the denial scale requires the interviewer to make inferences when rating denial behavioral characteristics of the subject.

In an attempt to eliminate interviewer bias and provide objective data, this researcher has modified the Hackett-Cassem Denial Scale into a self-administered denial scale. Permission to modify the Hackett-Cassem Denial Scale was granted to the researcher by Dr. Thomas P. Hackett. Statements 2, 3, 4, 5, 6, 8, 9, 11, 13, 15, 17, 18, and 19 on the Self-Appraisal Inventory are modified statements from items 1, 7, 8, 10, 4, 17, 11, 14, 23, 2, 25, and 27, respectively, from the Hackett-Cassem Denial Scale. For example, in this scale item 8 refers to the patient admitting to a fear of death. This investigator modified the statement to read, "I have a concern about death."

The remainder in the statements were developed from the researcher's past experiences in working with myocardial infarction patients and from a review of the literature. During the instrument modification, input was received from two cardiovascular clinical nurse specialists. These two individuals reviewed sentence structure, word usage, readability, and accuracy of the items in the inventory.

The Self-Appraisal Inventory consists of 20 statements, with responses entered on a 4-point Likert-type scale. It requires 5 to 10 min to administer. Subjects are instructed to give their first reaction to how they feel about each statement (e.g., ""I don't really believe that there is anything wrong with my heart"). Subjects respond to each statement by selecting one of the following: (1) strongly agree, (2) agree, (3) disagree, or (4) strongly disagree.

A strength of this inventory is that it is a self-administered measurement. The individual completes the inventory without the involvement of others. However, readability of the items is a problem when an individual has considerable reading difficulties.

ADMINISTERING AND SCORING THE MEASURE

The Self-Appraisal Inventory was designed to be self-administering and to be given on an individual basis. It requires 5 to 10 min to administer to those individuals who have average or above average reading ability. Those with considerable reading difficulties will not be able to complete the inventory.

Although many of the items have face validity as measures of denial, the examiner should not use this term in administering the inventory. Rather, the inventory should consistently be referred to as the Self-Appraisal Inventory.

Complete instructions for the Self-Appraisal Inventory are printed on the test form. Participants are asked to read each item carefully. Then they are to circle the number of the answer that best indicates how they feel about the statement. It is important to emphasize that they are to give their first reaction to the item. There are no right or wrong answers. Subjects will generally respond more objectively and accurately if they are informed that their responses and names will be kept confidential.

Each Self-Appraisal Inventory item is given a weighted score of 1 to 4. A rating of 4 indicates the presence of a high level of denial for 10 items (e.g., "I am seriously ill," "I feel afraid when the monitor alarm goes off"). A high rating indicates low denial for the remaining 10 items (e.g., "When the pain first began, I did not feel the need to see a doctor," "I don't really believe that there is anything wrong with my heart"). The scoring weights for the high-denial items are the same as the circled numbers on the test form. The scoring weights for the low-denial items are reversed; that is, responses circled 1, 2, 3, or 4 are 4, 3, 2, or 1, respectively. The low-denial items for which the scoring weights are reversed on the inventory are 2, 3, 6, 7, 8, 12, 13, 17, 18, and 19.

To obtain scores for the inventory, add the weighted scores for the 20 items that make up the measure, taking into consideration the 10 scores that are reversed. Scores can range from a minimum of 20 to a maximum of 80.

METHODOLOGY FOR TESTING THE RELIABILITY AND VALIDITY OF THE MEASURE

Since the Self-Appraisal Inventory is a modified instrument, the use of the State-Trait Anxiety Inventory served as a test of the validity of the denial instrument. In validating the measure of denial, the primary concern was the extent to which the measure corresponded to situational (state) anxiety. Construct validity is supported if one finds a denier experiencing less state anxiety than a nondenier.

Developed by Spielberger in collaboration with Gorsuch, Lushene, Vagg, and Jacobs (1983), the State-Trait Anxiety Inventory (STAI Form Y) is a two-part self-administered test. The self-report scales measure the concepts of state and trait anxiety. Each scale consists of 20 phrases and requires only 5 to 10 min. to administer. The STAI Form Y contains explicit directions, so the scoring is standardized and not subject to influence by the researcher. The T-Anxiety (trait) scale directs subjects to describe how they generally feel, and the S-Anxiety (state) scale asks subjects to indicate how they feel right now. Scores range from a minimum of 20 to a maximum of 80 on both of the subscales.

The reliability of STAI Form Y has been established through the methods of test-retest correlation, measures of internal consistency using the Cronbach modified KR-20 formula (Waltz, Strickland, & Lenz, 1984), and item remainder correlations. Construct validity was established through administering the S-Anxiety scale to a sample ($N = 977$) of undergraduate college students. Under normal conditions the students scored lower than under exam conditions. Both of the critical ratios and correlation coefficients were highly statistically significant (Spielberger et al., 1983).

In a previous methodological study using the Self-Appraisal Inventory, this researcher tested the hypothesis that with trait anxiety controlled, there is a significant negative relationship between denial and state anxiety levels of second-day postmyocardial infarction male subjects. Even though the hypothesis was rejected (one-tailed test, $p = .069$), the relationship between denial and state anxiety variables went in the predicted direction: as denial scores increased, state anxiety scores decreased. The alpha reliability of the denial scale was .65. The study involved 30 male subjects with a mean age of 48 years. The State-Trait Anxiety Inventory Form X, utilized to measure anxiety levels of the subjects in the study, served as a test of the validity of the denial instrument (Robinson, 1982).

A recent attempt was made by this investigator to streamline the denial instrument and increase the reliability by conducting an item-to-item correlation and a cluster analysis on the original data set of 30. Item-to-item correlations ranged from .276 to .743. Cluster analysis revealed five subscales within the Self-Appraisal Inventory. The first cluster contained items 1, 3, 6, 12, 13, and 20 with an R^2 ratio of .313 to .932. R^2 ratio gives the ratio of next highest to own cluster. A small ratio indicates a well-separated cluster (Anderberg, 1973). Items in the first cluster mainly refer to the subject feeling fine and not believing that he has had a myocardial infarction. The second cluster included items 9, 11, and 18, which involve the need for reassurance that everything is fine. The ratio ranged from .030 to .048, which indicated a well-separated cluster. The third cluster was composed of items 2, 10, and 17, with a ratio of .007 to .136. These items allude to denial of chest pain when it first occurred and then fear that it might recur. The fourth cluster contained items 4, 8, and 16, which involve worry about health and death. The R^2 ratio was .003 to .366. The fifth and last cluster included items 5, 7, 14, 15, and 19 with an R^2 ratio of .238 to .798. these items refer to the subject worrying about being an invalid, family more worried than he, and the need by the patient to learn more about myocardial infarctions. After analyzing these recently obtained results, this researcher concluded that a larger sample size was needed to streamline and increase the reliability of the denial instrument.

Statistical Analysis Procedures

The demographic data included age, education, number of prior heart attacks, and sedation that the subjects received prior to the administration of the questionnaires. This information was summarized by using descriptive statistics.

The hypothesis stated that with trait anxiety controlled, there is a significant negative relationship between denial and state anxiety levels of second-day postmyocardial infarction subjects. This hypothesis was tested by using multiple regression, with *F* tests performed at each step to determine the contribution of each variable.

Correlations and significant levels were determined between the variables of age, T-Anxiety, and S-Anxiety in relationship to denial. Internal consistency was computed on the denial scale by using the coefficient alpha method. In addition, a cluster analysis was conducted on the present data.

Results

The sample consisted of 26 second-day post-myocardial infarction patients. The ages of the patients ranged from 42 to 68 years; mean age, 57.12 years. There were 19 men and 7 women in the sample. One of the subjects had experienced a previous myocardial infarction. None of the group had received sedation.

The findings with regard to educational level were that 2 (7.7%) had gone only as far as the elementary level and 7 (26.9%) had completed some high school. Fifteen (57.7%) of the subjects had completed high school, and 2 (7.7%) had some college education.

The state-trait anxiety and denial scores were calculated for each of the 26 completed questionnaires. The S-Anxiety scores ranged from 26 to 53, with a mean score of 35.92 and a SD of 7.44. The T-Anxiety scores ranged from 28 to 52, with a mean score of 36.31 and a SD of 5.92. The denial scores ranged from 40 to 54, with a mean score of 47.50 and a SD of 4.84.

Multiple regression analysis was used in this methodological study to test the hypothesis. This analysis enables the researcher to consider the relationship between two or more predictor variables and one criterion variable (Waltz & Bausell, 1981). Table 3.1 presents a test of significant regression relationship between the variables S-Anxiety and denial when T-Anxiety was held constant.

Statistical results in Table 3.1 revealed that there was a significant negative relationship between the denial and state anxiety levels of the subjects when the trait anxiety was controlled, $F (1,23) = 21.33$, $B = -1.03$, $p = .0001$. The regression coefficient was -1.03 when S-Anxiety was regressed on denial, holding T-Anxiety constant.

Table 3.2 presents the stepwise regression procedure that was utilized. At each step of the analysis, *F* tests were performed to determine the con-

TABLE 3.1 Regression Results between the Variables of Denial and S-Anxiety with T-Anxiety Held Constant ($R^2 = .556$)

Sourse	df	SS[a]	MS[b]	F	p
Model	2	771.137	385.568	14.43	.0001
Error	23	614.709	26.726		
Corrected total	25	1385.846			
		Type III SS			
T-Anxiety	1	44.097		1.65	.2118
Denial	1	570.030		21.33	.0001

Parameter	Estimate	T for HO: Parameter = 0	p
Intercept	76.343	5.43	.0001
T-Anxiety	.234	1.28	.2118
Denial	−1.030	−4.62	.0001

[a] SS = Sum of square
[b] MS = Mean of square

tribution of each variable in the equation as if it were the last to enter. Results indicate that 52.5% of the variance in S-Anxiety is explained by denial, and this is significant at the 0.0001 level. When T-Anxiety was entered into the analysis, the multiple R^2 of .556 indicates that 55.6% of the variance in S-Anxiety can be predicted by denial and T-Anxiety, and this is significant at 0.0001.

Internal consistency reliability was computed on the denial scale by using the alpha coefficient method. The alpha value of the scale was .41 in the present study and .65 in a previous study. When the researcher removed those items with a variance greater than 1.046, the alpha value increased to .62 in the present study. This involved removing items 3, 5, 6, 7, and 17 from the inventory.

Additional findings revealed that age was not a significant variable in relation to S-Anxiety scores; sample correlation, −0.104; $p = .612$. T-Anxiety was revealed to be a signifigant variable in relation to S-Anxiety scores; sample correlation, .381; p, .05. As expected, findings indicated that the higher the T-Anxiety score, the higher the S-Anxiety score.

Findings revealed that age and S-Anxiety were significant variables in relation to denial scores; sample correlation, .427; (p, .029) and −.724 (p, = .0001), respectively. Findings indicated that the older the subject, the higher the denial score. It was also revealed that the lower the S-Anxiety score, the higher the denial score of the individual. Additional findings revealed that there was no significant relationship between the variable of T-Anxiety to denial scores; sample correlation, −.290; p, .150. However,

TABLE 3.2 Stepwise Regression Procedure for Dependent Variable
S-Anxiety

Variable entered on step number 1...Denial $(R^2 = .525)$				
	df	SS	MS	F	p
Regression	1	727.040	727.040	26.49	.0001
Error	24	658.806	27.450		
Total	25	1385.846			

	B value	STD Error	Type II SS	F	p
Intercept	88.809				
Denial	−1.113	.216	727.040	26.49	.0001

Variable entered on step number 2...T-Anxiety $(R^2 = .556)$				
	df	SS	MS	F	p
Regression	2	771.137	385.568	14.43	.0001
Error	23	614.709	26.726		
Total	25	1385.846			

	B value	STD Error	Type II SS	F	p
Intercept	76.343				
T-Anxiety	.234	,182	44.097	1.65	.212
Denial	−1.030	.223	570.030	21.33	.0001

the direction of the relationship between the two variables of T-Anxiety
and denial was as anticipated in that as denial scores increased, T-Anxiety
scores decreased.

INTERPRETATIONS/IMPLICATIONS

The findings in a study by Bigos (1981) substantiated the conclusions of this
and other studies that denial is effective in decreasing anxiety in
postmyocardial infarction patients (Gentry, Foster, & Haney, 1972; Hackett
et al., 1968). Bigos (1981) classified subjects as deniers and nondeniers, based
on their complaints of fear and apprehension during the coronary care unit
stay. Bigos reported that nondeniers had significantly higher scores than
deniers on the state subscale of the State-Trait Anxiety Inventory. Findings
of the present study reported that subjects with higher denial scores had
lower S-Anxiety scores when T-Anxiety was controlled. This relationship
was highly statistically significant ($p = .0001$).

Results showing age not to be a significant variable in relation to
S-Anxiety of postmyocardial infarction patients corresponded with results
by Rosen and Bibring (1966). As anticipated, T-Anxiety was revealed to
be a significant variable in relation to S-Anxiety. This finding supports
the results obtained by Spielberger (1972; Spielberger et al., 1983).

There was a significant positive correlation between age and the subject's use of denial. It was determined that the older the subject, the higher the denial score. However, this finding does not support the results obtained by other researchers (Croog, Shapiro, & Levine, 1971; Hackett, et al., 1968).

Findings of the present study revealed that there was no significant relationship between the variable of T-Anxiety to denial scores at the .05 level of significance. The results indicate that S-Anxiety of the individual is a much better predictor of the level of denial than is the T-Anxiety pattern.

Internal consistency reliability is frequently used for cognitive measures when the concern is with the consistency of performance of one group of individuals across the items on a single measure. The alpha coefficient, the preferred index of internal consistency reliability, measures the extent to which performance on any one item on an instrument is a good indicator of performance on any other item in the same instrument (Waltz, et al., 1984). The Self-Appraisal Inventory has shown promise in a previous study, with an alpha value of .65. The resulting alpha value of .41 in the present study indicates that the test has a low degree of internal consistency reliability, that is, that the item intercorrelations are low. As a result, performance on any one item is not a good predictor of performance on any other item. However, it is important to note that when the researcher removed the five items from the inventory with a variance greater than 1.046, the alpha value increased to .62.

Cluster analysis on the original data set of 30 revealed five subscales within the Self-Appraisal Inventory. In the case of tests designed to measure more than one attribute (e.g., those with subscales or components), alpha should be determined for each scale or subset of homogeneous items rather than for the test as a whole (Waltz et al., 1984). In the present study the alpha value was computed only for the entire instrument. This researcher is attempting to conduct a cluster analysis on the present data set of 26 and to determine the alpha value of each subscale. Some difficulties with the process have occurred, and it is presently felt that a large sample size is required.

The possibility of the sample being too homogeneous, in that 96.2% of the subjects had just experienced their first myocardial infarction, should be considered when discussing the low alpha value of the denial instrument. In addition, denial scores ranged only from 40 to 54. The ages of the group ranged from 42 to 68 years. According to Waltz et al. (1984), when alpha is utilized with a group of subjects homogeneous in the attribute being measured, the alpha value will be lower than when a heterogeneous group is measured.

It is important for the reader to remember that the focus of the present study was on the further development, refinement, and validation of an instrument to measure denial. In validating the measure of denial, the primary concern was with the extent to which the measure corresponded to S-Anxiety. Since statistical results revealed a significant negative relationship, one could conclude that the construct validity of the denial instrument was established at 0.0001 level of significance.

Implications drawn from the conclusions indicated the need for further study in developing, refining, and improving measurements such as the Self-Appraisal Inventory to measure denial levels. The Self-Appraisal Inventory had previously shown promise with an alpha reliability of .65, but the present study revealed an alpha value of .41. The value increased to .62 after five items were removed from the inventory. Based on the results of the study, an attempt must be made to refine the instrument and increase the reliability. Items 3, 5, 6, 7, and 17 should be looked at closely in terms of modification or permanent deletion from the inventory. After revision of the measurement, this researcher would recommend that a similar study be replicated using a larger sample size.

An inventory such as the Self-Appraisal Inventory would provide the nurse with objective data in regard to the presence and degree of denial in the post-myocardial infarction patient. With this information, the nurse would be in a better position to make a nursing diagnosis of denial and to identify specific nursing interventions for the patient.

Acknowledgements: The author wishes to express sincere appreciation to Ada Sue Hinshaw, Ph.D., R.N., F.A.A.N., and to the health care personnel at St. Agnes Hospital, Moorhead, MN, and St. Luke's Hospitals – Meritcare Fargo, ND.

REFERENCES

Anderberg, M. R. (1973). *Cluster analysis for applications*. New York: Academic Press.

Bigos, K. M. (1981). Behavioral adaptation during the acute phase of a myocardial infarction. *Western Journal of Nursing Research, 3*(2), 150-171.

Cassem, N. H., & Hackett, T. P. (1971). Psychiatric consultation in a coronary care unit. *Annals of Internal Medicine, 75*, 9-14.

Croog, S. H., Shapiro, D. S., & Levine, S (1971). Denial among male heart patients. *Psychosomatic Medicine, 33*, 385-397.

Freud, A. (1946). *Ego and mechanisms of defense*. New York: International Universities Press.

Gentry, W., Foster, S., & Haney, T. (1972). Denial as determinant of anxiety and perceived health status in the coronary care unit. *Psychosomatic Medicine, 34*, 39-44.

Hackett, T. P., & Cassem, N. H. (1969). Factors contributing to delay in responding to the signs and symptoms of acute myocardial infarction. *The American Journal of Cardiology, 24*, 651-658.

Hackett, T. P., & Cassem, N. H. (1974). Development of a quantitative rating scale to assess denial. *Journal of Psychosomatic Research, 18*, 93-100.

Hackett, T. P., Cassem, N. H., & Wishnie, H. A. (1968). The coronary care unit: An appraisal of its psychological hazards. *New England Journal of Medicine, 279*, 1365-1370.

Polit, D. F., & Hungler, B. P. (1978). *Nursing research: Principles and methods*. Philadelphia: J. B. Lippincott.

Robinson, K. R. (1982). *Denial and anxiety in second day myocardial infarction patients*. Unpublished master's thesis, Texas Woman's University, Denton, TX.

Rosen, J. L., & Bibring, G. L. (1966). Psychological reactions of hospitalized male patients to a heart attack. *Psychosomatic Medicine, 28,* 808-821.

Scalzi, C. (1973). Nursing management of behavioral responses following an acute myocardial infarction. *Heart and Lung, 2,* 62-69.

Spielberger, C. D. (1972). *Anxiety-current trends in theory and research.* New York: Academic Press.

Spielberger, C. D., Gorsuch, R. L., Lushene, R., Vagg, P. R., & Jacobs, G. A. (1983). *Manual for the state-trait anxiety inventory.* Palo Alto, CA: Consulting Psychologists Press.

Waltz, C. F., & Bausell, R. B. (1981). *Nursing research: Design, statistics and computer analysis.* Philadelphia: F. A. Davis.

Waltz, C. F., Strickland, O. L., & Lenz, E. R. (1984). *Measurement in nursing research.* Philadelphia: F. A. Davis.

SELF-APPRAISAL INVENTORY*

Directions: A number of statements which people have used to describe how they feel are given below. Please carefully read each statement. Circle the number of the answer which best indicates how you feel about these statements. Please give your *first reaction* to the statement. There are no right or wrong answers.

Please answer according to the following key:

> 1 – strongly agree
> 2 – agree
> 3 – disagree
> 4 – strongly disagree

1.	I am seriously ill.	1	2	3	4
2.	When the pain first began, I did not feel the need to see a doctor.	1	2	3	4
3.	Since being in the hospital, I feel that my doctor has placed too many restrictions on me.	1	2	3	4
4.	I have a concern about death.	1	2	3	4
5.	I worry that I will be an invalid.	1	2	3	4
6.	Since I feel fine, I think that my doctor should send me home.	1	2	3	4
7.	Since being in the hospital, I have not been worried about anything.	1	2	3	4
8.	In the past when I have been ill or faced any sort of danger, I have not been worried.	1	2	3	4
9.	I feel afraid when the monitor alarm goes off.	1	2	3	4
10.	I am afraid that the chest pain will come back.	1	2	3	4
11.	I wish that the doctors and nurses would tell me more often that I am doing well.	1	2	3	4
12.	I don't really believe that there is anything wrong with my heart.	1	2	3	4
13.	The proverb, "let sleeping dogs lay" reflects my attitude toward life.	1	2	3	4
14.	I feel the need to learn more about heart attacks.	1	2	3	4
15.	I, myself, decided that I needed to see a doctor.	1	2	3	4
16.	At present my main worry is my health.	1	2	3	4
17.	Others helped me decide that I needed to see a doctor.	1	2	3	4
18.	To avoid worrying about the future, I put my life in the hands of fate.	1	2	3	4
19.	My family is more worried about my health than I am.	1	2	3	4
20.	I feel that I need to follow my doctor's instructions.	1	2	3	4

* Copyright © Karen Robinson, R.N., M.S., Veterans Administration Medical Center, 21st Avenue North and Elm Street, Fargo, North Dakota 58102.

4

Information Preferences and Information-Seeking in Hospitalized Surgery Patients

Sarah S. Strauss

The purpose of this study was to refine several tools available for measuring the information preferences of people seeking information on health. This was accomplished by establishing the reliability and validity of two existing measures – the Krantz Health Opinion Survey (KHOS) and the Attitude Toward Information Index (ATI) – and developing a valid coding system for a third (the Information-seeking Questionnaire).

REVIEW OF THE LITERATURE AND EXISTING TOOLS

The significance of information-seeking behavior related to health care decisions – that is, how and when people seek health-related information, their information sources, individual preferences for information, and relationships between preferences or patterns and information-seeking behavior – is of vital interest to nurses, who spend extensive time providing health-related information. Johnson and her colleagues and others (Hartfield & Cason, 1981; Hartfield, Cason, & Cason, 1982; Johnson, Fuller, Endress, & Rice, 1978; Johnson, Kirchhoff, & Endress, 1975; Johnson & Leventhal, 1971; Johnson, Rice, Fuller, & Endress, 1978; Padilla et al., 1981; Sime & Libera, 1985; Ziemer, 1983) have systematically pursued the premise that because humans use cognitive mediation to cope with stressful events (e.g., aversive procedures and surgery), provision of specific kinds of information (e.g., sensation vs. procedure information) permits individuals to cope more effectively with events. Furthermore, investigators such as Padilla et al. (1981) recommended additional study of whether congruence between the type of control strategies (cognitive versus behavioral) offered patients and the control preference of the patient reduced distress (p. 386). Specifically, Auerbach, Martelli, and Mercuri (1983) found that dental surgery outpatients with a preference for information demonstrated better adjustment behavior during the surgical procedure when they received specific as opposed to general information. To measure information preferences they utilized an instrument developed by Krantz, Baum, and Wideman (1980), the Krantz Health Opinion Survey (KHOS).

The KHOS was developed to measure the concept of information preferences and desire for behavioral involvement in health care. It represents a first step toward identification of information preferences as a concept separate from locus of control. Reliability and discriminant and predictive validity of the KHOS and its two subscales, Information Preference (I Subscale) and Behavioral Involvement (B Subscale) have been determined by Krantz et al. (1980) and Auerbach et al. (1983). Krantz et al. (1980) investigated construct validity using the known-groups method with 200 college students in an ambulatory health care setting. Auerbach et al. (1983) assessed construct validity for the scale using an experimental approach with 40 dental surgery outpatients. Based on their scores on the I-subscale of the KHOS, patients were classified into two groups, high or low information preferences. Individuals with high and low information preference then viewed one of two videotapes presenting specific (procedure) versus general (setting) information. During the surgical procedure, patients' behaviors were scored for tenseness, uncooperative responses, and verbal admission of pain. Patients having high information preferences demonstrated significantly better adjustment. This finding has great significance in preparation of patients for various aversive procedures. If the KHOS could be used to identify patients who prefer and whose adjustment would be facilitated by detailed information, nurses could better tailor preparatory information to meet patient needs.

Krantz et al. (1980), however, recommended further reliability and validity studies be developed to test the utility of the KHOS with groups of patients having serious health problems. Logically, in situations involving fear, uncertainty, and potential harm, factors often present in serious illness and/or hospitalization, an individual's desire for control and information may be significantly different from that of young adults and dental surgery outpatients in relatively benign health care situations. Therefore, a major objective of this project was to develop a methodology for establishing the reliability and validity of the KHOS in a health care situation involving hospitalization and some element of common risk, the surgical experience.

The KHOS taps information preferences for health care situations in general but not for specific health care situations such as the surgical experience. Therefore, a 5-item scale, the Attitude Toward Information Index (ATI), specifically tapping information preferences for patients undergoing surgery (Parrish, 1976), was selected as an addendum to the KHOS I-subscale. The inclusion of the ATI in this project also provided the opportunity to establish reliability and validity for this short but potentially useful instrument.

A second project objective included development of a valid, reliable coding system for interview data generated from the investigator-designed information-seeking questionnaire. Frequency of self-reported information-seeking behaviors and other risk reduction strategies used by hospitalized surgery patients could then be used to extend further the validity of the KHOS to patient populations with serious health problems.

CONCEPTUAL BASIS

Lazarus and Launier (1978) identified information-seeking as a mode of coping: therefore, coping was selected as the concept linking information preference, desire for behavioral involvement, and information-seeking behavior in health care situations involving risk.

Coping and Appraisal

Coping and appraisal are the two major processes mediating person-environment transactions in Lazarus's cognitive phenomenological theory of psychological stress, which views humans in a reciprocal relationship with their environments (Folkman & Lazarus, 1980; Lazarus & Launier, 1978). Folkman and Lazarus (1980) define coping as cognitive and behavioral efforts to master, reduce, or tolerate external and internal demands and conflicts. Problem-focused coping facilitates management of sources of stress through alteration of the troubled person-environment transaction. Emotion-focused coping regulates emotions arising as a result of the troubled transaction. Information-seeking, a cognitive strategy, may be used to actively problem-solve, thus reducing stress, or to allay anxiety arising from the stressful situation.

The process of appraisal involves evaluating the situation in terms of what is at stake (primary) and what resources for coping are available (secondary). The individual may appraise the situation as benign or stressful, that is, involving harm/loss, threat, or challenge. Individuals' perceptions of risk to situational threats can be attributed to (1) the particulars of a situation, (2) the individual's appraisal of that situation as stressful or nonstressful (irrelevant or benign), and (3) individual preferences or patterns that are a part of personality (Aldwin, Folkman, Schaefer, Coyne, & Lazarus, 1980).

Appraisal of the health care situation involving threat may generate emotions of fear and anxiety and a sense of uncertainty, depending on the degree of risk perceived by the patient. Duration, intensity, and type of emotion are contingent on the situation and the individual's preferred patterns. Lazarus and Launier (1978) suggest that input from the environment is filtered through a human system with relatively stable characteristics in terms of response to specific events. These "stable characteristics," or preferred patterns of coping in response to certain emotions triggered by environmental input, occur as a result of repeated reappraisals over time (Scott, Oberst, & Dropkin, 1980). Therefore, some individuals, because of the nature of their experience, may consistently use information-seeking as a mode of coping. Other modes or patterns of coping identified by Lazarus and Launier (1978) include direct action, inhibition of action, and intrapsychic processes.

Information-seeking as a mode of coping can be used to support direct action in problem-solving or to regulate the emotions, for example, to make the individual ""feel better" by making the stressful transaction seem more under control (Lazarus & Launier, 1978, p. 316). Therefore, information-seeking strategies may increase or decrease in health situations depending on the nature of the stressful appraisal (harm/loss, threat, or challenge) or the magnitude of the emotional response stemming from appraisal. A general preference for information and/or desire for behavioral control in the health care situation also may be modified by the nature of the stressful appraisal.

Fear, Uncertainty, and Perceived Risk

Emotional responses such as fear/anger are powerful intervening variables during stressful transactions related to health/illness. Fear is generated when a stressful appraisal involves harm/loss. The magnitude of the emotional response, however, may be a function of the degree of perceived risk. Cox (1967), in studying consumer behavior, viewed the degree of perceived risk to be a function of two factors: (1) the amount that would be lost if consequences of an act (e.g., surgery) were unfavorable and (2) the individual's subjective feeling of certainty that the consequences will be unfavorable. Cox identified six behaviors designed to minimize risk by decreasing the amount at stake and/or increasing subjective certainty: (1) reliance on past experience or past experience of others, (2) information-seeking, (3) taking precautionary measures, (4) choice avoidance, (5) goal avoidance, and (6) delegation of responsibility to others.

Several studies have examined the effect of fear and anxiety associated with surgery on patients' responses to informational interventions and recovery outcomes. Sime (1976) studied information-seeking (conceptualized as a coping process), desire for information, and preoperative fear and recovery indicators (e.g., frequency of pain medication and sedatives) and length of hospital stay in 57 female patients having abdominal surgery. No relationship between extent of information-seeking and the recovery indicators was found. A significant interaction between information and level of fear relative to recovery was found. Patients with the most information and high levels of fear needed fewer pain medications and recovered most quickly. Sime's participants also experienced significant self-reported negative affect postoperatively. Unfortunately, no reliability or validity was reported for instruments used to measure the variables: preoperative fear, preoperative coping (extent of information-seeking and information desired), preoperative information, and postoperative negative affect.

Johnson, Rice, Fuller, and Endress (1978) found that for cholecystectomy patients ($N = 58$) who were fearful preoperatively, the three information interventions employed – sensation, procedures, and preadmission exercise instruction (coping strategies) – significantly reduced negative mood states postoperatively (measured by the Mood Adjective Checklist). These findings, however, did not extend to patients undergoing hernia surgery. A replication study (Johnson, Fuller, Endress, & Rice, 1978) confirmed these findings. In conclusion, fear, the frequent emotional response to appraisal of a situation as threatening and hence stressful, is an important variable to tap in probing hospitalized patients' information-seeking strategies.

Information Preference and Desire for Control

Information preference as an individual difference variable has been used only in two information intervention studies; both utilized brief interventions for short duration procedures (Auerbach, et al., 1983; Padilla et al., 1981). The Auerbach et al. study discussed earlier was conceptualized as a validity study for the KHOS since scores on the I-subscale were predictive of better adjustment demonstrated during the surgical procedure by patients having a high information preference.

In the second study, Padilla et al. (1981) selected 50 patients undergoing nasogastric tube insertion. Independent variables were four interventions and preference for control. Patients were simply asked whether they wanted to "help" with what happened during the procedure or whether they preferred to leave the entire procedure up to the "professionals in charge" (p. 377). Dependent measures were self-reported measures of behavior, specifically, 15-point visual analog scales to measure pain, discomfort, and anxiety during the procedure. Patients also completed a Nasogastric Intubation Checklist, which required that they rate 10 sensations experienced during the procedure on a 4-point scale. They were also asked to rate their "perceived control" during the procedure. Results indicated that the procedure with sensory and coping behavior information was effective in decreasing discomfort, pain, and anxiety for control and no-control patients but was most effective in reducing intubation distress for patients preferring no control.

These findings suggest that individuals who prefer control may experience heightened distress (e.g., pain) during the procedure. Ziemer (1983) reported similar findings in her postoperative patients who received the procedure with sensation and coping strategy information and who utilized suggested coping strategies. These patients also reported significantly greater postoperative distress.

Information-seeking

Information-seeking can be defined as an active strategy to promote human adaptation by organizing transactions between individuals and their environment in order to increase control and predictability by decreasing the amount at stake and increasing subjective certainty. More specifically, information-seeking is a cognitive mode of coping utilized to assess (reappraise) and manage (cope with) situations appraised as stressful. Individuals who consistently use information-seeking as a coping strategy should also theoretically express a higher preference for information and perhaps a greater desire for behavioral control. Factors such as background, personality, and situations have been identified as influencing information-seeking behavior (Lenz, 1984). Background variables – for example, socioeconomic class and past experience combined – explained much variability in information-seeking behavior. Therefore, information-seeking may vary contingent upon the situation/context, cognitive appraisal (harm/loss, threat, or challenge), and individual preferences or patterns. Furthermore, it occurs in a matrix of other strategies used to decrease risk and enhance personal control, thus reducing fear and uncertainty.

Information-seeking behavior relative to health decision-making and information and control preferences for patients undergoing experiences in which harm/loss and threat to physical and psychosocial integrity are inherent remains largely unstudied. The ability to adequately study relationships between information-seeking, information preferences, and desire for behavioral control in health care situations and other intervening variables, specifically fear and anxiety, is contingent on the development of adequate instrumentation. Therefore, the following instruments were administered to patients before and after surgery: the KHOS, a measure of information preference and desire for behavioral control in health care situations; the ATI, a measure of information preference in surgery patients; the Profile of Mood States (POMS), which includes subscales measuring fear and anxiety; and analog scales to measure perceived risk. The Information-Seeking Interview Questionnaire, a semistructured interview designed to tap information-seeking and other coping strategies used by surgery patients to manage perceived risk and recovery, also was conducted before and after the surgical experience. Table 4.1 describes the relationships among the conceptual framework, the study design, and the instrumentation of concepts for this project.

INSTRUMENT TESTING PROCESS

Establishing Reliability and Validity for the KHOS and ATI

A norm-referenced model was used by Krantz et al. (1980) in development of the Krantz Health Opinion Survey (KHOS) (Table 4.2). There-

TABLE 4.1 Concepts, Measured Variables, and Instruments

Concept	Preoperative measured variable	Tool	Postoperative measured variable	Tool
Appraisal	Perceived risk	Analog scale "How concerned are you?"	Same as preoperative	Analog scales: progress and fit with expectations
Coping process	Strategies for decreasing amount at stake and increasing subjective certainty	Tape-recorded preoperative Information-Seeking Questionnaire, coded for six risk-reduction categories	Tape-recorded postoperative Information-Seeking Questionnaire	Taped postoperative interview
Coping pattern	Preference for information and behavioral involvement	KHOS: I-subscale B-subscale ATI	Same as preoperative	Same
Emotional response	Fear/anxiety and related emotions: fatigue, depression, confusion, anger	Profile of Mood States (POMS) (this week): tension/anxiety, vigor, fatigue, depression, confusion, anger Preoperative analog scale "How concerned are you?"	Same as preoperative	POMS and subscales
Other factors	Occupation Education SES Knowledge of health problem Type of surgery	Demographic data Preoperative Information-Seeking Questionnaire	–	–

fore, the norm-referenced model was also assumed for this project. Reliability and discriminant and predictive validity for the KHOS have been established by Krantz et al. (1980) and Auerbach et al. (1983). The ATI, however, has no established reliability or validity.

The procedures for establishing reliability and validity of the KHOS and ATI in an inpatient setting within the context of this study are described below. (Specific information regarding each instrument used in the study can be found in Table 4.3.)

TABLE 4.2 Krantz Health Opinion Survey

		Yes	No
1.	I usually don't ask the doctor or nurse many questions about what they're doing during a medical exam.	( )	( )
2.	Except for serious illness, it's generally better to take care of your *own* health than to seek professional help.	( )	( )
3.	I'd rather have doctors and nurses make the decisions about what's best than for them to give me a whole lot of choices.	( )	( )
4.	Instead of waiting for them to tell me, I usually ask the doctor or nurse immediately after an exam about my health.	( )	( )
5.	It is better to rely on the judgements of doctors (who are the experts) than to rely on "common sense" in taking care of your own body.	( )	( )
6.	Clinics and hospitals are good places to go for help since it's better for medical experts to take responsibility for health care.	( )	( )
7.	Learning how to cure some of your own illnesses without contacting a physician is a good idea.	( )	( )
8.	I usually ask the doctor or nurse lots of questions about the procedures during a medical exam.	( )	( )
9.	It's almost always better to seek professional help than to try to treat yourself.	( )	( )
10.	It is better to trust the doctor or nurse in charge of a medical procedure than to question what they are doing.	( )	( )
11.	Learning how to cure some of your illnesses without contacting a physician may create more harm than good.	( )	( )
12.	Recovery is usually quicker under the care of a doctor or nurse than when patients take care of *themselves*.	( )	( )
13.	If it costs the same, I'd rather have a doctor or nurse give me treatments than to do the same treatments myself.	( )	( )
14.	It is better to rely less on physicians and more on your own common sense when it comes to caring for your body.	( )	( )
15.	I usually wait for the doctor or nurse to tell me the results of a medical exam rather than asking them immediately.	( )	( )
16.	I'd rather be given many choices about what's best for my health than to have the doctor make the decisions for me.	( )	( )

Note. From Assessment of preferences for self-treatment and information in health care by D.S. Krantz, A. Baum, & M. Wideman, 1980, *Journal of Personality and Social Psychology, 39,* p. 980. Reprinted by permission of the publisher and author.

TABLE 4.3 Instrument Length, Response Format, Scoring and Availability

Instrument	Length/response format	Scoring

Krantz Health Opinion[a] Survey (2 subscales)
  I Scale (information preference)
  B Scale (preference for behavioral involvement
	16 items/binary response yes/no)
	7 items (1, 3, 4, 8, 10, 15, 16)
	9 items (2, 5, 6, 7, 9, 11, 12, 13, 14)
		Negatively worded items are reverse-scored; sum positive responses (yes); high scores are indicative of preference for information and desire for control

Attitude Toward Information Index[b]	5 items/5-point Likert scale. Item 1, baseline; definitely yes to	Item 1 scored as "definitely no", 0; "definitely yes", 4; items 2-5 scored, strongly *cont.*

TABLE 4.3 *(continued)*

Instrument	Length/response format	Scoring
	definitely no. Items 2-5, "strongly agree" to "strongly disagree"	agree, 4 points, strongly disagree, 0; scores on 2-5 only are summed for 16 possible points; items 3, 4, 5 are reverse-scored.
Profile of Mood States[c]	65 adjectives 6 mood factors (subscales) rated on 5-point Likert scale from not at all to extremely.	Sum responses for each mood factor; a few items are reverse scored; some items are weighted, therefore; see manual (McNair, Lorr & Droppleman, 1981) for details
Information-Seeking Questionnaire[d] (preoperative and postoperative interviews)	Semistructured 10-20 min interviews. Preoperative: Open-ended questions: "Tell me about your present health problem"; "When you learned you were coming to the hospital who what did you go to for information or questions about the hospital? surgery?" Analog scale, "How concerned are you right now about your surgery?" (Discussion of response) Postoperative: Two analog scales; "How do you feel you're progressing?" "How does this fit in with what you expected?" (discussion of responses)	Patient responses to open-ended questions and discussion of responses to analog scales scored according to risk-reduction coding protocol. 10-cm analog scales scored from 0 to 10, or from least amount of an emotion or feeling to the most amount, 10.

[a] Available from David Krantz, Ph.D., Department of Medical Psychology, Uniformed Services University of Health Sciences, 4301 Jones Bridge Road, Bethesda, MD 20014. Published in *Journal of Personality & Social Psychology 39*, 980.

[b] Available from John Parrish, M.S., 32 Oak Shadows Court, Katonsville, MD 21228. (see Parrish, 1976).

[c] Available from Educational and Industrial Testing Services, Box 7234, San Diego, CA 92107 (cost very reasonable).

[d] Available from Sarah Strauss, Box 567, MCV Station, Richmond, VA 23298.

Reliability

Preoperative (evening before surgery) and postoperative (3 to 4 days after surgery) administration of the KHOS provided the basis for examining test-retest reliability of instrument stability across the operative course for the ATI, the total KHOS, and its subscales (I and B), that is, just prior to a potentially harmful event and several days after this event. The Spearman rho coefficient was used to compute test-retest reliability. Internal consistency of the total KHOS and subscales was computed for both the preoperative and postoperative administrations using the KR-20 formula, a variation of alpha appropriate for testing internal consistency of instruments with a binary response format (Waltz, Strickland, & Lenz, 1984). Cronbach's alpha was used to test the internal consistency of the ATI, which uses a 5-point Likert response format. (See Table 4.3).

The Profile of Mood State (POMS), a 65-item adjective rating scale with six factor subscales (McNair, Lorr, & Droppleman, 1981), was administered before and after surgery along with the KHOS and the ATI. This instrument monitored a range of emotional states, specifically in the Tension-Anxiety, Fatigue, Vigor, Confusion-Bewilderment, Anger-Hostility, and Depression-Dejection subscales. Because it has established reliability and validity with groups with identified mental health problems and college students, it also served to further establish discriminant and convergent validity of the KHOS and its subscales. For example, patients scoring high on the Vigor subscale of the POMS preoperatively, might possess energy necessary to involve themselves in their care (high B-subscale and Vigor subscale correlations), whereas patients who were fatigued might score lower (lower correlations between the Fatigue subscale of the POMS and the B-subscale). Furthermore, measurement of mood states before and after surgery provided baseline data on a number of emotional responses that potentially influenced information-seeking behavior. Internal consistency for the POMS and its subscales was computed using Cronbach's alpha; test-retest reliability was ascertained by correlating pre- and postoperative scores using the Spearman rho coefficient.

Further discriminant and convergent validity for the KHOS was sought by documenting self-reported use of information-seeking and other risk-reduction strategies in the Information-Seeking Questionnaire, an investigator-developed semistructured interview questionnaire that alternated open-ended questions with analog scales (Table 4.3). Since the Information-seeking Questionnaire was an investigator-designed interview, it was reviewed by two other experts for clarity and fit with the conceptual framework. All interviews were conducted by the investigator to ensure consistency. Content analysis of verbatim transcripts of interviews was conducted using the steps outlined by Waltz et al. (1984, pp. 258-262).

1. Definition of universe of content: the self-reported operative experience was defined as the universe of content to be coded.

2. Identification of the concepts to be measured: Information-seeking was defined within a conceptual framework using coping as the major theme and within a matrix of several risk-reduction strategies identified by Cox (1967): reliance on past experiences, information-seeking, taking precautionary measures, choice and/or goal avoidance, and delegation of responsibility to others.
3. Selection of the unit of analysis: Themes within the tape-recorded interviews were designated as the units of analysis. These were risk-reduction behaviors. Other themes tentatively coded included evaluative statements, risk appraisal statements, and statements reflecting emotional status.
4. Sampling: The entire universe of content was coded; that is, entire interview sequences were transcribed.
5. Development of a scheme for categorizing content: Development of the scheme initially preceded deductively Cox's (1967) six categories of risk-reduction strategies. All phrases, statements, and passages reflective of use of risk-reduction strategies were coded.
6. Development of coding and scoring instructions: Category scores were derived from summed frequencies of risk-reduction strategies, for example, information-seeking for both the preoperative and postoperative interview. Two independent coders scored verbatim transcripts using an investigator-developed coding protocol in which Cox's risk-reduction strategies were defined and instructions for coding provided. Category scores were then to be correlated with the KHOS, ATI, and POMS scores.
7. Pretesting categories and coding instructions: Two coders rated four interviews using the protocol based on Cox's (1967) risk-reduction strategies. Although correlations between coders' category scores were planned as the method for computing interrater reliability, percent agreement was initially used as a rapid simple method for assessing problems. Percent agreements ranged from .54 to .84. In addition, risk-reduction strategies emerged that were not easily coded using Cox's categories.

Therefore, the coding scheme was reworked, using an inductive approach; that is, deriving categories from the data. All risk-reduction statements from four interviews were identified and agreed on by the coders. Statements were sorted into "similar" categories. Some categories (e.g., information-seeking) remained the same. Other labels were changed to reflect the broader scope of the category (Table 4.4). The categories remained compatible with the conceptual framework. The second four interviews were coded with an improved overall percent agreement of .77.

The first four interviews were then recoded using the revised protocol. Category scores ranged from a mean of 6.63 (SD = 7.60) for mental mechanisms to a mean of .88 for faith, hope, and trust (SD = 1.12). Category means for acceptance, information-seeking, and action were 4.0 (SD

TABLE 4.4 Revised Coding Protocol Categories for Information-Seeking Questionnaire

Category	Sample behavior
Help-seeking: Seeking help for problems.	"I went to the clinic when I realized I was sick."
Information-seeking: Actively seeking answers to questions/concerns from caregivers and others.	"That's when I went to another doctor, and he told me the same thing."
	"And we asked him [surgeon] how many procedures of this type he had done."
Acceptance: Unquestioning acceptance of information, reassurance, and/or care provided by caregivers or others.	"So, I'm not really concerned. . . Dr. X went over everything." "The doctor gave me this book, and I really enjoyed it."
	"I just bear with it – pain – I don't want to make them mad."
Mental maneuvering: Use of defensive and intrapsychic strategies to decrease the amount at stake and increase subjective certainty.	"You've got to give up something to get something."
	"If I'm not going to be in here that long, there really can't be that much to it."
Faith, hope and trust: Clear statement that faith and trust in others and hope for a positive outcome provides added security in threatening situations.	"One thing led to another, and I put my trust in him, and he brought me this far."
Direct action: Involves some direct action based on cognitive problem-solving and/or reading internal cues; often involves an element of challenge.	"The more you sit around, the worse you feel."
	"get up and walk in the hall . . . and that really helps."

= 2.5), 3.13 (SD = 3.7) and 2.75 (SD = 3.96), respectively.

Pearson correlation coefficients were then computed between category scores since two coders were used (Waltz et al., 1984, p. 141). They ranged from a low of .83 for the acceptance category to a .98 for the action category. Coefficients for mental mechanisms and information-seeking; faith, hope, and trust; and help-seeking were .97, .89, and .88, respectively. Therefore, all but acceptance met the .85 requirement for intercoder reliability.

Approach to Data Collection

A nonrandom sample of eight inpatients undergoing elective surgical procedures in a university health center hospital participated in this pilot project. Criteria for inclusion included (1) nonemergency surgical procedures with preplanned admission; (2) age 18 years and older; (3) ability to read questionnaires and respond appropriately in interview; (4) no severe visual, hearing, or learning impairments; (5) no specialized knowledge in health care. Eligible patients were identified from reviewing operative schedules, computerized patient status reports, and patient records. After informed consent was obtained, patients completed paper-and-pencil instruments the evening before surgery. The preoperative interview was then conducted. Postoperative data collection was conducted as soon as patients felt well enough to complete the instruments and participate in the postoperative interview. This varied from 2 to 4 days after the surgery, depending on type of surgery discharge plans.

SCORING THE KHOS, ATI, AND POMS

The KHOS utilizes a binary response format and is reverse-scored for negatively worded items (see Table 4.3). A total score of 16, with subscale scores of 7 (information) and 9 (behavior), is possible. High scores are indicative of preference for information and control in health care situations. The ATI, which consists of five questions excerpted by Parrish (1976) from Vernon and Bigelow (1974), was administered as an addendum to the KHOS, but it was scored separately. Questions were scored on a five-point Likert scale with a midpoint neutral or no opinion option. A score of 4 was given for strong agreement, 0 for strong disagreement, and 2 for neutral or no opinion. The scores for questions 2 through 5 were summed. The response to question 1 will be used as a reliability check for interview responses to Part II: Information Checklist.

Each of the 65 adjectives on the POMS is scored on a five-point Likert scale relative to how the person has been feeling during the past week, including today. Choices range from not at all (0) to extremely (4). Each factor was hand-scored using templates. Specific instructions for scoring are found on each template (see Table 4.2 for additional details on scoring).

RESULTS

Description of the Sample

Although an effort was made to balance men and women, seven women and one man participated. Surgical procedures included cholecystectomies, gastric stapling, hernia repair, colon reanastomosis, hysterectomies, and perineal repair. The mean sample age was 33.6 years (SD = 8.25). Education level ranged from 8 to 14 years (mean, 10.75; SD = 2.9).

Reliability of Instruments

To develop a better picture of this sample, descriptive statistics were calculated for the KHOS total scale, I-subscale, and B-subscale, and for the ATI. Since the scales were administered both preoperatively and postoperatively, differences between the scores for each scale and subscale were computed. Scores did not approximate a normal distribution; therefore, the Mann Whitney U-test was used to determine that no significant differences between preoperative and postoperative scores existed for the KHOS, its subscales, or the ATI. Therefore, the preoperative scores are the basis of subsequent statistics reported unless otherwise specified. Mean total KHOS score was only 6.63 (SD = 2.13). All but two patients scored a 5 or 6 on the I-subscale (mean, 4.88, SD = 1.36). Scores on the B-subscale were quite low (mean, 1.75; SD = 1.50). This may be reflective of the fact that patients do not have or desire a great deal of control in inpatient settings, which in turn may be a function of the more serious nature of their health situation that required hospitalization. The mean ATI score was 13 (out of a possible 16) (SD = 2.14).

Internal consistency figures for the KHOS and the B-subscale preoperatively were .51 and .55 (KR-20). Postoperative coefficients were higher (total KHOS, .66; B-subscale, .66). The KR-20 coefficients for the I-subscale were low (preoperative, .36; postoperative, .07). Alpha coefficients for the ATI were .49 before surgery and .80 after surgery. Waltz et al. (1984) suggest that when scores on a measure are not normally distributed, low internal consistency coefficients may result. Lack of a normal distribution of scores (small, nonrandom sample) undoubtedly contributed to low coefficients for the I-subscale. Only I-subscale items 2, 5, 6, and 7 had p levels between .30 and .70 (Waltz et al., 1984, p. 152). Internal consistency coefficients reported by Krantz et al. (1980) in their standardization study of 200 college student outpatients were total scale, .77, I-subscale, .74, and B-subscale, .76. Given this sample and score distribution, the KR-20 coefficients for the total KHOS and the B-subscale are encouraging.

Test-retest reliability (correlation of preoperative and postoperative scores using the Spearman rho formula) was total scale, .84, I-subscale, .72, and B-subscale, .59. These coefficients approach the figures of Krantz et al. (1980): total scale, .74; I-subscale, .71; and B-subscale, .59. ATI test-retest reliability was .53, giving it marginal stability for this sample. A total scale test-retest reliability coefficient for the KHOS of .84 suggests stability of the measure over the operative course. Although only 3 to 5 days elapsed between administration of the KHOS, the intervening events of anesthesia and surgery should have disrupted remembering preoperative responses to some extent.

Although score distributions for the KHOS subscales were skewed in opposite directions and internal consistency figures were low for the I-subscale, further testing with a larger sample should be done before attempting to revise the scale. Testing with a larger sample would also permit a factor analysis on the scale to validate the current subscale structure. Comments from the patients relative to the binary response format suggest that a forced choice on certain items – for example, item 9, "It's almost always better to seek professional help than to try to treat yourself," may not reflect actual behavior. Several participants indicated that their yes or no response did not accurately reflect their preference, specifically self-treatment for "colds and flu" and physician treatment for "serious illness." A 4-point Likert scale response format might allow for greater accuracy and variability in patient responses.

Revisions in the ATI should also await testing with a larger sample. Internal consistency figures are promising, and greater variability of scores should occur with increased sample size. In addition, the scale can be completed quickly in the clinical setting, and it is easily understood by patients.

POMS

For this small sample, internal consistency for the POMS and several of its subscales was good. Alpha coefficients for the total scale were .88 preoperatively and .83 postoperative. Preoperative coefficients for the subscales Tension-Anxiety (T/A), Vigor (V), Fatigue (F), and Depression/Dejection (D/D) were also good (T/A, .80; V, .83; F, .82; D/D, .75). Coefficients for the Anger-Hostility (A/H) and the Confusion-Bewilderment (C/B) subscales were low (.10 and .30, respectively).

Test-retest coefficients (correlations of pre- and postoperative test scores) for the POMS and subscales were as follows: total POMS, –.11; T/A, .16; D/D, .47; A/H, –.23; V, .87; F, –.18; C/B, .43). For this sample these figures indicate that only the Vigor subscale showed stability from preoperative to postoperative measurement. As expected, all other moods fluctuated.

Validity

Interscale correlations for the KHOS provide some evidence for discriminant and convergent validity in this sample (Table 4.5). The correlation between the I-subscale and the KHOS total scale for the preoperative administration was .62; B-subscale and the KHOS total scale correlation was very good (.86). The correlation between the I- and B-subscales was low (.20). This suggests that each subscale correlates well with the total scale, but the subscales measure different concepts.

Because the internal consistency coefficients for the I-subscale were low for this sample, validity coefficients (correlations between the KHOS and subscales, the POMS and subscales, and risk reduction categories) have limited meaning; therefore, a multimethod-multitrait matrix was not developed. Increased sample size in subsequent work will prove useful in examining the validity of the KHOS and its subscales.

High to moderate correlations of interest in the intercorrelation matrix

TABLE 4.5 Spearman Coefficients, Preoperative Scores, POMS, KHOS, Risk Reduction Categories

	I-Sub-scale	B-Sub-scale	ATI	POMS Total	T/A	D/D	A/H	V	F	C/B	ACPT	MM	FHT	IS	ACT	HLPSK
KHOS, total	.62	.86**	-.03	-.23	-.04	-.07	-.59	-.19	-.25	-.19	-.39	.48	-.02	.46	.34	-.23
I Scale		.20	-.30	.05	.21	-.07	-.09	.17	-.04	-.65*	-.29	-.06	.23	.77**	-.08	-.24
B Scale			.11	-.32	-.19	.04	-.56	-.47	-.30	.18	-.30	.65*	-.14	.25	.58	-.12
ATI				.15	-.05	-.19	-.36	-.16	.43	.36	-.22	-.19	-.33	-.31	-.57	-.44
POMS total					.30	.75**	.13	-.20	.32	.20	.85**	.02	.13	.26	.04	.58
Tension/Anxiety (T/A)						.63	-.28	.22	-.07	-.03	.50	.01	-.20	.07	-.05	.62*
Depression (D/D)							-.25	-.17	-.04	.40	.69**	.36	-.05	.02	.30	.54
Anger/Hostility (A/H)								-.24	.49	-.09	.35	-.32	.34	.30	.04	.00
Vigor (V)									-.46	-.47	-.40	-.31	-.31	-.36	-.42	.00
Fatigue (F)										.17	.23	-.31	.86**	.38	-.53	-.43
Confusion (C/B)											.27	.55	.24	-.22	.20	.00
Acceptance (ACTP)												-.10	-.05	.02	.24	.70**
Mental Mechanisms (MM)													.03	.31	.65*	.00
Faith, Hope, Trust (FHT)														.53	.49	-.70**
Information-seeking (IS)															.14	-.23
Action (ACT)																.51

* p, .10; ** p, .05.

(Table 4.4) include a .77 ($p = .02$) between scores on the I-subscale of the KHOS and the Information-Seeking category scores. Given the low internal consistency coefficient for the I-subscale, conclusions related to the relationship between self-reported information-seeking behavior and information preference in health care situations measured by the I-subscale are encouraging but premature.

Correlations between the B-subscale and the POMS subscales also represent an interesting pattern. For example, preoperative B-subscale scores have a moderate inverse correlation with preoperative Vigor subscale scores ($r = -.47$, $p = .24$) and a moderately high positive correlation with *postoperative* Fatigue subscale scores ($r = .64$, $p = .09$). The latter may represent greater behavioral involvement in postoperative recovery activities (e.g., walking) that would increase fatigue. The positive moderate correlation between the risk-reduction category, action ($r = .58$, $p = .14$), and the preoperative B-subscale score gives some support to this explanation.

Also of interest is the moderately high negative correlation ($r = -.65$, $p = .08$) between the I-subscale and the ATI preoperatively. It was expected that these two measures would be positively correlated if they were measuring the same construct, information preference. It may be that information preference as a general orientation in health care situations (measured by the I-subscale) and a desire for information relative to surgery (more situation-specific) measured by the ATI are different concepts, or different dimensions of the same concepts, for example, trait versus state.

DISCUSSION

No definitive conclusions can be drawn relative to the instruments used in this project, the KHOS, ATI, and POMS, because of the small sample size. Preliminary results based on analysis of data from eight surgery patients, however, suggests that extension of data collection using the methodology developed in this project may prove productive in identifying relatively simple tools for identifying variables that impact on recovery from surgical procedures.

There are no studies examining information and control preferences and use of risk-reduction strategies, specifically information-seeking, and emotional states. Establishing the reliability and validity of the KHOS and ATI would permit studying the relationship of preferences for information and involvement in health care on patients' subjective responses and objective outcomes following surgery.

A necessary prerequisite to development of an intervention study matching information and/or control preference with an intervention is development of reliable, valid instruments for measuring information and control preferences. It seems logical that individuals who have a high information and control preference actively seek information in health care situations. Specifically, do patients with different preferences for information and involvement in health care respond differently to different informational and care strategies. Greater knowledge about patient desire for and response to information could increase the efficacy of information provision for certain groups of patients, thus reducing costs and increasing nurse and patient satisfaction with information interventions.

REFERENCES

Aldwin, C., Folkman, S., Schaefer, C., Coyne, J., & Lazarus, R. (1980, September). *Ways of coping: A process measure.* Paper presented at the meeting of the American Psychological Association, Montreal.

Auerbach, S. M., Martelli, M. F., & Mercuri, L. G. (1983). Anxiety, information, interpersonal impact, and adjustment to a stressful health care situation. *Journal of Personality & Social Psychology, 44,* 2384-2396.

Cox, D. F. (1967). Risk-handling in consumer behavior - an intensive study of two cases. In D. F. Cox (Ed.), *Risk taking and information handling in consumer behavior* (pp. 34-82). Boston: Harvard University.

Folkman, S., & Lazarus, R. S. (1980). An analysis of coping in a middle-aged community sample. *Journal of Health and Social Behavior, 21,* 219-239.

Hartfield, M. J., & Cason, C. L. (1981). Effect of information on emotional responses during barium enema. *Nursing Research, 30,* 151-155.

Hartfield, M. J., Cason, C. L., & Cason, G. J. (1982). The effect of information about a threatening procedure on patient's expectations and emotional distress. *Nursing Research, 31,* 202-205.

Johnson, J. E., Kirchoff, K. T., & Endress, M. P. (1975). Altering children's distress behavior during orthopedic cast removal. *Nursing Research, 24,* 404-410.

Johnson, J., & Leventhal, H. (1971). Effects of accurate expectations and behavioral instructions on reactions during a noxious medical exam. *Journal of Personality and Social Psychology, 29,* 710-718.

Johnson, J. E., Fuller, S. S., Endress, M. P., & Rice, V. H. (1978). Altering patients' responses to surgery: An extention and replication. *Research in Nursing and Health, 1,* 111-121.

Johnson, J. E., Rice, V. H., Fuller, S., & Endress, M. P. (1978). Sensory information, instruction in coping strategy and recovery from surgery. *Research in Nursing and Health, 1,* 4-17.

Krantz, D. S., Baum, A., & Wideman, M. (1980). Assessment of preferences for self-treatment and information in health care. *Journal of Personality and Social Psychology, 39,* 977-990.

Lazarus, R. S., & Launier, R. (1978). Stress-related transactions between person and environment. In L. A. Pervin & M. Lewis (Eds.), *Perspectives in Interactional Psychology* (pp. 287-327). New York: Plenum Press.

Lenz, E. R. (1984). Information seeking: A component of client decisions and health behavior. *Advances in Nursing Science, 6,* 59-72.

McNair, D. M., Lorr, M., & Droppleman, L. F. (1981). *Profile of mood states.* San Diego, CA: Edits.

Padilla, G. V., Grant, M. M., Rains, B. L., Hensen, B., Bergstrom, N., Wong, D., & Hanson, R. (1981). Distress reduction and the effects of preparatory teaching films and patient control. *Research in Nursing and Health, 4,* 375-387.

Parrish, J. (1976). *Individual coping styles, level of state anxiety, stress relevant information, and recovery from surgery associated with cancer.* Unpublished master's thesis, Virginia Commonwealth University, Richmond, VA.

Scott, D. W., Oberst, M. T., & Dropkin, M. J. (1980). A stress-coping model. *Advances in Nursing Science, 3,* 9-22.

Sime, A. M. (1976). Relationship of preoperative fear, type of coping and information received about surgery to recovery from surgery. *Journal of Personality and Social Psychology, 34,* 716-724.

Sime, A. M., & Libera, M. B. (1985). Sensation information, self-instruction and responses to dental surgery. *Research in Nursing and Health, 8,* 41-47.

Vernon, D. T., & Bigelow, D. A. (1974). Effect of information about a potentially stressful situation on response to stress impact. *Journal of Personality & Social Psychology, 29,* 50-79.

Waltz, C. F., Strickland, O. L., & Lenz, E. R. (1984). *Measurement in nursing research,* Philadelphia: F. A. Davis.

Ziemer, M. M. (1983). Effects of information on post surgical coping. *Nursing Research, 32,* 282-287.

5

The Measurement of Compliance as a Nursing Outcome

Gail Hilbert

This chapter discusses the Compliance Questionnaire, a measure of patient compliance with therapeutic regimens.

PURPOSE

The purpose of this chapter is to examine a number of issues related to the measurement of compliance: definitions of compliance, congruence of various definitions of compliance with nursing conceptual frameworks, calculation of meaningful compliance scores, methods of determining compliance, reliability of those methods, and finally, ethical issues surrounding reported noncompliance. These issues will be addressed in relation to an investigation of compliance of myocardial infarction (MI) patients (Hilbert, 1983). The instrument used in this study was a self-report questionnaire with a Likert-type scale. Content validity and interrater reliability were obtained. Triangulation of data from three different sources (subject, spouse, and investigator) was further support for the validity of the tool.

CONCEPTUAL BASIS AND REVIEW OF THE LITERATURE

Overview of the Compliance Study

The study for which the compliance questionnaire was developed focused on the influence of spouse support on the compliance of 60 male patients ages 38 to 73 who were at least 3 months post-MI. The theoretical framework was based on both the social support and compliance literatures. Spouse support was assumed to be a specific category of social support that has been linked with the ability to cope with stress, as well as being positively related to a variety of health outcomes (House, 1981).

This chapter includes content previously published in "Accuracy of Self-Reported Measures of Compliance," *Nursing Research, Vol. 34,* pp. 319-320.

Spouse support was defined as the degree to which the spouse of an MI patient engaged in activities directed toward providing her husband with physical assistance, intimate interaction, social participation, material aid, guidance, and feedback (Barrera & Ainlay, 1983). The study on which this chapter is based used home interviews of subject and spouse to test the hypothesis that spouse support was positively related to compliance. However, the focus of this chapter will be on approaches and issues related to the measurement of compliance.

Definition of Compliance

A number of decisions have to be made concerning compliance as a nursing outcome. The first important decision facing the researcher is to select a theoretical definition of compliance that is congruent with the conceptual and theoretical frameworks on which the study is based. A commonly used definition of compliance is that of Sackett (1976): "the extent to which the patient's behavior coincides with the clinical prescription" (p. 1).

One crucial question is left unanswered by this definition: whose prescription? Early compliance studies made the assumption that it was the physician's prescription. However, nursing has been moving away from the medical model toward a nursing model. The literature concerning compliance reflects this change and the struggles to come to terms with compliance within a nursing model that concerns itself with holism and the nursing management of interaction between the patient and the environment to promote healing or health (Fawcett, 1984; Flaskerud & Halloran, 1980).

As early as 1974 there was concern about the connotations of the word *compliance*, which suggests a dictatorial process in which the clinician does not involve the patient. At that time an interdisciplinary group at the Workshop/Symposium on Compliance with Therapeutic Regimens at McMaster University expanded the definition of compliance to "the extent to which the patient's behavior coincides with the clinical prescription *regardless of how the latter was generated*" (Sackett, 1976, p. 1). They went on to say that the term *compliance* describes the extent to which the patient yields to health instructions and advice "whether declared by an autocratic, authoritarian clinician or developed as a consensual regimen through negotiation between a health professional and a citizen" (p. 2).

In 1979 an interdisciplinary group (Barofsky, Sugarbaker, & Mills) described a social control continuum with three points: compliance, adherence, and therapeutic alliance. They stated that any patient-provider relationship has had or does have elements of all three types of relationships. Compliance describes a standard external to both parties. Adherence is a more appropriate term when both patient and provider expect a particular pattern of behavior, and it implies less social control due to interaction between the two. Therapeutic alliance implies negotiations that have resulted in acceptance of the regimen. A therapeutic alliance should develop over time if the patient is able to negotiate with the health care provider and assume responsibility for self-care.

By 1982 a number of articles by nurses addressed the issue of whether compliance and noncompliance were appropriate terms for nursing. Dracup and Meleis (1982) described these terms using an interactionist approach. They stated that there is a false assumption underlying the medical model that describes noncompliance in terms of the characteristics of the patient alone, rather than focusing on characteristics of both patient and health professional and on the interaction between them.

Approaching the term *noncompliance* from the standpoint of nursing diagnosis, Stanitis and Ryan (1982) viewed noncompliance as reflecting hierarchical values in which the health care provider is "one up" and the client is "one down." They did not suggest a more appropriate approach to the problem, but an editor's note stated that the Fifth National Conference on Nursing Diagnoses agreed that a less value-laden term be developed.

An issue of *Nursing Clinics of North America* addressed the topic of patient compliance in September 1982. Conway-Rutkowski (1982), editor of that issue, noted the paucity of research about the negotiation process in which the nurse and patient participate to select an appropriate therapeutic plan. In that some issue Moughton (1982) suggested the use of the term *therapeutic alliance* and advocated involving the patient in the nursing care plan.

The study in which the present compliance questionnaire was used was initiated in 1979, when the issue of the therapeutic alliance was not considered by the researcher in the choice of a theoretical definition. The definition chosen was that previously quoted from Sackett (1976, p. 1): "the extent to which the patient's behavior coincides with the clinical prescription." The prescription with which the subject was complying was that of the health team, as recalled by the subject. During semistructured interviews with the MI patients and their spouses it became apparent that very little "tailoring of the consensual regimen," a phrase coined by Fink (1976), had taken place.

There are several implications for future research that may be drawn from this section. First, researchers need to choose a definition of compliance that is congruent with their theoretical framework and specify with whose recommendations the compliance is concerned. Second, there is a need to examine the therapeutic alliance as it pertains to nursing. Little research has been done on the extent to which nurses consider the needs and life-styles of patients and negotiate with them in planning for therapeutic regimens.

Are patients with this kind of interaction more likely to be successful? O'Brien (1983), in her longitudinal study of hemodialysis patients, discovered that those who expired earliest demonstrated highest compliance, and those surviving longest had the lowest compliance. She used the term "reasoned compliance" to describe the noncompliers. This type of compliance behavior was more particularly suited to personal needs, such as the need for energy, the need to feel normal, and the need to share a meal or a particular kind of food with others as a social event. This interesting finding suggests the need for longitudinal studies that examine the relationships among compliance behaviors, quality of life, and disease outcomes.

METHODOLOGY

Description of the Compliance Questionnaire

The second important decision facing the researcher is the choice of the instrument for specifying the operational definition of compliance. It was assumed that it is preferable to select an existing instrument that has established validity and reliability.

A review of the compliance literature located three studies dealing with compliance of MI patients. Johnson (1974) interviewed 225 married males under 75 years of age who had experienced a first MI. Marston (1969) conducted interviews of 28 male MI patients between the ages of 44 and 64. Bille (1975) did telephone interviews of 24 males aged 32 to 75. Although all of these studies of MI patients examined different independent variables, all used compliance as the outcome measure and all used variations of the same compliance questionnaire.

Johnson (1974)[1] adapted an instrument used by Davis (cited in Marston, 1969). Johnson's instrument included seven areas of recommendations: medications, diet, weight loss, physical activity, smoking, alcohol use, stress, exercise, sexual intercourse, and work. Subjects were asked to describe the physician's recommendations in each area and any difficulties encountered, and to rate themselves as to how well they had been able to follow each recommendation. The rating categories were "all of the time," "most of the time," "less than half of the time," and "very little or not at all."

Marston (1969) added the categories of weight loss and work to this questionnaire and eliminated sexual intercourse. She used the same format, in terms of questioning for additional information and a similar rating scale, separating out "very little" and "not at all" into two categories. She also added a numerical value (ranging from 4 for "all of the time" to 0 for "not at all").

Bille (1975) used the same categories and rating scale as Marston (1969). He conducted telephone interviews and developed guidelines for placing subjects in categories when discrepant information was obtained. For example, when a subject rated himself low on medication compliance because he did not take a prn medication, he would be placed in the "all of the time" category.

The present instrument (Hillbert, 1983) added caffeine use to the ten categories of compliance used in the instruments described above. The

[1]This instrument was developed in 1964 but not published until 1974.

respondent was instructed to recall recommendations made by the health team, rather than the physician. This was based on the assumption that nurses, dietitians, and other members of the health care team are involved in instructing MI patients about their therapeutic regimens. The subjects were also instructed to limit their recall of how well they had carried out the instructions to the previous week. This was because the researcher was interested in recent compliance and because it was thought that this would allow for more accurate recall. For the present instrument, subjects indicated their compliance using the Likert-type scale of Marston (1969) ranging from 4 for "all of the time" to 0 for "none of the time."

Validity

Content validity of the questionnaire was determined by a panel of three nurses with master of science degrees in nursing who had expertise in the area of coronary rehabilitation. The 11 categories of compliance were also consistent with the information found in the protocol of the teaching plan for one of the cardiac rehabilitation programs from which the subjects were obtained (Widemer, 1979). The category of sexual advice was later removed when it was found that none of the 60 subjects had been given specific advice in this area. All subjects had been told to resume whatever was normal for them or had been given no advice in this area. The final instrument contained the following categories: medication, diet, weight reduction, stress reduction, exercise, physical activity, smoking cessation, alcohol and caffeine use, and work (Hilbert, 1983).

Scoring

To allow comparison of results from several studies and for the purpose of replication, it is necessary to specify the manner in which compliance scores have been derived. The first decision that must be made by the researcher is whether to use a continuous or a dichotomous score. Although a continuous score allows for more powerful statistical manipulation, some types of compliance are categorical by their nature. For example, receiving an immunization would be categorized into "yes" and "no." Other times a subject may be placed in a category based on the distribution of scores, such as a median split or quartiles. Gordis (1979) recommends using a biologic rationale, such as the level of compliance required to achieve a therapeutic response for dichotomizing patients into compliers and noncompliers. In the absence of such information, it is possible to select an arbitrary level of compliance as adequate.

Second, the researcher must decide whether or not to use a composite score when there is more than one area of compliance to be measured. In the present study it was possible that a subject would have some recommendations that would not apply – for example, the individual who was of normal weight at the time of the MI and thus had no recommendation regarding weight loss. This was handled by having a "not applicable" option. A total compliance score was then derived by totaling the scores for all recommendations that were applicable and dividing by the total possible score, resulting in a percentage score. It was deemed important to use separate areas of compliance, as well as the total score, in hypothesis testing because there was no evidence that the individual scores would be highly intercorrelated. As shown in Table 5.1, some individual compliance items were moderately correlated, but this was not true for all items.

A third decision regarding the calculation of compliance scores is whether or not to weight scores based on information that may be obtained in addition to the subject's self-report. One possible approach is to weight each item of the regimen according to the importance of that item. Davis (cited in Marston, 1969) developed a composite index based on the physician's actual recommendation, patient's and physician's independent estimates of the degree of compliance, and a weighting factor derived from the physician's evaluation of the relative importance of various components of the regimen.

Another approach to deriving a score would be to examine the degree of change by comparing present behavior with previous behavior for each recommendation. This is based on the assumption that 100% compliance with a particular recommendation may indicate a great deal of change for one patient and little for another. For example, a patient who smoked two packs of cigarettes per day before the MI and then stopped has had to change more than the person who smoked five cigarettes. No study

TABLE 5.1 Pearson Correlation Coefficients among Self-Reported Compliance Items

	Diet	Weight loss	Physical activity	Exercise	Stress	Smoking	Alcohol	Caffeine	Work
Medication	.002	.193	.163	.014	−.054	.165	.053	−.117	.319
Diet		.073	−.242	−.088	.070	−.056	−.093	−.006	−.069
Weight loss			.206	.396**	.291*	378**	−.039	.156	−.104
Physical activity				.128	.215*	.043	.395**	.010	.624**
Exercise					.153	.113	.014	.068	−.040
Stress reduction						.197	.138	.000	.301*
Smoking cessation							.118	.069	.219
Alcohol use								−.138	.302
Caffeine use									.255

* $p = < .05$; ** $p = < .01$.

that used this method was located, but it is something that should be considered as a possibility in order to allow for more meaningful comparative scores.

Still another approach is to consider the amount of difficulty involved in achieving the recommendation. Although for some subjects the amount of difficulty may be synonomous with the amount of change, there is no empirical evidence to support this assumption. Difficulty might be considered by looking at the success rate for each recommendation across subjects. Those recommendations with low compliance means would be considered more difficult than those with higher mean achievement, thus allowing a weighting formula to be developed. It is also possible to obtain the subjects' estimates of the relative difficulty in achieving each recommendation and devise a weighting schema based on that information.

Methods of Determining Compliance

Another dilemma facing the researcher is whether an indirect or a direct measure of compliance will result in greater validity and reliability. Outcome criteria, self-report of subjects, and ratings by family members and clinicians are examples of indirect measures of compliance. Outcome criteria, such as blood pressure reduction for those on antihypertensives, tend to be unreliable because of individual differences in response to treatment (Gordis, 1979). Self-report is the most commonly used indirect measure of compliance, mainly because of the relative ease in obtaining such a measure. There is little evidence that subjects will falsify information. However, all self-reports of deviant behavior tend to be underreported and nondeviant behavior overreported (Erickson & Smith, 1974).

Ratings by clinicians have been shown to be as inaccurate as self-report (Dunbar & Stunkard, 1979). A number of researchers have stated that ratings by family members are useful for such behaviors as food choice (Brownell, 1981), smoking (Lichtenstein, 1979), and drinking (Miller, 1981).

Direct measures of compliance, such as pill counts and biochemical assessment, are also problematic because patients may fail to return unused pills or may deviate from dosage schedules (Dunbar & Stunkard, 1979). Some types of drug compliance lend themselves to biochemical assessment, but this may be misleading due to individual physiologic variations.

Collection of Compliance Data

A decision was made to use self-reports obtained during home interviews for the present study. The interview allowed the investigator to assess the subject's recall of recommendations and discuss any problems encountered in carrying them out. It also allowed the investigator to note discrepancies between self-report and environmental evidence, such as the presence of foods that were not allowed on the subject's diet. It was not assumed that the subject was noncompliant in such cases. However, the investigator was then able to question whether or not the subject usually included such foods in his diet on a regular basis. It was also noted that a number of subjects smoked during the interview, verifying their noncompliance in that area.

In a manner similar to the husband, the wife was asked to describe her understanding of her husband's recommendations and any difficulties he encountered in carrying them out. She then rated her perceptions of her husband's compliance in each area for the previous week. Husband and wife were interviewed separately, and all interviews were tape-recorded.

The investigator also determined a judged compliance score, which was based on her detection of discrepancies within the self-reports. For example, if a subject had given himself a "4" or "all of the time" rating but made statements about not complying all of the time – missing doses of medication, drinking caffeinated coffee when instructed not to do so, exceeding the recommended amounts of alcohol, eating foods not allowed on a low-sodium or modified-fat diet, engaging in activities forbidden by the doctor, exceeding the calorie limit, smoking or not meeting the exercise recommendations – the judged score was lower than the subject's self-reported score.

If a subject had rated himself lower than would be expected – for example, had rated himself low on medication but the medication was related to need and did not have to be taken everyday, or he was allowed some caffeine or alcohol and had not exceeded the limit – the judged score was higher than the self-report score. The judged compliance score for each subject and each category might be the same as the self-report, higher, or lower.

Reliability

Interrater reliability was determined by having a second rater listen to the tapes and record compliance scores for the first five interviews and every tenth interview thereafter. The interrater reliability was .96 for both the self-reported compliance scores and wife's rating and .84 for the judged compliance scores.

FINDINGS AND RESULTS

The judged ratings and the self-reported ratings were correlated significantly for all 10 aspects of the regimen, ranging from .531 to .994 ($p <$ .001). Husbands and wives also had significantly correlated ratings (from .297 to .972) at the .001 level, with the exception of alcohol use (.419 at

$p < .05$), physical activity (.101), and stress reduction (.247), which were not significantly correlated. These findings from triangulation of data lent further support to the validity and reliability of the tool.

The investigator found that subjects were able to admit to considerable noncompliance, as shown in Table 5.2. For example, a number of subjects rated themselves low for diet, weight loss, and stress reduction. As might be expected, weight reduction was a difficult area in which to achieve compliance, with subjects reporting a mean compliance of 64%, based on the ratio of the reported scores to the highest possible score. Of the 33 subjects who were smoking at the time of the MI, six were still smoking and did so during the interviews.

It was concluded that subjects rate themselves accurately in direct interviews conducted by an investigator who has established rapport and communicates concern. An introductory comment about understanding how difficult it is to comply and that most patients are not completely compliant sets the right atmosphere.

The interview format allows the investigator to find out the subjects' recall of recommendations, thus stimulating their memories. Questions can focus on prescriptions, diet pamphlets, and teaching programs, as well as the day-to-day manner in which the subject attempts to carry out the recommendations. The interview format also allows for gentle probing if there are any discrepancies. For example: "Think back to the past week and tell me how many doses of your medication you think you missed" or "What do you do about your diet if you are eating in a restaurant?"

Although no method of assessing compliance is ideal and the optimal method will vary with the type of compliance being assessed, interview methods incorporating the previous suggestions should allow researchers to place greater confidence in the validity of the data obtained.

TABLE 5.2 Mean, Standard Deviation, and Percent Compliance for Self-Reported Compliance

Recommendation	Number of cases	Mean	SD	% Compliance
Medication	57	3.807	.398	95
Diet	57	3.018	.834	75
Weight loss	39	2.564	1.294	64
Limits on physical activity	46	3.717	.584	93
Exercise	59	3.051	1.209	76
Stress reduction	51	3.078	.668	77
Smoking cessation	33	3.588	1.598	90
Alcohol use	31	3.548	.961	89
Caffeine use	52	3.341	1.132	84
Work	46	3.913	.354	98
Total self-reported compliance	60	82.22	12.27	82

Ethical Issues

Another dilemma facing the researcher who studies compliance is the ethical dilemma of how to deal with subjects who report potentially dangerous noncompliance. This is an issue unique to studies of deviant behavior, such as noncompliance with therapeutic regimens, unethical behaviors, and illegal acts. In the present study there was the case of a subject who had considerable heart damage and had stopped taking his medication. Several other subjects were pushing the limits of physical activity by lifting heavy objects and chopping wood.

The dilemma arises because the subject has been assured confidentiality as part of the protection of human subjects. The consent form states that information will not be shared with the physician or anyone connected with the subject's care. However, the researcher in this study was also a nurse and was committed to promoting health and prolonging useful life.

There is little in the literature to guide the researcher who is confronted with such a situation. Two sources that addressed the problem were located. Treece and Treece (1982) state that in such situations confidentiality must be maintained. Bush (1985) gives examples of this type of problem but offers no solutions. The present researcher dealt with the dilemma by doing health teaching, referring subjects back to the health team for further counseling, and involving the spouse (with the consent of the subject).

CONCLUSIONS

This chapter has addressed a number of issues relevant to compliance as a nursing outcome, as well as describing the development of an instrument that measures compliance for 10 aspects of the MI regimen. Researchers are urged to give careful consideration to decisions relating to their choice of both theoretical and operational definitions of compliance.

Questions to be considered include the following:

Is the theoretical definition congruent with the nursing conceptual framework?

With whose prescriptions is the subject complying?

How will compliance scores be calculated for maximum utility in terms of comparability with other subjects and studies and for statistical analysis?

Should self-report scores be used, or are more objective means available?

How can one protect noncompliant subjects from loss of confidentiality while at the same time ensuring that they will not endanger their health?

It was concluded that compliance as it has traditionally been defined is not congruent with nursing conceptual frameworks. It is more appropriate for nurses to consider the therapeutic alliance and examine the interaction between caregiver and client as it relates to outcomes. Ideally, such clients should be complying with the negotiated regimen.

Several suggestions are made in regard to the calculation of compliance scores. When there are a number of items in the therapeutic plan, scores should be calculated for each aspect as well as for the total plan. Scores based on weighted composites of a number of factors have been suggested, such as importance of each item, amount of change required, difficulty in achieving each recommendation. Consideration of these factors may result in a more valid measurement of compliance.

The issue of the accuracy of self-reported compliance has been discussed. The study of compliance of MI patients suggested that subjects do admit to noncompliance if the investigator establishes rapport and communicates acceptance of less than perfect compliance. Home interviews using gentle probing will help the subject recall deviations from the prescribed regimen.

The ethical dilemma of subjects reporting dangerous noncompliance has been discussed. It is suggested that family members be involved, if the subject gives his consent, and that subjects be referred back to caregivers for further education.

Finally, an instrument for measuring compliance of MI patients has been described. Content validity and interrater reliability has been established for this instrument. Concurrent ratings by the researcher and the subject's spouse yielded further evidence of the validity of the instrument.

It is hoped that this chapter has stimulated your thinking about these issues. The decisions are not always easy, but thoughtful consideration of the choices should enable nurses to conduct compliance research that is both theoretically and methodologically sound.

REFERENCES

Barofsky, I., Sugarbaker, P. H., & Mills, M. E. (1979). Compliance and quality of life assessment. In J. Cohen (Ed), *New directions in patient compliance* (pp. 59-74). Lexington, MA: D. C. Heath.

Barrera, M., & Ainlay, S. L. (1983). The structure of social support: A conceptual and empirical analysis. *Journal of Community Psychology, 11,* 133-143.

Bille, D. A. (1975). *Structured vs. unstructured teaching format and body image, compliance with post-hospitalization prescriptions and knowledge about life following heart attack.* Unpublished doctoral dissertation, University of Wisconsin, Madison.

Brownell, K. D. (1981). Assessment of eating disorders. In D. H. Barlow (Ed.), *Behavioral assessment of adult disorders* (pp. 329-404). New York: The Guilford Press.

Bush, C. T. (1985). *Nursing Research*. Reston, VA: Reston Publishing.

Conway-Rutkowsky, B. (1982). Foreword to Symposium on patient compliance. *The Nursing Clinics of North America, 17*(3), 440-450.

Dracup, K. A., & Meleis, A. I. (1982). Compliance: An interactionist approach. *Nursing Research, 21,* 37-42.

Dunbar, J. M., & Stunkard, A. N. (1979). Adherence to diet and drug regimen. In R. Levy, B. Rifkind, B. Dennis, & N. Ernst (Eds.), *Nutrition, lipids, and coronary heart disease* (pp. 391-423). New York: Raven Press.

Erickson, M. L., & Smith, W. B. (1974). On the relationship between self-reported and actual deviance: An empirical test. *Humboldt Journal of Social Relations, 2,* 106-113.

Fawcett, J. (1984). *Analysis and evaluation of conceptual models of nursing*. Philadelphia: F. A. Davis.

Fink, D. L. (1976). Tailoring the consensual regimen. In D. L. Sackett & R. B. Haynes (Eds.), *Compliance with therapeutic regimens* (pp. 110-118). Baltimore: The Johns Hopkins University Press.

Flaskerud, J. H., & Halloran, E. (1980). Areas of agreement in nursing theory development. *Advances in Nursing Science, 3*(1), 1-7.

Gordis, K. (1979). Conceptual and methodologic problems in measuring patient compliance. In R. B. Haynes, D. W. Taylor, & D. L. Sackett (Eds.), *Compliance in health care* (pp. 23-45). Baltimore: The Johns Hopkins University Press.

Hilbert, G. K. (1983). *The relationship between spouse support and compliance of the myocardial infarction patients*. Unpublished doctoral dissertation, University of Pennsylvania, Philadelphia.

House, J. S. (1981). *Work, stress and social support*. Reading, MA: Addison-Wesley.

Johnson, W. L. (1974). *Adjustment to the crisis of coronary heart disease*. New York: National League for Nursing.

Lichtenstein, E. (1979). Social learning, smoking and substance abuse. In N. A. Krasnegor (Ed.), *Behavioral analysis and treatment of substance abuse* (NIDA Monograph 25) (pp. 113-127). Washington, DC: U.S. Governmen Printing Office.

Marston, M. V. (1969). *Compliance with medical regimens as a form of risk-taking in patients with myocardial infarctions*. Unpublished doctoral dissertation, Boston University, Boston.

Miller, P. M. (1981). Assessment of alcohol abuse. In D. H. Barlow (Ed.), *Behavioral assessment of adult disorders* (pp. 271-300). New York: Brunner/Mazel.

Moughton, M. (1982). The patient – a partner in the health care process. *The Nursing Clinics of North America, 17,* 3.

O'Brien, M. E. (1983). *The courage to survive*. New York: Grune & Stratton.

Sackett, D. L. (1976). Introduction. In D. L. Sackett & R. B. Haynes (Eds.). *Compliance with therapeutic regimens* (pp. 1-6). Baltimore: The Johns Hopkins University Press.

Stanitis, M. A., & Ryan, J. (1982). Noncompliance: An unacceptable diagnosis? *American Journal of Nursing, 82,* 941-942.

Treece, E. W., & Treece, J. W. (1982). *Elements of research in nursing*. St. Louis: C. V. Mosby.

Widemer, N. (1979). *Inpatient cardiac education*. Philadelphia: Albert Einstein Medical Center, Daroff Division.

Compliance Questionnaire

HUSBAND

Instructions: The questions you will be asked have to do with recommendations you have been told to follow by the health team (nurses, doctors, physical therapists, dietitians, etc.).

I.   Let's start with **MEDICATIONS**.

A. Are you taking medicine of any kind?

	Type	Frequency
1.		
2.		
3.		
4.		

B. Have you had any difficulty with taking any of these? What kind of difficulty (e.g., remembering, inconvenience, cost, side effects, etc.)?

C. For the drugs mentioned: Would you estimate that you have been taking it (in the past week):

Judged score

—   __ (4) all of the time
—   __ (3) most of the time
—   __ (2) about half of the time
—   __ (1) very seldom
—   __ (0) none of the time

D. Do you think you have missed any doses in the past week? How many?

E. What has been helpful in regard to your taking the medications as directed?

What has not been helpful?

II.   Let's go to **DIET** other than weight reduction.

A. Are you on a diet?   What kind?

B. Did anyone on the health team (doctor, nurse, dietitian, physical therapist, etc.) make suggestions regarding your eating patterns (e.g., reduce the amount of salt and salty foods, reduce the amount of fat, change the kind of fat, reduce or eliminate certain foods)?

If so, what was recommended? Were you given diet sheet? Have you read books, pamphlets?

C. Who prepares this? Who does the food shopping?

D. Have you had any difficulty with following your dietary recommendations? If so, what kind of difficulty? What about eating out, going to parties, etc.?

E. Would you estimate that you have been able to follow your diet (in the past week):

Judged score

___   ___ (4) all of the time

___   ___ (3) most of the time

___   ___ (2) about half of the time

___   ___ (1) very seldom

___   ___ (0) none of the time

F. What has been helpful for you in regard to carrying out these recommendations?

What has not been helpful?

III.   Let's go to **WEIGHT LOSS**.

A. Did anyone on the health team make any recommendations concerning loss of weight?

If so, what were you told?

___ lose weight   ___maintain same weight

Who made the recommendation?

B. If you were told to lose weight, how much were you told to lose?

C. What method was recommended?

D. Over how long a period of time were you to have lost this?

E. Have you lost weight, maintained same weight, or gained weight?

F. How much have you lost or gained?

G. Have you had any difficulty in following the recommendations for weight loss?

H. What kind of difficulty?

I. In the past week, how much of the time have you followed the recommendations regarding your weight reduction?

Judged score

  —   __ (4) all of the time

  —   __ (3) most of the time

  —   __ (2) about half of the time

  —   __ (1) very seldom

  —   __ (0) not at all

J. What has been helpful in regard to carrying out these recommendations?

What has not been helpful?

IV.   Let's go to **PHYSICAL ACTIVITY** in terms of activity that could be considered harmful.

A. Did any member of the health team suggest that you limit your activity in any way (e.g., avoiding strenuous activity, avoiding working or exercising in very hot or very cold weather, avoiding isometric exercise, lifting a maximum amount of weight, mowing the lawn, shoveling snow)?

How?

Who made the recommendation?

B. have you had any difficulty in following these recommendations?

C. What kind of difficulty have you had?

D. Would you estimate that you have been able to follow these recommendations (in the past week):

Judged score

  —   __ (4) all of the time

  —   __ (3) most of the time

  —   __ (2) about half of the time

  —   __ (1) very seldom

  —   __ (0) none of the time

E. What has been helpful in carrying out these recommendations?

What has not been helpful?

V.   Let's go to **EXERCISE** that could be considered helpful.

A. Did any member of the health team suggest that you engage in an exercise program (daily walks, using an exercycle, using a treadmill, swimming, etc.)?

What recommendations were made? How often did you go to the rehab program? If done at home, optimal pulse rate.

Who made them?

B. Have you had any difficulty in following these recommendatinos?

C. What kind of difficulty?

D. Would you estimate that you have been able to follow these recommendations:

Judged score
—   __ (4) all of the time
—   __ (3) most of the time
—   __ (2) about half of the time
—   __ (1) very seldom
—   __ (0) none of the time

E. What has been helpful in carrying out these recommendations?

What has not been helpful?

VI. Let's go to **STRESSFUL SITUATIONS**.

A. Did any member of the health team recommend that you try to avoid stressful situations or make changes in your life to better deal with stress when it arises (e.g., set practical goals, lighten your load of responsibility, discuss problems with someone, set aside a time each day for relaxation, etc.)?

Who made the suggestions?

What suggestions were made? Was anything specific said?

B. Have you had any difficulty in following this advice?

C. What kind of difficulty have you had?

D. Would you say that you have been able to avoid stressful situations or deal with stress in specific ways (in the past week):

Judged score
—   __ (4) all of the time
—   __ (3) most of the time
—   __ (2) about half of the time
—   __ (1) very seldom
—   __ (0) not at all

    E. What has been helpful in carrying out these recommendations?

       What has not been helpful?

VII.   Let's go to **SMOKING**.

    A. Did you smoke prior to your illness?

       If yes, how much of each of the following per day?

       cigarettes __ cigars __ pipe __

    B. Did anyone of the health team suggest that you cut down or eliminate smoking?

       If so, who made the recommendation?

       Did anyone suggest a method for stopping smoking?

    C. Have you had any difficulty in following this advice?

    D. What kind of difficulty have you had?

    E. How much of the time have you followed these recommenda-
       tions in the past week:
Judged score
—   __ (4) all of the time
—   __ (3) most of the time
—   __ (2) about half of the time
—   __ (1) very seldom
—   __ (0) not at all

    F. How much do you smoke now? cigarettes __ cigars __ pipe __

    G. What has been helpful in carrying out these recommendations?

       What has not been helpful?

VIII.   Let's go to **ALCOHOL USE**.

    A. Did you drink alcoholic beverages before your illness? if yes, how much per week? beer __   wine __   hard liquor __

B. Did anyone on the health team make any recommendations to you about alcohol use?

What were you told?

By whom?

C. Have you had any difficulty in following this advice?

D. What kind of difficulty have you had?

E. How much of the time have you followed these recommendations in the past week?

Judged score

___   ___ (4) all of the time

___   ___ (3) most of the time

___   ___ (2) about half of the time

___   ___ (1) very seldom

___   ___ (0) not at all

F. How much do you now drink per week?

G. What has been helpful in regard to following the recommendations about alcohol use?

What has not been helpful?

IX.   Let's go to **CAFFEINE INTAKE**.

A. Did you drink beverages containing caffeine, such as coffee, tea, or colas, before your illness?

B. If so, how much per day? coffee ___ tea ___ colas ___

C. Did anyone on the health team make any recommendations about intake of beverages containing caffeine (coffee, tea, colas)?

Who made the recommendations?

What was recommended?

D. Have you had any difficulty in following these recommendations?

E. If so, what kind of difficulty have you had?

F. How often in the last week would you estimate that you have been following the recommendations about caffeine intake?

Judged score
—   __ (4) all of the time
—   __ (3) most of the time
—   __ (2) about half of the time
—   __ (1) very seldom
—   __ (0) none of the time

   G. How much are you now drinking of beverages containing caf-
       feine per day? coffee __ tea __ colas __

   H. What has been helpful in carrying out these recommendations?

       What has not been helpful?

X.   Let's go to **SEXUAL ACTIVITY.**

   A. Did anyone on the health team make recommendations about
       sexual activity (positions, relationship to meals and alcoholic
       beverages, using nitroglycerin, etc.)?

   B. What recommendations were made?

       Who made them?

   C. What changes have occurred in your sexual relationship with
       your wife since your illness?

       What are your thoughts about factors that have contributed to
       these changes?

   D. Have you had any difficulties in carrying out the recommenda-
       tions of the health team about sexual activity? (If recommenda-
       tions applied to a limited period and no longer applies, skip D
       and E.)

   E. In the past month how much of the time have your carried out
       the recommendations about sexual activity?

Judged score
—   __ (4) all of the time
—   __ (3) most of the time
—   __ (2) about half of the time
—   __ (1) very seldom
—   __ (0) none of the time

   F. What has been helpful in adjusting sexually since your
       illness?

       What has not been helpful?

XI.   Let's go to **WORK**.

        A. What was your occupation before you became ill?

        B. Did anyone on the health team suggest any changes be made in regard to your work?

            Who made the recommendation?

            What was recommended?

        C. Have you returned to work? If so:

            __ same job as before   __ different job
            __ same job but with   __ totally different
                fewer demands   __ somewhat different
            __ same job but with   __ slightly different
                shorter hours

            If you are in a different job, what are you now doing?

        D. If you have *not* returned to work, do you plan to return to work?

            If yes, how will you decide on a future job?

            __ own judgment   __ other, specify
            __ health team advice

        E. If anyone on the health team made recommendations regarding changes in work, have you had difficulty in following these recommendations?

            If yes, what kinds of difficulty?

        F. How much of the time are you currently following recommendations in regard to work?

Judged score

    —   __ (4) all of the time
    —   __ (3) most of the time
    —   __ (2) about half of the time
    —   __ (1) very seldom
    —   __ (0) none of the time

        G. What has been helpful in adjusting to the changes you have had to make in regard to work?

            What has not been helpful?

Compliance Questionnaire

WIFE

Instructions: The questions you are being asked refer to the recommendations your husband has been told to follow by the health team (nurses, doctors, physical therapists, dietitians, etc.).

I.   Let's start with **MEDICATIONS**.

   A. Is your husband taking medications of any kind?

	Type	*Frequency*
1.		
2.		
3.		
4.		
5.		

   B. Has he had any difficulty with taking any of these? What kind of difficulty (remembering, inconvenience, cost, side effects, etc.)?

   C. For the drugs mentioned, would you estimate that your husband has been taking them (in the past week):

Judged score
—   __ (4) all of the time
—   __ (3) most of the time
—   __ (2) about half of the time
—   __ (1) very seldom
—   __ (0) dont know

   D. Do you think he has missed any doses in the past week? If yes, how many?

   E. How did you find out about this recommendation?

   Were you told directly?   Who told you?

II.   Let's go to **DIET**.

   A. Is your husband on a diet other than weight reduction? What kind?

B. Did anyone on the health team make suggestions regarding your husband's eating patterns (reduce the amount of salt or fat, reduce or eliminate certain foods)?

If so, what was recommended? Were you given a diet sheet? Have you had books or pamphlets?

C. Who prepares it? Who does the food shopping?

D. Has your husband had any difficulty with following the dietary recommendations? If so, what kind of difficulty?

E. Would you estimate that he has been able to follow his diet (in the past week):

Judged score

—	__ (4) all of the time
—	__ (3) most of the time
—	__ (2) about half of the time
—	__ (1) very seldom
—	__ (0) none of the time
—	__ don't know

F. How did you find out about the dietary recommendations?

Were you told directly?

Who told you?

G. What do you do to try to help him follow the dietary recommendations?

III.   Let's go to **WEIGHT LOSS**.

A. Did anyone on the health team make any recommendations to your husband concerning loss of weight?

If so, what was he told?

__ lose weight   __ maintain weight

Who made the recommendation?

B. What method of weight loss was recommended?

C. Has your husband had any difficulty in following these recommendations?

D. What kind of difficulties?

E. In the past week, how much of the time has your husband fol-

Judged score

lowed the recommendations regarding weight reduction?

___   ___ (4) all of the time
___   ___ (3) most of the time
___   ___ (2) about half of the time
___   ___ (1) very seldom
___   ___ (0) not at all

F.   How did you find out about the weight loss recommendations?

Were you told directly?

Who told you?

G.   What do you do to try to help your husband follow the weight loss recommendations?

IV.   Let's go to **PHYSICAL ACTIVITY** (in terms of activity that could be considered harmful).

A.   Did any member of the health team suggest to your husband that he limit his activity in any way (e.g., avoiding strenuous activity, avoiding working or exercising in very hot or very cold weather, avoiding isometric exercise, lifting a maximum amount of weight, mowing the lawn, shoveling snow)?
How?

Who made the recommendation?

B.   Has your husband has any difficulty in following these recommendations?

C.   What kind of difficulty has he had?

D.   Would you estimate that he has been able to follow these recommendations (in the past week):

Judged score

___   ___ (4) all of the time
___   ___ (3) most of the time
___   ___ (2) about half of the time
___   ___ (1) very seldom
___   ___ (0) none of the time
___   ___   don't know

E.   How did you find out about the activity recommendations?

Who told you?

Were you told directly?

    F. What do you do to try to help your husband follow the physical activity recommendations?

    V. Let's go to **EXERCISE** that could be considered helpful.

    A. Did any member of the health team suggest that your husband engage in an exercise program (daily walks, using an exercycle, using a treadmill, swimming, etc.)?

    What recommendations were made?

    Who made them?

    B. Has your husband had any difficulty in following these recommendations?

    C. What kind of difficulty?

    D. Would you estimate that he has been able to follow these recommendations (in the past week):

Judged score
—	__ (4) all of the time
—	__ (3) most of the time
—	__ (2) about half of the time
—	__ (1) very seldom
—	__ (0) none of the time
—	__ don't know

    E. How did you find out about the exercise recommendations?

    Who told you?

    Were you told directly?

    F. What do you do to try to help him follow the exercise recommendations?

VI.   Let's go to **STRESSFUL SITUATIONS**.

    A. Did any member of the health team recommend that your husband try to avoid stressful situations or make changes in his life to better deal with stress when it arises (set practical goals, lighten his load of responsibility, discuss problems with someone, set aside a time each day for relaxation, etc.)?

    Who made the suggestions?

    What suggestions were made? Was anything specific said?

    B. Has your husband had any difficulty in following this advice?

C. What kind of difficulty has he had?

D. Would you say that he has been able to avoid stressful situations or deal with stress in specific ways (in the past week):

Judged score
—   __ (4) all of the time
—   __ (3) most of the time
—   __ (2) about half of the time
—   __ (1) very seldom
—   __ (0) not at all
—   __   don't know

E. How did you find out about the recommendations regarding
stressful situations?

Who told you?

Were you told directly?

F. What do you do to try to help him deal with the recommendations regarding stressful situations?

VII.   Let's go to **SMOKING**.

A. Did your husband smoke prior to his illness? How much? cigarettes __   cigars __   pipe __

B. Did anyone on the health team suggest that he cut down or
eliminate smoking?
If yes, who made the recommendation?

C. Has your husband had any difficulty in following this advice?

D. What kind of difficulty has he had?

E. How much of the time has your husband followed these recommendations in the past week?

Judged score
—   __ (4) all of the time
—   __ (3) most of the time
—   __ (2) about half of the time
—   __ (1) very seldom
—   __ (0) not at all
—   __   don't know

F. How much does your husband now smoke in a day?
cigarettes __   cigars __   pipe __

G. How did you find out about the recommendations regarding smoking?

Who told you?

Were you told directly?

H. How do you try to help your husband carry out the recommendations about smoking?

VIII. Let's go to **ALCOHOL USE**.

A. Did your husband drink alcoholic beverages before his illness?

If yes, how much per week? beer ___ wine ___ hard liquor ___

B. Did anyone on the health team make any recommendations to your husband about alcohol use?

What was he told?

By whom?

C. Has your husband had any difficulty in following this advice?

D. What kind of difficulty has he had?

E. How much of the time has your husband followed these recommendations in the past week?

Judged score
___   ___ (4) all of the time
___   ___ (3) most of the time
___   ___ (2) about half of the time
___   ___ (1) very seldom
___   ___ (0) not at all
___   ___   don't know

F. How much does your husband drink now per week?

G. How did you find out about the recommendations regarding drinking?

Who told you?

Were you told directly?

H. What do you do to try to help your husband carry out the recommendations about alcohol?

IX.   Let's go to **CAFFEINE INTAKE**.

A. Did your husband drink beverages containing caffeine (coffee, tea, colas) before his illness?

B. If so, how much per day? coffee ___ tea ___ cola ___

C. Did anyone on the health team make any recommendations to your husband about intake of beverages containing caffeine (coffee, tea, colas)?

Who made the recommendations?

What was recommended?

D. Has your husband had any difficulty with this recommendation?

E. What kind of difficulty has he had?

F. How often in the last week would you estimate that your husband has followed the recommendations about caffeine intake?

Judged score
—   ___ (4) all of the time
—   ___ (3) most of the time
—   ___ (2) about half of the time
—   ___ (1) very seldom
—   ___ (0) none of the time
—   ___ don't know

G. How many cups a day of caffeinated beverages is your husband now drinking? coffee ___ tea ___ colas ___

H. How did you find out about the recommendations regarding use of beverages containing caffeine?

Who told you?

Were you told directly?

I. What do you do to try to help your husband carry out the recommendations about caffeine intake?

X.   Let's go to **SEXUAL ACTIVITY**.

A. Did anyone on the health team make recommendations about sexual activity (positions, relationship to meals and alcoholic beverages, using nitroglycerin, etc.)?

B. What recommendations were made?

   Who made them?

C. What changes have occurred in your sexual relationhip with your husband since his illness?

   What are your thoughts about factors that have contributed to these changes?

D. Have you had any difficulties in carrying out the recommendations of the health team about sexual activity? (If recommendations no longer apply because they were limited to a specific period, skip D and E)

   What difficulties have you had?

E. In the past month how much of the time have you carried out the recommendation about sexual activity?

Judged score

—   __ (4) all of the time
—   __ (3) most of the time
—   __ (2) about half of the time
—   __ (1) very seldom
—   __ (0) none of the time

F. How did you find out about the recommendations regarding sexual activity?

   Who told you?

   Were you told directly?

G. What do you do to help your husband in the area of your sexual relationship?

6

Measuring Health Goal Attainment in Patients

Imogene M. King

This chapter discusses the Criterion-Referenced Measure of Goal Attainment Tool, a measure of funcitonal abilities and goal attainment.

Standards of nursing practice are generated for the purpose of measuring outcomes of nursing care. Among these outcomes are those that indicate attainment of a functional state of health consistent with an individual's and a family's ability to function in their usual roles, such as teacher, administrator, mother, and father. Determining whether or not a standard is met is contingent on evaluating the outcome(s) associated with a standard. The criteria used for outcome evaluation are written in terms of behavioral performance expected in individuals and families.

A review of the nursing, management, community health, and community mental health literature revealed a paucity of instruments to measure goal attainment. This provided the impetus for the project undertaken during a 2-year continuing education program sponsored by the University of Maryland and the Division of Nursing, Special Projects Branch. This report presents the purpose, the conceptual basis for the instrument, the method used, the instrument, and implications for use of the instrument in clinical nursing situations. Implications for use of the instrument in nursing research to test hypotheses generated by King's theory of goal attainment are addressed.

PURPOSE

The primary purpose to be achieved in this measurement project was to develop an instrument that could be used to measure goal attainment in nursing situations. Since a goal-oriented nursing record was proposed to implement goal setting and goal attainment (King, 1981), data from the use of this instrument would provide documentation of nursing care in the permanent record of the patient. Documentation provides the information that determines effectiveness of nursing care.

A second purpose was to develop a reliable and valid tool that could be used to conduct research related to a theory of goal attainment in nursing situations. Instruments must be developed from a nursing perspective to test theoretical ideas.

CONCEPTUAL BASIS FOR MEASUREMENT TOOL

Several reliable and valid tools have been developed and used to assess functional abilities of individuals. An evaluation of at least four instruments in current use – Katz Index of ADL (Kane & Kane, 1981, pp. 45-47), Barthel Index (Kane & Kane, 1981, pp. 48-50) and LORS-II (Carey & Posavac, 1982) – were judged to be somewhat limited from a nursing perspective and were norm-referenced tools. A norm-referenced tool is defined as one that "evaluates the performance of a subject relative to the performance of other subjects in some well-defined comparison or norm group. A key feature of a norm-referenced measure is variance" (Waltz, Strickland, & Lenz, 1984, p. 4). Most instruments that deal with averages within groups are norm-referenced. Although norm-referenced tools are helpful in some situations, they do not provide information about an individual's status as a basis for planning nursing care. A rating scale to assess movement from dependence to independence indicated movement toward a criterion-referenced measure in nursing (Williams, 1960).

In contrast, a criterion-referenced measure is defined as one that is used "to ascertain an individual's status with respect to a well-defined behavioral domain" (Popham, 1978, p. 93). Since a philosophy of individualized care has pervaded nursing's history, a criterion-referenced measure seemed to be conceptually congruent with assessment of functional abilities of patients to gather data from which to make decisions about individualized plans of care.

The conceptual framework for nursing was a theory of goal attainment (King, 1981). This theory for nursing identified both process and outcome variables. Process variables included mutual goal setting and nurse and patient verbal and nonverbal communication behaviors relevant in the interactions that lead to transactions. Outcome variables were the goals attained by patients as a result of mutual goal setting and transactions made. In an initial study to identify the process of nurse-patient interactions that lead to transactions and goals, direct observations of nurse-patient interactions in a natural environment of a hospital unit provided data for analysis. This small study resulted in a classification system to study interactions that lead to transactions. This process facilitates mutual goal setting that leads to goal attainment by patients as an outcome of nursing care. Outcome variables were the goals attained by patients as a result of mutual goal setting and transactions made by nurse and patient.

In designing an instrument to measure goal attainment, one problem in nursing was addressed. Nurses have always set goals for nursing care but have not always stated them in terms of expected patient performance behavior that is observable and/or measurable. Mager's (1965) framework was selected for writing goals in terms of patient performance. The goal statements were based on the functional-abilities assessment scales that were part of this project.

METHOD

Several factors are considered essential in the development of a criterion-referenced instrument. Waltz and associates (1984) noted "the primary goal of criterion-referenced measurement is to accurately determine the status of some objects in terms of a well-defined domain" (p. 164). A clear definition of the content domain was an essential factor that was considered in developing the instrument.

The content domain for this criterion-referenced tool is described clearly as functional abilities of individuals and as goal attainment behaviors. Functional abilities were defined more specifically as the physical ability of individuals to perform activities of daily living and the behavioral response of individuals to the performance of activities of daily living. Goal attainment was defined as mutual goal setting by nurse and patient on the basis of data from the assessment of functional abilities and from the nurse-patient interactions in which they share information about the presenting conditions and/or problems to be solved.

Subsequent to defining the content domain of the criterion-referenced measure, a homogeneous collection of items was written that accurately assess the content domain. A distinguishing feature of a criterion-referenced measure is that it is based on a specified domain rather than on a specified population or group. Performance standards that defined the domain status were determined. Evaluation of the performance of individuals relative to these standards determined a person's status. The method used to develop a criterion-referenced measure of goal attainment relates to the objectives of the domain measured, the item specifications, directions for use, scoring, reliability, and validity.

Domain Objectives

The criterion-referenced measure was designed to measure outcomes, that is, the ability of individuals to perform activities of daily living. The domain objectives were

1. To assess physical ability of individuals to perform activities of daily living related to personal hygiene, movement, and human interaction.

2. To assess the behavioral response of individuals in the performance of activities of daily living related to personal hygiene, movement, and human interaction.
3. To select a goal and to measure goal attainment in performing activities of daily living related to personal hygiene, movement, and human interaction.

A criterion-referenced instrument was constructed that consisted of three scales representing the domain objectives: physical abilities, behavioral response, and goals. Each scale was composed of three subscales: (1) personal hygiene, (2) movement, and (3) human interaction. Multiple items within each subscale were written. The personal hygiene subscale consisted of eight items representative of essential tasks in performing actions related to hygiene. Six items were written that were representative of the movement subscale. The human interaction subscale included 12 items representative of sensory perceptions, verbal and nonverbal communication, and interactions and transactions.

Item Specification

A clear specification of the behaviors to be measured was characterized by an essential and behavioral response of the patient in a nursing situation. Data from these assessment scales were used to identify a feasible goal for patients and to measure their attainment of the goal. Measurement of goal attainment may be used to determine effectiveness of nursing care.

Each of the three scales was developed to clearly describe the behaviors of patients. The goal scale was written to specify outcomes that are the performance standards to be attained by patients.

Several rules were identified to create the items in the personal hygiene, movement, and human interaction subscales. First, a decision was made to construct a 4-point scale. Second, items in each of the subscales were developed to assess a range of behaviors from dependence to independence in the performance of activities of daily living. Third, consistency in the terms used to indicate specific behaviors at each level of performance was essential in item writing. Fourth, a sufficient number of items within each subscale were developed to sample the essential behaviors expected in patients' performance of activities of daily living. This instrument was designed to be used by registered professional nurses. The following example illustrates the *general description* for a measure of physical ability to perform mouth care: "Brushes teeth/dentures without assistance." The following example illustrates the *general description* for a measure of behavioral response to perform mouth care: "Assumes responsibility for daily oral hygiene." The following example illustrates the *general description* for a measure of goal attainment: "Given the equipment, health reasons for mouth care, a demonstration of techniques, patient performs mouth care a minimum of two times a day."

Sample Item

This section of the three subscales included items related to personal hygiene. Select only one statement in each of the scales. Place a check mark in the box to the left of the statement.

Physical ability to perform activity	*Behavior response to perform activity*
Personal hygiene 　Mouth care	Personal Hygiene 　Mouth care
☐ Unable to brush teeth/dentures	☐ Rejects assistance in brushing teeth/dentures
☐ Requires assistance with equipment and brushing teeth/dentures	☐ Tolerates assistance with mouth care
☐ Requires supervision with equipment and brushing teeth/dentures	☐ Seeks assistance in brushing teeth/dentures
☐ Brushes teeth/dentures without assistance	☐ Assumes responsibility for oral hygiene

Goal setting and goal attainment

Personal hygiene
　Mouth care

☐ Oral hygiene provided by caregiver with demonstration of technique and health reasons for mouth care given to patient

☐ Patient demonstrates adequate mouth care under supervision of care giver

☐ Patient demonstrates proper technique in performing mouth care once a day

☐ Patient uses appropriate technique in performing mouth care a minimum of two times a day

The first draft of the instrument was analyzed by ten graduate students in clinical nursing of adults. Suggestions for clarity were given and several items were revised, but none were discarded. The next step in the process was to write clear directions for using the instrument and for scoring.

Directions for Using the Instrument

The purpose of the criterion-referenced measure is to assess patients' functional abilities in performance of activities of daily living. Using the assessment data, nurses set goals with patients and measure goal attainment by scoring the differences between goals set and goals attained. The initial assessment takes about 15 min. and serves as baseline data for comparison with future assessments. *Direct observations of patients'* ability to perform the functions of daily activities are required to assess patients.

Only registered professional nurses are responsible for using the instrument for goal setting and for measuring goal attainment. This is a professional nursing function within which decisions are made for nursing care. This criterion-referenced instrument measures each individual's attainment of goals. Data from the assessment scales and from the goal attainment scale will be placed on the permanent patient record to be used by professional nurses in planning, implementing, and evaluating effectiveness of care. The results are used to determine status of patients based on performance standards specified in the domain.

Scoring

The assessment scale was designed to evaluate the functional ability of individuals related to activities of daily living. The 4-point scale contains items that are ordered from dependence to independence. Definitions for functional dependence and independence are as follows:

1. Completely dependent: patient needs help with the activity.
2. Requires assistance by caregiver or mechanical aid in performance of the activity.
3. Requires supervision of activity; patient is independent of caregiver but needs monitoring of performance of activity.
4. Independent of caregiver; patient can perform the activity with or without mechanical aids.

If the nurse gives the patient a score of 1 on physical ability to brush teeth, the goal to be attained may be set at 3. The highest goal attainment score for anyone is 4. If goal is set at 3 and the patient attains 3, this is equal to 0, or congruence between goal set and goal attained. The score for patients can range from −3 to +3. For example, if the goal is set at 3 and the patient achieves 1, the expected goal is not attained and a score of −3 is recorded. If goal is set at 1 and the patient achieves 4, then the score is +3 and exceeds expected performance. The standard score is set for each individual on a scale of 1 to 4; for example, 1 equals dependence in functioning, and 4 equals independence in functioning. In some instances a percentage score may be used in a criterion-referenced instrument as a measure of absolute performance. The formula to convert a raw score to a percentage score is:

$$\text{Percentage Score} = \frac{\text{subject's raw score on measure}}{\text{maximum possible raw score}} \times 100$$

If the raw score on goal attainment is 3, then performance score is 3/4 × 100, or 75%.

Validity

An initial draft of the instrument was analyzed by 10 graduate students, who offered excellent suggestions for clarity and consistency. The draft was revised to be consistent with Mager's (1965) suggestions for writing objectives that are measurable. Each goal scale should contain three elements: (1) describe the respondent (who is the patient), (2) describe the behavior the respondent will demonstrate when the goal is achieved, (3) describe the conditions under which the respondent demonstrates goal attainment.

In determining content validity each item represented a measure of the content domain; that is, the representativeness of the total collection of items (or behavior) is a measure of content domain. The judgment of two content specialists in nursing was used to assess the validity of the items within three major categories of functional abilities related to personal hygiene, movement, and human interaction. The two judges were given the domain objectives, the set of items, and a form for recording their rating of the relevance of each item to a domain. For example, 1 = not relevant; 2 = somewhat relevant; 3 = quite relevant; 4 = very relevant. Content validity is the proportion of items rated as quite/very relevant (3 or 4) by both judges. A content validity index (CVI) of .88 was obtained.

Waltz and associates (1984) defined content validity as "a representative collection of items that measured a specific content domain" (pp. 193-194). Content validity was also achieved in the systematic way the tool was developed. A content analysis was done on four tools currently used to assess functional abilities. A category system was developed from this analysis, resulting in the three subscales. The categories also represented elements in King's theory of goal attainment and definition of health.

The measurement literature indicated that terms used to describe validity for criterion-referenced measures were different from those used for norm-referenced measures. For example, Popham (1978) used the terms *descriptive* and *functional* validity. He noted that descriptive validity was related to content validity. When items are congruent with domain objectives, congruency percentages of 90 or higher are satisfactory. He described functional validity as the accuracy with which a criterion-referenced measure satisfies the purpose for its use. This is like criterion-related validity if accurate predictions can be made.

Another type of validity for criterion-referenced measures is decision validity, in which appropriate decisions result from scores on a measure. Data from the two assessment scales were used to make decisions about goal setting and goal attainment. This instrument has content validity and decision validity.

Reliability

Estimates of interrater reliability were determined. Two nurses with master of science degrees in nursing volunteered to use the instrument to assess 20 patients in a nursing home setting. These nurses were equally familiar with the patients. Since there was minimal variability in this homogeneous group of patients, percentage of interrater agreement was determined rather than product-moment correlations. The interrater agreement for the total score was 85%. Interrater agreement on each of three subscales was 83% for physical ability, 84% for behavior response, and 87% for goal attainment. Percentage of agreement was obtained for each item and ranged from 63% to 100%.

A second sample of 20 patients was assessed by two nurses with BSN degrees in a critical care unit of a large metropolitan hospital. Product-moment correlation coefficients of interrater reliability were determined for this sample, which was more heterogeneous than the nursing home sample. Estimates of interrater reliability for the instrument were .99 for the three scales and for the three subscales:

1. Physical ability: personal hygiene, .99; movement, .95; and human interaction, .92.
2. Behavior response: personal hygiene, .99; movement, .97; and human interaction, .92.
3. Goal attainment: personal hygiene, .99; movement, .97; and human interaction, .92.

Item correlations ranged from .70 to 1.00 with sleep and written communication below .70 (.54 and .68).

Interscale relationships were determined between physical ability and behavior response, between physical ability and goal attainment, and between behavior response and goal attainment. Correlations between the physical scale and the behavior scale on the three subscales were as follows: personal hygiene, .99; movement, .98; and human interaction, 1.00. Correlations between the physical scale and the goal scale were as follows: personal hygiene, .99; movement, .99; and human interaction, 1.00. Correlations between the behavior and the goal scale were as follows: personal hygiene, .99; movement, .99; human interaction, 1.00. Since the interscale correlations yielded by the two nurses were not significantly different, the interscale correlations represent the averages of the correlations from the two nurses.

MAJOR FINDINGS AND RESULTS

The purpose of this project, which was to develop a criterion-referenced measure of goal attainment that could be used by nurses in clinical nursing practice and in research, has been achieved. This instrument, which has a CVI of .88 and reliability of .99 provides a tool for nurses to assess functional abilities of patients, to make decisions about goal setting with and for patients, and to measure goal attainment. Goals set and goals attained provide a measure of effectiveness of care. The reliability and validity of this instrument augur well for its use in nursing research that tests hypotheses generated from King's theory of goal attainment.

One of the results of developing this criterion-referenced measure was the demonstration of a need to develop many more tools for use in nursing research and practice. This instrument was limited to measurement of functional abilities and goal attainment of individuals within three subscales of personal hygiene, movement, and human interaction. The format can be used to develop instruments to measure goal attainment in other areas of nursing practice.

MAJOR IMPLICATIONS FOR NURSING

The development of instruments from a nursing perspective is essential if research is to provide knowledge for the discipline of nursing. This project is an initial attempt to provide a valid and reliable instrument for use in nursing practice and research. This has implications for doctoral students who may wish to develop tools to measure goal attainment in specialized areas of nursing practice. If practicing nurses use this criterion-referenced measure to assess patients, the data provide reliable information for planning nursing care. In addition, using the ideas from the theory of goal attainment, practicing nurses may implement King's (1981) goal-oriented nursing record system. This provides a permanent patient record of goals set and goals attained. Such a record system simplifies any quality assurance program since the information one evaluates in a nursing audit is recorded. Use of this tool provides valid and reliable data which should result in decisions for care that are consistent from nurse to nurse and from situation to situation.

Implications for use of this criterion-referenced measure in nursing research are numerous. For example, in a study designed to test King's theory of goal attainment, a hypothesis could examine the relationship between mutual goal setting and functional abilities of patients. This valid and reliable criterion-referenced measure will be used to collect data related to this hypothesis. This instrument can be used to measure functional abilities of patients in a variety of areas of nursing, such as care for the elderly, rehabilitation nursing, and care for individuals with chronic illness. This instrument can also be used in studies related to the transfer of patients from one unit of care to another and from hospital to other agencies. The format used to design the instrument can serve as a model for designing additional instruments to observe/measure goal attainment in specialty areas of nursing practice.

In conclusion, it is hoped that this project will provide an incentive for professional nurses to use valid and reliable instruments to collect assessment data for decision making in clinical practice. Interested doctoral students and nurse researchers may also use the format to develop instruments to measure goal attainment in specialized areas of practice.

REFERENCES

Carey, R. G., & Posavac, E. J. (1980). *Manual for the level of rehabilitation scale*. Park Ridge, Il: Lutheran General Hospital.

Carey, R. N., & Posavac, E. J. (1982). Revised level of rehabilitation scale (LORS-II). *Archives of Physical Medicine Rehabilitation, 63*, 367-370.

Kane, R., & Kane, R. (1981). *Assessing the elderly: Practical guide to measurements*. Lexington MA: Lexington Books.

King, I. M. (1981). *A theory for nursing: Systems, concepts and process*. New York: John Wiley.

Mager, R. R. (1965). *Preparing instructional objectives*. Palo Alto, CA: Fearon Publishers.

Popham, W. J. (1978). *Criterion-referenced measurement*. Englewood, NJ: Prentice Hall.

Waltz, C., Strickland, O., & Lenz, E. (1984). *Measurement in nursing research*. Philadelphia: F. A. Davis.

Williams, M. (1960). The patient profile. *Nursing Research, 9*, 122-124.

A Criterion-Referenced Measure of Goal Attainment: Assessment of Functional Abilities and Goal Attainment Scales

Scale 1: Physical ability to perform activity	Scale 2: Behavior response to perform activity	Scale 3: Goal to be attained by patient

PERSONAL HYGIENE

Mouth care

Unable to brush teeth/ dentures	Rejects assistance in brushing teeth/dentures	Oral hygiene provided by caregiver with demonstration of technique and health reasons for mouth care given to patient
Requires assistance with equipment and brushing	Tolerates assistance with mouth care	Demonstrates adequate mouth care under supervision of care giver
Requires supervision with equipment and brushing teeth/dentures	Seeks assistance in brushing teeth/dentures	Demonstrates proper technique in performing mouth care once a day
Brushes teeth/dentures without assistance	Assumes responsibility for oral hygiene	Uses appropriate technique in performing mouth care a minimum of two times a day

Bathing

Unable to bathe self	Rejects assistance with complete bath	Permits caregiver to give bath
Requires assistance with bathing except for hands and face	Tolerates assistance in bathing but washes face and hands	Permits caregiver to bathe back, legs, and torso
Requires supervision when bathing self	Seeks assistance in bathing self	Bathes self when assisted into tub/shower
Bathes self without assistance	Assumes responsibiity for daily bath	Takes shower/bath safely once a day without assistance

Eating

Unable to feed self	Rejects assistance with eating and drinking	Permits caregiver to feed him/her
Requires assistance with eating and drinking	Tolerates assistance with eating and drinking	Asks to select food and liquids and eats and drinks with assistance
Requires supervision when eating and drinking	Seeks assistance when eating and drinking	Given food selected by patient, eats slowly and in small amounts 4 times a day
Eats and drinks without assistance	Assumes responsibility for eating and drinking without assistance	Selects appropriate food, eats and drinks 3 times a day without assisance

Dressing

Unable to dress self	Rejects assistance in dressing	Permits caregiver to dress him/her
Requires assistance with dressing	Tolerates assistance in dressing	Assists caregiver in dressing self
Requires supervision when dressing self	Seeks assistance in dressing self	Dresses self with supervision 50% of the time
Dresses self without assistance	Assumes responsibility for dressing self each day	Dresses self without assistance 100% of the time

Grooming

Unable to perform grooming activities	Refuses to perform grooming activities	Permits caregiver to perform grooming activities
Requires assistance with grooming activities	Tolerates assistance with grooming	Assists caregiver with grooming
Requires supervision with grooming activities	Seeks assistance with grooming activities	Performs grooming with supervision 50% of the time
Performs grooming activities without assistance	Assumes responsibility for grooming activities	Performs basic grooming activities 100% of the time

Bladder

Unable to pass urine	Rejects chemical/ mechanical aids	Accepts use of chemical/ mechanical aids to pass urine
Requires assistance in use of chemical/mechanical aids to pass urine	Tolerates assistance in use of chemical/mechanical aids	Cooperates with care-giver in use of aids
Requires supervision in	Seeks assistance in use of	Seeks supervision in use

use of chemical/mechanical aids to pass urine	chemical/mechanical aids	of aids
Passes urine with or without chemical/ mechanical aids	Assumes responsibility for using aids when necessary	Maintains adequate urinary elimination daily with or without aids

Bowels

Unable to have bowel movement	Refuses chemical/ mechanical aids	Accepts use of aids
Requires assistance in use of chemical/ mechanical aids	Tolerates use of chemical/mechanical aids	Cooperates with caregiver in use of aids
Requires supervision in use of chemical/mechanical aids	Seeks assistance in use of aids	Seeks supervision in selection of aids to use
Defecates with or without assistance of chemical/ mechanical aids	Assumes responsibility for using aids when necessary	Maintains adequate bowel elimination with or without aids based on pattern of defecation once a day

Continence

Total incontinence relative to urination/defecation	Unaware of incontinence	Aware of incontinence by verbalizing discomfort
Partial incontinence with urination/defecation	Expresses fear and embarrassment due to incontinence	Cooperates with care in planning to control incontinence
Partial/total control by catheter, enemas, or regular toilet times	Seeks assistance in controlling incontinence	Seeks supervision in establishing patterns of elimination to control incontinence
Urination/defecation controlled by self	Assumes responsibility for control of incontinence	Controls incontinence with or without chemical/ mechanical aids 100% of the time

MOVEMENT

Walking

Unable to walk	Rejects mechanical or caregiver assistance in trying to walk	Permits caregiver to move legs and arms and sits up in bed
Requires mechanical or caregiver assistance to walk from bed to chair	Tolerates mechanical or caregiver assistance in walking from bed to chair	Assists caregiver in walking 10 feet
Requires mechanical or	Seeks mechanical or	Walks 100 feet using

caregiver supervision in walking 100 feet

caregiver assistance in walking 100 feet

supportive aids under supervision of caregiver

Walks without caregiver assistance

Walks within physical limits with mechanical aids

Walks safely with or without mechanical aids

Wheelchair

Unable to transfer to wheelchair from bed

Rejects assistance in transfer from bed to wheelchair

Given a demonstration of techniques for transfer, patient is able to perform arm, leg, and body movements in bed

Requires caregiver or mechanical assistance to transfer from bed to wheelchair and wheelchair to bed

Tolerates assistance in transfer from bed to wheelchair and wheelchair to bed

Demonstrates transfer from bed to wheelchair and wheelchair to bed with caregiver assistance

Requires supervision to transfer from bed to wheelchair and wheelchair to bed

Seeks asistance in transfer from bed to wheelchair and wheelchair to bed

Transfers safely to and and from bed to wheelchair with caregiver supervision

Transfers safely without assistance from caregiver

Assumes responsibiity for transferring safely from bed to wheelchair and wheelchair to bed

Transfers safely from bed to wheelchair and wheelchair to bed independently 100% of the time

In Bed

Unable to turn, sit up, or get in or out of bed

Rejects assistance in turning and sitting up in bed

Permits caregiver to turn and to sit up in bed

Requires assistance to turn, sit up, and get in or out of bed

Tolerates assistance in turning and sitting up in bed

Demonstrates techniques in turning and sitting up in bed with caregiver assistance

Requires supervision in getting in and out of bed

Seeks assistance in getting in and out of bed

Moves in and out of bed with caregiver assistance

Moves in and out of bed with or without mechanical support

Assumes responsibility within physical limits to move in and out of bed

Moves safely in and out of bed without caregiver assistance

Exercises

Unable to exercise

Rejects assistance in exercising

Permits 15 min of passive exercise a day

Requires complete assistance in active exercises

Tolerates passive exercises and assistance with active exercises

Demonstrates active exercises in arms and legs for 10 min a day

Requires partial assistance in active exercise

Seeks assistance in active exercises

Demonstrates active exercises in extremities in walking 15 min a day

Exercises without caregiver assistance	Assumes responsibility for daily exercises	Exercises consistently in moderation a minimum of 15 min a day

Range of motion

Unable to move extremities	Rejects assistance to move legs and arms	Permits caregiver to put extremities through full range of motion
Requires caregiver assistance to move legs and arms	Tolerates assistance in moving legs and arms	Demonstrates partial range of motion with assistance twice a day
Requires caregiver to supervise movement of legs and arms	Seeks assistance of caregiver in moving legs or arms	Demonstrates full range of motion in extremities with assistance twice a day
Moves legs and arms independently	Expresses satisfaction in ability to move extremities	Demonstrates full range of motion in extremities without assistance twice a day

Sleep

Unable to sleep at night	Rejects all forms of assistance by caregiver	Verbalizes long-term use and effects of sleeping pills
Requires chemical assistance to sleep at night	Tolerates assistance with relaxation techniques to accompany use of medications	Demonstrates to caregiver the use of two relaxation techniques
Requires supervision with relaxation techniques	Seeks assistance to use relaxation techniques	Demonstrates to caregiver use of two relaxation techniques learned from pamphlets, AV materials, and caregiver's demonstration
Able to sleep without chemical assistance	Expresses satisfaction in ability to sleep without chemical assistance	Performs relaxation technique each evening prior to bedtime

HUMAN INTERACTION

Consciousness

Unable to arouse (comatose)	No response to painful or noxious stimuli	Demonstrates no response to painful or noxious stimuli
Requires use of strong verbal and tactile stimuli (stuporous or semiconscious)	Responds lucidly to verbal stimuli followed by irrational response	Demonstrates lucid response to verbal stimuli 50% of the time

Requires assistance with complex mental activity (confused)

Responds slowly to sensory stimuli and simple mental activity; oriented to time, place, and some persons

Demonstrates slow response during interactions with individuals in environment 100% of the time

Able to interact in time and place with individuals

Responds to sensory stimuli, oriented to time, place, and persons

Demonstrates orientation to time, place, persons through appropriate interactions with individuals 100% of the time

Hearing

Unable to hear or read lips

No response and unable to read lips

Demonstrates ability to place hearing aid in ear with 100% accuracy

Requires complete assistance with use of mechanical aid

Tolerates mechanical aid

Demonstrates ability to adjust hearing aid to environment with 100% accuracy

Requires partial assistance with use of mechanical aid

Seeks assistance if necessary

Demonstrates use of hearing aid with 100% accuracy

Can distinguish sounds and hears conversation with or without mechanical aid

Expresses satisfaction in use of mechanical aid

Demonstrates ability to engage in normal conversations with hearing aid with 100% accuracy

Vision

Unable to see without glasses

Refuses help from caregivers in movement in the environment and with personal hygiene

Accepts caregiver's assistance with activities of daily living

Requires assistance in the environment without glasses

Tolerates partial assistance with personal hygiene and movement in limited environment

Performs personal hygiene and moves about room with assistance of caregiver

Requires supervision to get used to glasses in moving around in the room

Tolerates glasses and moves cautiously in limited environment

Demonstrates use of special glasses and cares for self without assistance

Performs activities of daily living independently and moves around in familiar surroundings with glasses

Expresses satisfaction in taking walks in the environment

Performs activities of daily living and moves around in familiar surroundings without assistance

Smell

Unable to detect noxious odors

Rejects help in detecting differences in odors

Permits caregiver to present a variety of odors to learn differences

Requires assistance to differentiate one odor from another	Tolerates assistance in differentiating between normal odors and harmful odors	Practices differentiating pleasant from harmful odors
Requires supervision to differentiate one odor from another	Seeks feedback and reinforcement in differentiating odors	Demonstrates discrimination of odors with 70% accuracy
Discriminates odors without assistance	Responds slowly in differentiating odors	Demonstrates discrimination of odors with 100% accuracy

Taste

Unable to distinguish between sweet, sour, salty, bitter tastes and temperature	Rejects help to distinguish different taste sensations	Tastes different kinds of foods and liquids to try to distinguish between various taste sensations and temperatures
Requires assistance to determine differences in taste sensations and temperature	Tolerates assistance in distingushing taste sensations and temperatures	Demonstrates differences between sweet, sour, salty, bitter foods, and hot and cold liquids with 50% accuracy
Requires supervision in differentiating taste sensations and temperature	Seeks assistance in distinguishing taste sensations and temperatures	Demonstrates differences between sweet, sour, salty, bitter foods, and hot and cold liquids with 75% accuracy
Differentiates tastes and temperature without assistance	Verbalizes satisfaction in distinguishing tastes and temperatures	Demonstrates with 100% accuracy ability to differentiate between sweet, sour, bitter, salty, hot and cold taste sensations

Touch

Unable to detect sensation of light touch, heat, or cold	Rejects assistance in detecting sensation of light touch, heat, or cold	With assistance from caregiver practices touching objects and describing cutaneous sensation
Requires assistance to sense light touch, heat, and cold	Tolerates assistance in differentiating between light touch, heat, and cold	Demonstrates discrimination between sensations of light touch, heat, and cold with 50% accuracy
Requires supervision with objects that are hot or cold	Seeks assistance in differentiating between heat and cold	Demonstrates with 75% accuracy discrimination between sensation of light touch, heat, and cold
Discriminates between	Expresses satisfaction in	Demonstrates with 100%

sensations of light touch, heat, and cold	ability to differentiate cutaneous sensations	accuracy discrimination between cutaneous sensations of light touch, heat, and cold

Communication, Verbal

Unable to speak	Rejects assistance in using words	Demonstrates use of simple words correctly 100% of time
Speaks words slowly with cues from others	Tolerates assistance in using words to communicate to caregiver	Demonstrates use of sentences correctly 100% of time
Speaks sentences slowly with cues from others	Seeks assistance to reinforce use of words in sentences	Demonstrates ability to speak slowly and clearly 100% of time
Uses sentences appropriately when interacting with other human beings	Expresses satisfaction in ability to carry on a conversation with others	Demonstrates ability to engage in a conversation with others 100% of the time

Listening

Unable to comprehend spoken word	Rejects assistance by caregiver to repeat messages slowly	Demonstrates comprehension of simple words when spoken slowly and clearly
Responds to spoken messages with assistance from therapist/caregiver	Tolerates spoken messages	Demonstrates comprehension of spoken sentences 100% of time when delivered slowly and clearly
Responds to spoken messages with minimal assistance from therapist/caregiver	Seeks reinforcement that message is understood	Demonstrates comprehension of verbal messages 100% of time
Comprehends spoken messages	Expresses pleasure in listening to persons, to TV, and to radio	Demonstrates ability to listen and respond appropriately 100% of the time

Reading

Unable to read	Refuses to read	Demonstrates ability to read menu and select food
Requires assistance in reading menu	Tolerates assistance with reading menu and instructions for diagnostic tests	Demonstrates ability to read diet instructions 100% of time
Requires supervision in reading about diet and medications	Seeks assistance to understand what is read about diet and medications	Demonstrates ability to read and understand instructions for diagnostic

		tests, diet, and medications 100% of the time
Able to read magazines and books	Expresses pleasure in reading anything in the environment	Demonstrates abiity to read and comphrehend articles, books, and directions within educational background with 100% accuracy.

Writing

Unable to write	Rejects assistance in writing simple words	Demonstrates use of pad and pencil to write simple words
Requires assistance in writing words	Tolerates assistance in writing sentences	Demonstrates ability to write clear sentences 100% of time
Requires supervision in writing sentences	Seeks assistance to write clear messages	Demonsrates ability to write clear messages 75% of time
Writes sentences that clearly communicate messages	Expresses satisfaction when written messages are understood by others	Demonstrates ability to communicate clearly in writing 100% of the time

Communication, Nonverbal

Unable to interact with gestures	Rejects assistance to purposefully interact nonverbally	Uses several meaningful gestures to interact with caregiver
Requires assistance to use meaningful gestures	Tolerates assistance to use meaningful gestures	Demonstrates use of gestures that clearly communicate 100% of the time
Requires partial assistance with gestures	Seeks feedback and reinforcement for clear nonverbal interactions	Demonstrates clear communication through use of nonverbal techniques 100% of the time
Interacts clearly and appropriately with gestures	Responds with satisfaction when nonverbal gestures communicate messages clearly	Interacts clearly with appropriate nonverbal techniques 100% of the time

Transactions (decisions)

Unable to make transactions with caregiver	Rejects participation in decision making about care	Demonstrates beginning acceptance of responsibility for decisions about health status

Requires assistance in decision making that leads to transactions	Tolerates assistance in making decisions	Demonstrates ability to make some decisions that lead to transactions
Requires supervision by caregiver in making transactions that lead to goals	Seeks feedback and reinforcement in decision making that leads to transactions	Demonstrates ability to make transactions that lead to goal attainment 75% of the time
Able to make decisions that lead to transactions and goal attainment	Expresses satisfaction with transactions that lead to goal attainment	Makes transactions with relevant others that lead to goal attainment 100% of the time

7

The Self-Administered ADL Scale for Persons with Multiple Sclerosis

Elsie E. Gulick

This chapter discusses the MS Self-Care ADL Scale, a measure of self-care requisites in persons with multiple sclerosis.

Alterations in the performance of daily activities of living (ADL) among persons with chronic disease such as multiple sclerosis (MS) generally require many adjustments by the patient and family during the course of the disease. A patient's self-awareness of his/her ADL strengths and deficits, together with an understanding of the nature of the disease, facilitates this adjustment. Awareness of one's strengths and deficits can be enhanced through periodic, structured ADL self-assessments. Structured self-assessments can provide information to the patient, the family, and the nurse or other health personnel as the basis for determining the effectiveness of self-care or treatments, needed services, and change in ADL functioning over time.

REVIEW OF THE LITERATURE

Studies have shown that patients are capable of and responsible for performing self-assessments. Accurate self-assessments of health, when compared to health assessments performed by health care professionals, have been demonstrated among elderly community residents (Fillenbaum, 1979; Maddox & Douglas, 1973) and spinal cord-injured patients undergoing rehabilitation (Stephens, Norris-Baker, & Willems, 1983). Further-

This research was supported by Grant No. 9918 from the Robert Wood Johnson Foundation's Research and Development Program to Improve Patient Functional Status. Tool development was facilitated through the Measurement of Clinical and Educational Nursing Outcomes Project sponsored by the University of Maryland, School of Nursing, and funded by the Division of Nursing, Special Projects, Department of Health & Human Services.

more, patients who are encouraged to participate in self-care demonstrate a greater number of health behaviors (Dodd, 1984; Vickery et al., 1983). Increased self-care behavior has been effective in reducing the number of ambulatory visits and decreasing health care costs in an HMO population (Vickery et al., 1983). Encouraging patients to perform self-assessments and health monitoring promotes health control and health responsibility within the individual and decreased dependency on others.

The unusual disease characteristics of MS render the use of existing ADL assessment scales inadequate. MS, which primarily affects young adults, is characterized by exacerbations or continued disease progression, resulting in limb paresis, sensory disturbance such as paresthesia and position sense, bowel and bladder dysfunction, and visual impairment (Poser, 1979). More severely disabled persons may have slurred speech, memory and concentration deficits, and mood alteration (Albion, 1983; Pavlou, 1979). These multiple disabilities generally affect the MS person's ability to perform ADL. ADL is defined as those everyday behaviors performed by individuals in eating, dressing, transfer, walking, travel, urination, bowel elimination, work, recreation and socialization, sensory input and communication, and intimate relationships.

A review of existing scales to measure ADL were found to lack sensitivity and comprehensiveness of daily activities particularly important to MS persons. A number of functional scales for measuring ADL are available for the elderly (Duke University, 1978; Katz, Ford, Moskowitz, Jackson, & Jaffee, 1963), chronically ill persons (Katz et al., 1963; Mahoney & Barthel, 1965; Seltzer, Granger, & Wineberg, 1982), physically disabled persons (Crewe & Athelstan, 1981; Iversen, Silberberg, Stever, & Schoening, 1973; Sarno, Sarno, & Levita, 1973), and specific diseases including cancer (McCorkle & Benoliel, 1981), arthritis (Meenan, Gertman, Mason, & Dunaif, 1982), and multiple sclerosis (Kurtzke, 1981). The types of activities, number of items per activity, and scaling formats vary among these scales. Most of the scales require administration by health personnel. Standardization of these scales is minimal or absent (Kaufert, 1983; Keith, 1984).

The ADL scale for MS, known as the Incapacity Status Scale, developed by the International Federation of Multiple Sclerosis Societies (1984), requires administration by a trained interviewer. The scale format reflects a five-point progressive decline on single rather than multiple behaviors within an ADL activity. At best, the scale provides a global ADL rating. Sensitivity to small changes in ADL functioning is unlikely to be determined by this scale.

It was clear that existing scales did not meet the sensitivity, comprehensiveness, and self-administered scale requirements needed for MS persons and their family members to participate directly in the assessment and monitoring of the MS person's daily functioning.

THEORETICAL FRAMEWORK

Self-assessment is an aspect of self-care. It involves self-observation, symptom perception, labeling, and making judgments of severity of the condition (Levin, Katz, & Holst, 1979). Orem (1980) notes that individuals evaluate their own state of health each day, sometimes more frequently. Orem proceeds to indicate that individuals with chronic disease or who undergo certain diagnostic tests or therapies "must learn to collect data as a basis for judging their own human functioning" (p. 123). This self-assessment provides information for determining "an individual's view of self as a self-care or dependent-care agent and the freedom with which the individual accepts and acts with responsibility for self-care or dependent care" (p. 124). Self-assessment includes developing the ability to assess strengths and goals realistically and to determine whether those strengths are sufficient to meet goals with or without assistance (Nowakowski, 1980).

ADL deficits that render a person or family incapable of providing self-care give rise to the need for nursing systems. Nursing systems, according to Orem (1980), are formed when nurses use their abilities to prescribe, design, and provide nursing for patients.

Nursing systems may be needed by MS persons and their families as a result of the progression of MS manifestations during the course of the disease. Disease manifestations frequently alter the MS person's ability to obtain the universal self-care requisites identified by Orem (1980). The universal self-care requisites include maintaining sufficient intakes of water, food, and air; providing for elimination; maintaining a balance between rest and activity; maintaining a balance between social interaction and solitude; preventing hazards to human life; and promoting human functioning and development within social groups. The universal self-care requisites translate into essential ADL: eating, dressing, walking, transfer, travel, bathing, urine and bowel elimination, work, recreation and socializing, sensory input and communicating, and intimate relationships. The ADL Self-Care Scale described below is a mechanism by which self-care deficits among essential ADL functions and therapeutic self-care demands can be identified and monitored. The ADL Self-Care Scale includes two complementary checklists: Assistive Devices and MS-Related Symptoms.

Specific objectives in this phase of instrument development included determination of internal consistency of subscale items, stability of the subscales, and construct validity as determined by the relationships among the ADL Self-Care Scale, Assistive Devices Checklist, and MS-Related Symptoms Checklist.

INSTRUMENT DEVELOPMENT

Initial work on the development of the ADL Self-Care Scale for use by MS persons and health professionals commenced June 1981. An attempt was made to modify the Social Dependency Scale (McCorkle & Benoliel,

1981) by altering the existing Guttman-type scale statements in a manner that would reflect ADL especially relevant to MS persons. Structured interview guidelines were used to conduct either in-person or telephone interviews. Because of the difficulty in determining differences between interquartile scale items, a problem reported by others (Jeffreys, Millard, Human, & Warren, 1969; Kaufert et al., 1983), together with the extensive time required to administer and score the scale, a self-administered matrix-type scale was developed.

A number of assumptions and essential scale requirements guided scale development. The assumptions pertaining to self-assessments presented below are congruent with the propositions and presuppositions contained in Orem's (1980) theory of self-care.

1. Individuals want to function at their highest potential level;
2. Individuals routinely assess the effects of their behavior on their level of functioning;
3. Individuals will explore alternate behaviors to determine those behaviors that enhance their level of functioning.

The seven essential scale requirements presented below focus on the appropriateness and measurement of ADL content specific to persons with MS. They represent an attempt to ensure content validity by providing guidelines for obtaining a representative collection of items and a "sensible" method of test construction (Nunnally, 1978).

1. Inclusion of essential activities encountered by all persons in everyday life that are especially important to MS persons.
2. Determination of what functions the MS person *presently performs*, not what the person *can perform*, together with the frequency with which those functions are performed.
3. Determination of those functions for which the MS person requires help from other persons and the frequency with which that help is used.
4. An equal number of subscale items within each activity.
5. Scale sensitivity toward changing functional abilities.
6. Self-administration or scale administration by a family member or other health personnel.
7. A reliable and valid measure of the MS person's capabilities, deficits, and dependency needs in ADL.

Scale Content

The scale consists of 12 subscales that represent essential ADL. The 12 ADL activities include the following subscales: Eating, Dressing, Transfer, Walking, Travel, Bathing, Urination, Bowel Elimination, Recreation and Socializing, Sensory and Communication, Work, and Intimacy. The selection of the subscale categories and five behavioral items within each subscale was based on direct work with persons with MS, review of literature pertaining to MS, scales designed to measure ADL of the population focus, and experience from the initial MS scale construction. The scale was given to three client service coordinators affiliated with the National Multiple Sclerosis Society for the purpose of determining content representativeness, clarity of items, and appropriateness of the scale format. Two of the experts were clinical nurse specialists with master's degrees, and the third had more than ten years of clinical experience in working with MS clients. Minor modifications of various items were made, resulting in agreement by the clinical experts as to content, clarity, and scale format. The scale was given to five MS persons who indicated that the items were clear and who reported being able to complete the scale without difficulty.

Scale Scoring

Each subscale consisting of five items is presented twice, with the exception of intimacy. Responses to the first listing, Self-Care, determine the respondent's present self-care ability; the second listing, Help from Others, determines the MS person's dependency on other persons for ADL functioning. Both are completed by the individual with MS. A Likert-type scale consisting of six categories – Never, Almost Never, Occasionally, Usually, Almost Always, and Always – is used. Scores range from 0 (Never) to 5 (Always), with a total subscale score range between 0 and 25. Score values are reversed for all items in the Urination and Bowel Elimination subscales and in the fifth item in the Transfer subscale to reflect positive or less invasive self-care behavior. The higher the score obtained on the Self-Care subscales, the higher the level of ADL self-care ability. Higher scores obtained on the Help from Others subscales indicate a higher level of dependency on other persons in the MS individual's performance of his/her ADL. A difference score between Self-Care and Help from Others can be obtained by subtracting scores obtained from the Help from Others subscales from scores obtained from the matching Self-Care subscales. The difference score can be graphed and numerically recorded on a Self-Care ADL Profile. Large positive scores are expected for persons with minimal disability or for those with disability in which assistive devices can compensate for the physical handicap in maintaining the related ADL. The presence of small positive or negative difference scores may suggest the need to determine if excessive dependency, insufficient use of assistive devices, or deterioration in health exists. The total Self-Care score ranges between 0 and 300; the total Help from Others score ranges between 0 and 275.

Scale Administration

The scale can be self-administered or administered by members of the family or health personnel. Brief instructions for responding to the items accompany the scale. Respondents are asked to check the frequency with which they perform or require help from other persons to perform each item. The amount of time required to complete the scale varies from 15 to 30 min. depending on the respondent's ability to manipulate pages and hold a pen.

Scale Pilot

The scale was piloted among 28 persons diagnosed with MS to determine alpha reliability and test-retest reliability. Mean age of the respondents was 51.6 years, mean education was 13.4 years, mean age when initial symptoms of MS appeared was 29.0, and mean age when MS was diagnosed was 37.9 years. Seventy-five percent of the respondents were female and 25% were male.

Cronbach alpha reliability coefficients for the Self-Care subscales ranged between .60 and .98, with the exception of the subscales Walking, Work, Sensory and Communication, and Intimacy. Those four subscales used a format other than the Likert type described earlier. The total scale alpha correlation coefficient was .76. Alpha correlation coefficients for the Help from Others subscales ranged between .77 and .97, with a total scale *r* of .85. The subscales Walking, Work, Sensory and Communication, and Intimacy were not included in the analyses due to the different scale format used for them. The subscales for those four activities have been redeveloped to conform to the other subscales.

Test-retest conducted over a period of 1 to 4 weeks for all subscales (except Walking, Work, Sensory and Communication, and Intimacy) resulted in a correlation coefficient range between .66 and .91 for Self-Care and a range of .33 to .91 for Help from Others. The total scale test-retest correlations were .86 and .90 for Self-Care and Help from Others, respectively.

Further Scale Revision and Related Scale Development

Items reflecting less than .30 in the inter item correlation matrix were either rewritten or replaced with new items and subjected to a panel of three MS patient service coordinators for judgment on item appropriateness and clarity. The scales Walking, Work, Sensory and Communication, and Intimacy were revised to reflect five items that used the six-response Likert scale format previously described.

Development of an Assistive Devices Checklist and MS-Related Symptoms Checklist was undertaken to provide a mechanism to test construct validity of the ADL Self-Care Scale. The checklists may also provide useful information to health care providers who work with MS clients as well as the MS person and his/her family. The Assistive Devices Checklist includes a list of 37 devices commonly used by MS persons as determined from the literature and from direct observation of MS clients. The assistive devices are listed under the ADL subscale headings for which they were generally used, such as Eating, Walking, and so on. Subjects are asked to rate the frequency that each assistive device is used on a Likert-type scale similar to the scale format used in the ADL Self-Care Scale. A total score, ranging between 0 and 185, may be computed. It is anticipated that as self-care ability decreases, the frequency of use of assistive devices will increase. As the scores for Help from Others approach or become greater than the Self-Care score, a decrease in the number of assistive devices might be expected. The latter situation may suggest the need for increased use of assistive devices to reflect less dependency on other persons. For example, clinical experience shows that MS persons are initially reluctant to use a cane or walker and prefer the arm of another person for assistance in walking.

The MS-Related Symptoms Checklist consists of 26 signs or symptoms commonly experienced by MS persons as determined from the literature and from direct observation of MS clients. A frequency rating for each symptom is determined by the same procedure used for the ADL scale. The total score ranges between 0 and 130. High scores on the MS-Related Symptoms Checklist are expected to be associated with deficits in related self-care activities and reflect small difference scores. This information may suggest the need for relevant health care services such as information, counseling, assistive devices, and medical referral.

Content validity in part was established for the Assistive Devices Checklist and the MS-Related Symptoms Checklist by having three MS client service coordinators reach agreement on the representativeness and clarity of the checklist items. The checklists take the respondent approximately five to ten minutes to complete.

METHOD

The ADL Self-Care Scale and the Assistive Devices and MS-Related Symptoms checklists were self-administered by 629 MS persons, either independently or with the assistance of a spouse or significant other. The subjects were randomly selected from lists of MS persons from two New Jersey chapters of the National Multiple Sclerosis Society that had a combined membership of approximately 2,500. No subjects residing in nursing homes were included in the study. Initial telephone calls were made to all subjects by two trained research assistants, explaining and answering questions about the study and describing the extent of the subject's participation in the study. Following verbal consent to participate in the study, a packet, consisting of a cover letter on chapter stationery, a consent form, the ADL Self-Care Scale, a Personal Data Inventory, and a self-addressed and stamped envelope for returning the completed materials, was sent to each subject. No difficulty by subjects in completing the ADL scale was apparent from their responses, except for the Work subscale which is discussed below.

No differences in demographic characteristics, such as age and duration of MS, or ADL scores for MS persons were observed between the two MS chapter samples. Therefore, the total sample of 629 subjects was combined for data analysis and reporting. The subjects ranged in age from 20 to 84 years, with a mean of 48.5 years. The range in age for onset of MS symptoms was 10 to 73 years, with a mean of 31. The range in age for diagnosis of MS was 10 to 75 years, with a mean of 35.9. The duration of MS disease ranged between 1 and 49 years, with a mean of 12.5. Educational level ranged between 5 and 22 years of schooling, with a mean of 13.2 years. Seventy-five percent of subjects were female and 25% were male. Seventy-three percent of the subjects were married, 10.1% were separated or divorced, and the remainder were never married, divorced or widowed. Forty-five percent had one or more preschool or school-age children, which reflects the young adult group that MS primarily targets.

Construct Validity and Internal Consistency of Items

Three aspects of construct validity proposed by Nunnally (1978) were conducted. First, the domain of items related to ADL self-care behavior was specified in the initial identification of subscale items. The second aspect consisted of factor analysis of the ADL Self-Care Scale items. A third aspect included determining the relationship between the ADL scale factors and checklist factors.

Factor analysis was conducted separately for the 60-item Self-Care ADL scale, the 37-item Assistive Devices Checklist, and the 26-item MS-Related Symptoms Checklist. The SPSSX software package was used for performing statistical analyses. Alpha factoring was initially conducted to extract the number of factors with items loading .30 or higher on one factor and all or most of the items with higher loadings on the first factor than on subsequent factors. Next, items in the extracted factors were subjected to Varimax rotation to maximize factor variance on as few of the items as possible, with little of the variance loading on the remaining items (Zeller & Carmines, 1980). Items on each rotated factor were refactored by the principal-component procedure to obtain theta reliability coefficients (Zeller & Carmines, 1980). Theta coefficients have the advantage over alpha coefficients of taking into account intercorrelations among items, an important consideration when highly heterogeneous intercorrelations among items exist.

Six factors were extracted from the items contained in the ADL Self-Care Scale on factor analysis in which Varimax rotation was employed (Table 7.1). All items in four of the ADL subscales – Dressing, Bathing, Transfer, and Eating – loaded above .38 on the first factor. The items represent ADL behaviors involving the upper part of the body, so Factor 1 was labeled "Upper Torso." The second factor was labeled "Lower Torso" because the two ADL subscales, Walking and Travel, primarily

TABLE 7.1 Factor Loadings from Varimax Rotation and Theta Coefficients Derived from Principal Component Analysis for the ADL Self-Care Scale (*N* = 629)

Factor and subscale items	Factor loading	Eigenvalue	Theta coefficient
Upper Torso		13.45	.97
Dressing			
Put on underwear	.90		
Put on trousers/dresses	.90		
Remove clothes	.89		
Put on socks	.88		
Work buttons	.76		
Bathing			
Get in/out of bathroom	.84		
Get bath supplies	.83		
Wash hard to reach parts	.82		
Wash all of body	.79		
Get in/out of tub/shower	.75		
Transfer			
One sitting position to another	.77		
Sitting to standing	.76		
Lying to sitting	.62		
Turning side to side	.60		
Use of mechanical lift	.38		
Eating			
Open containers	.66		
Cut food	.66		
Pour liquids	.65		
Transfer food	.59		
Feed self	.55		
Lower Torso		5.09	.95
Walking			
On uneven surfaces	.81		
Outside house	.77		
Up and down ramps	.75		
Ascend/descend stairs	.63		
Inside house	.51		
Travel			
Travel freely as desired	.60		
Travel long distances	.54		
Get in and out of buidings	.49		
Get to and from vehicle	.41		
Get on and off vehicles	.39		
Intimacy		3.63	.91
Exchange tender touches	.93		
Intimate conversations	.92		
Exchange loving glances	.91		
Satisfactory sexual activities	.67		
Share confidential matters	.52		

cont.

TABLE 7.1 (*continued*)

Recreation and Socializing		3.23	.86
Visitors in home	.76		
Social activities with family	.69		
Recreation activities in home	.63		
Social activities outside home	.63		
Recreation activities outside home	.61		
Sensory and Communication		2.50	.75
Speak so others understand	.64		
Use a telephone	.59		
Hear at normal speaking tones	.53		
Read printed/written material	.45		
Write clearly	.35		
Bowel elimination		1.89	.63
Use laxatives	.74		
Use special foods to promote elimination	.51		
Use suppositories	.48		
Use enemas	.35		

require performance from the lower part of the body. Four items from the Lower Torso factor had slightly higher loadings on the Upper Torso factor. These items were "Walk inside the house" (.67), "Get on and off vehicle" (.61), "Get to and from vehicle" (.58), and "Get in and out of buildings" (.50). The remaining four factors – Intimacy, Recreation and Socializing, Sensory and Communication, and Bowel Elimination – consist of the ADL items for which they are named. All factor loadings were higher on the identified factor compared to factor loadings on other factors. One item in the ADL subscale, Bowel Elimination, failed to load .30 or higher. The names of the items and factor loadings for each factor, together with the theta coefficients derived by the principal-component procedure, are presented in Table 7.1. Theta coefficients for the first 5 factors reflect moderately high to high internal consistency among the items. The smaller number of items contained in the sixth factor influences its lower correlation coefficient. Two items on the Urination subscale and no items on the Work subscale had factor loadings of .30 or higher. The Urination subscale items were reworked and tested on a sample of 94 additional MS persons and yielded a Cronbach alpha reliability coefficient of .71. Cronbach alpha reliability coefficients for the ADL Self-Care, Help from Other, and difference scales were .96, .97, and .97, respectively.

Five factors were extracted from among the 37 items contained within the Assistive Devices Checklist. The first factor was labeled "Dressing" because the three items were related to that name. The second factor was

TABLE 7.2 Factor Loadings from Varimax Rotation and Theta
Coefficients Derived from Principal Component Analysis for the
Assistive Devices Checklist (*N* = 629)

Factor and subscale items	Factor loading	Eigenvalue	Theta coefficient
Dressing		1.87	.70
Elastic waistband	.78		
Pullover	.65		
Velcro closures	.46		
Eating		1.85	.69
Special cup	.72		
Plate guard	.60		
Spoon instead of fork	.39		
Bathing		1.68	.61
Shower hose	.79		
Tub or shower seat	.47		
Long-handled brush	.37		
Mobility restricted		1.55	.53
Wall	.60		
Walker	.48		
Bar	.39		
Mobility, increased restrictions		1.52	.52
Wheelchair	.58		
Transfer board	.47		
Railing	.41		

labeled "Eating" and consisted of three items related to that area. The
third factor, labeled "Bathing," consisted of three related items. The
fourth and fifth factors, each with three items, represented differing levels of mobility restrictions. The names of items, together with their factor
loadings for each factor and theta coefficients, are presented in Table 7.2.
The factors extracted from the Assistive Devices Checklist, except for
Dressing and Eating, reflect low theta coefficients, primarily due to the
small number of items loading on the factors and lower factor loading.
The Cronbach alpha reliability coefficient for the 37-item Assistive
Devices Checklist was .75.

Four factors were extracted from among the 26 items contained within
the MS-Related Symptoms Checklist. The first factor was labeled
"Skeletal" because the eight items pertained primarily to skeletal functions. The second factor, "Kinesthetic," was named for four sensory items
and one sleep item. The third factor, "Emotions," consisted of the three
related emotional behaviors. The fourth factor, labeled "Head," reflected
four items related to visual, memory, and swallowing functions. The
names of the items, together with their factor loadings for each factor
and theta coefficients, are presented in Table 7.3. All factors extracted
from the MS-Related Symptoms Checklist reflect moderately strong theta
coefficients. The Cronbach alpha reliability correlation coefficient for the
26-item MS-Related Symptoms Checklist was .87.

TABLE 7.3 Factor Loadings from Varimax Rotation and Theta Coefficients Derived from Principal Component Analysis for the MS-related Symptoms Checklist (*N* = 629)

Factor and subscale items	Factor loading	Eigenvalue	Theta coefficient
Skeletal		3.45	.81
Spasms	.64		
Leg weakness	.64		
Knee locking	.61		
Tremors	.53		
Falling	.52		
Balance	.51		
Arm weakness	.46		
Fatigue	.39		
Kinesthetic		2.42	.73
Numbness	.65		
Pins and needles sensation	.63		
Burning sensation	.54		
Pain	.53		
Inability to sleep	.34		
Emotions		2.15	.80
Depression	.85		
Anxiety	.69		
Loneliness	.65		
Head		2.03	.68
Double vision	.65		
Blurred vision	.65		
Forgetfulness	.45		
Difficulty swallowing	.40		

Descriptive statistics for each ADL subscale is presented in Table 7.4. Descriptive statistics are also presented for the factors extracted from the Assistive Devices and MS-Related Symptoms checklists. Because of the unequal number of items among the checklist factors, each mean factor score was derived by summing the individual items and dividing by the number of items in that factor. Total ADL scale mean and total checklist means represent summing over all individual items contained within the scales.

Factor Stability

Test-retest analysis was performed on data from 87 randomly selected subjects from the larger sample. Pearson product-moment correlation coefficients ranged between .73 and .93 for the ADL Self-Care subscales. Correlation coefficients ranged between .72 and .92 for the ADL Help from Others subscales. Correlation coefficients for the Assistive Devices factors ranged between .68 and .85 and between .80 and .84 for factors extracted from the MS-Related Symptoms Checklist. Test-retest correlation coefficients for the total ADL Self-Care Scale (not including Work)

TABLE 7.4 Descriptive Statistics for ADL Self-Care, Assistive Devices, and MS-Related Symptoms (*N* = 629)

Scale	Mean	Standard deviation	Score range
ADL Self-Care			
Upper Torso			
Eating	18.74	7.52	0 - 25
Dressing	19.55	8.47	0 - 25
Bathing	19.13	8.60	0 - 25
Transfer	19.10	7.52	0 - 25
Lower Torso			
Walking	12.10	9.48	0 - 25
Travel	14.34	8.83	0 - 25
Intimacy	14.84	7.94	0 - 25
Recreation and Socializing	15.27	6.67	0 - 25
Sensory and Communication	20.96	4.27	4 - 25
Bowel Elimination	19.88	4.46	5 - 25
Total ADL Scale score excluding Work	178.88	53.58	40 - 250
Assistive Devices factor			
Eating	.30	.66	0 - 5
Dressing	1.80	1.42	0 - 5
Bathing	1.19	1.43	0 - 5
Mobility restricted	1.47	1.31	0 - 5
Mobility, increased restrictions	.84	1.04	0 - 5
Total Assistive Devices score	30.24	17.19	0 - 96
MS-Related Symptoms Factor			
Skeletal	2.35	.98	0 - 5
Kinesthetic	1.74	1.04	0 - 5
Emotions	1.68	1.09	0 - 5
Head	1.19	.94	0 - 5
Total MS-Related Symptoms score	46.45	17.95	3 - 116

was .86; total ADL Help from Others Scale was .92; for Assistive Devices Checklist, .76; for MS-Related Symptoms Checklist, .89. Specific correlation coefficients for each ADL subscale and checklist factor are presented in Table 7.5.

Construct Validity

Correlations between the ADL Self-Care Scale and checklist factors were determined by the Pearson product-moment correlation procedure. Only correlation coefficients that were beyond the .000 probability level and were equal to or greater than .20 are reported. The Assistive Devices factor Mobility had low to moderate correlations with all ADL Self-Care factors. The Assistive Devices factor, Eating, had low to moderate correlations with four ADL Self-Care factors: Upper Torso, Lower Torso, Recreation and Socializing, and Sensory and Communication.

The MS-Related Symptoms factor, Skeletal, reflected low to moderate

TABLE 7.5 **Test-Retest Pearson Product-Moment Correlations for ADL Subscales and Checklist Factors (N = 87)**

Subscale	Self-Care r	Help from Others r	Checklist r
ADL Scale			
Upper Torso			
Dressing	.93	.92	
Bathing	.92	.81	
Transfer	.91	.85	
Eating	.90	.87	
Lower Torso			
Walking	.93	.72	
Travel	.82	.83	
Intimacy	.88	–	
Recreation and Socializing	.82	.80	
Sensory and Communication	.73	.81	
Bowel Elimination	.81	.89	
Total ADL Scale except Work	.86	.92	
Assistive Devices			
Dressing			.68
Eating			.85
Bathing			.84
Mobility restricted			.85
Mobility, increased restrictions			.82
Total Assistive Devices Checklist			.76
MS-Related Symptoms			
Skeletal			.84
Kinesthetic			.80
Emotions			.81
Head			.84
Total MS-Related Symptoms Checklist			.89

correlations with all ADL Scale factors except Intimacy. The Emotions factor, had low correlations with two ADL Scale factors: Recreation and Socializing and Sensory and Communication.

Several factor correlations between the checklists were observed. The Skeletal factor from MS-Related Symptoms correlated with all Assistive Devices factors. Correlation coefficients for each factor pair described above is presented in Table 7.6.

ADL Difference Scores

Correlations between the ADL difference scores (obtained by substracting the Help from Others score from the Self-Care score) and factor scores from the checklists were determined. Only statistically significant correlation coefficients that were beyond the .000 probability level and were equal to or greater than .20 are reported. Z scores were used in these analyses in order to standardize scores for all variables.

TABLE 7.6 Pearson Product-Moment Correlations Between Factors
(N = 1.29)

First factor	Second factor	r
ADL Self-Care	Assistive Devices	
Upper Torso	Eating	−.48
Upper Torso	Mobility, increased restrictions	−.66
Lower Torso	Dressing	−.24
Lower Torso	Eating	−.40
Lower Torso	Mobility, increased restrictions	−.71
Lower Torso	Mobility, restricted	−.29
Intimacy	Mobility, increased restrictions	−.20
Recreation & Socializing	Eating	−.21
Recreation & Socializing	Mobility, increased restrictions	−.30
Sensory & Communication	Eating	−.31
Sensory & Communication	Mobility, increased restrictions	−.28
Bowel Elimination	Mobility, increased restrictions	−.30
ADL Self-Care	MS-Related Symptoms	
Upper Torso	Skeletal	−.37
Lower Torso	Skeletal	−.46
Recreation & Socializing	Skeletal	−.34
Recreation & Socializing	Emotions	−.23
Recreation & Socializing	Head	−.22
Sensory & Communication	Skeletal	−.35
Sensory & Communication	Emotions	−.23
Sensory & Communication	Head	−.38
Bowel Elimination	Skeletal	−.23
Assistive Devices	MS-Related Symptoms	
Dressing	Skeletal	.22
Eating	Skeletal	.27
Mobility, increased restrictions	Skeletal	.32
Mobility, restricted	Skeletal	.31

Assistive devices used for eating and mobility correlated moderately high with all ADL difference scores except Intimacy. Assistive devices used for dressing showed a low correlation with the ADL Walking difference score. Skeletal symptoms correlated moderately high with all ADL difference scores except Intimacy. Emotional symptoms showed low correlations with the ADL Travel and Sensory and Communication difference scores. The specific correlations are presented in Table 7.7. The scores for Self-Care and Help from Others, plotted in Figure 7.1, illustrate the difference between ability and dependent care needs for the aggregate sample.

DISCUSSION

A self-administered instrument designed to assess an MS person's ADL self-care ability and dependency on others for ADL functioning was demonstrated using the self-care theory proposed by Orem (1980). Testing

TABLE 7.7 Pearson Product-Moment Correlations Between ADL
Difference and Checklist Scores (*N* = 629)

Subscale	Factor	*r*
ADL difference score	Assistive devices	
Eating	Eating	−.44
Eating	Mobility, increased restrictions	−.56
Dressing	Eating	−.46
Dressing	Mobility, increased restrictions	−.63
Walking	Eating	−.31
Walking	Mobility, increased restrictions	−.55
Walking	Dressing	−.27
Walking	Mobility restricted	−.47
Transfer	Eating	−.46
Transfer	Mobility, increased restrictions	−.64
Travel	Eating	−.40
Travel	Mobility, increased restrictions	−.66
Travel	Dressing	−.22
Travel	Mobility restricted	−.28
Bathing	Eating	−.44
Bathing	Mobility, increased restrictions	−.67
Bowel Elimination	Eating	−.36
Bowel Elimination	Mobility, increased restrictions	−.54
Recreation & Socializing	Eating	−.27
Recreation & Socializing	Mobility, increased restrictions	−.44
Recreation & Socializing	Mobility restricted	−.26
Sensory & Communication	Eating	−.31
Sensory & Communication	Mobility, increased restrictions	−.30
ADL difference score	MS-related symptoms	
Eating	Skeletal	−.39
Dressing	Skeletal	−.35
Walking	Skeletal	−.45
Transfer	Skeletal	−.37
Travel	Skeletal	−.45
Travel	Emotional	−.20
ADL difference score	MS-related symptoms	
Bathing	Skeletal	−.35
Bowel Elimination	Skeletal	−.30
Recreation & Socializing	Skeletal	−.44
Recreation & Socializing	Head	−.22
Sensory & Communication	Skeletal	−.33
Sensory & Communication	Emotional	−.24
Sensory & Communication	Head	−.37

the ADL Self-Care Scale supported construct validity, internal consistency, and test-retest reliability for all subscales except Work and Urination. Factor analysis determined that there were five factors comprising 15 of the original 37 items in the Assistive Devices Checklist and four factors comprising 20 of the 26 items contained in the MS-Related Symptoms Checklist.

The ADL subscale Work failed to emerge as an independent factor. Respondents who did not perform their usual work reported difficulty in

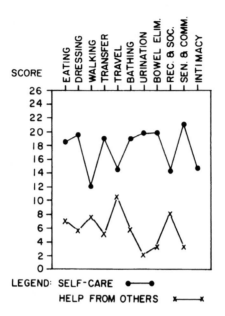

FIGURE 7.1 MS Self-Care ADL Profile illustrating the aggregate level of self-care and help from others (N = 629).

completing the subscale. Some of the items may not have been applicable to persons who no longer perform their usual work. This may have interfered with responding to the subscale. Others may have been reluctant to disclose their true work capability due to fear of jeopardizing their insurance benefit claims. In either case, the Work subscale requires revision. It may be best to present an open-ended question for subjects to respond to with respect to their work, chores, or related activities.

Three items from among the remaining 55 ADL scale items failed to load at or above .30. Two items were from the Urination subscale and one was from the Bowel Elimination subscale. The Urination item "Use an indwelling catheter" is not representative of a self-care behavior, and "Perform daily self-catheterization" is a behavior that is not widely practiced. The item from the Bowel Elimination subscale, "Have bowel accidents," failed to correlate positively with the other subscale items. Item substitution was made on the Urination subscale and retested on 94 additional subjects. A Cronbach alpha reliability coefficient of .71 was obtained. The revised Urination subscale has become part of the Self-Care ADL Scale.

Relationships among the ADL scale factors, checklist factors, and ADL difference scores were observed. Negative correlations between checklist factor scores and both the ADL factor scores and ADL difference scores suggest that increased independent ADL self-care is associated with decreased use of assistive devices. Also, the fewer the MS-related symptoms reported by the MS subjects, the higher their ADL Self-Care factor scores and larger the ADL difference scores. The frequency with which the assistive devices used for eating and maintaining mobility were associated with both the Upper and Lower Torso factors can be explained by the high correlation ($r = .77$) between these factors. The central nervous system pathology arising from MS tends to produce concurrent deficits in both fine motor skills such as finger dexterity and gross motor skills such as walking. These deficits are reflected in the skeletal symptoms, which showed moderate correlations with all ADL functional areas except Intimacy.

The aggregate ADL profile presented in Figure 7.1 is instructive in terms of what ADL activities reflect decreased self-care ability and increased dependent care required from other persons. Small score differences between the activities requiring lower torso functioning, such as walking and travel, recreation and socializing, are clearly evidenced. These are areas where particular programs and/or services by MS client service coordinators may need to be developed for the aggregate population. Additionally, an individual's ADL profile is useful in depicting his/her specific strengths and deficits. The analysis of self-care deficits used in conjunction with information from the Assistive Devices Checklist and MS-Related Symptoms Checklist scores can be used for designing appropriate ADL behaviors and obtaining necessary assistive devices or services to increase the MS person's self-care ability.

The findings from this study support the ADL Self-Care Scale for persons as an instrument worthy of further investigation. Orem's (1980) theory of self-care appears to offer an adequate base for self-assessment of ADL among persons diagnosed with MS. The work subscale is currently undergoing revision.

IMPLICATIONS FOR FUTURE RESEARCH

Additional testing of the ADL Self-Care Scale is currently in progress. The assessment of memory change on the accuracy of self-assessment is being conducted, together with comparisons among ADL ratings performed by the MS person, his/her significant other, and his/her health professional. The determination of criterion validity by comparing scores from the ADL Self-Care Scale with scores obtained from the Disability Status Scale (Kurtzke, 1981) is in progress. A study to determine whether MS persons who monitor their ADL functioning over time by performing periodic ADL self-assessments compared to MS persons who do not perform periodic assessments is also in progress. The latter study may provide additional construct validity for the ADL Self-Care Scale.

The scale can be adapted for use with microcomputers placed in office or clinic waiting rooms to permit ADL self-assessment. This information could be a valuable adjunct to the health appraisal performed by nurses and other health personnel as well as provide an ADL status report to the client.

REFERENCES

Albion, J. H. (1982). Multiple Sclerosis: A chronic-care focus. *Nurse Practitioner,* *8*(4), 29-35.

Crewe, N. M., & Athelstan, G. T. (1981). Functional assessment in vocational rehabilitation: A systematic approach to diagnosis and goal setting. *Archives in Physical Medicine and Rehabilitation, 62,* 229-305.

Dodd, M. J. (1984). Measuring informational intervention for chemotherapy knowledge and self-care behavior. *Research in Nursing and Health, 7,* 43-50.

Duke University Center for the Study of Aging and Human Development. (1978). *Multidimensional functional assessment: The OARS methodology* (2nd ed.). Durham, NC: Author.

Fillenbaum, B. B. (1979). Social context and self-assessments of health among the elderly. *Journal of Health and Social Behavior, 20,* 45-51.

International Federation of Multiple Sclerosis Societies. (1984). *Minimal record of disability in multiple sclerosis.* New York: National Multiple Sclerosis Society.

Iversen, I. A., Silberberg, N. E., Stever, R. C., & Schoening, H. A. (1973). *The revised Kenney self-care evaluation. A numerical measure of independence in activities of daily living.* Minneapolis, MN: Sister Kenney Institute, Abbott Northwestern Hospital. (Publication 722P).

Jeffreys, M., Millard, J. M., Human, M., & Warren, M. D. (1969). A set of tests for measuring motor impairment in prevalence studies. *Journal of Chronic Diseases, 22,* 303-319.

Katz, S., Ford, A. B., Moskowitz, R. W., Jackson, B. A., & Jaffee, M. W. (1963). Studies of illness in the aged. The index of ADL: A standardized measure of biological and psychosocial function. *Journal of the American Medical Association, 185,* 303-319.

Kaufert, J. M. (1983). Functional ability indices: Measurement problems in assessing their validity. *Archives of Physical Medicine and Rehabilitation, 64,* 260-267.

Keith, R. A. (1984). Functional assessment measures in medical rehabilitation current status. *Archives in Physical Medicine and Rehabilitation, 65,* 74, 78.

Kurtzke, J. F. (1981). A proposal for a uniform minimal record of disability in multiple sclerosis. *Acta Neurological Scandinavica, 64* (Suppl. 87), 110-129.

Levin, L. S., Katz, A. H., & Holst, E. (1979). *Self-care lay initiatives in health* (2nd ed.). New York: Prodist.

Maddox, G. L., & Douglas, E. B. (1973). Self-assessment of health: A longitudinal study of elderly subjects. *Journal of Health and Social Behavior, 14*(1), 87-93.

Mahoney, F. I., & Barthel, D. W. (1965). Functional evaluation: The Barthel Index. *Maryland State Medical Journal, 14*(2), 61-65.

McCorkle, R., & Benoliel, J. Q. (1981). *Cancer patient responses to psychosocial variables.* Seattle, WA: University of Washington, Community Health Care Systems Department.

Meenan, R. F., Gertman, P. M., Mason, J. H., & Dunaif, R. (1982). The arthritis impact measurement scales. Further investigations of health status measure. *Arthritis and Rheumatism, 25*(9), 1048-1053.

Nowakowski, L. (1980). Health promotion/self-care programs for the community. *Topics in Clinical Nursing, 2*(2), 21-27.

Nunnally, J. C. (1978). *Psychometric theory* (2nd ed.). New York: McGraw-Hill.

Orem, D. E. (1980). *Nursing: Concepts of practice* (2nd ed.). New York: McGraw-Hill.

Pavlou, M. (Ed.). (1979). *Variety and possibility in multiple sclerosis.* Chicago: Bio Service Corp.

Poser, C. M. (1979). A numerical scoring system for the classification of multiple sclerosis. *Acta Neurologica Scandinavica, 60,* 100-111.

Sarno, J. E., Sarno, M. T., & Levita, E. (1973). The functional life scale. *Archives of Physical Medicine and Rehabilitation, 54,* 214-220.

Seltzer, B., Granger, C. V., & Wineberg, D. (1982). Functional assessment: Bridge between family and rehabilitation medicine within an ambulatory practice. *Archives of Physical Medicine and Rehabilitation, 63,* 453-457.

Stephens, M. A. P., Norris-Baker, C., & Willems, E. P. (1983). Patient behavior monitoring through self-reports. *Archives of Physical Medicine and Rehabilitation, 64,* 167-171.

Vickery, D. M., Kalmer, H., Lowry, D., Constantine, M., Wright, E., & Loren, W. (1983). Effect of self-care education program on medical visits. *Journal of the American Medical Association, 250,* 2952-2956.

Zeller, R. A., & Carmines, E. G. (1980). *Measurement in the social sciences.* New York: Cambridge University Press.

ADL Self-Care Scale for Persons with Multiple Sclerosis*

Developed by Elsie E. Gulick with contributions from chapter staff and members of the National Multiple Sclerosis Society

ACKNOWLEDGMENTS

The ADL Self-Care Scale was developed as a result of contributions from research personnel, MS client service coordinators and many MS persons. Dr. Gulick contributed research acumen and experience from caring for MS persons residing in the community as well as first-hand experience gained from her husband, who was diagnosed with MS in 1969.

Ms. Sally Hennessey has coordinated client services for the Mid-Jersey Chapter, National Multiple Sclerosis Society, for a period of 11 years. Ms. Patricia Price assisted Ms. Hennessey in the coordination of client services for 3 years. Both Ms. Hennessey and Ms. Price assisted with initial scale development and piloting.

Many MS persons, together with agency staff from the Mid-Jersey, Bergen-Passaic, and Northern New Jersey chapters of the National Multiple Sclerosis Society, assisted with the refinement of the scale items through scale pilot testing. The agency staff included Sally Hennessey, RN; June Halper, MSN, RNC; and Constance Booth, MSW, all client service coordinators. Jacqueline Schachter, an MS Self-Help Group facilitator, provided assistance in piloting the scale.

Dr. Gulick's participation in the Measurement of Clinical And Educational Nursing Outcomes Project 1984-1985, sponsored by the University of Maryland, School of Nursing, together with grant support she received from the Robert Wood Johnson Foundation's Research and Development Program to Improve Patient Functional Status provided valuable resources for further scale development and scale testing.

MS SELF-CARE ADL SCALE

ID NUMBER: _____

Date: _____

Agency: _____

Scale Completed By:

__ MS Person   __ Relative/Friend

__ Spouse   __ Agency Staff

* Submitted for copyright 1986

Directions: Twelve activities of daily living, such as dressing, walking, toileting, and so forth, are each described by five statements. Please rate each statement according to *what you presently do.* You will then be asked to rate the questions again according to how much *help from others* you receive in performing each activity, with the exception of two of the activities. One will be rated only once and one asks for a short written response.

Rate each activity according to what you do on a *typical* day. The ratings include

Never	Almost never	Occasionally	Usually	Almost always	Always
0	1	2	3	4	5

Checklists for Assistive Devices and MS-Related Symptoms are included. Check the frequency that you use assistive devices and the frequency that you experience any of the symptoms. A Self-Care ADL Profile with instructions is attached for persons who wish to plot their own functional level among 11 activities. Thank you.

Eating

	Self-Care					
Do you:	Never	Almost Never	Occas.	Usually	Almost Always	Always
Prepare meals and/or transfer food from one place to another	___	___	___	___	___	___
Cut your own food	___	___	___	___	___	___
Pour liquids	___	___	___	___	___	___
Open milk cartons or similar containers	___	___	___	___	___	___
Feed yourself	___	___	___	___	___	___

	Help from Others					
Do you need help from other persons to:	Never	Almost Never	Occas.	Usually	Almost Always	Always
Prepare meals and/or transfer food from one place to another	___	___	___	___	___	___
Cut your own food	___	___	___	___	___	___
Pour milk or other liquids	___	___	___	___	___	___
Open milk cartons or similar containers	___	___	___	___	___	___
Feed yourself	___	___	___	___	___	___

Dressing

	Self-Care					
Do you:	Never	Almost Never	Occas.	Usually	Almost Always	Always
Put on underwear						
Put on socks/stockings/ shoes/braces						
Work buttons/zippers/ laces						
Put on trousers/dresses, shirts coats, or other items						
Remove your own clothes						

	Help from Others					
Do you need help from other persons to:	Never	Almost Never	Occas.	Usually	Almost Always	Always
Put on underwear						
Put on socks/stockings/ shoes/braces						
Work buttons/zippers/ laces						
Put on trousers/dresses, shirts coats, or other items						
Remove your own clothes						

Walking

	Self-Care					
Do you:	Never	Almost Never	Occas.	Usually	Almost Always	Always
Walk inside the house						
Walk outside the house (minimum of one block)						
Walk on uneven ground surfaces						
Walk up or down a ramp						
Climb and descend one flight of stairs						

	Help from Others					
Do you need help from other persons to:	Never	Almost Never	Occas.	Usually	Almost Always	Always
Walk inside the house						
Walk outside the house (minimum of one block)						

Walk on uneven ground
surfaces
Walk up or down a ramp
Climb and descend one
flight of stairs

Transfer

	Self-Care					
Do you:	Never	Almost Never	Occas.	Usually	Almost Always	Always
Turn from side to side while in a lying position						
Get into a sitting position from lying and vice versa						
Get from sitting to standing and vice versa						
Get from sitting position to another sitting position						
Transfer only with assistance of mechanical devices such as a patient lift						

	Help from Others					
Do you need help from other persons to:	Never	Almost Never	Occas.	Usually	Almost Always	Always
Turn from side to side while in a lying position						
Get into a sitting position from lying and vice versa						
Get from sitting to standing a vice versa						
Get from sitting position to another sitting position						
Transfer by using mechanical devices such as a patient lift						

Travel

Check (✓) the type of travel you use most frequently:
__ car   __ bus   __ train   __ airplane   __ wheelchair   __ other, describe

	Self-Care					
Do you:	Never	Almost Never	Occas.	Usually	Almost Always	Always
Get to and from your present method of travel (car, bus, other)						

Get on and off your present method of travel (car, bus, other) _____ _____ _____ _____ _____ _____

Get into, through, and out of buildings _____ _____ _____ _____ _____ _____

Travel long distances _____ _____ _____ _____ _____ _____

Travel freely as desired _____ _____ _____ _____ _____ _____

	Help from Others					
Do you need help from other persons to:	Never	Almost Never	Occas.	Usually	Almost Always	Always
Get to and from your present method of travel (car, bus, other)	_____	_____	_____	_____	_____	_____
Get on and off your present method of travel (car, bus, other)	_____	_____	_____	_____	_____	_____
Get into, through, and out of buildings	_____	_____	_____	_____	_____	_____
Travel long distances	_____	_____	_____	_____	_____	_____
Travel freely as desired	_____	_____	_____	_____	_____	_____

Bathing

	Self-Care					
Do you:	Never	Almost Never	Occas.	Usually	Almost Always	Always
Get in and out of the bathroom	_____	_____	_____	_____	_____	_____
Get in and out of the tub or shower	_____	_____	_____	_____	_____	_____
Get water and supplies	_____	_____	_____	_____	_____	_____
Wash "hard to reach" body parts	_____	_____	_____	_____	_____	_____
Wash all body parts (total bath)	_____	_____	_____	_____	_____	_____

	Help from Others					
Do you need help from other persons to:	Never	Almost Never	Occas.	Usually	Almost Always	Always
Get in and out of the bathroom	_____	_____	_____	_____	_____	_____
Get in and out of the tub or shower	_____	_____	_____	_____	_____	_____
Get water and supplies	_____	_____	_____	_____	_____	_____
Wash "hard to reach" body parts	_____	_____	_____	_____	_____	_____
Wash all body parts (total bath)	_____	_____	_____	_____	_____	_____

Toileting – Urination

Do you:	Self-Care					
	Never	Almost Never	Occas.	Usually	Almost Always	Always
Limit the amount of fluid you drink to control urine accidents	___	___	___	___	___	___
Take medication to control urine problems	___	___	___	___	___	___
Apply hand pressure over the bladder to assure complete emptying	___	___	___	___	___	___
Experience leaking or dribbling of urine	___	___	___	___	___	___
Use an absorbent pad or external catheter or sheath because of urine leakage	___	___	___	___	___	___

Do you need help from other persons to:	Help from Others					
	Never	Almost Never	Occas.	Usually	Almost Always	Always
Control the amount of fluid you drink	___	___	___	___	___	___
Take medication to control urine problems	___	___	___	___	___	___
Apply hand pressure over the bladder to assure complete emptying	___	___	___	___	___	___
Assist with care following loss of urine should it occur	___	___	___	___	___	___
Use an absorbent pad or external catheter or sheath	___	___	___	___	___	___

Toileting – Bowel

Do you:	Self-Care					
	Never	Almost Never	Occas.	Usually	Almost Always	Always
Use special foods to promote normal bowel movements	___	___	___	___	___	___
Use laxatives or other medicines	___	___	___	___	___	___
Use suppositories	___	___	___	___	___	___
Have bowel accidents	___	___	___	___	___	___
Use enemas	___	___	___	___	___	___

	Help from Others					
Do you need help from other persons to:	Never	Almost Never	Occas.	Usually	Almost Always	Always
Prepare or serve special foods that promote normal bowel movements	___	___	___	___	___	___
Take laxatives or other medicines to make your bowels move	___	___	___	___	___	___
Administer suppositories	___	___	___	___	___	___
Help you prevent bowel accidents and/or assist with care if they occur	___	___	___	___	___	___
Administer enemas	___	___	___	___	___	___

Recreation and Socializing

	Self-Care					
Do you:	Never	Almost Never	Occas.	Usually	Almost Always	Always
Participate in social activities outside the home	___	___	___	___	___	___
Participate socially with visitors in the home	___	___	___	___	___	___
Participate socially with family members in the home	___	___	___	___	___	___
Participate in receational activities outside the home	___	___	___	___	___	___
Participate in recreational activities inside the home	___	___	___	___	___	___

	Help from Others					
Do you need help from other persons to:	Never	Almost Never	Occas.	Usually	Almost Always	Always
Participate in social activities outside the home	___	___	___	___	___	___
Participate in social activities inside the home	___	___	___	___	___	___
Participate socially with family members in the home	___	___	___	___	___	___
Participate in recreational activities outside the home	___	___	___	___	___	___
Participate in recreational activities inside the home	___	___	___	___	___	___

Sensory and Communication

Do you:	Self-Care					
	Never	Almost Never	Occas.	Usually	Almost Always	Always
Read printed or written material	____	____	____	____	____	____
Hear what other persons are saying at normal speaking tones	____	____	____	____	____	____
Speak so other persons can easily understand what you say	____	____	____	____	____	____
Use a telephone	____	____	____	____	____	____
Write clearly	____	____	____	____	____	____

Do you need help from other persons to:	Help from Others					
	Never	Almost Never	Occas.	Usually	Almost Always	Always
Read printed or written material	____	____	____	____	____	____
Hear what others are saying at normal speaking tones	____	____	____	____	____	____
Speak so other persons can easily understand what you say	____	____	____	____	____	____
Use a telephone	____	____	____	____	____	____
Write clearly	____	____	____	____	____	____

Intimacy

Do you:	Self-Care					
	Never	Almost Never	Occas.	Usually	Almost Always	Always
Confide in someone regarding personal matters	____	____	____	____	____	____
Exchange loving glances with someone special	____	____	____	____	____	____
Exchange tender touches with someone special	____	____	____	____	____	____
Share intimate conversations with someone special	____	____	____	____	____	____
Experience satisfactory sexual activity with someone special	____	____	____	____	____	____

Work or Chores

1. Please describe the work or chores that you do.

2. What makes it difficult for you to do your work or chores?

3. What makes it easier for you to do your work or chores?

ASSISTIVE DEVICES

Check how frequently you use the Following aids due to MS	Never	Almost Never	Occas.	Usually	Almost Always	Always
Bathing						
Tub or shower seat						
Hand-held shower hose						
Long-handled brush						
Toileting						
Catheter (condom)						
Catheter (intermittent use)						
Catheter (remains in bladder)						
Badpan or urinal						
Commode						
Dressing						
Pullover sweaters/shirts						
Elastic waistbands						
Velcro closures						
Buttoning aid						
Shoehorn						
Elastic shoelaces						
Eating						
Spoon instead of fork						
Enlarged fork handle						
Rocker knife						
Nonskid plate or guard						
Special cup						
Sensory and Communication						
Glasses						
Magnifying glass						
Hearing aid						
Voice amplifier						

Transfer/Walking/Travel

Transfer board	
Grab bars	
Bed rails	
Furniture or walls	
Walker	
Rocker shoes	
Leg brace	
Cane	
Crutches	
Wheelchair	
Stair glide	
Ramp	
Motorized chair or cart	
Lift	

MS-RELATED SYMPTOMS

Check how frequently you experience the following symptoms	Never	Almost Never	Occas.	Usually	Almost Always	Always
Fatigue						
Arm weakness						
Leg weakness						
Spasms						
Tremors						
Knee locking or collapsing						
Balance problems						
Falling						
Double vision						
Blurred vision						
Difficulty swallowing						
Forgetfulness						
Inability to sleep						
Loneliness						
Depression						
Anxiety						

Pain	
Burning sensation	
Numbness	
Pins and needles sensation	
Increased urinating fre- quency (day)	
Increased urinating fre- quency (night)	
Trouble making toilet on time (day)	
Trouble making toilet on time (night)	
Difficulty in starting to urinate	
Urinary infection	

MS SELF-CARE ADL PROFILE

To: MS Person

Scale Completed By: _____
Date: _____

Place a circle around any of the activities listed above the graph that you would like to discuss with an agency staff member.

Would you like a copy of the completed Self-Care ADL Profile? __ Yes   __ No

If you wish to complete the Self-Care ADL Profile, you are encouraged to do so. The directions follow:

Summarize the 5 ratings for each Self-Care and Help from Others scale that you previously chcked.

Place an (o) on the graph that corresponds to the activity and rating score obtained for Self-Care.

Place an (x) on the graph that corresponds to the activity and rating score obtained for Help from Others.

Subtract the Help from Others score from the Self-Care score to obtain the difference score and record below the graph for each activity.

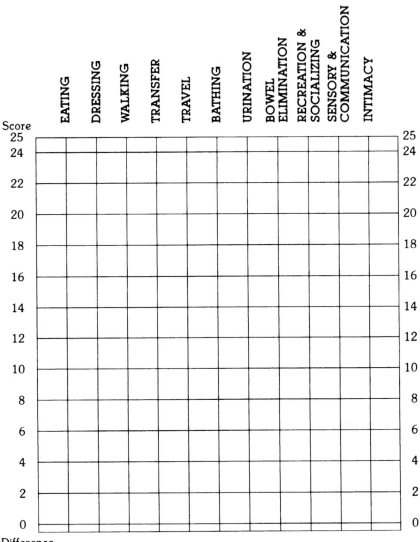

Score

| | EATING | DRESSING | WALKING | TRANSFER | TRAVEL | BATHING | URINATION | BOWEL ELIMINATION | RECREATION & SOCIALIZING | SENSORY & COMMUNICATION | INTIMACY | |

Difference
Score: ___ ___ ___ ___ ___ ___ ___ ___ ___ ___ ___

8

Measuring the Clinical Outcomes of the Patient with Chronic Pain

Gail C. Davis

This chapter discusses the McGill Comprehensive Pain Questionnaire, a measure of physical pain.

Pain is a common problem addressed within the realm of nursing practice. With pain as the common element, acute pain and chronic pain are two distinctly different entities to be addressed. "Alteration in Comfort: Pain" was identified as a nursing diagnostic category by the National Conference for Classification of Nursing Diagnosis in 1978 and accepted in 1980 (Kim & Moritz, 1982). Although this group has not yet divided the pain diagnosis into acute and chronic pain, Carpenito (1983) does make this division for purposes of application to clinical practice. Acute pain is defined as "pain that can last from one second to as long as 6 months. It subsides with healing or when the stimulus is removed" (p. 117). Chronic pain is "persistent or intermittent pain that lasts for more than six months" (p. 122). Although duration is noted as the key element of difference in most definitions of pain, the increased complexity of effects experienced by the chronic pain patient is another major difference. It is the prolonged and unknown duration that leads to other patient responses. This pain that "exists without a known time limit ... becomes a constant companion, to be controlled if possible but always to be lived with" (Johnson, 1977, p. 141).

In order for nurses to adequately assess and treat chronic pain, its characteristics (effects) and the desired outcomes of treatment need to be identified. A tool is needed that will not only provide an effective and efficient approach to assessment as a basis for nursing intervention but will also provide an approach to gathering information for the further research needed to establish the reliability and validity of the identified characteristics and outcomes of chronic pain. The major purpose of this study was to determine the adequacy of the McGill Comprehensive Pain

Questionnaire (MCPQ) (Monks & Taenzer, 1983) for use in assessing the clinical outcomes of the patient with a nursing diagnosis of Alteration in Comfort: Pain (Chronic).

REVIEW OF LITERATURE

Definition of Pain

The literature is in agreement about the difficulty of defining pain (Jacox, 1977; Johnson, 1977; McCaffery, 1979; Sternbach, 1974). A group of individuals concerned with the consistent use of terminology related to pain worked from 1976 to 1978 to arrive at a taxonomy that could provide a common operational framework and a basis for further development. This Subcommittee of the Association for the Study of Pain (IASP Subcommittee on Taxonomy, 1979) defined pain as "an unpleasant sensory and emotional experience associated with actual or potential damage, or described in terms of such damage" (p. 250). This definition reflects a conscious effort to "call pain something which is part of the subjective experience of an individual. Actual changes in tissue and in the nervous system are not pain" (Merskey, 1982, p. 13).

Approaches to Pain Measurement

The measurement of pain is necessary if the treatment and the relief of pain are to be evaluated. Since pain is highly subjective, clinical evaluation is focused on the measurement of an individual's pain over time. Stewart (1977) reports three basic approaches to the measurement of clinical pain: "(1) eliciting the person's subjective report of pain, either through verbal or written accounts, (2) observing a person's behavior – for example, restlessness, agitation, grimacing, or crying; and (3) using instruments to measure autonomic signs of pain, such as increase in blood pressure and pulse or excessive perspiration" (pp. 107-108).

Several researchers support the concept of combining verbal and physiological measurement; this combination provides a fourth approach. Bromm (1984) points out that the verbal report is the most important measure of pain in man but adds that this subjective report should be objectified by also measuring pain related to physiological variables. "In general, reported strengths of sensation are objectified through the measurement of simultaneously occurring physiological reactions to the same stimulus" (p. 8). Such physiological measurement might include such measures as "peripheral nerve activity, withdrawal reflexes, skin resistance reactions, evoked potentials, and change in the electroencephalogram" (p. 12). Physiological techniques have received little attention in the study of chronic pain. In some cases, reflex mechanisms may contribute to the development of chronic pain (Zimmermann, 1984). Noting that chronic pain could possibly be relieved through local anesthesia, Zimmermann supports further study of the "theoretical and practical aspects" of some chronic pain. "At the present time, there seems to be an appreciation of the concept of chronic pain as being more complex than that which can be encompassed by neurophysiological concepts or which can be treated by using only traditional medical procedures" (Bellissimo & Tunks, 1984, pp. 67-68).

CONCEPTUAL BASIS FOR MEASUREMENT TOOL

The conceptual basis that supports the selection of the MCPQ (Monks & Taenzer, 1983) for evaluation of its adequacy in measuring the clinical outcomes of chronic pain is a comprehensive interpretation of chronic pain. Such an interpretation is founded on the belief that pain is a complex individual experience that can be subjectively reported by the patient. One's total pain experience is modulated by the interplay of a variety of factors: perception, personality structure, biological variables, and social variables (Sternbach, 1968). Adequate assessment of chronic pain should be aimed at meeting the following goals: "identify biological (organic) pain generators and/or sources of impairment; identify significant psychosocial problem areas; delineate strengths and resources of the individual and his milieu; facilitate treatment outcome; and allow testing of research hypotheses" (Monks & Taenzer, 1983, p. 233).

RESEARCH QUESTIONS

The approach to pain measurement selected for further investigation in this study was the patient's subjective report of pain. The tool that provides the comprehensive approach necessary to measuring chronic pain is the MCPQ. Its adequacy for measuring the outcomes of chronic pain was tested through study of the following research questions:

1. Is the MCPQ valid for evaluating clinical outcomes of patients with a nursing diagnosis of Alteration in Comfort: Pain (Chronic)?
2. Do the tool's quantitative components – present pain intensity (PPI), pain rating index (PRI), number of words chosen (NWC), dimension subscales: Sensory, Affective, Evaluative, Miscellaneous – discriminate between two groups of patients, for example, those with acute pain (postsurgical) and those with chronic pain (rheumatoid disease)?
3. Is there a good correlation between the patient's pain intensity score when measured concurrently by the pain intensity scale of the MCPQ and the visual analog scale?
4. Is there a good relationship between the intensity of pain associated with toothaches, headaches, and stomachaches as rated on the

MCPQ by the acute patient group preoperatively and postoperatively?

5. What areas of daily living (work, leisure, sleep, weight, habits, mood, attitudes) are most affected by chronic pain?

METHODOLOGY

Sample

The major sample population was composed of patients with a nursing diagnosis of Alteration in Comfort: Pain (Chronic). Thirty subjects were selected through a purposive, nonrandom sampling procedure. These subjects met the following criteria for selection:

1. Had a nursing diagnosis of Alteration in Comfort: Pain (Chronic).
2. Had a medical diagnosis of rheumatoid disease.
3. Were at least 21 years of age.
4. Had a medical treatment plan for rheumatoid disease.

Figure 8.1 illustrates the composition of the chronic pain group according to their medical diagnosis within the broad category of rheumatoid disease. These patients had experienced pain within a time range of 1 to 30 years, with an average of 11.4 years.

A second sample group was selected from patients admitted to the hospital for general surgery. Figure 8.2 shows a categorization of the surgical experiences of this group. Again, a purposive, nonrandom sampling procedure was used to select 30 patients who met the following criteria: (1) had a potential nursing diagnosis of Alteration in Comfort: Pain (Acute) related to a general surgical procedure; and (2) were at least 21 years of age.

The demographic data describing the two groups are shown in Figure 8.3.

Instrumentation

Discussion of the instrument used relates to both the McGill Pain Questionnaire (MPQ) and the MCPQ. The original MPQ was developed by Melzack (1983b) at McGill University, and its focus is on pain description (see Figure 8.4). The first paper describing its scoring properties was published by Melzack in 1975. The first testing of the tool indicated that it provided "quantitative information that can be treated statistically, and is sufficiently sensitive to detect differences among different methods to relieve pain" (Melzack, 1975, p. 277). The MCPQ has expanded the MPQ and its pain description by adding additional questions related to pain history, past medical history, medication, pain modifiers, effects of pain, personal history, and patient expectations. Most of these are open-ended questions, providing qualitative data not appropriate for statistical testing.

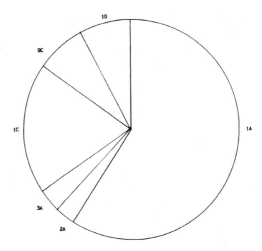

FIGURE 8.1 Chronic pain (rheumatoid disease). 1A, rheumatoid arthritis (56.7%); 2A, ankylosing spondylitis (3.33%); 3A, osteoarthritis (3.33%); 1C, lupus erythematosus (23.3%); 9C, bursitis and/or tendonitis (6.67%); 10, miscellaneous (palindromic rheumatism).

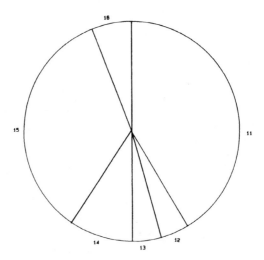

FIGURE 8.2 Acute pain (pre- and postsurgery). 11, hysterectomy (36.7%); 12, hernia repair (6.67%); 13, mastectomy (6.67%); 14, general abdominal (10.0%); 15, orthopedic (33.3%); 16, urological (6.67%).

The major difference in the two tools is the increased comprehensiveness of the patient's data base (Monks & Taenzer, 1983).

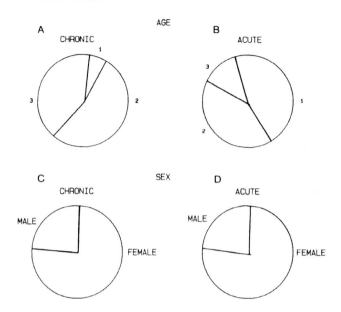

FIGURE 8.3 Demographic data. A: 1, young adult (24-39 years), 3.33%; 2, middle adult (40-64 years), 53.3%; 3, older adult (65-81 years), 43.3%. B: 1, young adult, 40.0%; 2, middle adult, 40.0%; 3, older adult, 20.0%. C: female, 76.6%; male, 23.3%. D: female, 76.7%, male, 23.3%.

MCPQ

The MCPQ was further modified for this study. This modification consisted primarily of combining two parts of the original MCPQ: (1) the patient questionnaire and (2) the interview guide. The original version of the tool is organized so that the questionnaire (Part 1) can be sent to the patient for completion prior to being seen in the Pain Center of the Montreal General Hospital, where Part 2 (the interview portion) is used (Monks & Taenzer, 1983). In addition to the combining of items, the tool was shortened by eliminating some items. Most items relating to past personal and medical history were omitted, as the primary focus was placed on assessment of the present health-related status of the patient. Some personal items were also eliminated, keeping a focus on those areas in which the nurse might intervene.

MPQ

More information is available about the MPQ (or quantitative portion of the MCPQ). One of the advantages provided by the MPQ is that it provides quantitative information that can be treated statistically (Melzack, 1975). Three different types of quantitative data are available: (1) pain rating index (PRI), obtained by adding the rank order value for each dimension and dividing the sum by the total possible dimension score

(Kremer, Atkinson, & Ignelzi, 1982); (2) the total number of words chosen
(NWC), which refers to the total number of words selected in the sensory,
affective, and evaluative dimensions; and (3) present pain intensity, based
on a scale of 0 to 5, with 0 representing "no pain" and 5 representing
"excruciating pain." The MPQ is a "start... toward the measurement of
clinical pain and permits research on the effects of experimental and therapeutic procedures on pain in clinical rather than laboratory conditions"
(Melzack, 1975, p. 294).

The MPQ "permits measurement of the sensory, affective, and evaluative dimensions of pain," and "it also provides information on the relative
intensity of each, as well as several measures of the patient's evaluation
of the overall intensity of the pain" (Melzack, 1983a, p. 4). This tool has
probably been the one that is most clinically useful in measuring qualitative and quantitative pain experiences (Torgerson & BenDebba, 1983).
The word descriptors for the PRI were drawn from an earlier study by
Melzack and Torgerson (1971). This study classified words into three
quality categories to describe the pain experience: (1) sensory – temporal,
spatial, pressure, thermal, and other properties; (2) affective – tension,
fear, and autonomic properties that are part of the pain experience; and
(3) evaluative – words describing overall intensity.

The MPQ is reported to have good reliability and validity. Reading
(1983) reports the results of two different studies with cancer patients.
He reports that "repeated administrations of the questionnaire to cancer
patients have yielded a consistency index of 75% (range 35 to 90%)
between the first two administrations" (p. 56). Over the course of weekly
administrations, the consistency "decreased to 66% and then increased to
80%." In another study, "the consistency of word choice by 10 cancer
patients over 3 days ranged from 50 to 100%, with a mean of 70.3%."
Although more factor-analytical studies of the word groupings are needed
to answer some of the questions related to the distinct differences of the
descriptive scales, a study by Prieto et al. (1980) demonstrated that three
factors were evident and that the Affective and Evaluative categories were
distinctly different. Face validity of the tool is indicated by the fact that
it has been selected as the instrument of measurement in a number of
different studies. A study by Kremer and Atkinson (1983) addressed the
issue of construct validity. They demonstrated that "the affective dimension of the MPQ was systematically related to an independent measure of
affective distress [Brief Symptom Inventory (BSI)] in chronic pain
patients" (p. 119).

VAS

The visual analog scale (VAS) was also used. The VAS is a line (vertical
or horizontal) with clearly defined boundaries (Figure 8.5). Usually the
line is 10 cm in length, and the patient is asked to make a mark on the
line at a point that describes the intensity of his pain. The distance of the

McGill Pain Questionnaire

PATIENT'S NAME ______________ DATE ________ TIME ______ am/pm

PRI: S ______ (1-10) A ______ (11-15) E ______ (16) M ______ (17-20) PRI(T) ______ (1-20) PPI ______

1 FLICKERING, QUIVERING, PULSING, THROBBING, BEATING, POUNDING
2 JUMPING, FLASHING, SHOOTING
3 PRICKING, BORING, DRILLING, STABBING, LANCINATING
4 SHARP, CUTTING, LACERATING
5 PINCHING, PRESSING, GNAWING, CRAMPING, CRUSHING
6 TUGGING, PULLING, WRENCHING
7 HOT, BURNING, SCALDING, SEARING
8 TINGLING, ITCHY, SMARTING, STINGING
9 DULL, SORE, HURTING, ACHING, HEAVY
10 TENDER, TAUT, RASPING, SPLITTING
11 TIRING, EXHAUSTING
12 SICKENING, SUFFOCATING
13 FEARFUL, FRIGHTFUL, TERRIFYING
14 PUNISHING, GRUELLING, CRUEL, VICIOUS, KILLING
15 WRETCHED, BLINDING
16 ANNOYING, TROUBLESOME, MISERABLE, INTENSE, UNBEARABLE
17 SPREADING, RADIATING, PENETRATING, PIERCING
18 TIGHT, NUMB, DRAWING, SQUEEZING, TEARING
19 COOL, COLD, FREEZING
20 NAGGING, NAUSEATING, AGONIZING, DREADFUL, TORTURING

PPI
0 NO PAIN
1 MILD
2 DISCOMFORTING
3 DISTRESSING
4 HORRIBLE
5 EXCRUCIATING

BRIEF	RHYTHMIC	CONTINUOUS
MOMENTARY	PERIODIC	STEADY
TRANSIENT	INTERMITTENT	CONSTANT

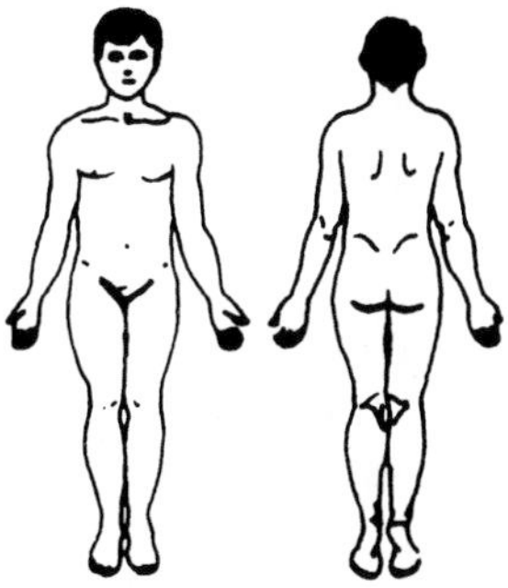

E = EXTERNAL
I = INTERNAL

COMMENTS:

FIGURE 8.4 McGill Pain Questionnaire. The descriptors fall into four major groups: sensory, 1 to 10; affective, 11 to 15; evaluative, 16; and miscellaneous, 17 to 20. the rank value for each descriptor is based on its position in the word set. The sum of the rank values is the pain rating index (PRI). The present pain intensity (PPI) is based on a scale of 0 to 5. Copyright 1970 Ronald Melzack.

No pain ——————————————————————————————— My pain is
at all   as bad as it
                                                                              could possibly
                                                                              be
FIGURE 8.5 Visual analog scale.

mark from the end of the line represents the pain intensity score. Several studies have shown the VAS to provide a reliable method of measurement (Aitken, 1969; Huskisson, 1983). High correlation has also been shown between the analog scale and other methods of measuring pain (Ohnhaus & Adler, 1975; Scott & Huskisson, 1976; Woodforde & Merskey, 1972). A major weakness of the VAS, however, is that it is a one-item tool, which makes its scores highly susceptible to measurement error.

Data collection

The investigator administered the VAS and the modified version of the MCPQ, using the interview method, to all 30 subjects in the chronic pain group. The subjects were interviewed within one of three different settings: (1) an arthritis clinic in a public hospital, (2) a private arthritis clinic, or (3) in the home setting. The names of those patients interviewed at home were provided, with their permission, by the local Arthritis Foundation office. Each interview took approximately 1 hr.

The investigator and another nurse administered the quantitative portion (MPQ) of the MCPQ to the 30 subjects in the acute pain group. The sample was selected from patients admitted to a 650-bed private hospital for surgery. The same nurse administered the questionnaire to the patient prior to surgery and again on the second postoperative day. This time interval was selected on the basis of a study by Hunter, Philips, and Rachman (1979), which reports that "The Melzack Pain Questionnaire can be used with confidence to assess pain that was experienced up to 5 days before the assessment was carried out" (p. 45). An assumption is made, then, that any reported change in pain is valid. The VAS was also used with this group to evaluate pain intensity preoperatively and postoperatively.

RESULTS

The student's t-test was used to test for significant differences ($p < .05$) between the chronic and acute pain groups in relation to all of the quantitative data (see Table 8.1). The study demonstrated that one of the word description subscales, the Affective dimension, discriminated between the chronic and acute pain patients. The Affective subscale discriminated significantly, using both scale scores and z scores. In addition, a discriminant analysis of the 4 subscales was done using Wilks's method. This analysis

TABLE 8.1 Comparison of
Quantitative Data Between Groups

Variable	t-value
Present pain intensity (PPI)	0.50
Number of words chosen (NWC)	1.22
Word descriptor groups	
1	1.15
2	1.00
3	0.63
4	1.08
5	0.08
6	0.42
7	2.15*
8	3.29**
9	1.72
10	0.63
11	1.34
12	0.83
13	2.60**
14	1.32
15	1.35
16	0.37
17	0.44
18	0.24
19	2.22*
20	0.78
Word descriptor subscales	
Sensory	0.80
Affective	2.24*
Evaluative	0.37
Miscellaneous	0.72

$*p < .05; **p < .01$

yielded one canonical function (Affect) that approached significance ($p = .059$). Specific words that also discriminated between the two groups were "hot," "tingling," and "fearful"; these were used by the chronic pain group to describe their pain.

The present pain intensity scale of the MCPQ and the VAS were compared using the Pearson product-moment correlation procedure. This comparison ($r = .5753$) demonstrates a moderate level of concurrent validity for measuring pain intensity at a given time.

The Pearson r was also used to test the reliability of the MCPQ's pain intensity rating scale. The acute pain patients were asked to rate the pain intensity related to their "worst toothache," "worst headache," and "worst stomachache." This scale is the same one used to measure present pain intensity ("mild" to "excruciating"). The findings, pain correlation coefficients ranging from 0.86 to 0.92, demonstrated a strong relationship between the preoperative and postoperative ratings, indicating reliability of the pain intensity rating scale.

TABLE 8.2 Qualitative Indicators Identified by Chronic Pain Group

Items identified according to category	%
Location of pain	
Joint	77
Time element	
Continuous, steady, constant	83
Leisure	
Hobbies, etc. – no longer can do because of pain	75
Still participate in hobbies, etc., which can still do	89
Have not begun new activities since pain began	79
Habits	
Do not drink alcohol	75
Attitude	
There are people with whom pain can be discussed	82
Religion helps cope with pain problem	84
Modifiers that increase pain	
Standing	82
Walking	76
Fatigue	83
Modifiers that decrease pain	
Heat	80
Enjoying things	80
Talking with others	77
Rest	83
Modifiers that have no effect	
Collars	80

TABLE 8.3 Word Descriptors Selected by Chronic Pain Group

Word	Dimension	%
Exhausting	Affective	53
Sharp	Sensory	50
Throbbing	Sensory	43
Shooting	Sensory	43
Burning	Sensory	37
Penetrating	Miscellaneous	37
Nagging	Miscellaneous	37
Cramping	Sensory	33
Aching	Sensory	33
Tender	Sensory	33
Tiring	Affective	33
Fearful	Affective	33
Numb	Miscellaneous	33

The qualitative data were studied for the indications they might provide for further refinement of the instrument. Descriptive statistics – frequencies and percentages – were used for analysis. Those qualitative areas that demonstrated an occurrence of at least 75% are summarized in Table 8.2. These would seem to give direction for areas of further tool development. In addition, the word descriptors were evaluated to determine which were selected by the chronic pain patients at least one-third of the time (Table 8.3).

DISCUSSION

The major purpose of this study was to determine the adequacy of the MCPQ for use in evaluating the clinical outcomes of the patient with a nursing diagnosis of chronic pain. The tool's various quantitative components were evaluated for discriminant validity, concurrent validity, and reliability. Qualitative portions were studied in order to determine those indicators that occurred most frequently in relation to chronic pain.

The Affective subscale of the MCPQ's word descriptors discriminated between the acute and chronic pain groups. The Affective dimension includes 5 word groups, 11 through 15. This finding, in relation to the outcomes of earlier studies, supports the discriminant validity of the MCPQ's word scales. Reading (1983) reported that "women experiencing pelvic pain showed that acute pain patients displayed greater use of sensory word groups... in contrast, chronic pain patients used affective and evaluative groups with greater frequency" (p. 58). This finding is also consistent with a review of pain language and affective disturbance (Kremer & Atkinson, 1983) which indicated that "affective distress influences pain language in a systematic fashion, and that the MPQ is a reliable, valid and unobtrusive measure of emotional disorder in chronic pain patients" (p. 120). Several researchers (Kremer & Atkinson, 1983; Lindsay & Wyckoff, 1981; Philips, 1983) have questioned whether the affective distress experienced by the person with chronic pain might be indicative of depression and/or anxiety. Sternbach (1978) states that the association between chronic pain and depression has "not been adequately investigated because there is no good animal model of chronic pain which has been studied... and it has not been possible to produce laboratory manipulations of depression" (p. 243). McCreary (1983) further questions whether the affective pain description indicates that anxiety and depression occur as state or trait measures.

Chapman (1978) discounts the association of anxiety with chronic pain, stating that "patients with chronic pain have relatively low anxiety levels" (p. 179). The uncertainty and surprise of pain has dissipated for the person for whom pain is constant. Exceptions to this might be the cancer patient for whom pain recurrence could indicate the spread of disease or to the cardiac patient for whom successive onset of pain might indicate a fatal heart attack. These exceptions would more likely involve intermittent rather than constant pain.

The MCPQ's pain intensity rating demonstrated moderate reliability with the VAS, indicating acceptable concurrent validity of these two pain measurements. This is consistent with previous studies, which have shown correlations from 0.39 to 0.10 between the MPQ and verbal and visual analog rating scales (Reading, 1983). Instructions to the patient for how to respond to either the MPQ or the VAS is necessary for completion. When five patients were asked to respond with only written instructions, only one was able to accomplish this task without asking for further direction. The horizontal VAS was used in this study, and some patients had difficulty visualizing the continuum. This might be more obvious if the vertical line, rather than the horizontal, were used. These problems encountered by the patients using the written instructions with the VAS also emphasizes the need to use caution when using such one-item scales.

The pain intensity rating scale of the MCPQ was reliable when used by the acute pain group to measure the pain intensity of toothaches, headaches, and stomachaches. The strong correlations indicate that patients can use this scale consistently. Although the person's memory capacity might be a confounding factor, this finding does provide evidence that one can report pain retrospectively. This ability to consistently recall pain intensity could be important to the nurse who is making pain assessments in the clinical setting.

The length of the interviews (approximately 1 hr) reinforced the purpose of developing an efficient and effective tool for the clinical measurement of chronic pain. The qualitative data were carefully examined to determine (1) what areas seemed related to the chronic pain patient with rheumatoid disease and (2) where reorganization of these data might occur within the tool as modified for this study. In further evaluating these data, a question that deserves further consideration is whether one tool can efficiently assess the chronic pain of patients with differing medical diagnoses.

Eighty percent of the acute pain patients and 83% of the chronic pain group described their pain as being "constant." In light of questions that have been raised concerning anxiety and depression in chronic pain patients, the pain time element (constant, intermittent, or transient) should be retained as a part of measurement even though it did not discriminate between the two groups of patients in this study.

A number of relative qualitative areas were identified within the Effects of Pain portion of the tool. The areas of work and leisure were important to the individual. In this study, 67% were not working. The tool could efficiently determine why (retired, quit due to pain, unable to perform physical activities, etc.) and how the person is using leisure time. Eighty-nine percent stated that they still participated in hobbies and social activities that they were still able to do, and 21% had started participating in new activities since their pain had begun. If, indeed, depression is related to chronic pain in some cases, the individual's level of involvement might provide an indicator for further assessment.

Sleep did not appear to be a strong indicator; 54% had trouble falling asleep, and 46% did not. Many patients, though, indicated that they felt worse, not refreshed, in the morning. This question might be made more specific, especially for the patient with rheumatoid disease who may experience joint stiffness upon arising.

Appetite does not appear to be strongly affected by chronic pain; 21% described their appetite as "too good" and 68% as "good." Weight does appear to be highly related. When patients' weights were compared to normals using the Metropolitan Life chart, none were underweight, 36% were within normal limits, and 64% were overweight. The majority also stated that they had either lost weight or had not experienced any real weight change, indicating that overweight was a problem for them when the pain began.

Habits did not seem highly related to the chronic pain experience. A few brief questions could be retained to determine whether there are habits that are assisting the person in coping with pain. For such information, observation would probably be preferable to self-report.

Some indication of the patient's own perception of mood was possible with this tool. The majority (74%) were "happy" most of the time, and only 1 person described himself as "unhappy." The remaining 22% stated that their moods varied. Major self-description of mood, in addition to admitted anger and irritability, was information that patients seemed willing to discuss. Again, this area would seem critical to study in order to gain information for further assessment of the patient. Using the interview technique also seems important here to assess whether some discrepancy exists between the patient's answers and behavior.

In their responses to influences on pain attitude, patients noted several indicators. A majority (61%) thought about their pain at least several times daily. Having someone with whom they could discuss their pain was important to 82%. Religious faith assisted 84% in coping with pain. Sixty-seven percent stated that their pain had not affected their feelings about themselves as persons.

The Pain Modifiers section emerges as an important one. The format facilitated data collection, and some of the other indicators throughout the questionnaire could probably be reorganized and placed within this section. Those modifiers that increased or decreased pain for at least 75% of the patients are noted in Table 8.2. Some of these – standing, walking, heat – might be specific to the rheumatoid disease diagnosis. Those modifiers within the social realm would more likely relate to all patients experiencing chronic pain.

The first three sections as presently organized within the MCPQ – pain history, present medical history, and medication – are not viewed as essential elements of a nursing assessment tool. Information from these sections that was viewed as providing background essential to the nursing assessment included the following:

1. How long the patient has experienced pain.
2. Any other current health problems, such as high blood pressure, ulcer, diabetes, etc.
3. Names of medications currently being taken.
4. Location of the pain as illustrated on the body map.

With the arthritis patients experiencing pain in several joints, it was also helpful to have them rank the pain (worst to least) in the various body parts. This was helpful in interpreting their responses to many of the questions.

The major implication of this study is that the MCPQ provides a good beginning measure of the outcomes of chronic pain. It provides a valid and reliable measure of pain intensity, and the word descriptors differentiate chronic from acute pain. The qualitative portion of the tool identifies those areas of the patient's daily living that are most affected by chronic pain. These indicators can be further tested to determine whether they are indeed the characteristics (or outcomes) that should guide the measurement of chronic pain.

Further study is needed to make the tool more efficient in providing adequate measurement of patient outcomes. Revision of the tool will be aimed at organizing relevant questions (those identified as indicators) into more objective questions for quantification. Reliability and validity testing will then need to be done for the revision prior to actual use in evaluating outcomes related to various interventions. Such testing should include evaluation of construct validity and the possible relationship of chronic pain to depression.

REFERENCES

Aitken, R. C. B. (1969). Section of measurement in medicine: A growing edge of measurement of feelings: Measurement of feelings using visual analogue scales. *Proceedings of the Royal Society of Medicine, 62,* 989-993.

Bellissimo, A., & Tunks, E. (1984). *Chronic pain: The psychotherapeutic spectrum.* New York: Praeger.

Bromm, B. (1984). The measurement of pain in men. In B. Bromm (Ed.), *Pain measurement in man* (pp. 3-13). New York: Elsevier.

Carpenito, L. J. (1983). *Nursing diagnosis: Application to clinical practice.* Philadelphia: J. B. Lippincott.

Chapman, C. R. (1978). Perception of noxious events. In R. A. Sternbach (Ed.), *The psychology of pain* (pp. 169-202). New York: Raven Press.

Hunter, M., Philips, C., & Rachman, S. (1979). Memory for pain. *Pain, 6,* 35-46.

Huskisson, E. C. (1983). Visual analogue scales. In R. Melzack (Ed.), *Pain measurement and assessment* (pp. 33-37). New York: Raven Press.

IASP Subcommittee on Taxonomy. (1979). Pain terms: A list with definitions and notes on usage. *Pain, 6,* 249-252.

Jacox, A. K. (1977). Sociological and psychological aspects of pain. In A. K. Jacox (Ed.), *Pain: A sourcebook for nurses and other health professionals* (pp. 57-87). Boston: Little, Brown.

Johnson, M. (1977). Assessment of clinical pain. In A. K. Jacox (Ed.), *Pain: A sourcebook for nurses and other health professionals* (pp. 139-166). Boston: Little, Brown.

Kim, M., & Moritz, D. A. (Eds.). (1982). *Classification of nursing diagnoses: Proceedings of the third and fourth national conferences.* New York: McGraw-Hill.

Kremer, E. F., & Atkinson, J. H., Jr. (1983). Pain language as a measure of affect in chronic pain patients. In R. Melzack (Ed.), *Pain measurement and assessment* (pp. 119-127). New York: Raven Press.

Kremer, E., Atkinson, J. H., & Ignelzi, R. J. (1982). Measurement of pain: Patient preference does not confound pain measurement. *Pain, 10,* 241-248.

Lindsay, P. G., & Wyckoff, M. (1981). The depression-pain syndrome and its response to antidepressants. *Psychosomatics, 22,* 571-577.

McCaffery, M. (1979). *Nursing management of the patient with pain* (2nd ed.). Philadelphia: J. B. Lippincott.

McCreary, C. (1983). Pain description and personality disturbance. In R. Melzack (Ed.), *Pain measurement and assessment* (pp. 137-141). New York: Raven Press.

Melzack, R. (1975). The McGill Pain Questionnaire: Major properties and scoring methods. *Pain, 1,* 277-299.

Melzack, R. (1983a). Concepts of pain measurement. In R. Melzack (Ed.), *Pain measurement and assessment* (pp. 1-5). New York: Raven Press.

Melzack, R. (1983b). The McGill Pain Questionnaire. In R. Melzack (Ed.), *Pain measurement and assessment* (pp. 41-47). New York: Raven Press.

Melzack, R., & Torgerson, W. S. (1971). On the language of pain. *Anesthesiology, 34,* 50-59.

Merskey, H. (1982). Body-mind dilemma in chronic pain. In R. Roy & E. Tunks (Eds.), *Chronic pain: Psychosocial factors in rehabilitation* (pp. 10-19). Baltimore: Williams & Wilkins.

Monks, R., & Taenzer, P. (1983). A comprehensive pain questionnaire. In R. Melzack (Ed.), *Pain measurement and assessment* (pp. 233-237). New York: Raven Press.

Ohnhaus, E. E., & Adler, R. (1975). Methodological problems in the measurement of pain: A comparison between the verbal rating scale and the visual analogue scale. *Pain, 1,* 379-384.

Philips, C. (1983). Chronic headache experience. In R. Melzack (Ed.), *Pain measurement and assessment* (pp. 97-103). New York: Raven Press.

Prieto, E. G., Hopson, L., Bradley, L. A., Byrne, M., Geisinger, K. F., Midax, D., & Marchisello, P. J. (1980). The language of low back pain: Factor structure of the McGill Pain Questionnaire. *Pain, 8,* 11-19.

Reading, A. E. (1983). The McGill Pain Questionnaire: An appraisal. In R. Melzack (Ed.), *Pain measurement and assessment* (pp. 55-61). New York: Raven Press.

Scott, J., & Huskisson, E. C. (1976). Graphic representation of pain. *Pain, 2,* 175-184.

Sternbach, R. A. (1968). *Pain: A psychophysiological analysis.* New York: Academic Press.

Sternbach, R. A. (1974). *Pain patients: Traits and treatment.* New York: Academic Press.

Sternbach, R. A. (1978). Clinical aspects of pain. In R. A. Sternbach (Ed.), *The psychology of pain* (pp. 241-264). New York: Raven Press.

Stewart, M. L. (1977). Measurement of clinical pain. In A. K. Jacox (Ed.), *Pain: A source book for nurses and other health professionals* (pp. 107-137). Boston: Little, Brown.

Torgerson, W. S., & BenDebba, M. (1983). The structure of pain descriptors. In

R. Melzack (Ed.), *Pain measurement and assessment* (pp. 49-54). New York: Raven Press.

Woodforde, J. M., & Merskey, H. (1972). Some relationships between subjective measures of pain. *Journal of Psychosomatic Research, 16,* 173-178.

Zimmermann, M. (1984). Neurobiological concepts of pain, its assessment and therapy. In B. Bromm (Ed.), *Pain measurement in man* (pp. 15-35). New York: Elsevier.

McGill Comprehensive Pain Questionnaire*

Date of Interview _____ Administrator _____
Patient Name (or Number Assigned) _____
Date of Birth _____ Male or Female _____
Physician _____ Medical Diagnosis _____

1. *Pain History*
    a. When did this pain begin?   Year _____ Month _____
    b. Did this pain begin?:   Gradually _____ Suddenly _____
    c. How did this pain begin? Please check (✓). Then give any specific details on the lines below.
        1) Accident at work __   4) Following surgery __
        2) Accident at home __   5) Pain just began __
        3) Following an illness __
                                        5) Other (e.g., car accident) __
        Details: _____

    d. Were there any changes in your life during the year before this pain began? (For example: job change, buying or selling a home, death or loss of a friend or family member, marital problems)
    _____
    _____

    e. Is the pain the same now as it was when it began? Yes __ No __
    f. If No, elaborate on any change in location, sensation, intensity, and time pattern frequency. _____
    _____

    g. Have you had any length of time, since the pain began when you have been free of pain? Yes __ No __
        1) If Yes, date(s) of episode(s) _____
        2) Why do you feel that you had relief at this time? (i.e., any physical, psychological, or environmental changes)
        3) Why do you feel the pain returned? _____
        4) Has this been a pattern? Yes __ No __

2. *Present Medical History*
    a. Please list any illnesses or health problems (other than the pain problem) you may have *now* (i.e., high blood pressure, ulcer, etc.). Briefly note how it is being treated.

    * MCPQ adapted (shortened) for the purpose of this study.

    Developed by Richard C. Monks, M.D., and Paul Taenzer, Ph.D. Used and modified with permission of R. C. Monks, M.D.

Problem	Present Treatment

b. Does this problem (these problems) have any effect on the pain problem?
   Yes __ No __
   If Yes, Please describe briefly.

_____

_____

_____

3. *Medication*
   Please list *all* drugs you are *now* taking for any reason, including drugs that
   may or may not be prescribed by a physician (include home remedies, over-
   the-counter medications, birth control pills).

Name of Drug	Dosage	How Many Times Per Day Per Week	Reason for Taking

4. *Pain Description*
   Using the body figures shown in Figure 8.6, please mark in with a pencil the
   areas where you feel the pain.

   a. Using the body map *filled in by the patient*, add the following
      information:
      1) Mark the palce where pain is with a (*). If a whole area hurts, shade
         in that area with light pencil strokes.
      2) If the pain radiates anywhere else, use a dotted line and arrow to
         show how this usually occurs.
      3) If the pain is internal (inside the body), put "I" beside the spot or
         area. If the pain is external (surface), put "E" beside the spot or area.
         If both, put "EI."
      4) If there are areas of increased or decreased sensation, indicate this
         by putting "IS" or "DS" next to the area involved.
      5) Areas of peculiar sensations other than pain may be indicated by
         putting "PS" next to the area indicated.
      6) Any areas where touching can begin, increase, or decrease the pain
         (trigger zones) can be indicated by the letter "T."

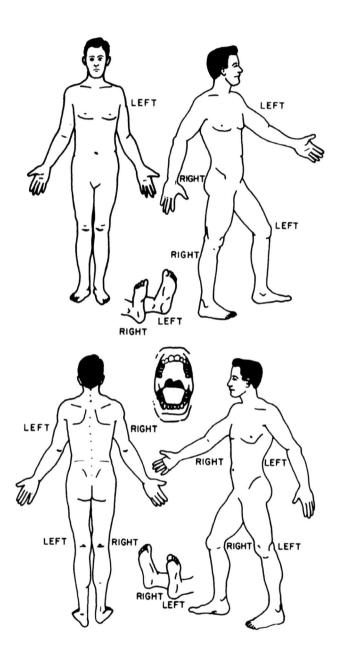

FIGURE 8.6 Body maps for pain description.

b. Does the pain feel as if it is located in: Check (✓)
Bone __ Joint __ Muscle __ Nerve __ Skin __
Other: _____

c. If pain is widespread, are there any areas that are free of pain?
_____

d. Choose *one* word group. Check (✓)
__ Continuous, steady, constant
__ Rhythmic, periodic, intermittent
__ Brief, momentary, transient

e. The following words represent pain of increasing intensity:
1. Mild   2. Discomforting   3. Distressing   4. Horrible
5. Excruciating
Choose the number of the word which best describes:

__ Your pain right now   __ The worst toothache you ever
__ Your pain at its worst   had
__ Your pain at its least   __ The worst headache you ever had
__ Your pain most of the time   __ The worst stomachache you ever
                                  had

f. Tell me which words best describe your present pain. Leave out any word
group that is not suitable. Use only a single word in each appropriate
group – the one that applies *best*. Indicate answer with a check (✓).

1	2	3	4
__ 1. FLICKERING	__ 1. JUMPING	__ 1. PRICKING	__ 1. SHARP
__ 2. QUIVERING	__ 2. FLASHING	__ 2. BORING	__ 2. CUTTING
__ 3. PULSING	__ 3. SHOOTING	__ 3. DRILLING	__ 3. LACERATING
__ 4. THROBBING		__ 4. STABBING	
__ 5. BEATING		__ 5. PIERCING	
__ 6. POUNDING			

5	6	7	8
__ 1. PINCHING	__ 1. TUGGING	__ 1. HOT	__ 1. TINGLING
__ 2. PRESSING	__ 2. PULLING	__ 2. BURNING	__ 2. ITCHY
__ 3. GNAWING	__ 3. WRENCHING	__ 3. SCALDING	__ 3. SMARTING
__ 4. CRAMPING		__ 4. SEARING	__ 4. STINGING
__ 5. CRUSHING			

9	10	11	12
__ 1. DULL	__ 1. TENDER	__ 1. TIRING	__ 1. SICKENING
__ 2. SORE	__ 2. TAUT	__ 2. EXHAUSTING	__ 2. SUFFOCATING
__ 3. HURTING	__ 3. RASPING		
__ 4. ACHING	__ 4. SPLITTING		
__ 5. HEAVY			

13	14	15	16
__ 1. FEARFUL	__ 1. PUNISHING	__ 1. WRETCHED	__ 1. ANNOYING
__ 2. FRIGHTFUL	__ 2. GRUELLING	__ 2. BLINDING	__ 2. TROUBLESOME
__ 3. TERRIFYING	__ 3. CRUEL		__ 3. MISERABLE
	__ 4. VICIOUS		__ 4. INTENSE
	__ 5. KILLING		__ 5. UNBEARABLE

17	18	19	20
__ 1. SPREADING	__ 1. TIGHT	__ 1. COOL	__ 1. NAGGING
__ 2. RADIATING	__ 2. NUMB	__ 2. COLD	__ 2. NAUSEATING
__ 3. PENETRATING	__ 3. DRAWING	__ 3. FREEZING	__ 3. AGONIZING
__ 4. PIERCING	__ 4. SQUEEZING		__ 4. DREADFUL

5. *Effects of Pain*
   a. *Work*
      1) At what age did you start working? _____
      2) How many jobs have you had? _____
      3) What is the longest length of time you've had a job? _____
      4) What type of work do you do or did you do last (include Housewife):
         _____
         Where? _____
         For how long? _____
         Number of hours per week?
         Duties (particularly physical activities, body postures, emotional stresses)? _____

      5) Has the pain caused any change in your work? Yes __ No __ If Yes, do the changes include:
         Change in number of hours worked? Yes __ No __
         From: _____ hours per week before
         To: _____ hours per week now.
         Change of type of work? Yes __ No __
         From: _____ To _____
         Satisfaction with work?   More __ Same __ Less __
         Efficiency at work?   More __ Same __ Less __
         Change in how you get/got along with co-workers, clients, etc. If Yes, please specify: _____

      6) *If you are not presently working*, please answer:
         If you did not have a pain problem, would you go back to work?
         Yes __ No __
         What job would you really like to have? _____

   b. *Leisure*
      1) Are there any hobbies, sports, recreational and social activities that you no longer do because of the pain? Yes __ No __
         If Yes, what activities? _____

      2) What hobbies, social activities, etc. can you still do?
         _____
         _____
         Do you? __ Yes __ No
         If Yes, which ones? _____
      3) Do any of your present activities help take your mind off the pain?
         __ Yes __ No
         If Yes, which ones? _____

4) Are there any *new* activities that you have begun since the pain began? __ Yes __ No
If Yes, what activities? _____
_____

c. *Sleep*
   1) When do you usually go to bed at night? _____
   2) Approximately how long does it take you to fall asleep? _____
   3) Do you have trouble falling asleep? Yes __ No __
   4) What body position do you use to sleep? _____
   5) Do you awaken in the night?   Yes __ No __
      How many times? _____
      Do you empty your bladder?   Yes __ No __
      Do you take medication?   Yes __ No __
      Do you awaken others?   Yes __ No __
      If Yes, what do they do? _____
   6) When do you usually finally awaken for the day? _____
   7) Do you feel refreshed or worse in the morning? _____
   8) Was your sleep pattern different before the pain? __ Yes __ No If Yes, please specify: _____
d. *Weight/Diet*
   1) How is your appetite?
      __ Too good   __ Good   __ Poor   __ Very poor
   2) Has your weight changed since the pain began? __ Yes __ No
      If Yes: From __ lbs. or __ kilos to __ lbs. or __ kilos
                Were you following a diet? __ Yes __ No
   3) Are you following a diet now? __ Yes __ No
   4) What is your weight now? _____ Your height? _____
e. *Habits*
   1) Do you smoke? __ Yes __ No
      If Yes, what? _____ and how much? _____
   2) Please indicate the number of cups/bottles you drink of the following each day:
      Coffee _____ Tea _____ Cola _____
   3) Do you drink alcohol? __ Yes __ No
      If Yes, what type of alcoholic beverages? _____
      Do you drink to: (Please check)
      __ Relieve the pain   __ Relax
      __ Sleep   __ Socialize
   4) Have you had any problems because of alcohol (i.e., physical, legal, psychological, social)? __ Yes __ No
      If Yes, please explain (i.e., loss of or difficulty with friends, family, job; liver disease, blackouts, passing out, seizures, fits, hallucinations, etc.). _____
      _____

f. *Mood*
   1) Has your mood changed since the pain began? __ Yes __ No
      If yes, how? _____
   2) What is your mood, on the whole, these days? _____
      _____
   3) Do you feel better in the A.M. __ P.M. __ Same __?
   4) Do you have crying spells? __ Yes __ No

If Yes, how often? _____
5) Do you feel life is not worthwhile? __ Yes __ No
6) Do you have any thoughts of harming yourself? __ Yes __ No
   If Yes, elaborate on method, immediacy, etc. _____

_____

7) Do you feel irritable more often these days? __ Yes __ No
   If Yes, in what situations? _____

_____

8) Tell me how you express your anger. (Clarify whether the patient recognizes the emotion, how soon, and how it is dealt with.)

_____

_____

g. *Attitude Toward Pain*
   1) What do *you* feel is the cause of your pain? _____

_____

   2) How has your pain been explained to you? _____

_____

   3) How often in a day do you think about your pain? _____

_____

   4) Are there situations where you find that you are often thinking about pain? if so, describe: _____

_____

   5) Are there people with whom you discuss your pain problem? __ Yes __ No
      If Yes, with whom? _____ How often? _____
      How do they respond? _____
   6) Has this pain problem affected your feelings about yourself? __ Yes __ No. If Yes, in what way? _____

_____

   7) Does religious faith help you to cope with the pain problem? __ Yes __ No. If Yes, in what way? _____

_____

   8) Are there thoughts, memories, or fantasies that you can think about which help you cope with your pain? __ Yes __ No If Yes, could you describe them? _____

_____

   9) What other methods do you use to help you cope with the pain problem? _____

_____

6. *Patient's Expectations*
   What are your life goals at this time? (Give at least 3-5 if possible.)

_____

_____

_____

7. *Pain Modifiers*
   a. For each of the following:
      Please mark with a "+" if it increases the pain.
      Please mark with a "−" if it decreases the pain.
      Please mark with an "0" if it has no effect on the pain.

__ BRIGHT LIGHTS	__ HEAT	__ STANDING
__ CASTS	__ HOUSEWORK	__ VIBRATOR
__ COLD	__ LOUD NOISES	__ VIGOROUS EXERCISE
__ COLLARS	__ LYING DOWN	__ WALKING
__ CORSETS	__ MASSAGE	__ WEATHER
__ COUGHING, SNEEZING	__ MILD EXERCISE	__ WORK RELATED
__ GOING TO TOILET	__ SITTING	__ OTHERS

b. Using the same signs (+, −, or 0) as in the question above, please indicate how any of the following feelings and social situations affect your pain.

__ ANGER	__ ENJOYING THINGS	__ HAPPINESS
__ CONTENTMENT	__ FATIGUE	__SADNESS
__ BEING WITH	__ FRUSTRATION	__ TALKING WITH
OTHERS		OTHERS
		__ WHEN OTHERS ARE
		SYMPATHETIC

c. If parts of your body (i.e. stomach or muscles) are tense or tight, does the pain get worse? __ Yes __ No
Which parts of your body get tense or tight? _____

d. Have you found that the pain changes when you are with certain people (i.e., relatives, boss, etc.)? __ Yes __ No
If Yes, please specify: _____

e. Does rest decrease your pain? __ Yes __ No
How many hours do you rest? _____
Where and how do you usually rest? _____

f. Have you learned *specific* ways to relax yourself when the pain is bad?
__ Yes __ No. If Yes, what do you do? _____
_____
_____

g. How do people around you know that you are in pain? _____
_____

Acknowledgment: I gratefully acknowledge the assistance of Peggy M. Mayfield, M.S.N., R.N., C., A.N.P., for her assistance in the data collection.

9

Client Risk for Pressure Sores

Davina J. Gosnell

This chapter discusses the Pressure Sore Risk Assessment tool, a measure of client risk for pressure sores.

Despite dramatic advances in medical science, the problem of pressure sores continues to plague mankind. Effective means of prevention, care, and treatment of pressure sores is a goal that has proved difficult to attain. A major area of concern is the ability of nurses to assess a patient's risk for pressure sores so that adequate preventive measures will be implemented. The focus of this study was the development and testing of an instrument to assess a client's potential risk for pressure sore formation.

The incidence of pressure sores is extensive and varies greatly, reportedly from as low as 1.5 to 3% of all general hospital admissions (Gearson, 1975; Petersen & Bittman, 1971; Rubin, Dietz, & Abruzzese, 1974) to 25 to 30% in elderly hospitalized (Barton, 1977; Norton, McLaren & Exton-Smith, 1962; Williams, 1972) to as great as 80 to 85% of spinal cord-injured patients (Kosiak, 1959; Spence, Burke, & Rae, 1967). According to Shannon (1982), "five to ten percent of the approximately one million Americans hospitalized every year develop pressure sores: 50,000 to 100,000 persons" (p. 357). Richard Meir (1984), founder of the Center for Tissue Trauma Research, notes that "the bedsore or decubitus ulcer accounts for two-thirds of all tissue trauma or three and one half (3.5) million cases requiring treatment annually: about $8.5 billion in treatment. Statistics indicate that prevention would cost 1/214th of what it costs to treat" (p. 13). In addition to the monetary aspect, the physical and emotional cost to patient, family, and others is very great.

Manley (1978), in a survey of 800 patients in an acute care setting, found that 9.7% of the total population had pressure sores. However, of those 60 to 70 years of age, 17.5% had pressure sores. In addition, 30% of semicomatise patients had pressure sores.

In a study conducted by Clark, Barbanel, Jordan, and Nicol (1978), 24.8% of patients classified as chairfast and totally helpless had pressure sores, 18.6% of those classified as bedfast and totally helpless also had pressure sores, and 20.7% of the incontinent patients had pressure sores.

In addition, 18.1% of hemiplegic patients, 21.6% of paraplegic patients, and 23.1% of quadriplegic patients were afflicted with pressure sores.

Williams (1972), Gosnell (1973), Norton (1975), and others have all documented a relationship between a debilitated health state, chronic illness, longevity, and the occurrence of pressure sores. Given the current trends of increased life span and the accompanying increase in chronic illnesses, it seems apparent that the incidence of pressure sores will continue to increase unless greater attention and more rigorous research efforts are directed toward examining how this devastating condition can be prevented and/or reduced.

RISK FACTORS

Investigation of the etiology and pathology of pressure sore formation has provided only a basic understanding of causative factors. Excessive pressure between bony prominences and an external object, resulting in anoxia and anemia of the underlying tissue and depriving it of vital nourishment, has been shown to be the primary cause of pressure sore formation. More specifically, both the intensity and duration of traumatic pressure are known to be crucial to the formation of a pressure sore.

Secondary factors that seemingly further predispose one to a pressure sore include circulatory impairment, impaired sensation, decreased mobility, advanced age, poor nutrition, malnutrition, obesity or low body weight, depressed levels of consciousness, infection, diminished body responses due to such things as medications, and disturbed autonomic functioning. The extent to which any of these factors or combinations of factors predisposes one to pressure sore formation is unknown.

Research to determine the cause of pressure sores has been ongoing for more than 50 years. Findings indicate that the primary cause of pressure sores is extended ischemia due to sustained supracapillary pressure, which results in devitalization of deep tissue. In addition, limitation of body sensation and movements, a debilitated state of health, advanced age, and diminished physiological and psychosocial responses all contribute to the incidence of pressure sores.

After an extensive study of the effects of pressure on tissue, Husain (1953) concluded that "a combination of pressure and tissue of 'changed character' due to increased nitrogen loss provide the greatest potential for the development of pressure sores" (p. 357).

Rudd (1962) identified four factors that contribute to pressure sore formation: sustained pressure, reduction of bodily movements, devitalization of deep tissue, and reduced general resistance.

While it is agreed that all four items are important factors, the research findings of Exton-Smith and Sherwin (1961), Husain (1953), Miller and Sachs (1974), and Trimble (1930), and others all indicate that sustained pressure is the primary cause for tissue breakdown.

Pressure

Research by Husain (1953) has shown that the median pressure for normal existence is 1.5 lb/sq in. of body surface with even distribution. If it is not evenly distributed and the pressure differs more than 1 lb/sq in. (50 mmHg) from the normal, the shape of tissue will alter and induce pathological changes.

Kosiak (1961) reports microscopic changes in the muscles of animals 24 hr after application of 1.4 lb (70 mmHg) of constant pressure for 2 hr. His research studies of 40 rats also indicated that alternating pressure applied at 5-min intervals caused considerably less damage to tissue than when the same amount of pressure was constantly applied over a time interval. He identified the critical time interval in which pathological changes occur to be 1 to 2 hr.

Trimble (1930) calculated that if a person's weight was equally distributed over the entire body surface available for weight bearing in the recumbent position, it would amount to less than 1/3 lb/sq in. (17 mmHg). One knows, however, that weight is not borne evenly and that when in the recumbent position the body's weight is borne primarily by areas of bony prominence. The ischeal tuberosities are such a bony prominence and bear up to 75% of the total body weight when a person is in a sitting position. Kosiak (1961) reports that average pressures under the ischeal tuberosities and surrounding areas generally exceed 3 lb pressure (150 mmHg) when an individual assumes a sitting position. This is clearly in excess of reported tissue tolerance and is tolerated without incidence only when there is alternating distribution of the pressure.

Decreased Mobility

A healthy person's spontaneous movements are constantly redistributing the pressure of body weight and thus enable the body to tolerate greater amounts of pressure. Conditions that limit or inhibit spontaneous body movements, however, allow for uneven distribution of pressure for extended periods of time. Reduction of body movement was identified by Rudd (1962) as contributing to pressure sore formation.

Clay (1968) has reported that the healthy person changes position about 50 to 150 times per night while asleep and thus, is frequently redistributing pressure on his body. One changes position in response to nervous stimuli. When these stimuli receptors are dulled or damaged, the individual changes position much less frequently. Exton-Smith and Sherwin (1961), in a study of the significance of spontaneous bodily movements in a laboratory animal experiment, found that low pressure for long periods of time resulted in more tissue damage than did high pressure for short periods; the time factor, then, is of greater significance than is pressure intensity. When an individual does not have spontaneous body movements, either due to lack of perceived stimulti or absence of the ability to move one's body, there is a very great possibility that the limit of tissue tolerance will be exceeded unless a planned schedule of repositioning is maintained.

Tissue destruction due to shearing forces and friction have also been cited by Reichel (1958), Dinsdale (1974), and Berecek (1975) as increasing the risk potential for pressure sores. Moisture, in the form of perspiration due to excessive body or environmental temperatures or other discharge including urine, feces, or drainage, are also thought to predispose one to pressure sores (Irvine, 1961; Norton et al., 1962; Rubin et al., 1974). Adams and Hunter (1969) found that friction increased by nearly 50% in the presence of moisture, and Shannon (1982) states that "both shearing force and friction are increased in the presence of moisture" (p. 370).

Devitalized State of Health

Rudd (1962) identified devitalization of deep tissue as an important factor in the development of pressure sores. Compressed or necrosed deep tissue is more prone to secondary bacterial invasion via the blood stream. He reported that multiple thromboses of small vessels, with subsequent necrosis, are consistent pathological findings in pressure sores. Schnell and Walcott (1966) have identified an increased metabolic rate due to fever as a cause of cellular metabolic deficiency. Barton (1977) and Shannon (1982) also identify infection as an important risk factor for pressure sore formation. Reddy (1983) suggests that "decubitus ulcers are among the most common causes of fever of unknown origin in the elderly and may cause significant loss of body proteins, leading to progressive weakness and debilitation."

Reduced general resistance and a debilitated state of health are also identified by Rudd (1962) and others as predisposing one to pressure sores. Malnutrition, anemia, vitamin deficiencies (especially of vitamin C), and a negative nitrogen balance can all be causes for decreased resistance to trauma resulting from excessive pressure. Tissue of malnourished persons is known to be increasingly more liable to breakdown. Mulholland's (1943) studies showed healing only when patients were in a state of positive nitrogen balance, a state that requires the maintenance of an adequate nutritional level. This is accomplished primarily by having a protein intake that exceeds the protein output. Studies have shown that protein anabolism is mandatory for wound healing. When a state of negative nitrogen balance exists, there is serum protein wasting; anemia results, yielding a lack of oxygen supply to the cells and subsequent lack of nutrition. As an end result, there is necrosis of tissue. Protein metabolism is thus an important factor in determining resistance. In addition, muscle tissue is the largest store of protein in the body. When muscle tissue is damaged, a vital protein source is destroyed ("Tissue protein," 1969).

More recently, Natow (1983) provided an in-depth examination of the nutritional requirements necessary for prevention and treatment of decubitus ulcers. She suggested "a diet high in carbohydrates, high in protein, and moderate in fat, vitamin C and zinc supplement" (p. 44).

Increasing Age

Numerous studies suggest a direct relationship between advancing age and the occurrence of pressure sores. Gearson (1975), in a study of more than 5,000 patients admitted to three acute care hospitals, found that the average age of the patients who developed pressure sores was 67.6 years; the average age of those who did not develop pressure sores was 49.5 years. Petersen and Bittman (1971), in a comprehensive survey in Denmark, also found that there was an increase in pressure sores with age, especially after age 50. Manley (1978), in a survey of 800 patients confined to an acute care hospital, found a dramatic increase in the incidence of pressure sores with increasing age. Whereas 9.7% of the total population had pressure sores, 17.5% of those aged 60 to 70 had pressure sores and 32% of those aged 70 and over had pressure sores. In a survey of an entire healthy district involving more than 10,000 patients in Great Britain, Clark and associates (1978) also found a dramatic increase in the incidence of pressure sores with age. Six percent of the patients 69 years old or younger had pressure sores, but 11.6% of those 70 or older had pressure sores. In a study of 250 hospitalized elderly patients (Norton et al., 1962), it was found that almost twice as many patients over age 85 developed pressure sores, as did those under age 75. These studies were done with different populations and different methodologies, but nonetheless, the findings suggest that the occurrence of pressure sores increases dramatically with age.

Medical Diagnosis

The medical diagnosis of a patient also seems to be related to the formation of a pressure sore. Petersen and Bittman (1971) report arteriosclerosis, cerebral hemorrhage, cardiac failure, cancer, renal disease, fractures (especially of the femur), and neurological disorders as the diseases most common in their 246 subjects who developed pressure sores. Rubin and associates (1974) found malignancies, orthopedic problems, and debilitation other than malignancy, including diabetes, to be the most frequently occurring diagnoses. Gearson (1975) found that over 60% of all patients who had pressure sores could be classed into one of three diagnostic categories: neoplasms, diseases of the circulatory system, and accidents (mostly fractures of the femur). Clark and associates (1978) reported eight diagnoses as being prominent in their survey: multiple sclerosis, paralysis agitans, cerebral paralysis, arthritis and rheumatism, malignant neoplasms, diseases of the skin and subcutaneous tissues, diseases of the circulatory system, and diabetes mellitus. Manley (1978) found that carcinoma, renal and urinary diseases, and diabetes were often found in those with pressure sores. There appears to be a consistent pattern among these studies; medical diagnoses often associated with elderly chronically debilitated individuals predominate in patients who develop pressure sores.

A group of patients in whom an exceedingly low incidence of pressure sores has been found to occur are those with amyotrophic lateral sclerosis (ALS) (Furukawa & Toyokura, 1976; Parish, Smith, & Collins, 1978). Forrester (1976) suggests that this finding might be due to the fact that constricted blood vessels are harder to occlude than large dilated vessels.

Other Potential Risk Factors

An area where there is little reported research is that of the relationship of medications to the occurrence of pressure sores. There are numerous medications given routinely, especially to persons hospitalized, that create situations that depress the patient's physical and mental activity, thus creating the potential for greater risk. Gosnell (1973) reported that "when the four persons who developed a pressure sore were compared with the 26 subjects who did not, all four persons were found to be receiving analgesics, cardiotonics, and tranquilizers, and two were receiving two different types of tranquilizers. . . . Moreover, three of the four subjects who developed pressure sores were also receiving sedatives in contrast to only one-half of the subjects with intact skin" (p. 58). No other studies have been found that report the nature of medication regimens for patients developing pressure sores.

In a study of 35 elderly residents of long-term care facilities, Gosnell (1983) found that six were at high risk for pressure sores. Of the six, two developed pressure sores, and of the four who did not, all had diastolic blood pressures greater than 60 mmHg. This is consistent with Gosnell's (1973) previous findings that all patients who developed pressure sores had diastolic blood pressures of less than 60 mmHg. Gosnell's findings and the early work of Trimble (1930) support Shannon's (1982) suggested hypothesis that "increased and sustained resistance to the compressibility of blood vessels as measured by diastolic blood pressure greater than 60 mmHg prevents the development of pressure sores" (p. 365).

The quest for prevention of pressure sores has existed since antiquity, and considerable research as to the causative factors has been undertaken. Still, many of the findings are inconclusive. Sustained pressure resulting in tissue trauma is known to result in a pressure sore. Considerable knowledge regarding the etiology of such occurrence is available. There are numerous other variables, however, that in both isolation and combination predispose one to greater risk for pressure sores. Research findings to date have delineated what these most crucial variables might be but are as yet quite inconclusive as to their actual effect or the extent of combined effect in predisposing someone to risk for pressure sore formation.

PURPOSE

Nurses assume primary responsibility for maintaining skin integrity; thus, the need for clinical research of pressure sore prevention is especially crucial for nursing practice. What are the contributing factors to pressure sore formation? What are the most significant predisposing situations? Are there physiological indicators that could be predictors of the degree of risk for pressure sore formation? Answers to such questions are needed if there is to be effective intervention for prevention of pressure sores.

The specific purposes of this study were twofold:

1. To develop a "preclinical" instrument for detection of risk factors before a pressure sore becomes clinically evident.
2. To test the reliability and validity of the instrument with a select patient population in an acute care setting.

METHOD

Instrument Development

The initial and now classic work in the area of instrument development to assess one's risk for pressure sore formation is that of Norton and associates (1962). Now commonly referred to as the Norton Scale, the instrument was initially used in a survey of 250 patients in a geriatric hospital ward in England. Five items – physical condition, mental condition, activity, mobility, and incontinence – are rated on a scale of 1 to 4. Total scores can range from 5 to 20; the lower the score, the poorer one's health status and the greater one's risk is believed to be for development of a pressure sore. In that study 48% of the patients scoring less than 12 developed a pressure sore, in contrast to only 5% with scores of 18 or greater.

In 1970 a study was conducted of 30 geriatric patients in four nursing homes to determine their potential risk for pressure sore development (Gosnell, 1973). The instrument used was developed by the author and adapted from the Norton Scale. A nutrition item was substituted for physical condition; specific criteria guidelines for rating the five items were delineated; additional categories were added to the instrument – including vital signs; skin appearance, tone, and sensation; and medications; and there was provision made for multiple ratings. Although no reliability or validity data were available, the instrument was found to be easy to use and versatile, since it had potential use for research purposes as well as a clinical assessment tool. Following publication of the study, numerous requests and correspondence regarding use of the instrument were received. The extent to which the instrument or adaptations thereof are in use is impossible to estimate; however, there are at least two drug companies, Knoll Pharmaceutical and Squibb, who publish assessment tools that are modifications of the instrument. In addition, many hospitals have devised specific assessment tools or portions thereof that are based on the instrument. No reliability or validity data exist for any of these instruments. In addition, it should be noted that although these instruments are being used extensively in acute care settings for the entire adult population, the work of both Norton and associates (1962) and Gosnell (1973; 1983) was done with elderly clients in long-term care settings.

The instrument used in the present study is a revision of the original Gosnell (1973) instrument. Changes were made based on findings of the author's studies (Gosnell, 1973, 1983), literature review, and pilot testing. They were as follows:

- A reverse order change in the scoring of the five rated variables was made so that the higher the score, the greater the risk for pressure sore formation.
- There was further refinement of the criteria guidelines.
- The skin appearance category was revised, and specific descriptors were delineated for four specific characteristics: color, moisture, temperature, and texture.
- Provision was made for more detailed information regarding the category of medications to include dosage, frequency, and route.
- A diet category was added to provide more specific information about the nature and quality of nutrition, since the rated nutrition category provides quantitative data.
- A "24-hour fluid balance – intake and output" category was added to provide more detail regarding the hydration state of the subject.
- An "interventions" category was added to provide information about whether or not any preventive device, measure, or nursing care activity was being used.

(A copy of this revised instrument with category guidelines can be found at the end of this chapter.)

The instrument is of a criterion-referenced nature, since the variables (risk factors) to be examined are primarily related to the subjects' physiological status and assessed by direct observation. The specific domain of reference is that of pressure sore occurrence and prevention. For the purposes of this study a pressure sore is defined as an insult with break in skin integrity caused directly by the application of excessive force (pressure) to the body surface that results in destruction of skin tissue.

Scoring

Scoring for the present instrument calls for numerical ratings of each of five major variables: mental status (1-5), continence (1-4), mobility (1-4), activity (1-4), and nutrition (1-3). A total score for the five variables can range from 5 to 20. The higher the score, the greater the pressure sore risk factor. This scoring is similar to the original Norton Scale except for the reverse order of intensity of the assigned score.

All other items included in the instrument are to be quantified descriptively. With more reliable and valid data it is planned that rating scores will be assigned to other factors found to be either consistently present or of specific intensity in persons who eventually develop pressure sores. All factors included in the descriptive portion of the instrument were added on the basis of either previous research and/or the literature. Guidelines for numerical rating of the five variables and classifying the descriptive data accompany the instrument.

Data Collection

Data have recently been gathered on 80 subjects by nurse data collectors who were oriented to the instrument and the data collection procedure. The data collectors were staff members of the two community hospitals that were the study sites, and the data were gathered in the course of their regular nursing activities.

Since the author (Gosnell, 1973, 1983) found in her previous study that initial ratings alone did not adequately identify those at risk, data were gathered within the first 24 hr after admission and then on an every-other-day basis during the entire period of hospitalization or for a 30-day period, whichever was the lesser. The rationale for selection of this time interval for data collection was that Norton and associates (1962) noted that the majority of patients developed pressure sores within the first 2 weeks of admission. It was believed that data gathered every 48 hr in an acute care setting where patients' conditions change rapidly would be advantageous in providing a descriptive pattern for examination.

Criteria for selection of subjects were as follows:

- Admitted to the hospital within past 24 hr.
- Admitted to a unit included in the study during the period of data collection.
- Free of pressure sores at the time of admission.
- Age 65 years or older.
- Medical diagnosis in the categories of neoplasm, malignancy, chronic illness, orthopedic condition, or neurological condition. The data are currently being analyzed.

Reliability

Because of the nature of the instrument, test-retest and parallel form procedures to determine reliability are not appropriate. Therefore, reliability measures used for this instrument include interrater reliability, intrarater reliability, and internal consistency. Interrater and intrarater reliability was established at a .90 level of percent agreement.

Validity

Content validity for this criterion-referenced instrument was established by a panel of three content experts. Two were nurse faculty members with clinical expertise in gerontology and considerable experience in maintaining skin integrity, and one was an enterostomal therapist. These experts were asked to examine both instrument format and content items, and in addition, empirical interrater agreement was sought. The experts received reference literature to provide them with background information and rationale for selection of the specific items included on the instrument and a copy of the instrument with guidelines. They were given a form on which to rate each content item as to its relative importance in identifying persons at greatest risk for pressure sore development, and they were asked to respond in narrative regarding the instrument format and adequacy of the guideline definitions. On the basis of their ratings and comments, no changes in content items were deemed necessary, and the format was slightly modified to facilitate ease of data recording.

Initial construct validity was determined in the following manner. On a clinical unit comparable to those used in the study, nurses were asked to identify the five patients they believed to be at least risk and the five at greatest risk for pressure sore formation. These patients were then assessed with the study instrument. The average total score for the low-risk group was 6; that of the high-risk group was 13.8. As more data become available, we will eventually be able to determine the cut/standard scores via analysis of the score pattern of those who develop pressure sores and those who do not.

Criterion-related validity is of particular importance here since the purpose of this instrument is to identify accurately (predict) those persons at greatest risk for the development of a pressure sore. Therefore, determination of the predictive validity of the instrument is crucial. In this situation the criterion measure will be the occurrence of a pressure sore within 30 days of admission. At present, the predictor is the score(s) received on the five rating items, that is, mental status, mobility, activity, continence, and nutrition. The correlation coefficient and item analysis of all categories – that is, both the rated and descriptive items as well as discriminant analysis procedures – are being used in analysis of current data. Depending on the findings, possibly other factors will be assigned numerical rating scores for the next phase of instrument refinement.

FUTURE DIRECTIONS

Shannon (1982) suggests that "nurse-researchers must concentrate their efforts on defining and evaluating measures that contribute to prevention of pressure sores, on devising and evaluating tools for identifying patients likely to develop pressure sores and on developing and refining valid instruments for use in assessing and evaluating the effect of nursing care on prevention and/or treatment of the patient with pressure sores" (p. 377). The purpose of this study is indeed congruent with Shannon's directive and should yield vital data that will assist in the quest for prevention of pressure sores. As McCance and Reiber (1982) have noted, "The first step in the process of prevention is a comparison of certain characteristics in subgroups of human populations... to determine whether the risk is greater among groups of individuals with some characteristics in common than in others" (p. 85).

The instrument described in this chapter is far from final in form. There is much work yet needed to identify and validate each of the factors of consequence and to develop a rating system that will render an accurate predictive measure of clients' risk for pressure sore formation. The value of an instrument with predictive validity for delineating clients at risk for pressure sore development is great. With greater numbers of aged and chronically ill individuals, the increased incidence of pressure sores seems inevitable unless more aggressive preventive nursing care is undertaken. Only with specific delineation of the causative factors or combination of factors can truely effective preventive care be provided. Dickoff and James (1968) cite the need for predictive theories that can guide nursing practice. Findings from studies such as those described in this chapter can contribute to such ends.

REFERENCES

Adams, T., & Hunter, W. S. (1969). Modification of skin mechanical properties by eccrine sweat gland activity. *Journal of Applied Physiology, 26,* 417-419.

Barton, A. A. (1977). Prevention of pressure sores. *Nursing Times, 73,* 1593-1595.

Berecek, K. H. (1975). Etiology of decubitus ulcers. *Nursing Clinics of North America, 10,* 157-170.

Clark, M. O., Barbanel, J. C., Jordon, M. M., & Nicol, S. M. (1978). Pressure sores. *Nursing Times, 74,* 363-366.

Clay, E. (1968). Operation pressure sores. *Nursing Times, 68,* 393-394.

Dickoff, J., & James, P. (1968). A theory of theories: A position paper. *Nursing Research, 17,* 197-203.

Dinsdale, S.M. (1974). Decubitus ulcers: Role of pressure and friction in causation. *Archives of Physical Medicine and Rehabilitation, 55,* 147-152.

Exton-Smith, A. N., & Sherwin, M. A. (1961). The prevention of pressure sores: A significance of spontaneous bodily movements. *Lancet, 2,* 1123-1126.

Forrester, J. M. (1976). Amyotrophic lateral sclerosis and bedsores. *Lancet, 2,* 970.

Furukawa, T., & Toyokura, Y. (1976). Amyotrophic lateral sclerosis and bedsores. *Lancet, 1,* 862.

Gearson, L. W. (1975). The incidence of pressure sores in active treatment hospitals. *International Journal of Nursing Studies, 12,* 201-204.

Gosnell, D. J. (1973). An assessment tool to identify pressure sores. *Nursing Research, 22,* 55-59.

Gosnell, D. J. (1983). *A descriptive study of physiological factors in elderly patients at risk for pressure sore formation.* Unpublished manuscript, Kent State University, Kent, OH.

Husain, T. (1953). An experimental study of some pressure effects on tissue with reference to the bedsore problem. *Journal of Pathological Bacteriology, 66,* 347-358.

Irvine, R. F. (1961). Norethandrolone and prevention of pressure sores. *Lancet, 2,* 1333.

Kosiak, M. (1959). Etiology and pathology of ischemic ulcers. *Archives of Physical Medicine and Rehabilitation, 40,* 62-69.

Kosiak, M. (1961). Etiology of decubitus ulcers. *Archives of Physical Medicine and Rehabilitation, 42,* 19-29.

Manley, M. T. (1978). Incidence, contributory factors, and costs of pressure sores. *South African Medical Journal, 53,* 217-222.

McCance, K. L., & Reiber, G. E. (1982). Prevention: Implications for nursing research. *Advances in Nursing Science, 3*(2), 79-87.

Meir, R. (1984, June). DRG's spur increased interest in prevention of decubitus ulcers. *Health Care Systems,* pp. 12-18, 24.

Miller, M. E., & Sachs, M. L. (1974). *About bedsores: What you need to know to prevent and treat them.* Philadelphia: J. B. Lippincott.

Mulholland, J. (1943). Protein metabolism and bedsores. *Annals of Surgery, 118,* 1015-1023.

Natow, A. B. (1983). Nutrition in prevention and treatment of decubitus ulcers. *Advances in Nursing Science, 4*(4), 39-44.

Norton, D. (1975). Research and the problems of pressure sores. *Nursing Mirror, 140*(7), 65-67.

Norton, D., McLaren, R., & Exton-Smith, A. B. (1962). *An investigation of geriatric nursing problems in hospitals.* London: Nuffield Lodge, Regents' Park.

Parish, L., Smith, G., & Collins, E. (1978). Decubitus ulcers and amyotrophic lateral sclerosis. *Lancet, 1,* 658-659.

Petersen, N. C., & Bittman, S. (1971). The epidemiology of pressure sores. *Scandinavian Journal of Plastic Reconstructive Surgery, 5,* 62-66.

Reddy, M. P. (1983). Decubitus ulcers: Principles of prevention and management. *Geriatrics, 38*(7), 55-61.

Reichel, S. M. (1958). Shearing force as a factor in decubitus ulcers in paraplegics. *Journal of American Medical Association, 166,* 762-763.

Rubin, C. F., Dietz, R. R., & Abruzzese, R. S. (1974). Auditing the decubitus ulcer problem. *American Journal of Nursing, 74,* 1820-1821.

Rudd, T. N. (1962). Pathogenesis of decubitus ulcers. *Journal of American Geriatric Society, 10,* 48-53.

Schnell, V., & Walcott, I. (1966). The etiology, prevention, and management of decubitus ulcers. *Missouri Medicine, 63,* 100.

Shannon, M. (1982). Pressure sores. In C. M. Norris (Ed.), *Concepts classification in nursing* (pp. 357-382). Rockville, MD: Aspen Systems.

Spence, W. R., Burk, R. D., & Rae, J. W. (1967). Gel support for prevention of decubitus ulcers. *Archives of Physical Medicine and Rehabilitation, 48,* 283-288.

Tissue protein turn-over rate. (1969). *Nutrition Reviews, 27*(6), 181-182.

Trimble, H. C. (1930). The skin tolerance for pressure and pressure sores. *Medical Journal of Australia, 2,* 724.

Williams, A. (1972). A study of factors contributing to skin breakdown. *Nursing Research, 21,* 238-243.

Pressure Sore Risk Assessment

I.D. _____   Medical Diagnosis:
Age _____ Sex _____   Primary _____
Ht. _____ Wt. _____   Secondary _____
Date of Admission _____   Nursing Diagnosis:
Date of Discharge _____   _____
                                 _____

Instructions: Complete all categories within 24 hours of admission and every other day thereafter. Refer to the accompanying guidelines for specific rating details.

DATE	Mental Status	Continence	Mobility	Activity	Nutrition	
	1 Alert	1 Fully controlled	1 Full	1 Ambulatory	1 Good	
	2 Apathetic		2 Slightly limited	2 Walks with assistance	2 Fair	
	3 Confused	2 Usually controlled				
	4 Stuporous		3 Very limited	4 Bedfast	3 Poor	
		3 Minimally controlled	4 Immobile	3 Chairfast		
		4 Absence				TOTAL
	5 Unconscious	of control				SCORE

_____

_____

_____

_____

_____

_____

_____

_____

_____

_____

_____

_____

_____

_____

_____

_____

_____

_____

_____

	Vital Signs				24-Hour Fluid Balance		Color	Moisture	Temperature	General Skin Appearance Texture	Interventions	
							1. Pallor					
							2. Mottled					
							3. Pink			1. Smooth		
							4. Ashen			2. Rough		
							5. Ruddy	1. Dry	1. Cold	3. Thin/transp		
							6. Cyanotic	2. Damp	2. Cool	4. Scaly		
							7. Jaundice	3. Oily	3. Warm	5. Crusty		
Date	T P R BP	Diet		Intake	Output		8. Other	4. Other	4. Hot	6. Other	No Yes Describe	

For any item marked "other" please describe.

If any signs of pressure, etc. on bony prominences or other body parts are observed, please describe in detail the location, color, temperature, moisture, texture, and size and any other pertinent items.

PRESSURE SORE RISK ASSESSMENT MEDICATION PROFILE

Medication	Dosage	Frequency*	Route	Date Begun	Date Disc

*If PRN record pattern past 48 hr.

GUIDELINES FOR NUMERICAL RATING OF THE DEFINED CATEGORIES

Ruling	1	2	3	4	5
Mental status	Alert	Apathetic	Confused	Stuporous	Unconscious
An assesment of one's level of response to his environment	Oriented to time, place, & person. Responsive to all stimuli and understands explanations	Lethargic, forgetful, drowsy, passive, & dull; sluggish, depressed; able to obey simple commands possibly disoriented to time	Partial and/or intermittent disorientation to TPP; purposeless response to stimuli; restless, aggressive, irritable, anxious, & may require tranquilizers or sedatives	Total disorientation; does not respond to name, simple commands, or verbal stimuli	Nonresponsive to painful stimuli
Continence	Fully controlled	Usually controlled	Minimally controlled	Absence of control	
The amount of bodily control of urination & defecation	Total control of urine and feces	Incontinent of urine &/or of feces not more often than once q48 hr; *OR* has Foley catheter and is incontinent of feces	Incontinent of urine or feces at least once q24 hr	Consistently incontinent of both urine & feces	
Mobility	Full	Slightly limited	Very limited	Immobile	
The amount and control of movement of one's body	Able to control and move all extremities at will; may require the use of a device but turns, lifts, pulls, balances, and attains sitting position at will	Able to control and move all extremities but a degree of limitation is present; requires assistance of another person to turn, pull, balance, &/or attain a sitting position at will but self-initiates movement or request for help to move	Can assist another person who must initiate movement via turning, lifting, pulling, balancing &/or attaining a sitting position (contractures, paralysis may be present)	Does not assist self in any way to change position; is unable to change position without assistance; is completely dependent on others for movement	
Activity	Ambulatory	Walks with help	Chairfast	Bedfast	
The ability of an individual to ambulate	Is able to walk unassisted. Rises from bed unassisted; with the use of a device such as cane or walker is able to ambulate without the assistance of another person	Able to ambulate with assistance of another person, braces, or crutches; may have limitation of stairs	Ambulates only to a chair, requires assistance to do so *OR* is confined to a wheelchair	Is confined to bed during entire 24 hr of the day	
Nutrition					
The process of food intake	Eats some food from each basic foot category every day and the majority of each meal served *OR* is on tube feeding	Occasionally refuses a meal or frequently leaves at least half of a meal	Seldom eats a complete meal and only a few bites of food at a meal		

Vital signs	The temperature, pulse, respiration, and blood pressure to be taken and recorded at the time of every assessment rating.
Skin appearance	A description of observed skin characteristics: color, moisture, temperature, and texture.
Diet	Record the specific diet order.
24-hr fluid balance	The amount of fluid intake and output during the previous 24-hr period should be recorded.
Interventions	List all devices, measures, and/or nursing care activity being used for the purpose of pressure sore prevention.
Medications	List name, dosage, frequency, and route for all prescribed medications. If a PRN order, list the pattern for the period since last assessment.
Comments	Use this space to add explanation or further detail regarding any of the previously recorded data, patient condition, etc. *OR* Describe anything you believe to be of importance but not accounted for previously.

10
Measuring Children's Fears of Medical Experiences

Marion E. Broome, Astrid Hellier,
Thayer Wilson, Sandra Dale, and
Cathryn Glanville

This chapter discusses the Child Medical Fear Scale, a measure of children's concerns about health care.

Children's responses to hospitalization and medical experiences have been a concern to health care providers for several decades (Levy, 1951; Vernon, Foley, Sipowitz, & Schulman, 1965; Winer, 1982; Wolfer & Visintainer, 1979). Some nursing research has been directed toward a better understanding of children's negative responses to hospitalization and medical experiences in order to decrease these stressful events (Johnson, Kirchoff, & Endress, 1975; Menke, 1981; Timmerman, 1983). Preparation for medical events is one variable that may affect the outcome of a child's response (Johnson et al., 1975). It is not well documented in the literature whether or not preparation is needed for all children or just those children who demonstrate fear of a particular procedure. Therefore, it would be helpful to identify those children who are more fearful of medical experiences and who would benefit from preparation for the event. Unfortunately, there is limited empirical evidence reported in the literature that reflect ways to measure children's fears of hospitalization and medical experiences.

PURPOSE

The purpose of this research project was to develop an instrument that could enable nurses and other health care professionals to identify how individual children vary in their degree of fearfulness of medical experi-

The authors would like to thank the School of Nursing, Medical College of Georgia, for funding for this project.

ences. Such an instrument could provide nurses with information related to the type and intensity of children's fears. The nurse could then use the data generated from the instrument to better individualize and focus a preparation or teaching program and nursing care for each child. In research situations such an instrument could be used as one among many methods to measure a child's response to hospitalization, medical procedures, and illness.

An instrument that could measure the type and intensity of medical fears in children could improve the efficiency and evaluation of nursing practice in pediatric settings. The information derived from using the tool as either an interview or questionnaire (depending on the age of the child) would facilitate a nurse's focusing his/her teaching/preparation program for a child who will be hospitalized or experience some medical procedure.

REVIEW OF THE LITERATURE

Children's General Fears

The study of children's fears spans several decades (Bauer, 1976; Croake, 1967; Jersild & Holmes, 1935). Researchers have investigated the types of fears reported by children and the prevalence of these fears across age groups. Children generally decrease in fearfulness as they grow older, and the intensity of particular types of fear varies according to the age of the child (Baver, 1976; Miller, 1979). It has been hypothesized, however, that a decrease in fears across age groups may not be so much a decrease in experienced fears as a decrease in the expression of them. Older children may better control the way they exhibit fear (Winer, 1982).

Researchers have described children's fears in categories of political, supernatural, home, and personal fears (Miller, 1979). The most frequently mentioned fears in the political category are war and Communists taking over. The importance of political fears to 8- to 12-year-old children may be attributed to the Vietnam War, television, and the increase in mass communication (Croake, 1967). Supernatural fears include ghosts and spooks and are prevalent fears in children ages 7 to 12 years (Bauer, 1976; Jersild, & Holmes, 1935; Marreu, 1965). The fear of animals and bodily injury are major fears of school-age children (Bauer, 1976; Croake, 1967; Jersild & Holmes, 1935; Marreu, 1965). Three studies utilizing the Fear Survey Schedule II lend support to the finding that concern with bodily injury is a prominent fear of children 8 to 11 years old (Cost, 1977; Geer, 1965; Lego, 1971; Swanson, 1975).

Children's Medical Fears

Hospitalization is an event that is assumed to enhance children's fears of both general and medical experiences. These are fears of loss of control, injections, the unknown, pain, and death. The descriptive studies that are available in the nursing literature support these assumptions to varying degrees (Menke, 1981; Timmerman, 1983). In each of these studies hospitalized school-age children were asked to indicate what event, procedure, or individuals they perceive as "stressful" or frightening.

A game consisting of plastic cards, each with a colored drawing of a stimulus, was used by Menke (1981) to elicit children's perceptions of stress in the hospital from a sample of 50 school-age children. The cards included stimuli that could be perceived as both stressful and nonstressful (baby, toy, needle). The hypodermic needle was perceived as stressful by 86% of the sample. The dog was perceived as stressful by 38% of the sample, the doctor and food by 36%, and the hospital gown by 32%.

In another study, the fears of 16 children, ages 10 to 12, having surgery for the first time, were assessed using an interview method (Timmerman, 1983). The children were interviewed postoperatively. The most commonly recalled categories of preoperative fears were loss of control, the unknown,
injections, and pain or discomfort. Only 13% of the children recalled a fear of death. Forty-five percent reported a fear of destruction of bodily image.

Unfortunately, neither of these studies included a control group of nonhospitalized children of the same age. Thus, one is unsure whether the responses reflect the "stress of hospitalization" or children's fears in general. Also, the descriptive format used to report the data did not allow the investigator the opportunity to explore additional variables in the child's environment that may influence his/her degree of fearfulness.

Several researchers have used general fear surveys that include a subscale for "medical" fears in studies of both well and hospitalized children (Astin, 1971; Elkins & Roberts, 1984; Roberts, Wurtele, Boone, Ginther, & Elkins, 1981; Scherer & Nakamura, 1968). Reports of reliability coefficients for internal consistency for the subscales are not discussed in these studies. All studies that do not report current estimation of the reliability of the measures used should be viewed with caution (Lynn, 1985). In addition to the lack of reported reliability and validity, an analysis of the literature reveals another weakness in the available tools that measure children's fears of medical experiences. In most studies these instruments have not differentiated between the concepts of fear and anxiety.

In this study, fear and anxiety have been defined so that a distinction based on specificity of the feeling attached to each is made. Anxiety is defined as an unpleasant, transitory, emotional state or condition characterized by feelings of tension and diffuse apprehension (May, 1950; Speilberger, 1975). Fear is a temporary reaction and an emotional response to specific real or unreal danger (May, 1950; Wolman, 1978). Medical fears are defined as "any experience that involves medical personnel, or procedures involved in the process of evaluating or modifying health status in traditional health care settings" (Steward & Steward, 1981, p. 70).

Medical Fear Instruments

There are a limited number of instruments that have been used to measure children's fears of medical experiences. In fact, there are three reported in the literature; the Medical Fear Subscale of the Fear Survey Schedule for Children (FSS-FC) (Scherer & Nakamura, 1968), the Hospital Fear Scale, and the Hospital Fear Questionnaire (HFQ) (Melamed, Meyer, Gee, & Soule, 1976). These instruments have been used in a number of studies, but the estimates of reliability and validity on these instruments are not well documented.

The Medical Fear Subscale (FSS-FC) is a scale containing eight items:

Sharp objects
Having to go to the hospital
Getting a shot from the nurse or doctor
Going to the dentist
Going to the doctor
Getting a haircut
Deep water or the ocean
Getting carsick

These items evolved as a subscale after many items related to general fears were factor-analyzed from the FSS-FC, developed by Scherer and Nakamura (1968). The purpose of this research was to develop a fear scale for children in which items were grouped into subscales by means of factor analysis.

The items for the FSS-FC were selected on a conceptual basis under the following categories: School, Home, Social, Physical, Animal, Travel, Classical Phobia, and Miscellaneous. Some items were devised in consultation with graduate students and school personnel familiar with children's fears. Each item was rated on a scale of none, a little, some, much, very much. Two types of fear scores could be obtained: (1) the total number of fear items reported without regard to the degree of rated fear and (2) total degree of fear based on scoring of none = 1... very much = 5. Items were randomly assigned to odd-even positions within the scale.

The instrument was administered to 99 school-age children in the classroom setting on the same day by one investigator. The reported estimate of reliability coefficient for the overall FSS-FC was .94, indicating a high internal consistency reliability. No estimates of internal consistency for the individual subscales were reported. There was no test-retest reliability reported nor any estimates of validity.

The Hospital Fear Scale is a self-report measure that contains 25 items (Melamed et al., 1976). Eight items on the scale are from the Medical Fear Subscale of the FSS-FC, eight items assess hospital fears, and nine items were unrelated filler items. Each item was rated on a "fear thermometer" ranging from 1 (not afraid at all) to 5 (very afraid). Face validity for the eight items assessing hospital fears was reported, but there were no other estimates of reliability or validity included.

The Hospital Fear Questionnaire (HFQ) contains eight items that are a source of stress to children during hospitalization:

Nurses
Taking medicine
Having an operation
Being in strange places
Strangers
Being alone
Getting hurt

These items were developed by Roberts et al. (1981), who state that the instrument has face validity but do not report any other estimates of reliability or validity. A personal communication with the first author revealed that there was no psychometric testing of this instrument done prior to its use in this study.

The FSS-FC subscale and the HFQ were used in a study evaluating the effectiveness of a slide/audiotape program used to reduce school-age children's fears of hospital and medical procedures (Roberts et al., 1981). The sample consisted of 36 children, ages 7 to 12 years, in grades 2 to 5. The overall results showed a significant reduction in reported medical fears.

The HFQ was also used by Elkins and Roberts (1984) in a study evaluating the effectiveness of an innovative program about hospitalization. Children who received a prehospital orientation reported fewer medical fears than did those who did not participate. The reports of neither of these studies included any estimations of the reliability or validity of the FSS-FC subscale for medical fears or the HFQ. Therefore, it is difficult to assess the reliability and validity of their use with this sample.

These tools were also used with 30 surgical patients aged 4 to 12 years who were studied to determine their knowledge about medical instruments and their reported anxiety (Siaw, Stephens, & Holmes, 1986). The Medical Fear Subscale of the FSS-FC and the HFQ were utilized to assess the subjects' anxiety. Face validity of the HFQ was established by three pediatric nurses and a psychologist. No estimates of reliability or validity were reported on either instrument used in this study.

In summary, the major weakness of these three instruments is that the items used were not generated empirically but rather were generated from the literature. Children's perceptions of their own fears were not obtained prior to the development of the instruments. The instruments have few items and there is a strong possibility that they may not cover all fears that children may have pertaining to medical events. Finally, another major weakness is that the instruments were developed and used without initial psychometric testing (i.e., test-retest, criterion validity). When the instruments were used in subsequent studies, very little additional psychometric testing is reported.

CONCEPTUAL BASIS

There are several theoretical perspectives that shed light on the epigenesis of childhood fears. These include traditional psychoanalytic theory (Freud, 1935), social learning theory (Bandura, 1977), Piaget's theory of cognitive development (Piaget, 1967), and developmental theories in general (Werner, 1957; Witkin, 1974). Initially, it appears that these theoretical perspectives propose different explanations of why children develop and maintain fears. However, in-depth examination reveals several important commonalities among the theories that provided a basis for the development of a tool to measure children's fears, as shown below.

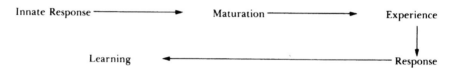

Fear as an innate response requires a certain level of maturation and differentiation in the organism. A response is elicited when the organism is confronted with a threatening experience. It was expected that school-age children would have had some actual or vicarious experiences related to health care. These experiences would have produced some impression on the child that he/she could describe to someone asking what he/she thought about illness, health professionals, and hospitals.

From a developmental viewpoint, it was expected that fears change with age, as do cognitive and perceptual development. Fears generally decrease in frequency with an increase in age and become better articulated, more varied, and more realistic as children develop (Bauer, 1976).

RESEARCH QUESTIONS

The research questions that guided the development of the Child Medical Fear Scale (CMFS) were the following:

1. Do children have fears they report that are specifically related to experiences in health care settings?
2. Can children's fears of medical experiences be categorized?
3. Can children's fears of medical experiences be quantified?

METHODOLOGY

Two studies were conducted during the development and testing of the CMFS. The first study was exploratory and involved interviewing school-age children about their fears of experiences related to health care. The purpose of this study was to generate items to measure children's fears from what the children themselves identified as concerns. In the second study, a different sample of school-age children was used, and their responses to the 29-item Medical Fear Scale were used to obtain various measures of psychometric properties of the scale.

Study 1: Exploration of Children's Fears

One hundred forty-six children were interviewed using an open-end, unstructured interviewing technique recommended by Lofland (1971). The sample was a convenience sample, using children from an elementary school. Letters were sent to all parents with children in kindergarten through grade five explaining the study and asking them to consent to having their child participate. All children of those parents who returned the consent were interviewed. The purpose of the interviews was to obtain information about the children's concerns and fears related to experiences involving illness and the health care system. The children in this phase of the study ranged in age from 6 to 11 years ($\overline{X}$ = 7.3). Forty-eight percent of the children were males, and 71% of the sample were white. The children were equally distributed over the five grades in school.

The questions the children were asked were as follows:

1. Tell me how you feel when you are sick/hurt. What do you like about being sick? What don't you like?
2. Tell me how you feel when you go to see the doctor/nurse. What do you like about seeing the doctor/nurse going to his/her office? What don't you like?
3. Tell me how you feel (or would feel) about going to the hospital. What do you like about the hospital? What don't you like?

Each interview took approximately 10 to 15 min. Responses by the child were clarified when necessary. If a child had not experienced a specific event (e.g., hospitalization), the interviewer asked the child to respond to what he/she "thought it would be like."

Item and Scale Development

Analysis of the taped interviews revealed a number of concerns and fears of children related to four themes identified by two individuals who listened to the tapes.

1. Their own bodies
2. Interactions with health care professionals
3. Medical procedures
4. Health care environment

The four themes were used as an organizational framework for the clusters of items drafted from content analysis of the children's specific concerns. Interrater agreement on how specific items were related to each category was not calculated. The themes were based on previous descriptions of children's fears found in the literature (Steward & Steward, 1981). Instead, each rater assessed whether the items seemed to logically fall into one of the four categories. The 29 items generated were divided among the four subscales as follows: intrapersonal fears ($N = 4$), interpersonal fears ($N = 9$), procedural fears ($N = 9$), and environmental fears ($N = 7$) (see Table 10.1).

Scoring and Administration

The items for the CMFS were written in a structured, three-point forced-choice format. The child was asked to indicate whether he/she was not at all, a little, or a lot afraid of each of the items. "I am afraid of getting a shot" *not at all* or *a little* or *a lot*. The items are scored so that *not at all* = 1 point, *a little* = 2, and *a lot* = 3. Therefore, the scale scores could range from 29 to 87, with low scorers reflecting children who are low in their fearfulness of medical experiences. The instrument was administered in an interview format for purposes of psychometric testing. This enabled the interviewer to clarify any confusing questions for the child. However, the tool could be used as a questionnaire for children in the third grade and above. In either case, the child would indicate if he/she is not at all, a little, or a lot afraid of the item. Items marked "not at all" receive 1 point, items marked "a little" receive 2 points, and those marked "a lot" receive 3 points. The points are added up to provide a total fear score for the child.

TABLE 10.1 Intercorrelations among Child Medical Fear Scale, Fear Survey Schedule, and CMFS Subscales

Assessment tool	CMFS 1	CMFS 2	FSS	Intra-personal	Inter-personal	Environ-mental	Proce-dural
CHFS 1 (Child Medical Fear Scale)	1.00	.84	.71	.96	.91	.94	.91
CMFS 2 (retest)							
FSS (Fear Survey Schedule)							
Subscales							
Intrapersonal				.72	.69	.69	
Interpersonal					.83	.72	
Environmental						.84	
Procedural							

$p < .001$

Study 2: Psychometric Testing of the CMFS

This phase of the project consisted of gathering data on the scale related to psychometric properties of the instrument. The items were randomly arranged so that no two items from the same subscale were sequentially placed.

The sample used for this phase consisted of 84 school-age children. The children were from a different school from those used in the exploratory phase and were interviewed at the school. All parents in the school were sent information about the study and encouraged to give consent for their child to participate in the study. All children whose parents gave consent were interviewed. The children ranged in age from 5 to 11 years ($\bar{X}$ = 7.2), 38% male and 62% female; 88% Caucasian and 11% Black. Forty-four percent of the children had been hospitalized at some time prior to the study, with the majority only experiencing one hospitalization.

RELIABILITY AND VALIDITY OF THE CMFS

Reliability: Coefficients of Internal Consistency and Stability

Internal Consistency

The coefficient of internal consistency conveys the degree of homogeneity of the items on the total test and subscales and was computed using responses to the CMFS from 84 children. The reliability coefficient of internal consistency using Cronbach's alpha was .93 for the total test. Subscale reliabilities were not computed due to the high correlations found between the four subscales (see Table 10.2). Each subscale was correlated with the other three at r = .69 or better (p < .001). They also correlated with the overall test at r = .85 or better (p < .001). This indicates that the test as a whole measured one factor and that subscales were not measuring different dimensions of children's fears of medical experiences.

Coefficient of Stability

A random sample of 22 children from the first testing of the CMFS were reinterviewed two weeks later. The Pearson product-moment coefficient was used to compute the degree of stability of the scale over time. It was obtained by correlating the individual scores of the children on each item at both points in time. The magnitude of the test-retest coefficient was .84, indicating a high degree of stability.

Validity: Content and Criterion

Content Validity

Evidence of content validity was provided by the grounding of the instrument in the children's responses to questions asked in the exploratory phase of this study. Three child health experts (head nurse in pediatrics,

TABLE 10.2 Items on Subscales of Child Medical Fear Scale

Procedural	Environmental	Intrapersonal	Interpersonal
I am afraid of getting a shot.	I am afraid of going to the doctor's office.	I am afraid of hurting myself.	I am afraid the doctor will tell me something is wrong with me.
I am afraid of having my finger stuck.	I am afraid of going to the hospital.	I am afraid of seeing blood come out of me.	I am afraid the doctor will not tell me what he/she is going to do to me.
I am afraid of the doctor or nurse looking in my ear.	I am afraid of lying down on the table in the doctor's office.	I am afraid to throw up.	I am afraid of missing school if I'm sick.
I am afraid of the doctor or nurse listening to my heart.	I am afraid if I went to the hospital I'd have to stay a long time.	I am afraid I will cry when I get hurt.	I am afraid my friends/family will catch something I have if I'm sick and play with them.
I am afraid of having the doctor or nurse look down my throat.	I am afraid I might die if I go to the hospital.		I am afraid the doctor will tell me what to do.
I am afraid of having my temperature taken using a thermometer.	I am afraid I will see lots of blood if I go to the hospital.		I am afraid the nurse will tell me something is wrong with me.
I am afraid of taking medicine.	I am afraid of being away from my family if I go to the hospital.		I am afraid the nurse will not tell me what he/she is going to do to me.
I am afraid of the doctor putting a wooden tongue blade in my mouth.			I am afraid the nurse will tell me what to do.
I am afraid I might have to have an operation if I go to the hospital.			I am afraid I will get behind in schoolwork if I'm sick.

pediatrician, and child mental health clinical nurse specialist) were also asked to review the instrument. The content specialists were given the objectives of the instrument and a list of all of the items. They were asked to rate whether each item was (1) not relevant, (2) somewhat relevant, (3) quite relevant, and (4) very relevant to the objectives. The content validity index (CVI) was defined as the proportion of items given a rating of quite or very relevant by both raters (Waltz, Strickland, & Lenz, 1984). The CVI for the CMFS was 78%.

The CVI was relatively low. One factor that could have influenced this might have been the differences in professional orientations of the raters. Two of the three worked with children with acute physiologic or psychologic dysfunction. In fact, there were two items that these raters did not think were at all relevant to children's medical fears. However, in the original interviews children themselves identified fear of contagion of family and friends and separation fears during hospitalization as two areas of concern. In the second set of interviews, the children again rated these items as moderately fearful.

Criterion Validity

Criterion-related validity establishes support that a measure functions as it should (Waltz et al., 1984). In this study, administration of the Medical Fear Subscale of the FSS-FC (Scherer & Nakamura, 1968) was concurrently given with the CMFS to 26 children in the sample to obtain concurrent validity. The FSS-FC is an 80-item Likert-type questionnaire that measures the type and effectiveness of fear cues that evoke emotional stimuli. Factor analytic procedures were used with a sample of 80 children to develop the 10 factors, one of which is the 11-item Medical Fear Subscale. It was expected that children who scored high on the FSS-FC Medical Fear Subscale would also tend to score high on the CMFS. The correlation coefficient calculated between the two measures was $r = .71$ ($p < .001$), indicating a moderately positive relationship and supporting the expectation. A second criterion measure used was age of the children. It was hypothesized that as children grew older their fears related to medical experiences would decrease, as they do for fears in general (Miller, 1979). In this sample ($N = 84$) there was no significant relationship found between age of a child and his/her score on the CMFS ($r = .04; p > .05$). No relationship between age and the Medical Fear Subscale of the FSS-FC was found either.

In summary, the CMFS does evidence a measure of validity and reliability. High estimates of internal consistency and test-retest reliability indicate that the items on the scale tend to measure the same attribute and that children's reports of how fearful they are of medical experiences are relatively stable over time. Content validity is based on the empirical nature of the initial interviews used to generate the items. An initial measure of criterion validity was obtained using the FSS-FC Medical Fear Subscale as a criterion indicating that the tool is measuring children's fears of medical experiences.

DISCUSSION

This investigation was a two-phase study designed to (1) explore children's concerns and fears of experiences related to illness and the health care system and (2) develop and test an instrument that would quantify a child's fearfulness of medical experiences. The interviews in the exploratory phase of this study yielded 29 concerns and fears verbalized by school-age children. These items were assembled in a 3-point forced-choice format and administered in interviews with 84 school-age children to obtain measures of psychometric properties of the instrument.

The high correlations found between items on the predetermined subscales and the total test indicated that the items as conceptually categorized were not in fact independent, and therefore these categories could not be said to be distinct attributes. Rather the same attribute, child medical fears in general, was being measured by the items from the four subscales.

None of the items was revised on the basis of the interviews during this testing. Most children at all ages had no difficulty understanding or responding to the items.

The somewhat surprising result indicating no relationship between the child's age and his/her degree of medical fears could be specific to this sample. One would expect medical fears to decrease over time, as general fears do. However, in this study that does not seem to be the case. Parents were asked to rate their perception of their children's general fearfulness on a scale of 1 to 5 prior to the testing of the child. There was no significant relationship found between the parent's rating of their child's general fearfulness and the child's self-report on the CMFS ($r = .13; p > .05$). It may be that children's medical fears are very specific and not strongly related to their general fearfulness, and hence, they may not decrease as the child grows older. This relationship needs further testing.

Further research on the CMFS is needed prior to widespread use in nursing. More data on different samples of children in varied age groups, preschool and adolescence as well as school age, need to be collected in order to establish norms for children's fears of medical experiences. Once norms are established, the instrument could be more effectively used in evaluation of the effectiveness of interventions used to decrease children's fears of medical experiences (i.e., hospitalization, surgery, etc.). Comparisons of chronically ill children's and well children's levels of fearfulness could be done to explore how the illness experience is related to medical fears. Nurse clinicians would find the tool especially helpful in determining which children are in greater need of intervention to reduce fears.

Currently, interviews with acutely ill children in the hospital setting are being conducted to determine what differences, if any, exist in sick children's reported medical fears. Another study is in progress in which the CMFS is used to measure changes across time of children hospitalized for surgery. In this study, an additional test of how preparation for surgery affects medical fears will be conducted.

Although medical fears are only one factor that can influence a child's response to health-related procedures, it is an important one. The CMFS will enable nurses to better understand why children respond differently and will help them to individualize care.

REFERENCES

Astin, E. W. (1971). Self-reported fears of hospitalized and non-hospitalized children aged ten to twelve. *Maternal-Child Nursing Journal, 6,* 17-24.

Bandura, A. (1977). *Social learning theory.* Englewood Cliffs, NJ: Prentice-Hall.

Bauer, D. H. (1976). An exploratory study of development changes in children's fears. *Journal of Child Psychology, Psychiatry, 17,* 69-74.

Cost, M. Y. (1977). *An investigation of the relationship between girls' perception of specific parental behavior and girls' fearfulness.* Unpublished doctoral dissertation, New York University, New York.

Croake, J. W. (1967). Fears of children. *Human Development, 12,* 239-247.

Elkins, P. D., & Roberts, M. X. (1984). A preliminary evaluation of hospital preparation for non-patient children: Primary prevention in a "Let's Pretend Hospital." *Children's Health Care, 12*(1), 31-35.

Freud, S. (1935). *A general introduction to psycho-analysis* (J. Riviere, Trans. & Ed.). New York: Liveright.

Geer, J. H. (1965). The development of a scale to measure fear. *Behavioral Research Therapy, 3,* 45-53.

Jersild, A., & Holmes, F. (1935). Children's fears. *Child Development Monographs, 20,* New York: Teachers College.

Johnson, J. E., Kirchoff, K. T., & Endress, M. P. (1975). Easing children's fright during health care procedures. *The American Journal of Maternal-Child Nursing, 4,* 206-210.

Lego, S. (1971). *An investigation of the showing of common fears between mothers and their eleven-year-old children in middle-class families.* Unpublished doctoral dissertation, New York University, New York.

Levy, D. M. (1951). Observations of attitudes and behavior in the child health center. *American Journal of Public Health, 41,* 182-190.

Lofland, J. (1971). *Analyzing social settings.* Belmont, CA: Wadsworth.

Lynn, M. R. (1985). Reliability estimates: Use and disuse. *Nursing Research, 34,* 254-256.

Marreu, A. (1965). What children fear. *Journal of Genetic Psychology, 106,* 265-277.

May, R. (1950). *The meaning of anxiety.* New York: Ronald Press.

Melamed, B. C., Meyer, R., Gee, C., & Soule, L. (1976). The influence of time and type of preparation of children's adjustment to hospitalization. *Journal of Pediatric Psychology, 1,* 31-37.

Menke, E. (1981). School-aged children's perception of stress in the hospital. *Journal of the Association of Children's Health, 9*(3), 80-86.

Miller, S. (1979). Children's fears, a review of the literature with implications for nursing research and practice. *Nursing Research, 28,* 217-223.

Piaget, J. (1967). *Six psychological studies.* New York: Random House.

Roberts, M. C., Wurtele, S. R., Boone, R. R., Gentber, L. J., & Elkins, P. D. (1981). Reductions of medical fears by use of modeling: A prevention application in a general population of children. *Journal of Pediatric Psychology, 6,* 293-300.

Scherer, M. W., & Nakamura, C. Y. (1968). A fear survey schedule for children (FSS-FC): A factor analytic comparison with manifest anxiety (CMAF). *Behavior Research and Therapy, 6,* 173-182.

Siaw, S., Stephens, L., & Holmes, T. (1986). Knowledge about medical instruments and reported anxiety in pediatric surgery patients. *Children's Health Care, 14,* 134-141.

Speilberger, C. D. (1975). *Anxiety: State-trait process. Stress and anxiety* (Vol. 1). Washington, DC: Hemisphere.

Steward, M. T., & Steward, D. (1981). Children's conceptions of medical procedures. In R. Bibace & M. Walsh (Ed.), *Children's conceptions of health, illness and bodily function* (pp. 67-84). San Francisco: Jossey-Bass.

Swanson, A. (1975). *An investigation of the relationship between a child's mother's anxiety. Self-differentiation and accuracy of perception of her child's general fearfulness.* Unpublished doctoral dissertation, New York University, New York.

Timmerman, R. R. (1983). Preoperative fears of older children. *AORN Journal, 38,* 827-834.

Vernon, D. T., Foley, J. M., Sipowitz, R., & Schulman, T. (1965). *The psychological responses of children to hospitalization and illness.* Springfield, IL: Charles C Thomas.

Werner, H. (1957). The concept of development from a comparative and organismic point of view. In D. Harris (Ed.), *The concept of development* (pp. 125-147). Minneapolis: University of Minnesota Press.

Winer, G. A. (1982). A review and analysis of children's fearful behavior in dental settings. *Child Development, 53,* 1111-1133.

Witkin, H. A. (1974). *Psychological differentiation: Studies of development.* New York: Erlbaum.

Wolfer, J. A., & Visintainer, M. A. (1979). Prehospital psychological preparation for tonsillectomy patients: Effects on children's and parents adjustment. *Pediatrics, 64,* 646-655.

Wolman, B. (1978). *Children's fears.* New York: Grosset & Dunlap.

Waltz, C., Strickland, O. L., & Lenz, E. (1984). *Measurement in nursing research.* Philadelphia: F. A. Davis.

11
Reliability and Validity of Selected Measures of Chemotherapy-Induced Nausea and Vomiting

Susan C. McMillan, Linda H. Johnston,
Kathy Tedford, and Candace Harley

This chapter discusses the Index of Nausea and Vomiting, the State-Trait Anxiety Inventory, the Motion Sickness Susceptibility Questionnaire, and the Morrow Assessment of Nausea and Emesis, measures of nausea and vomiting.

Nausea and vomiting are two of the most distressing and uncomfortable side effects of many of the drugs used to treat cancer (Cotanch, 1984; Rhodes, Watson, & Johnson, 1984a). Not only are nausea and vomiting distressing and uncomfortable for the cancer patient, but they put the patient at risk for nutritional deficits, dehydration, electrolyte imbalance, weakness, increased susceptibility to infection, and disruption of life-style (Cotanch, 1984). In addition, patients who have experienced severe nausea and vomiting may be reluctant to subject themselves to it a second or third time and may refuse further therapy. A recent survey of 56 cancer treatment centers revealed that up to 10% of patients refuse chemotherapy because of actual or feared chemotherapy-induced nausea and vomiting (Maule & Perry, 1983). Thus, nausea and vomiting represent a significant problem for patients receiving cancer chemotherapy. However, it is known that not all chemotherapeutic agents cause nausea and vomiting in all individuals. There is considerable variation, not only due to the drugs but also due to individual differences (Scogna & Smalley, 1979). Nursing does not have currently available methods for predicting which patients will experience the most severe symptoms. Nor are there widely available reliable and valid methods for systematic assessment of these problems. Therefore, the purpose of this measurement project is to evaluate the reliability and validity of selected measurement instruments in predicting and assessing chemotherapy-induced nausea and vomiting. An increased understanding of the phenomena of nausea and vomiting may assist oncology nurses in early identification of susceptible patients, more realistic and timely assessment of nausea and vomiting, and creative early intervention to minimize these prevalent problems.

REVIEW OF LITERATURE

As prevalent as nausea and vomiting are in a variety of nursing situations, it seems logical that the literature would abound with studies of these worrisome problems. Unfortunately, this is not the case. There are very few nursing studies that focus on nausea and/or vomiting. Therefore, most of the literature reviewed of necessity comes from other disciplines. Further, there are very few studies that focus on methods of measuring these variables. Most of the measurement tends to be informal or observational. For this reason, there is a limited number of tools from which to choose when beginning a study of nausea and vomiting.

Nausea tends to be linked to vomiting because it so often presages it. However, nausea frequently occurs without vomiting, and vomiting occasionally occurs without nausea. Although, physiologically, most attention is directed to vomiting, nausea as a source of serious discomfort to the patient who may or may not vomit should not be overlooked. Therefore, literature on nausea and vomiting are reviewed separately.

Nausea

Developing the concept of nausea is difficult because it is so rarely scrutinized alone. Most definitions link it to vomiting; for example, Frytak (1983) refers to it as an awareness of the need to vomit. Some studies measure nausea by the number of emetic episodes or the length of time until vomiting (Guignard & McCauley, 1982; Strum, McDermid, Opfell, & Reich, 1982; Stuart-Harris, 1983). Norris (1982), in reviewing the literature related to nausea and vomiting, commented on the dearth of research relevant to these events given their prevalence as health problems. She stated that nausea and vomiting are so loathesome that many would-be researchers are repulsed by rather than attracted to these problems and thus fail to study them.

Nausea may be induced by any number of physical causes: for example, morning sickness, motion sickness, poison, or anesthesia. However, causes of nausea are certainly not limited to physical ones. Events, sights, or sounds that are disgusting, revolting, shocking, or otherwise threatening to the psyche often cause feelings of nausea. The sight of blood, the smell of feces, or the sight of another person retching may cause nausea. The average American would be revolted to learn that meat being served at a meal was horse or skunk, and the result could well be nausea (Norris, 1982).

Nausea is a subjectively experienced distress of the stomach, which may be described as a feeling of heaviness, pressure, or a sinking feeling in the epigastric or sternal region. It is often associated with physical signs such as pallor, sweating, and feeling cold (Money, 1970). In addition, the individual may experience anorexia, epigastric awareness, increased salivation, increased peristalsis, and increased swallowing (Chinn & Smith, 1955; Norris, 1982).

Nausea may vary in intensity and severity. In measuring nausea, McClure, Lycett, and Baskerville (1982) had subjects rank the intensity of their nausea on a scale from 1 to 5 with "first feeling of stomach awareness" being ranked as one and "the feeling one had just prior to vomiting" being ranked as five (p. 255). Several other researchers have used a similar approach to measuring severity of nausea (Gathercole, Connolly, & Birdsell, 1982; Graybiel, Wook, Miller, & Cramer, 1968; Guignard & McCauley, 1982).

Vomiting

The term *vomiting* refers to the ejection of stomach contents through the mouth (Miller & Keane, 1972). During vomiting, the glottis closes and the breath is held midinspiration. This presumably protects the individual against aspiration of stomach contents. With the chest held in a fixed position, the abdominal muscles and diaphragm contract, resulting in increased intra-abdominal pressure. The relaxation of the esophagus and cardiac sphincter allow the contents of the stomach to be expelled (Frytak, 1983).

Vomiting is believed to occur when the emetic center, also known as the true vomiting center (TVC), in the dorsolateral reticular formation of the medulla has been stimulated (Frytak, 1983; Scogna & Smalley, 1979). Impulses from the mucosa of the upper gastrointestinal tract stimulate the TVC via visceral afferent pathways in the vagi and sympathetic nerves. The TVC may also be stimulated by the chemoreceptor trigger zone (CTZ) in the medulla.

Stimuli that cause the vomiting associated with radiation therapy, drugs, gastrointestinal involvement in malignant disease, and bacterial toxins are thought to operate through visceral afferent pathways. Drug- or chemical-induced vomiting is probably mediated by the CTZ. However, the precise manner in which antineoplastic agents produce vomiting is poorly understood (Borison, 1974; Frytak, 1983; Ganong, 1981; Scogna & Smalley, 1979). It is apparent that other afferents reach the TVC from the diencephalon and limbic system because of the important role that emotions play in induction of vomiting. The phrases "sickening sights" and "nauseating smells" exemplify this. Anticipatory nausea and vomiting probably operate through this pathway (Frytak, 1983; Ganong, 1981). The bony labyrinth, which is the culprit in motion sickness, also stimulates the vomiting center (Frytak, 1983).

Symptoms associated with vomiting are known to include tachycardia prior to vomiting and bradycardia during vomiting. In addition, subjects may experience a decrease in blood pressure, weakness or dizziness, pallor, and an increase in the depth and rate of respirations (Money, 1970).

Vomiting has been measured by researchers in a number of ways. It has been measured in some studies by counting the number of emetic episodes and by measuring the amount of emesis (Rhodes et al., 1984a; Strum et al., 1982). Some researchers, primarily physician-researchers, report using observation during hospitalization (Gralla et al., 1981) although Rhodes and associates (1984a) used the report of family members to validate the vomiting items of the Index of Nausea and Vomiting (INV). That is, patients used the INV to self-report their symptoms while a family member made independent observations for the purpose of studying construct validity. Vomiting has also been measured by patient report of the severity or intensity (Morrow, 1984; Rhodes et al., 1984a).

Motion Sickness

Motion sickness as a cause of vomiting has been studied extensively. Sharma (1980) describes motion sickness as a syndrome characterized by anorexia, nausea, dizziness, and vomiting in response to certain kinds of motion. Motion sickness has been reported after most forms of travel, including car, train, ship, airplane, wagon, and camel as well as after various amusement park rides. However, susceptibility to motion sickness varies widely among individuals (Chinn & Smith, 1955). Sharma (1980) reports that children are relatively resistant to motion sickness before the age of 6. The incidence of motion sickness after the age of 6 has been reported to be generally between 20 and 40% of the population (Chinn & Smith, 1955; Guignard & McCauley, 1982; Money, 1970; Sharma, 1980). The principal causes of motion sickness are visual, kinesthetic, and psychologic stimulation of the vestibular apparatus.

Treisman (1977) contends that vomiting that results from motion sickness is so disadvantageous to the animals and humans in whom it occurs that its development could not be accidental; there must be an explanation for its evolution. Treisman hypothesizes that motion sickness results when problems occur in the programming motions of the eyes or head caused by repeated and unpredictable interferences in the relationship between the spatial frameworks defined by the visual, vestibular, or proprioceptive inputs. Such interferences are often produced by certain types of motion, but ingested toxins may also cause disturbances in sensory input or motor control. The ingestion of toxins as a stimulus to motion sickness and ultimately emesis, would be important in nature, the main function of emesis being to rid the animal or person of the ingested toxins. Treisman states that the occurrence of emesis in response to motion is an accidental by-product of this protective mechanism.

In justifying his evolutionary hypothesis for motion sickness, Treisman (1977) points out that evolving species must have been under constant pressure to develop protection against ingested toxins. He states that there are three major lines of defense. The first line is rejection by taste. If this defense fails, there is emesis provoked by effects on the stomach lining or by stimulation of chemoreceptors during absorption. Failure of these first two lines of defense leaves the individual with the last line of defense which, according to Treisman, is early stimulation of the vestibular system, motion sickness, and emesis. Not only does this motion sickness and emesis provide protection during the initial encounter with the toxin, but it teaches the individual to avoid it in the future. Treisman calls this avoidance tactic aversion conditioning. This condition corresponds closely to the conditioned anticipatory nausea and vomiting seen in cancer patients treated with chemotherapy.

Support for Treisman's evolutionary hypothesis of motion sickness and emesis as a response to poisons can be found in the work of Money and Cheung (1983). These researchers removed the vestibular apparatus of seven dogs, which resulted in an impairment of the emetic response, not only to motion but also to several poisons that had previously caused vomiting in all seven animals. These results would seem to support the role of the vestibular apparatus as a last line of defense against circulating poisons. Since cancer chemotherapeutic drugs are known to be toxic, a logical argument could be made for questioning whether the vestibular apparatus plays a part in the chemotherapy-induced nausea and vomiting seen so frequently in cancer patients. A study reported by Morrow (1984) found a significant positive relationship between motion sickness susceptibility and chemotherapy-induced nausea and vomiting.

Anticipatory Nausea and Vomiting

Anticipatory nausea and vomiting is generally accepted to be a conditioned response to the experience of chemotherapy-induced nausea and vomiting. It does not appear before the first administration of chemotherapy but seems to be fully developed by the third or fourth administration (Morrow & Morrell, 1982; Nesse, Carli, Curtis, & Kleinman, 1980; Nicholas, 1982; Redd, Anderson, & Minagawa, 1982). Nicholas (1982) reports that approximately 45% of chemotherapy patients experience anticipatory nausea, and approximately 18% have anticipatory vomiting. In their sample of 500 patients, Morrow and Morell (1982) found anticipatory nausea and vomiting to have an overall prevalence of 25%.

Anxiety

It has long been recognized that anxiety may be associated with nausea; hence, the expression "sick with anxiety." Altmaier (1982) studied the psychologic functioning of patients with anticipatory nausea and vomiting and found that patients manifesting anticipatory vomiting tend to be characterized by psychosocial symptoms of anxiety and depression.

A pilot study of anxiety and chemotherapy-induced nausea and vomiting was reported by Rhodes, Watson, and Johnson (1984b). These nurse researchers attempted to determine the interaction of anxiety with nausea and vomiting in 36 individuals being treated with chemotherapy. Although the design did not control for variability introduced by using subjects receiving different drug protocols and different antiemetics, one interesting finding emerged; that is, the State Anxiety scores prior to the second cycle of chemotherapy predicted the post-therapy nausea, vomiting, and retching. This evidence, while inconclusive, suggests the need for further study of anxiety and its relationship to nausea and vomiting.

CONCEPT DEVELOPMENT

To measure concepts such as nausea and vomiting, it is necessary first to conceptualize them. This is the major purpose of the review of the literature. The abstract concepts of nausea and vomiting may become concrete or real through their characteristics. Therefore, based on the foregoing review of the literature, the following characteristics are identified.

Nausea and vomiting are both characterized by time. In order to assess these client problems, the nurse must focus on the time of onset, duration of the symptoms, and for vomiting, the frequency with which emesis occurs.

Nausea and vomiting are characterized by intensity. The severity of the symptoms may vary due to individual differences or treatment differences.

Nausea and vomiting are characterized by perception. Nausea is a type of distress that must be subjectively perceived; it cannot be observed by the nurse or others. Conversely, vomiting may be observed and measured by either researcher or health care provider.

Nausea and vomiting are characterized by causation; that is, there are a variety of etiologies for these two problems. A given client may have several reasons for experiencing nausea or may have none. In assessing nausea and vomiting, therefore, it is important for the nurse to look at antecedents. Therefore, this study looked at motion sickness susceptibility and anxiety as possible antecedents of chemotherapy-induced nausea and vomiting.

METHOD

The purpose of this study was to assess the reliability and validity of selected instruments used to measure the nausea and vomiting associated with cancer chemotherapy. Based on the foregoing review of literature, four instruments were selected for inclusion in the study: the Index of Nausea and Vomiting (INV), the State-Trait Anxiety Inventory (STAI), the Motion Sickness Susceptibility Questionnaire (MSS), and the Morrow Assessment of Nausea and Emesis (MANE).

Research Questions

The instruments were rated by means of the following questions:

1. To what extent is the INV a valid scale for assessing chemotherapy-induced nausea and vomiting?
2. How reliable is the INV?
3. To what extent is the STAI a valid scale for predicting severity of chemotherapy-induced nausea and vomiting?
4. To what extent is the STAI a valid scale for predicting incidence and severity of anticipatory nausea and vomiting?
5. To what extent is the MSS a valid scale for predicting severity of chemotherapy-induced nausea and vomiting?
6. To what extent is the MSS a valid scale for predicting incidence and severity of anticipatory nausea and vomiting?
7. How reliable is the MSS?

Sample

The sample consisted of outpatients receiving cancer chemotherapy with one of two drug protocols. These drug protocols were selected for the study because of their similarly high emetic potential. All patients were at least 18 years of age, well oriented, and able to read and understand English.

Drug Protocols

In order to study variance due to individual differences in response to chemotherapy, it was necessary to control variance due to differences in emetic potential of various drugs. Therefore, two chemotherapy protocols with similar emetic potential were included in the study. Subjects received either the CAV or the CAF (also known as FAC) protocol. CAF combines cyclophosphamide (Cytoxan®), doxorubicin (Adriamycin®), and 5-fluorouracil (5-FU) and is used largely in the treatment of breast carcinoma after mastectomy. CAV consists of Cytoxan, Adriamycin, and vincristine and is used primarily in the treatment of small cell bronchogenic carcinoma (Preston, Lyman, Weber, Sather, & Sleight, 1982).

The incidence of post-treatment nausea and vomiting with Cytoxan is known to be dose-related. It is estimated that 90% of patients receiving high-dose Cytoxan (greater than 1 g/m²) will experience nausea and vomiting. Both protocols require high-dose Cytoxan. Studies of the incidence of nausea and vomiting with Adriamycin suggest that its emetic potential is high. More than 75% of the subjects receiving Adriamycin experience nausea and/or vomiting. Vincristine is reported to have a low incidence of nausea and vomiting. 5-FU likewise is categorized as having low emetic potential, with an incidence of less than 20% (see Lasley & Ignoffo, 1981). Therefore, although somewhat different in composition, these two drug protocols may be said to be similar in emetic potential.

Instrumentation

Rhodes Index of Nausea and Vomiting

The Rhodes INV is an eight-item scale that purports to measure occurrence, severity, frequency, and duration of nausea, vomiting, and retching. This self-report measure is a five-point summated rating scale that requires subjects to circle the one sentence in each set of five that most clearly describes their own experience with nausea and vomiting (Rhodes et al., 1984a).

The INV was selected for use in the study because it matched the characteristics of nausea that had emerged from the literature. It was designed to be administered 12 and 24 hr after chemotherapy and thus took into account both time and antecedents. It is rated on a 5-point scale and also accounts for severity. It includes separate items on nausea and vomiting and thus treats these as two separate but related problems. And finally, it requires self-report by the patient, acknowledging the characteristic of perception.

The INV was also thought to be appropriate because of its usability with individuals who are sick from recently administered chemotherapy. Because it has only eight items and is confined to one page, the INV is not a cumbersome instrument to use with symptomatic individuals.

Reliability of the INV was estimated by using a split-halves procedure and Cronbach's alpha over 12 administrations of the INV ($N = 25$-32). Resulting reliability estimates ranged between $r = .83$ and $r = .99$. Validity was studied by using several techniques. Results of these assessments suggest that the INV has adequate validity for use as a tool to measure chemotherapy-induced nausea and vomiting (Rhodes et al., 1984a).

Motion Sickness Susceptibility Questionnaire

Mirabile (1982), developed a five-item self-report questionnaire to assess susceptibility to motion sickness in a study group of 1,525 adults. Evidence of concurrent validity was obtained by correlating scores with the number of revolutions it took in a rotating chair to cause motion sickness. A significant negative relationship ($r = -.45$, $p < .001$) was found. This suggests that the questionnaire and scoring method are able to provide a reasonably valid representation of motion sickness susceptibility as quantified by the amount of vestibular stimulation.

Reliability of the scale was estimated using test-retest on 45 normal subjects. A significant positive correlation ($r = .81$, $p < .001$) was found between the two administrations.

State-Trait Anxiety Inventory (STAI)

The STAI was developed to measure both state anxiety and trait anxiety (Spielberger, Gorsuch, & Lushene, 1970). State anxiety may be defined as a transitory emotional state that varies in intensity and fluctuates over time; it is characterized by subjective consciously perceived feelings of tension and apprehension. Trait anxiety is the relatively stable tendency toward subjective, consciously perceived feelings of tension and apprehension; that is, the tendency to perceive a wide range of situations as threatening. This self-report questionnaire consists of 40 items on a 4-point Likert-type summated rating scale. Each subscale (State and Trait) is made up of 20 items. Thus, the possible scores on each subscale range between 20 (low) and 80 (high). Validity and reliability data are available in the *STAI Manual* that accompanies the scale. Repeated studies have provided adequate evidence of reliability and validity for use with medical-surgical patients. However, the STAI has not previously been used to study anxiety as a method of predicting chemotherapy-induced nausea and vomiting.

Morrow Assessment of Nausea and Emesis (MANE)

The MANE is a self-report scale for measuring (1) anticipatory nausea, (2) anticipatory vomiting, (3) post-treatment nausea, and (4) post-treatment vomiting. The MANE assesses the frequency, severity, and duration of each of these four experiences (Morrow, 1984; Morrow, Arseneau, Asbury, Bennett, & Boros, 1982; Morrow & Morrell, 1982).

Psychometric properties of the MANE were studied, using a sample of 500 consecutive outpatients who received chemotherapy in three hospitals. Test-retest reliability coefficients ranged between $r = .72$ and $r = .96$. Construct validity was assessed by studying convergent and divergent validity. It was found that the MANE is more highly correlated with other measures of nausea and emesis than it is with measures of other chemotherapy-induced side effects (Morrow, 1984). This suggests that the MANE has adequate construct validity and therefore may be a useful tool for measuring anticipatory and post-treatment nausea and vomiting.

Procedures

This exploratory descriptive study involved utilizing selected measurement instruments with consenting subjects at the time of their first and fourth administrations of chemotherapy with CAV or CAF (see Figure 11.1). This schedule was necessary for two reasons. The subjects had to respond to their levels of anxiety and motion sickness susceptibility prior to their first treatment to avoid influencing their responses with symptoms that resulted from treatment with chemotherapy. The subjects had to respond to the MANE at the time of the fourth chemotherapy in order to allow anticipatory nausea and vomiting to develop fully before measurement of this phenomenon was attempted. At the time of the first chemotherapy the subject was asked to complete the MSS and the STAI prior to therapy. Following therapy the subject was given two copies of the INV with instructions to fill the first one out 12 hr after chemotherapy and the second one 24 hr after therapy. These INV forms were then mailed to the researcher. At the time of the fourth chemotherapy, the MANE and STAI (State only) were administered prior to therapy. Following therapy the subjects were again asked to fill out two INV forms, one at 12 hr and one at 24 hr.

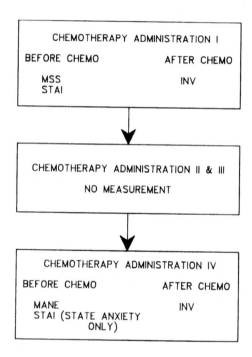

FIGURE 11.1 Schedule for administration of research instruments.

ANALYSIS OF DATA AND RESULTS

Data obtained from administration of the four measurement tools were analyzed in an attempt to answer the research questions.

To study the validity of the INV, scores from study subjects ($N = 30$) were compared with a group of normals ($N = 20$) using a t-statistic. Results showed a significant difference between groups ($t = 16.4$, $p < .001$). The ability of the INV to differentiate between chemotherapy recipients and working adults is an important piece of evidence of its construct validity.

A correlation of the INV with scores on the MANE was conducted. Specifically, items ($N = 27$) dealing with post-treatment nausea from the two measures were correlated, as were all items dealing with post-treatment vomiting. High positive correlations would provide evidence of the construct validity of the MANE as well as of the INV. Results revealed a moderate relationship between the nausea items ($r = .44$, $p < .02$), but the relationship between the emesis items on the two tools was small (.23) and nonsignificant.

The reliability of the INV was studied by assessing the internal consistency of the instrument using the alpha coefficient. The resulting alpha coefficient was .88. In addition to computing an alpha coefficient, a split-halves procedure was used. With correction for attenuation, the reliability coefficient was $r = .95$ ($p < .001$). These relatively high correlation coefficients support the reliability of the INV.

The validity of the STAI for predicting incidence and severity of chemotherapy-induced nausea and vomiting was studied by correlating STAI scores with scores on the INV. State Anxiety scores correlate at .37 ($p = .05$) with INV scores; the INV correlation with Trait scores was $r = .36$ ($p = .05$). A significant positive correlation offers evidence of predictive validity. However, these correlations, while significant, are probably not of any real practical importance since they suggest that anxiety accounts for only 13% of the variance in the INV scores.

The extent to which the STAI is valid for predicting severity of anticipatory nausea and vomiting was studied by correlating STAI scores with specific items on the MANE. The resulting correlations approached zero. This result might have occurred because there was so little incidence of anticipatory symptoms in the group of subjects, and thus there was almost no variance in these scores.

The ability of the MSS to predict incidence and severity of chemotherapy-induced nausea and vomiting was studied by correlating MSS scores with scores on the INV. A Significant positive relationship may be taken as evidence of predictive validity. Results indicated a moderate correlation ($r = .32$, $p < .05$) between MSS and INV. In like manner, the validity of the MSS for predicting incidence and severity of anticipatory nausea and vomiting was studied by correlating MSS scores with scores from specific items on the MANE. These correlations were very low, approaching zero. It is possible that this result occurred partly because of the relative infrequency of occurrence of MSS in the general population (20-40%) and partly because of the low incidence of anticipatory symptoms in the subjects.

The reliability of the MSS was studied using test-retest on a group of "normals." The resulting reliability coefficient ($r = .78$, $p < .01$) suggests adequate reliability. In addition, internal consistency was studied by correlating scores on two key items on the MSS. The designer of the MSS, Charles Mirabile (1982), stated that item 1 was designed to serve as a check on the accuracy of item 5, which requires the patient to graph his/her response. For this reason, a correlation between scores on these two items seems appropriate. Results ($r = .89$ for study subjects and $r = .79$, $p < .001$ for normals) suggest that the MSS has adequate internal consistency.

To explore the possibility that the MSS and the STAI together might better predict INV scores than either measure could used alone, a multiple regression was undertaken. The result suggested that only 15% of variance in INV scores could be accounted for by the use of the combined scores of the MSS and State Anxiety scores. Therefore, the MSS and STAI were not strong predictors of chemotherapy-induced nausea and vomiting in this group of subjects.

DISCUSSION

The purpose of this study was to assess the reliability and validity of instruments designed to measure chemotherapy-induced nausea and vomiting. Although no single study ever provides conclusive evidence, some interesting results emerged from this one. First, the INV was found to be valid and reliable for use as a measure of chemotherapy-induced nausea and vomiting. The fact that the INV was able to differentiate between two groups who were known to be different in their levels of nausea and vomiting (normals vs. study subjects) supports its validity. The low correlations with specific items on the MANE is probably attributed to a weakness in the MANE rather than to one in the INV; that is, clients responding to the MANE do so at their next visit for chemotherapy, or 4 weeks after the chemotherapy-induced nausea and vomiting have or have not occurred. So memory was a limiting factor in the use of the MANE in this study.

The two measures of internal consistency that were used to study the reliability of the INV, split halves and alpha coefficient, gave similarly good results. Therefore, as a result of this study, the INV appears to be a very usable instrument with excellent evidence of reliability and validity.

The other instruments in the study did not fare quite so well. Although it may be of interest to know the patient's level of anxiety just for anxiety's sake, it would be injudicious to attempt to predict chemotherapy-induced nausea and vomiting by using the STAI. The correlations, although positive and significant, were too weak to be of any real practical significance in a clinical setting.

The MSS was found to be acceptably reliable but not useful for predicting incidence or severity of nausea and vomiting after chemotherapy. Nor was it found to be valid for predicting anticipatory nausea or vomiting. The symptoms that patients experience in the car on the way to the treatment center may not, based on our data, be attributed to anything but conditioned response.

One unanticipated finding of the study was supremely encouraging for the nurses collecting the data. This result was that the subjects in the study had relatively mild symptoms of chemotherapy-induced nausea and vomiting. Only two of the study subjects (out of 29) had to be dropped from the study because of severe symptoms, necessitating hospitalization and more intensive antiemetic therapy. This happy result, along with the low to moderate scores on the INV, suggests that the antiemetic protocol that is in use with these patients is, for the most part, successful. That information alone made the study worthwhile. Through the use of the INV it may be possible for oncology nurses to identify patients who are having the most severe symptoms so that the antiemetic regimen can be altered within 24 hr after the first administration of chemotherapy. This should substantially reduce the risk of nutritional deficits, dehydration, electrolyte imbalance, weakness, and noncompliance – certainly a worthy nursing goal.

REFERENCES

Altmaier, E. M. (1982). A pilot investigation of the psychologic functioning of patients with anticipatory vomiting. *Cancer, 49,* 201-204.

Borison, H. L. (1974). Area postrema: Chemoreceptor trigger zone for vomiting – is that all? *Life Sciences, 14,* 1807-1817.

Chinn, H. I., & Smith, P. K. (1955). Motion sickness. *Pharmacological Reviews, 7,* 33-82.

Cotanch, P. H. (1984). Measuring nausea and vomiting in clinical nursing research. *Oncology Nursing Forum, 11,* 92-94.

Frytak, S. (1933). Management of nausea and vomiting in the cancer patient. In R. J. Gralla (Ed.), *Conference proceedings: Supportive care of the cancer patient.* New York: Memorial Sloan-Kettering Cancer Center.

Ganong, W. F. (1981). *Review of medical physiology.* Los Altos, CA: Lange.

Gathercole, F., Connolly, N., & Birdsell, J. (1982). The use of dexamethasone as an antiemetic in association with chemotherapy for neoplastic disease. *Oncology Nursing Forum, 9,* 17-19.

Copies of the instruments employed in this study may be obtained by writing to the following: For *the Index of Nausea and Vomiting (INV)*, write to Verna A. Rhodes, University of Missouri-Columbia, S314 School of Nursing, Columbia, MO 65211. For the *State-Trait Anxiety Inventory (STAI)*, write to Consulting Psychological Press Inc., 577 College Avenue, Palo Alto, CA 94306. For the *Motion Sickness Susceptibility Questionnaire (MSS)*, write to Charles S. Mirabile, Jr., M.D., Institute of Living, 400 Washington Street, Hartford, CT 06106. For the *Morrow Assessment of Nausea and Emesis (MANE)*, write to Gary R. Morrow, Ph.D., University of Rochester, Cancer Center, Box 74, Rochester, NY 14642.

Gralla, R. J., Itri, L., Pisko, S., Squillante, A., Kelson, D., Braun, D., Bordin, L., Braun, T. J., & Young, C. (1981). Antiemetic efficacy of high-dose metoclopramide:Randomized trials with placebo and prochlorperazine in patients with chemotherapy-induced nausea and vomiting. *New England Journal of Medicine, 305,* 905-909.

Graybiel, A., Wook, C. D., Miller, E. F., & Cramer, D. B. (1968). Diagnostic criteria for grading the severity of acute motion sickness. *Aerospace Medicine, 53,* 554-563.

Maule, W. F., & Perry, M. C. (1983). Management of chemotherapy-induced nausea and emesis. *American Family Physician, 27,* 226-234.

McClure, J. A., Lycett, P., & Baskerville, J. C. (1982). Diazepam as a motion sickness drug. *Journal of Otolaryngology, 11,* 252-259.

Miller, B. F., & Keane, C. D. (1972). *Encyclopedia and dictionary of medicine and nursing.* Philadelphia: W. B. Saunders.

Mirabile, C. S. (1982). A clinically useful polling technique for assessing susceptibility to motion sickness. *Perceptory Motor Skills, 54,* 987-991.

Money, K. E. (1970). Motion sickness. *Physiology Review, 50,* 1-39.

Money, K. E., & Cheung, B. S. (1983). Another function of the inner ear: Facilitation of the emetic response to poisons. *Aviation, Space, and Environmental Medicine, 54,* 253-257.

Morrow, G. R. (1984). The assessment of nausea and vomiting: Past problems, current issues, and suggestions for future research. *Cancer, 53,* 51-62.

Morrow, G. R., Arseneau, J. C., Asbury, R. F., Bennett, J. M., & Boros, J. (1982). Anticipatory nausea and vomiting with chemotherapy. *New England Journal of Medicine, 306,* 431-432.

Morrow, G. R., & Morrell, C. (1982). Behavioral treatment for the anticipatory nausea and vomiting induced by cancer chemotherapy. *New England Journal of Medicine, 307,* 1474-1480.

Ness, R. M., Carli, T., Curtis, G. C., & Kleinman, P. D. (1980). Pretreatment nausea in cancer chemotherapy. *Psychosomatic Medicine, 5,* 461-463.

Norris, C. M. (1982). Nausea and vomiting. In C. M. Norris (Ed.), *Concept Clarification in Nursing* (pp. 81-110). Rockville, MD: Aspen Systems.

Preston, J. D., Lyman, G. H., Weber, C. E., Sather, M. R., & Sleight, S. M. (1982). *Cancer chemotherapeutic agents: Handbook of clinical data* (2nd ed.). Boston: G. K. Hall.

Redd, W. H., Anderson, C. V., & Minagawa, R. Y. (1982). Hypnotic control of anticipatory emesis in patients receiving cancer chemotherapy. *Journal of Consulting and Clinical Psychology, 50,* 14-19.

Rhodes, V. A., Watson, P. M., & Johnston, M. H. (1984a, May). *Anxiety related to nausea and vomiting in chemotherapy.* Paper presented at the Oncology Nursing Society Congress, Toronto.

Rhodes, V. A., Watson, P. M., & Johnston, M. H. (1984b). Development of reliable and valid measures of nausea and vomiting. *Cancer Nursing, 7,* 33-41.

Scogna, D. M., & Smalley, R. V. (1979). Chemotherapy-induced nausea and vomiting. *American Journal of Nursing, 79,* 1562-1564.

See-Lasley, K., & Ignoffo, R. J. (1981). *Manual of oncology therapeutics.* St. Louis: C. B. Mosby.

Sharma, K. (1980). Susceptibility to motion sickness. *Acta Genetica Medicae et Gemellologiae, 29,* 157-162.

Spielberger, C. D., Gorsuch, R. L., & Lushene, R. E. (1970). *STAI Manual.* Palo Alto, CA: Consulting Psychologists Press.

Strum, S. B., McDermed, J. E., Opfell, R. W., & Reich, L. P. (1982). Intravenous metoclopramide: An effective antiemetic in cancer chemotherapy. *Journal of the American Medical Association, 247,* 2683-2686.

Stuart-Harris, R. (1983). Chlorpromazine, placebo, and Droperidol in the treatment of nausea and vomiting associated with cisplatin therapy. *Postgraduate Medical Journal, 59,* 500-503.

Treisman, M. (1977, July 29). Motion sickness: An evolutionary hypothesis. *Science,* 493-495.

12
Evaluation of Measures Assessing Family Response to Chronic Illness

Martha J. Foxall and Patrice Watson

This chapter discusses the Family Response to Chronic Illness Questionnaire, a measure to assess coping abilities in families where chronic illness is present.

The purpose of this research was to evaluate the reliability and validity of existing instruments which can be used to assess family response to chronic illness, specifically chronic obstructive pulmonary disease (COPD). The specific objective was to test the internal consistency and construct validity of six instruments:

Chronic Impact and Coping Instrument (CICI) (Hymovich, 1981, 1983)
Coping Scale (Felton, Revenson, & Hinrichsen, 1984)
Acceptance of Illness Scale (Felton, et. al. 1984; adapted from Linkowski, 1971)
Self-Esteem Scale (Rosenberg, 1965)
Affect Balance Scale (ABS) (Bradburn, 1969)
Social Adjustment Scale Self-Report (SAS-SR) (Weissman & Bothwell, 1976).

RATIONALE

A frequently cited problem in nursing research is the failure to determine the reliability and validity of measurements used to assess various constructs (Waltz, Strickland, & Lenz, 1984). This research was designed to assess the psychometric properties of six instruments on a previously untested population in an attempt to extend their usefulness as clinical nursing research measurements. Reliable and valid instruments are needed that assess stress of family members and how well they are coping

The assistance of Jeanette Y. Ekberg, M.S.N., R.N. is acknowledged for help in research project development and data collection.

in terms of social and psychological adjustment.

More than 10 million Americans have COPD, the fastest rising cause of disability and death in the United States (Lenfant & Moskowitz, 1984). The mortality rate of COPD increased 60% from 1968 to 1978 and accounted for 60,050 deaths in 1981 (American Lung Association, 1982). A significant portion of persons with COPD can be expected to develop respiratory distress and cardiovascular complications resulting in metabolic alterations, fatigue, and decreased physical and mental function. The estimated number of office, hospital, and nursing home visits and physician telephone calls related to COPD was 1,824,000 in 1981 (IMS America, 1981). The economic costs of COPD may go as high as $15 billion per year for health care, time lost from work, and lost wages (Public Services Laboratory, 1978).

The progressive nature of COPD and other associated disabilities requires adjustment by the spouse as well as the ill partner. The response of the spouse is one of the most important components in the adjustment of an ill partner. Dyk and Sutherland (1956) studied the adjustment of spouses of colostomy patients and determined that the spouse was the "significant other" most frequently indicated as the key to the patient's success or failure in personal adjustment. Few researchers have looked at coping behaviors used by both the ill partner and the spouse or at the relationship between coping and adjustment in these two groups. The complexity of the illness situation necessitates research which addresses the need for a wider range of reliable and valid assessment tools which are sensitive in determining patient and spousal responses to chronic illness.

LITERATURE REVIEW

Stress

In this study stress was conceptualized as the stimulus associated with the chronic illness that challenges the ill person's and spouse's adjustment capabilities (adapted from Lazarus, 1966). the term *stressors* referred to the sources of stress. Of the current research concerned with stressors, the association between non-illness-related stressful life events and a variety of physical and mental illnesses has received the greatest attention (Apley, 1974; Bell, 1977; Carter, 1979; Gorsuch & Key, 1974; Holmes & Rahe, 1967; Jalowiec & powers, 1981; Jenkins, 1971; Rabkin & Struening, 1976; Reeder, Scharama, & Dirken,1973; Stein & Charles, 1971, 1975; Zeldow & Pavlou, 1984).

The majority of studies which identified illness-related stressors have focused on the spouse of the ill partner and included factors related to the disease itself (period of convalescence, number of symptoms, level of severity, medical complaints, and possible death); factors related to the ill partner's behavior (attitudes, irritability, complaints, and regressive behavior); and factors related to self (feeling overburdened and need for information) (Brahm, Houser, Cline, & Posner, 1975; Bruhn, 1977; Croog & Fitzgerald, 1978; Grad & Sainsburg, 1968; Kobza, 1983; Sexton, 1985; Shambaugh & Kanter, 1969; Skelton & Dominian, 1973; Stevenson, 1977; Weisman & Sobel, 1979).

Few studies were found which described instruments used to measure sources of stress. In the available studies, the most frequently used instrument was the Social Readjustment Rating Scale (SRRS) (Holmes & Rahe, 1967) or its refined form, the Recent Life Changes (RLC) Questionnaire (Rahe, 1977). The SRRS lists 42 life events which are either indicative of or require some change and consequent coping behavior in the life of the individual. The RLC includes 76 stressful life events categorized into five major groups. While the SRRS and the RLC have been used in a variety of studies, the instruments have been criticized because they do not include chronic long-term disabilities or anticipated life stress (Dracup, 1982).

Subjective measurements of stress have also been reported. A frequently used instrument is the Subjective Stress Scale (SSS) (Bruhn, 1977; Croog & Fitzgerald, 1978; Graham & Reeder, 1972; Reeder, Scharama & Dirken, 1973; Sexton & Munro, 1985; Stevenson, 1977; Wishnie, Hackett, & Cassem, 1971). The SSS, developed by Chapman and colleagues (1966) in connection with studies of stress in heart patients, consists of four items related to the person's perceptions of herself before the husband's illness. While Schar, Reeder, & Dirken (1973) found that items in the SSS correlated positively with social stress items, Croog and Fitzgerald (1978) viewed subjective stress as part of general stress which did not correlate with perceived illness burdens. Jalowiec and Powers (1981) obtained subjective stress ratings by asking patients to rate their general levels of stress as low, medium, or high.

Other researchers have used a variety of measurements, including open-ended or semi-structured interviews, to determine stressors associated with chronic illness, including needs (Kobza, 1983; Leech, 1982; Skipper, Fink, & Hallenbeck, 1968) and current concerns (Weisman & Sobel, 1979).

Several studies indicated only the disease condition or illness situation as the stressor (Molumphy & Sporawski, 1984; Shambaugh & Kanter, 1969) or used other variables as indicators of stress without describing how the variable was operationalized (Schoeneman, Reznikoff, & Bacon, 1983: Skelton & Dominian, 1973).

Coping

For the purpose of this study, coping was conceptualized as the cognitive and behavioral efforts made to master, tolerate, or reduce stressors associated with chronic illness and the conflicts among them (adapted from Folman & Lazarus, 1980). The majority of studies on family coping have been in relation to childhood illnesses (Binger et al., 1969; Chodoff,

Friedman, & Hamburg, 1964; Friedman, Chodoff, Mason, & Hamburg, 1963; Hymovih, 1981, 1983; Kupst, Blatterbauer, Westman, Schulman, & Pard, 1977; McCubbin et al., 1983; Tropauer, Franz, & Dilgard, 1970; Venters, 1981; Videka-Sherman, 1982). Research on coping strategies utilized by chronically ill adults has included persons with psychiatric disorders (Bell, 1977; Fontana, Marcus, Noel, & Rakusin, 1972), paralytic conditions (Bulman & Wortman, 1977), long-term disability (Adams & Lindemann, 1977), physical health problems (Felton & Revenson, 1984; Felton et al., 1984), malignant conditions (Derogatis, Abeloff, & Melisaratos, 1979; Sanders & Kardinal, 1977; Weisman & Worden, 1976), and acute and chronic illness (Jalowiec & Powers, 1981; Viney & Westbrook, 1981, 1982).

Little research has investigated how people cope. Several researchers have categorized coping into similar units. Menninger, Mayman, and Pruyser (1963) classified coping strategies as direct behavior toward altering the circumstances, sidestepping the issue, and providing a solution. The researchers described many specific strategies. Self-discipline was one of the more commonly used, and talking was a universal strategy. Moos and Tsu (1977) defined seven categories of adaptive tasks and coping skills. They emphasized that specific techniques were either adaptive or maladaptive, depending on the situation in which they were used. Billings and Moos (1981) used a checklist of 19 coping strategies grouped into three major methods: active-cognitive coping, active-behavioral coping, and avoidance. Pearlin and Schooler (1978) asked individuals to explain how they dealt with problems in finance, marriage, work, and parenting. The responses were classified into a number of dimensions of coping style. Lazarus and Launier (1978) suggested that coping behaviors could be classified as problem-solving or emotion-regulating approaches. Fontana and colleagues (1972) delineated symptomatic and nonsymptomatic coping strategies in a study of 99 hospitalized mentally ill patients and their matched controls. Their model conceptualized behavior prior to hospitalization as well as during hospitalization was instrumental in the coping process. In a study of 89 chronically physically ill patients, Viney and Westbrook (1982) asked respondents to assess their own coping strategies. They concluded that some kinds of strategies may be better for coping with physical illness than others.

Many studies of the significance of coping behaviors have based their conclusions on clinical judgments (Pfeiffer, 1977; Sanders & Kardinal, 1977; Vaillant, 1971). Similarly, Hamburg and Adams (1967), in a review of literature related to stress and coping, determined that most studies were largely descriptive observations from interviews from which it was difficult to abstract general coping principles.

Reconceptualization of the nature of coping has led to the development of objectively scored measures (Coelho, Hamburg, & Adams, 1974; Moos, 1976). Two such measures were designed for administration to college students. Coelho, Silber, and Hamburg (1962) devised the Student TAT, a set of 10 ambiguous college situations (e.g., dating and sex, academic achievement pressures) presented in pictorial form to which the subject responded as to the Thematic Apperception Test. Protocols were scored in terms of solution (resolution or outcome), activity on the part of "hero," and favorableness of the resolution. The test differentiated among a clinically disturbed group, state university freshmen, and exceptionally competent freshmen. However, no attempt was made to assess process-strategies used to cope with the problem. Sidle, Adams, and Cady (1969) developed a two-part scale in an effort to identify general coping principles. The scale included problem situations and 10 strategies abstracted from various literature sources. They concluded that the strategies represented relatively independent ways of coping, and that there were sex differences in coping styles chosen.

A widely used inventory of coping behavior is the Ways of Coping Scale (Folkman & Lazarus, 1980). This 68-item measure includes a broad range of cognitive and coping strategies that may be used by an individual in a specific stressful episode. The strategies were derived from the framework suggested by Lazarus and his colleagues (Lazarus, 1966; Lazarus & Launier, 1978) and from suggestions offered in the coping literature (Mechanic, 1962, 1978; Sidle et al., 1969; Weisman & Worden, 1976). Items included are from the domains of defensive coping, information-seeking, problem-solving, palliation, inhibition of action, direct action, and magical thinking. The checklist is binary with response options of yes or no.

Utilizing 45 items from the Ways of Coping Scale (Folkman & Lazarus, 1980) and 10 items from the works of Pearlin and Schooler (1978), Felton and colleagues (1984) developed a 51-item coping scale to evaluate the utility of a stress and coping paradigm in 170 middle-aged and elderly adults representing four chronic diseases. The coping measure consists of six subscales describing qualitatively distinct coping strategies derived through factor analysis of the items. The researchers concluded that the effects of individual coping efforts on psychological adjustment were modest but that the stress and coping paradigm may be valuable in understanding the adjustment of chronically ill people.

Three coping measures were designed to determine strategies used by adults with chronic mental and physical health problems. Bell (1977) designed an 18-item coping tool to determine long- and short-term coping based on the reality-oriented constructive effort each person has in dealing with long-term stress. Several independent ways of coping were identified, based on works by Menninger and colleagues (1963) and Sidle and colleagues (1969). The tool was administered to 30 inpatient psychiatric patients and a matched control group and did differentiate these groups. The psychiatric group used more short-term coping methods than did the control groups.

In 1981 Jalowiec and Powers developed a rating scale to assess coping responses to stress in acute and chronic illness based on a critical and extensive review of the literature; 40 coping strategies emerged. Content validity for the coping scale was empirically supported by works of authorities in the field of coping (Coelho et al., 1974; Haan, 1977; Hamburg, 1974; Hamburg & Adams, 1967; Lazarus, 1976; Mechanic, 1978; Menninger et al., 1963; Moos, 1977; White, 1974). Coping strategies were differentiated as affective-oriented (handling the emotions evoked by the stressful situation) and problem-oriented (dealing with the situation itself) (Jalowiec & Powers, 1981) by having 20 volunteer judges familiar with behavioral research in stress and coping rate each of the 40 items as problem- or affective-oriented strategies. The researchers reported that classification of coping behaviors into these two categories was consistent with suggestions by Lazarus and Launier (1978). Results of the classification study yielded 15 problem-oriented and 25 affective-oriented ways of coping with stress. Overall agreement on classifying the 40 items was 85%. When this scale was used with patients, Jalowiec and Powers (1981) determined that chronically ill patients used significantly more problem-oriented coping methods than did acutely ill patients.

There is some agreement that strategies that are flexible and reality-oriented and that facilitate the expression of emotion are useful (Haan, 1977). A sense of control is thought to be important for some patients (Janis, 1958). Escape may not be a productive technique because it leaves the patient without important information about the threat (Haan, 1977).

Hymovich (1981, 1983) developed a tool to obtain parental perceptions of their child's chronic illness or disability and information on how parents cope with difficulties they encounter as a result of their child's condition. Following interviews with both parents of 63 children with a variety of health problems, coping strategies identified to manage stressors were grouped into subcategories using the critical incident technique. A closed-ended self-administered questionnaire was then developed.

Adjustment

In the present study, adjustment was conceptualized as the sociological and psychological outcomes of coping with stressors arising out of the interaction between the person and his environment within the context of chronic illness (adapted from Lazarus, 1981). Much of the research on adjustment to chronic illness has focused on either the person who was ill or the spouse and in the context of various settings. The few descriptive studies of COPD patients suggested that they experience deteriorating marital relationships and changes in social behavior and mood, including anxiety, depression, irritability, and paranoia (Agle & Baum, 1977; Barstow, 1974; Dudley, Glaser, Jorgensen, & Logan, 1980; Fishman & Petty, 1971; Hanson, 1982; Kent & Smith, 1977; Krop, Block, & Cohen, 1973; Lester, 1973; Lustig, Hass, & Castillo, 1972; McSweeny, Grant, Heaton, Adams, & Timms, 1982). Similar to coping research, the majority of studies on family adjustment to chronic illness have focused on parents of ill children.

Comparison of research related to family adjustment to chronic illness is difficult because of differences in the conceptualization of and methods used to operationalize adjustment. Several studies used open-ended questions or semistructured interviews to determine adjustment problems (Abram, Moore, & Westervelt, 1971; Bilodeau & Hackett, 1971; Comty, Leonard, & Shapiro, 1974; Cooper, 1984; Kobza, 1983; Shambaugh & Kanter, 1969; Skelton & Dominian, 1973). Most studies have used a single measurement with a predominantly psychological orientation – for example, the Minnesota Multiphasic Personality Inventory (Adsett & Bruhn, 1968; Canter, 1951; Covino, Dirks, Kinsman, & Seidel, 1982; Gilberstadt & Farkas, 1961; Honeyman, Rappaport, Reznikoff, Glueck, & Eisenberg, 1968; Shontz, 1955; Wender & Dominik, 1972), Zung Self-Rating Depression Scale and Taylor Manifest Anxiety Scale (Stern, Pascale, & Ackerman, 1977), the General Health Questionnaire (Livesley, 1981), the Self-Concept Instrument (Brooks & Matson, 1982; Matson & Brooks, 1977), the Interpersonal Dependency Inventory (Zeldow & Pavlou, 1984), the State-Trait Anxiety Inventory, and the Beck Depression Index (Schoeneman et al., 1983). Finally, various life satisfaction scales (Neugarten, Havighurst, & Tobin, 1961) have been used as a measure of adjustment or "morale" (Counte, Bieliauskas, & Pavlou, 1983; Fengler & Goodrich, 1979; Sexton, 1984). Laborde and Powers (1980) employed the Cantril Ladder (Cantril, 1965), an equal-interval, self-anchoring scale to determine "sense of well-being" in hemodialysis patients. Brown, Rawlinson, and Hilles (1981) used the Cantril Ladder to measure three areas of adjustment: life satisfaction, perceived health, and social activity. Harris, Hyman, and Woog (1982) utilized the Shantin's (1970) Situational Attitude Schedule as a measure of morale in preference to the Cantril Ladder because of ease of interpretation. The 10-item Situational Attitude Schedule was originally designed for and tested on chronic medical rehabilitation patients and was considered best suited for within- or between-group studies of changes in morale due to treatment.

Multiple measures have also been used to assess psychological adjustment. In a study of chronically ill persons and spouses, Klein, Dean and Bogdonoff (1967) employed two scales: the Psychophysiologic Distress Index, a 22-item symptom inventory designed to measure emotional disturbance, and the Role Tension Index, a 14-item measure of marital integration. Felton and colleagues (1984) utilized a battery of three tools to determine individual differences in psychological adjustment to four categories of chronic illness: a modified version of Linkowski's (1971) Acceptance of Illness Scale, Bradburn's (1969) Affect Balance Scale, and Rosenberg's (1965) Self-Esteem Scale. Linn, Hunter, and Perry (1979), in addition to 20 items selected from three well-known scales to measure self-esteem (Bown, 1961; Coopersmith, 1967; Rosenberg, 1965), employed the Life Satisfaction Index A and the Hopkin's Symptom Checklist. Linkowski and Dunn (1974) employed the Acceptance of Disability and Self Esteem Scale.

Using a variety of measurements, other researchers have focused on social functioning (Braham et al., 1975; De-Nour, 1982; Dimond,1979; Litman, 1964) and marital adjustment as an indicator of social functioning (Bradford, 1981; Skipper et al., 1968). Weissman and Bothwell (1976) developed a 42-item instrument which measured affective and instrumental performance in six major roles.

Several researchers have conceptualized adjustment as both psychological and sociological. Morrow, Chiarello, and Derogatis (1978) designed the Psychosocial Adjustment to Illness Scale with 45 items covering several domains derived from the authors' experience in clinical practice: health orientation, vocational environment, sexual environment, and psychological distress. Psychometric properties for this scale have been reported (DeVon & Powers, 1984), and it has been used in subsequent studies of chronically ill persons (De-Nour,1982; DeVon & Powers, 1984). In a study of 283 elderly, Linn and associates (1979) also defined adjustment by a combination of psychological and sociological variables: social participation, depression, social function, life satisfaction, and self-esteem. Dimond (1979) employed a 17-item Behavior Morale Scale (MacElveen, 1977) to assess "morale" and the Sickness Impact Profile (SIP) (Gilson, Gilson, & Bergner, 1975) to assess changes in social functioning. Psychometric properties were reported for these scales (Bergner, Bobbitt, Pollard, Martin, & Gilson, 1976). Others who have used the SIP as a measure of social adjustment include Ott and associates (1983) and Zeldow and Pavlou (1984).

CONCEPTUAL FRAMEWORK

The present research is guided by concepts from stress and coping theory, adjustment theory, and general systems theory in an attempt to explain family adjustment to a chronically ill member. The conceptual framework depicted in Figure 12.1 suggests that chronic illness results in stressors to both the person who is ill and to the spouse and that coping behaviors used by these two family members will predict psychological and sociological adjustment. This framework also suggests that the perception of stressors, coping behaviors, and adjustment of one family member influence the same factors among other family members.

Researchers have suggested that in order to understand adjustment to a stressful situation, such as a chronic illness, one should look at coping or responses to the stressors (Cohen & Lazarus, 1979; Moos & Tsu, 1977; Pearlin & Schooler, 1978). Stress and coping theory, as developed by Lazarus (1966), describes coping behavior as goal-directed and responsive to stress. Therefore, more coping behaviors will be evidenced when stress is high. The amount and type of coping behavior is influenced by the individual's cognitive appraisal of the situation (characteristics of the social environment and the nature of the stress), his repertoire of coping

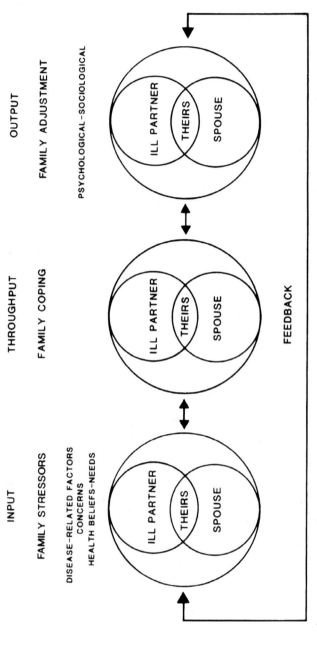

FIGURE 12.1 Conceptual model: family response to chronic illness.

behaviors, and his personal characteristics (Folkman & Lazarus, 1980; Katz, Weiner, Gallagher, & Hellman, 1970; Lazarus, 1966; Wolf & Goodell, 1968). To Lazarus (1966), cognitive appraisal is coping. One individual may cognitively appraise a stressful event as threatening, while another may view the same stressor as challenging. The stress-coping model provides for the wide range of coping styles evidenced in diverse human behavior. Although Lazarus's (1966) work pertains to well individuals, others have used the same or similar concepts to explain adjustment of chronically ill adults (Ben-Sira, 1983; Counte et al., 1983; De-Nour, Shanan, & Garty, 1977-1978; Felton et al., 1984; Matson & Brooks, 1977; Weisman & Worden, 1976) and parents of chronically ill children (Videka-Sherman, 1982).

Adjustment explains how and to what end a person deals with a stressful situation (Russell, 1981). Applied to chronic illness, adjustment is significant in assessing the effects of various coping behaviors in response to stressors produced by the illness (Moos & Tsu, 1977; Felton et al., 1984; White, 1974). Therefore, when stress is high, more coping behaviors are required, and adjustment is likely to be low. Once a person has adjusted to a stressful situation or when stress is low, adjustment is likely to be high and fewer coping behaviors will be required.

Conceptually, adjustment has been described in various ways. One school of thought views adjustment as a psychological state manifested in symptoms or a sense of psychic well-being (Lazarus, 1961), while others define adjustment in terms of social expectations (Weissman & Bothwell, 1976). While the two dimensions are interrelated, in research design they take different operational forms with potentially different results (Russell, 1981). A broad definition of adjustment that considers both behavioral and mental functioning provides a framework for examining the concept along several dimensions.

The term *adjustment* is often used for both the process through which the person goes in dealing with life demands and the outcome the person achieves (Russell, 1981). Seen as an outcome, success in coping with a chronic illness involves the person's acceptance of the illness (Bulman & Wortman, 1977; Cohen & Lazarus, 1979; Felton et al., 1984; Kerr & Thompson, 1972; Russell, 1981; Vash, 1975; Wright, 1960) and is related to one's overall self-esteem. When adjustment is achieved, the person does not deny the fact of illness and the difficulties it produces, nor does self-esteem become overly colored by the illness (Nickerson, 1971). Nickerson suggests that adjustment to an illness means being able to obtain satisfaction within limits imposed by the illness.

White (1974) also views the concept of adjustment as applied to chronic illness as a multiple construct and significant in assessing the positive or negative effects of various coping behaviors. Maintaining a balance of positive feelings toward one's life and the ability to contend with stress are important consequences of effective coping.

General systems theory emphasizes that anything that affects one part of a system affects every other part and the system as a whole (von Bertalanffy, 1968). Applied to the family, this theory implies that the family is an open system in which any condition or event, such as COPD, that affects one member may well affect all members. Essential aspects of application of systems theory are the interaction between the ill partner and spouse related to these variables. Thus, the adjustment of the ill partner and the spouse is not only influenced by each person's own perception of stress and coping behavior but by the partner's as well.

Within the systems model, stress sources are viewed as input variables into the family system and include disease-related factors, concerns, health beliefs, and help needs related to the chronic illness. Family response includes two dimensions: coping behavior and adjustment (psychological and sociological). Coping behavior is viewed as a throughput variable and adjustment as an output variable. Psychological and sociological adjustment is the overall effect of the interrelationship of stress and coping of family members to COPD.

OPERATIONAL DEFINITIONS

An extensive review of the literature led to identification of six instruments as appropriate to measure the concepts included in the study of family response to chronic illness.

> *Stress* was measured through three subscales (Concerns, Health Beliefs, and Help Needs) from the Chronic Impact and Coping Instrument (CICI) (Hymovich, 1981, 1983).
> *Coping* was measured through the Coping Scale (Felton et al., 1984).
> *Psychological adjustment* was measured through three instruments: the Acceptance of Illness Scale (Felton et al., 1984, adapted from Linkowski, 1971); the Self-Esteem Scale (Rosenberg, 1965); and two subscales [Positive Affect Scale (PAS) and Negative Affect Scale (NAS)] from the Affect Balance Scale (ABS) (Bradburn, 1969).
> *Sociological adjustment* was measured through the Sociological Adjustment Scale-Self Report (SAS-SR) (Weissman & Bothwell, 1976).

HYPOTHESES

Reliability was estimated by measuring the internal consistency of each scale or, where the scale was divided into subscales, each subscale. Internal consistency was assessed by testing the following hypothesis.

Hypothesis A: There will be a high internal consistency among items for each of the following subscales and scales: (1) the three CICI subscales; (2) the six Coping Scale subscales; (3) the five SAS-SR subscales; (4) the

Acceptance of Illness Scale; (5) the two ABS subscales; and (6) the Self-Esteem Scale.

Validity was approached in two ways. First, predictions were made about relations between scores, based on relations between constructs given in the conceptual framework. To the extent that these hypotheses were confirmed, the construct validity of the instruments would be supported. *Hypothesis B* predicted that

1. There would be positive correlations between the Coping Scale subscale and total scores, and subscale and total scores on the CICI.
2. There would be positive correlations between the Coping Scale subscale and total scores, and subscale and total scores on the SAS-SR.
3. There would be negative correlations between the Coping Scale subscale and total scores, and scores on the Acceptance of Illness Scale and the PAS.
4. There would be positive correlations between the Coping Scale subscale scores and total scores, and scores on the NAS and the Self-Esteem Scale.
5. There would be negative correlations between the CICI subscale and total scores, and scores on the Acceptance of Illness Scale and the PAS.
6. There would be positive correlations between the CICI subscale and total scores, and scores on the NAS and the Self-Esteem Scale.
7. There would be positive correlations between the CICI subscale and total scores, and subscale and total scores on the SAS-SR.
8. There would be negative correlations between the SAS-SR subscale and total scores, and scores on the Acceptance of Illness Scale and PAS.
9. There would be positive correlations between the SAS-SR subscale and total scores, and scores on the NAS and the Self-Esteem Scale.

The second approach to validity involved relationships among scores purporting to measure the same general construct. It was of interest to determine whether these interrelationships were so weak that they brought into doubt the construct validity of the tools or so strong that they implied redundancy. Thus, *Hypothesis C* stated that

1. There would be moderate positive correlations among the CICI subscale scores.
2. There would be moderate positive correlations among the Coping Scale subscale scores.
3. There would be moderate positive correlations between scores on the Acceptance of Illness Scale and the PAS, and between scores on the Self-Esteem scale and the NAS.

4. There would be moderate negative correlations between the NAS and Self-Esteem Scale scores, and scores on the PAS and the Acceptance of Illness Scale.
5. There would be moderate positive correlations among the SAS-SR subscale scores.

INSTRUMENTS TO BE TESTED

The following instruments were administered to the ill partners and spouses separately and simultaneously and resulted in ordinal level data. In addition, each subject completed a Health Information Form and a Demographic Information Form. The instruments took approximately 30 to 45 min to complete.

Chronic Impact and Coping Instrument (CICI)

This 51-item instrument was designed to assess the impact of a child's chronic illness on the family and coping patterns from the parents' perspective (Hymovich, 1983) with the intent to extend the use of the tool to populations of families in which there is a chronically ill adult (telephone conversation with Dr. Hymovich, 1984). The instrument was developed following critical incident analysis of interviews with 63 parents of children with chronic illness for themes about satisfying and problem areas (stressors) related to living with a chronically ill child and coping strategies used to solve identified problems. The CICI consists of six sections: the child with the condition, the parent completing the questionnaire, the spouse, other children, hospitalization, and "other". Within the sections are subscales concerning information related to stressors and coping. Internal consistency, using Hoyt's coefficient, was .94 for the stressor category and .93 for coping strategies (Hymovich, 1983). Content validity was established using a clinical psychologist, three master's-prepared registered nurses caring for families with chronic disorders, and a doctorally prepared nurse faculty member working with chronically ill adults. For the purpose of this study, three subscales (Concerns, Health Beliefs, and Help Needs) from the parent and spouse sections were adapted and used. The wording was adapted only so that the subscales could be used with chronically ill persons and spouses.

Scoring

The Concerns subscale has items rated on a 5-point continuum from "none/does not apply" to "a great deal"; the Health Beliefs subscale uses a 3-point "agree-disagree" continuum, and the Help Needs subscale a 3-point "no-not sure" continuum. A total score and three subscale scores are obtained, with higher scores indicating higher stress.

Coping Scale

The Coping Scale was developed by Felton and colleagues (1984) to measure coping in a longitudinal study of 151 middle-aged and elderly adults with one of four chronic illnesses (hypertension, diabetes mellitus, cancer, and rheumatoid arthritis). The instrument consists of two open-ended items that ask about the positive and negative effects of chronic illness and six subscales describing qualitatively distinct coping strategies (Cognitive Restructuring, Emotional Expression, Wish-Fulfilling Fantasy, Self-Blame, Information-Seeking, and Threat Minimization) derived through factor analysis of 55 self-report items. Content validity for the scale is supported because 45 of the items were drawn from the Ways of Coping Scale (Folkman & Lazarus, 1980), and 10 items were adapted from the work of Pearlin and Schooler (1978). Cronbach's alpha coefficient reliabilities for the six subscales ranged from .65 to .80.

Scoring

Each item on the scale is rated on a 5-point "never-mostly" continuum to ensure greater variability than the true-false format originally proposed by Folkman and Lazarus (Felton & Revenson, 1984). This scale yields a total score and six subscale scores, with higher scores indicating more frequent use of the strategy. For purposes of this study, only data from the multiple choice items were analyzed.

Acceptance of Illness Scale

This 8-item scale was adapted by Felton et al. (1984) from Linkowski's (1971) Sickness Impact Scale for use in a study of 151 chronically ill adults. It measures success in feeling accepted and valuable despite the disability, dependency, and feelings of uselessness which illness occasions. Felton and Revenson (1984) reported internal consistency alpha coefficients of .83 on initial interview and .81 at 7 months, and test-retest reliability of $r = .69$. Concurrent validity of the original 50-item scale with the Attitudes Toward Disabled scale was demonstrated ($r = .81$) in a study of 46 rehabilitation patients (Linkowski, 1971). Linkowski and Dunn (1974) indicated construct validity by clearly differentiating between two samples of subjects at contrasting points in their rehabilitation.

Scoring

Scale items are rated on a 5-point "agree-disagree" continuum. Higher scores indicate higher acceptance of illness.

Self-Esteem Scale

This 10-item Guttman sale measures overall sense of being capable, worthwhile, and competent (Rosenberg, 1965). Rosenberg reported a coefficient of reproductivity of 0.86 and a coefficient of scalability of

0.59. Felton and colleagues (1984) reported a coefficient alpha of .81 in a sample of chronically ill adults. This scale has been used extensively and found to have high construct validity across diverse samples (Robinson & Shaver, 1973).

Scoring

Items are rated on a 5-point "agree-disagree" continuum. Higher scores indicate lower self-esteem.

Affect Balance Scale (ABS)

This 13-item scale measures positive and negative mood states over recent months (Bradburn, 1969). For the purpose of this study, only data from the 5-item Positive Affect (PAS) and Negative Affect (NAS) subscales were analyzed. The wording was adapted only so that the subscales could be used with chronically ill persons and spouses. Felton and Revenson (1984), in a study of chronically ill adults, obtained internal consistency alpha coefficeints of .72 and of .71 for the PAS and .64 and .63 for the NAS on initial interview and at 7 months, respectively. Test-retest reliability of the PAS was $r = .67$; of the NAS, $r = .64$. Convergent validity was demonstrated in a study of 172 outpatients through high correlations of the PAS with the EASI-III Temperament Survey subscales of Sociability, Tempo, and Vigor and of the NAS with the EASI-III subscales of General Emotionality, Fear, Anger, and Inhibition of Impulse (Costa & McCrae, 1980).

Scoring

Items are rated with 2 points for Yes and 1 point for No. Higher scores indicate higher mood state in the category.

Social Adjustment Scale Self-Report (SAS-SR)

This 52-item scale measures affective and instrumental performance in six major roles: Work Outside the Home, Work at Home, Student, Spare Time, Family, and Children (Weissman & Bothwell, 1976). Each role includes assessment of performance at tasks, interpersonal relationships, inner feelings and satisfaction in roles. The period assessed is two weeks to facilitate recall and accurate reporting of behavior. Edwards, Yarvis, Mueller, Zingale, and Wagman (1978) demonstrated acceptable internal consistency (alpha coefficient .74) and test-retest stability of .80. A comparison of patients and nonpatients indicated that the scale differentiated between these two groups (Weissman, Sholomskas, & John, 1981). Using 25 patients, Weissman and colleagues (1981) demonstrated acceptable criterion validity between the SAS-SR and a Community Adjustment Profile System Questionnaire. Nonsignificant relationships between subscales indicated the differences in emphasis placed on adjustment categories by the two scales. For the purpose of this study, items pertaining to the student role and to single persons were omitted, as these items were considered inappropriate to the study subjects. Wording on the remaining 42 items was adapted only so that they could be used with chronically ill persons and spouses.

Scoring

The SAS-SR is scored on a 5-point Likert scale and yields a total score and six subscores. Higher scores indicate great impairment.

Other Instruments Used

The Health Information Form developed by Felton and colleagues (1984) consists of individual items related to the person's illness in several areas including length of illness, current health status, medical care, treatment demands and adherence, perceived susceptibility and severity of illness, and limitations associated with the illness.

The Demographic Information Form was used to collect demographic information on each subject to supplement data from the scales.

The instruments were combined and presented as a battery to facilitate administration. Two versions of the combined scales resulted and were titled Family Response to Chronic Illness (Ill Partner Version) and Family Response to Chronic Illness (Spouse Version). Copies of the two versions are found at the end of this chapter.

METHODS

Subjects

A convenience nonprobability sample of 18 families (18 ill partners with COPD and 18 spouses) were selected to participate in the study. The specific criteria for inclusion were (1) ill partner 21 years of age or over, (2) ill partner and spouse living together, (3) husband or wife (not both) diagnosed as having COPD (emphysema, chronic bronchitis, and/or asthma, physician-diagnosed) of at least 6 months duration from the date of interview, (4) absence of other significant pulmonary disease (i.e., tuberculosis, fibrosis, or neoplasm) in the ill partner, (5) absence of an acute cardiac disorder (myocardial infarction) in the past 3 months in the ill partner, (6) absence of any physical or mental health problem that would hinder participation (i.e., arthritis, retardation, etc.) in either partner.

Data Collection

A comprehensive COPD treatment center within a large medical center was used to select the study sample. Prior to data collection, trained researchers went to the site to identify and screen potential subjects.

Potential subjects were contacted by telephone to ascertain their willingness to participate. The purpose and protocol for the study were explained to the ill partners and spouses. All potential subjects who indicated a willingness to participate received a packet containing a consent form and a cover letter that outlined the purpose of the study, gave general instructions, and assured confidentiality and anonymity. A copy of the questionnaire and a stamped, addressed return envelope were also included. Thirty-six packets were mailed to the final sample which consisted of 36 subjects: 18 ill persons with COPD and their 18 spouses. The same instruments were used to collect data from patients and spouses using the appropriate version.

Data Analysis

All analyses were done separately for each of the study groups, ill persons and spouses of ill persons. Demographic variables and instrument scores were analyzed using medians, percentages, and ranges to allow description of the study groups. All statistical tests were performed using alpha = .05.

Reliability

The internal consistency reliability of each subscale of the CICI – the Coping Scale, the SAS-SR, and the ABS – and of the Acceptance of Illness Scale and the Self-Esteem Scale was assessed by Cronbach's alpha. The results of these analyses were used to evaluate Hypothesis A, that internal consistency would be high.

Validity

Two sets of hypotheses relating to the validity of the instruments were given: those concerning relationships between conceptual variables (hypotheses B1-B9) and those concerning relationships within conceptual variables (hypotheses C1-C5). Hypotheses B1-B9 and C4-C5 were assessed by Spearman's rho correlation coefficient, which is an appropriate statistic for data assumed to be measured on an ordinal scale. Hypotheses C1-C3 involve determining relationships among additive subscores. Cronbach's alpha coefficients were calculated for each set of subscores (those from the CICI, the Coping Scale, and the SAS-SR), using subscale scores as items, to give an overall index of the degree of consistency among subscale scores.

RESULTS

The 18 ill persons consisted of 15 males and 3 females, aged 34 to 76 years (mean, 67 years). Four had completed high school, and 11 indicated some type of formal education beyond high school. Reported illness duration ranged from 1 to 22 years (mean, 7.5 years); 8 reported having other illnesses or health problems, and 13 rated their health as fair or poor. All ill persons rated their COPD as serious or somewhat serious. The 18 spouses ranged in age from 32 to 79 years (mean, 63.8 years). Five had completed high school, and 11 indicated some type of formal education beyond high school. The majority of couples were Caucasian ($N = 17$) and reported their annual household income as \$21,000 to \$30,000 per year ($N = 12$). The mean length of marriage was 36.9 years.

Descriptive statistics for all instruments for each of the two groups of subjects can be found in Table 12.1.

Reliability

Hypothesis A1 – internal consistency of the scales. Cronbach's alpha coefficients were obtained for each of the CICI subscales, the Coping Scale subscales, the SAS-SR subscales, the Acceptance of Illness Scale, the PAS and NAS subscales, and the Self-Esteem Scale. These values can be found in Table 12.2.

The CICI subscale reliabilities were similar for ill persons and spouses; coefficients for both groups were high for the Concerns subscale, moderate for the Help Needs subscale, and low for the Health Beliefs subscale.

The Coping Scale subscale reliabilities were all moderate in size for the spouses. For the ill person, the coefficients were moderate to high for three of the subscales, and low for the Information-Seeking, Emotional Expression, and Threat Minimization subscales.

The SAS-SR subscale reliabilities were moderate to high for four of the five subscales for the spouses; the coefficient was low only in the Work Outside of Home subscale. For the ill persons, the coefficients were moderate in three of the five subscales nd low in the Spare Time and Family subscales.

The Acceptance of Illness scale and the Self-Esteem scale reliability coefficients were moderate for both ill persons and spouses. The reliability coefficients of the PAS and NAS were low for both spouses and ill persons.

Validity

Hypotheses B1-B4 – relationships between the Coping Scale scores and scores on the CICI, SAS-SR, and psychological adjustment scales. In Hypothesis B1, positive relationships were predicted between measures of coping (Coping Scale subscale and total scores) and stress (CICI subscale and total scores). Significant correlation coefficients are presented in Table 12.3. Notably, there are few significant relationships for the ill persons; there are low positive correlations between Wish-Fulfilling Fantasy Coping and CICI Concerns and Health Beliefs, and a low negative correlation between Threat Minimization Coping and CICI Concerns. More and slightly stronger significant relationships were found for the spouses, including two negative correlations. No significant relationships were

TABLE 12.1 Maximum Possible Score, Actual Range, Mean, and Standard Deviation of the Subscale and Total Scores of All Instruments for Chronically Ill Persons and Spouses

Scale	Maximum possible score	Actual Range I[a]	Actual Range S[b]	Mean I	Mean S	SD I	SD S
CICI (Hymovich, 1981, 1983)							
Concerns	95	0-65	13-95	43.7	50.2	19.5	19.8
Health Beliefs	30	11-24	11-23	16.4	17.7	3.2	3.1
Help Needs	50	11-41	15-41	34.0	27.6	7.2	6.1
Total	175	39-122	50-134	90.61	95.4	21.1	21.8
Coping (Felton et al., 1984)							
Cognitive Restructuring	65	23-57	27-51	37.2	38.7	9.7	6.8
Emotional Expression	40	12-33	8-26	21.2	15.8	5.0	4.9
Wish-Fulfilling Fantasy	35	11-31	7-30	21.9	19.2	6.7	5.9
Self-Blame	35	11-28	7-21	17.6	11.2	4.9	3.7
Information Seeking	25	7-15	5-21	11.1	10.4	2.5	3.7
Threat Minimization	55	20-44	15-39	31.5	28.9	5.4	6.7
Total	255	101-178	81-167	140.7	124.4	21.4	21.3
SAS-SR (Weissman & Bothwell, 1976)							
Work Outside Home	38	0-16	3-16	9.2	9.7	3.5	3.5
Work at Home	38	0-19	0-12	4.1	6.0	5.2	4.3
Spare Time	77	9-27	11-52	17.7	18.2	4.3	9.3
Family	68	7-25	14-29	19.2	20.1	4.7	4.6
Children	51	0-19	1-22	7.6	8.0	4.7	6.0
Total	272	37-80	36-115	59.2	63.5	11.0	17.8
Acceptance of Illness (Felton et al., 1984)	40	11-35	5-34	21.8	24.9	5.2	8.4
ABS[c] (Bradburn, 1969)							
PAS	10	5-10	5-10	7.0	8.3	3.1	2.0
NAS	10	5-8	5-9	5.6	5.9	1.6	1.4
Self-Esteem (Rosenberg, 1965)	50	29-46	22-41	36.9	35.4	4.6	5.0

[a]Ill person.
[b]Spouse.
[c]1 ill person and 1 spouse did not respond to all items on the ABS.

found between total Coping Scale scores and CICI scores; the CICI total score was significantly related to only one Coping Scale score (Self-Blame subscore, spouse group only).

In Hypothesis B2, positive relationships between measures of coping (Coping Scale subscale and total scores) and sociological adjustment (SAS-SR subscale and total scores) were predicted. Significant correlations coefficients are presented in Table 12.3. Few significant relationships were found for ill persons: total Coping Scale score was not related to any of the SAS-SR scores, and the total SAS-SR score was related

TABLE 12.2 Internal Consistency Reliability: Coefficient Alpha of All Instruments

	Alpha Value	
Scale	Ill Persons	Spouses
CICI (Hymovich, 1981, 1983)		
Concerns	.90	.93
Health Beliefs	.56	.50
Help Needs	.78	.84
Coping (Felton et al., 1984)		
Cognitive Restructuring	.90	.84
Emotional Expression	.58	.82
Wish-Fulfilling Fantasy	.88	.80
Self-Blame	.73	.73
Information-Seeking	.22	.77
Threat Minimization	.62	.72
SAS-SR (Weisman & Bothwell, 1976)		
Work Outside Home	.84	.49
Work at Home	.83	.82
Spare Time	.58	.91
Family	.60	.71
Children	.71	.87
Acceptance of Illness (Felton et al., 1984)	.72	.88
ABS (Bradburn, 1969)		
PAS	.62	.42
NAS	.18	.64
Self-Esteem (Rosenberg, 1965)	.76	.87

(negatively) only to one Coping Scale subscore, Threat Minimization; two low positive correlations were found between Coping Scale subscores and SAS-SR subscores. Among the spouses, there were many low to moderate significant correlations between Coping Scale scores and SAS-SR scores; all were positive.

In Hypothesis B3, negative correlations were predicted between measures of coping (Coping Scale subscale and total scores) and two measures of psychological adjustment (the Acceptance of Illness Scale score and the PAS score); and in hypothesis B4, positive correlations were predicted between the measures of coping and scores on the Self-Esteem Scale and the NAS. Significant correlations related to these hypotheses are presented in Table 12.3. Among ill persons, three significant coefficients were found, and all were positive; the correlation between the PAS score and one of the subscales was in the opposite direction from that predicted, but the correlation between the Self-Esteem Scale scores and two of the subscales was in the predicted direction. Among spouses, 10 significant coefficients were found, and all were in the predicted direction. Negative correlations were found between Acceptance of Illness score and Coping Scale scores; positive correlations were found between the NAS and Self-Esteem Scale scores and Coping Scale scores.

Hypotheses B5-B7 – relationships between CICI scores and scores on the SAS-SR and psychological adjustment scales. In these hypotheses, negative correlations were predicted between measures of stress (CICI subscale and total scores) and two measures of psychological adjustment (Acceptance of Illness Scale score and PAS score); positive correlations were predicted between measures of stress and scores on the SAS-SR, the Self-Esteem Scale, and the NAS. Significant correlation coefficients relevant to these hypotheses are found in Table 12.4. No significant correlations were found between CICI scores and scores on the PAS or the Self-Esteem Scale. Positive correlations between one of the CICI subscores and the NAS were found in each group (Concerns for the ill and Help Needs for the spouse), as predicted. Negative correlations were found between CICI scores and Acceptance of Illness Scale score in the ill group, consistent with predictions, but a positive correlation was found in the spouse group, contrary to prediction. There was no significant correlation between CICI total score and SAS-SR scores; nor between SAS-SR total scores and any CICI scores. There were a few low positive correlations among subscores on the CICI and SAS-SR, and no negative ones, consistent in direction with predictions.

Hypotheses B8-B9 – relationships between measures of sociological and psychological adjustment. In the hypotheses, negative correlations were predicted between scores on the SAS-SR and scores on the Acceptance of Illness Scale and the PAS. Positive correlations were predicted between SAS-SR scores and scores on the NAS and the Self-Esteem Scale. Significant correlation coefficients relevant to these hypotheses are found to be significantly correlated with SAS-SR total scores; they were negatively correlated (consistent with prediction) with the SAS-SR Spare Time subscore for ill persons and with the SAS-SR Work Outside Home subscore for spouses. The PAS scores were not significantly correlated with spouses' SAS-SR scores, but they were positively correlated with SAS-SR Work Outside Home (contrary to prediction) and negatively correlated with SAS-SR Spare Time (as predicted) for ill persons. The NAS scores were not significantly correlated with ill persons' SAS-SR scores, but they were positively correlated (as predicted) with SAS-SR Spare Time, Family, and total scores. Self-Esteem scale scores were significantly correlated with SAS-SR Children and total scores (positively, as predicted) for the spouses; they were significantly correlated with SAS-SR Spare Time in both groups (positively, as predicted).

Hypotheses C1-C3 – relationships among subscales. Contrary to prediction, the subscales of the CICI were not found to be positively interrelated, as indicated by the Cronbach's alpha coefficients (calculated using subscale scores as items) of .01 for ill persons and .03 for spouses. Among the subscale scores of the Coping Scale there were many moderate-sized, positive intercorrelations, reflected in Cronbach's alpha coefficients of .60 for ill persons and .72 for spouses. This finding was consistent with predictions. Relations among the subscale scores on the SAS-SR differed between ill persons and spouses, and findings for the spouse group were more consistent with predictions than findings for the ill group. Intercorrelations among subscale scores of the ill persons were low, and many were negative; this results in a Cronbach's alpha coefficient of .17. For spouses, intercorrelations among subscale scores were moderate and mostly positive; Cronbach's alpha was .53.

Hypotheses C4-C5 – relationships among psychological adjustment scales. There were several correlations of low to moderate significance ($p < .05$) among these scores, and all were in the predicted directions. The Acceptance of Illness Scale scores were positively correlated with PAS scores ($r = .56$ in each group and negatively correlated with Self-Esteem Scale scores ($r = -.55$ for ill persons and $4 = -.41$ for spouses). The PAS scores were negatively correlated with Self-Esteem Scale scores ($r = -.78$) only for the ill persons.

DISCUSSION

Reliability

Results of this study suggest that two of the CICI stress subscales (Concerns and Help Needs) were reliable for ill persons and spouses. Because the Health Beliefs subscale showed low internal consistency for both

TABLE 12.3 Significant Spearman rho Correlations Between the Coping Scale Scores and Scores on the CICI and the Adjustment Measures: SAS-SR, Acceptance of Illness Scale, ABS Scale, and Self-Esteem Scale

Scale	Cognitive restructuring		Emotional expression	
	I[a]	S[b]	I	S
CICI (Hymovich, 1981, 1983)				
Concerns	–	–	–	.44*
Health Beliefs	–	–.42*	–	–
Help Needs	–	–	–	–
Total	–	–	–	–
SAS-SR (Weissman & Bothwell, 1976)				
Work Outside Home	–	–	–	.49*
Work at Home	–	–	–	–
Spare Time	–	–	.45*	.60*
Family	–	–	–	.43*
Children	–	–	–	.48*
Total	–	–	–	.59*
Acceptance of Illness (Felton et al., 1984)	–	–	–	–.60*
ABS (Bradburn, 1969)				
PAS	–	–	–	–
NAS	–	–	–	.40*
Self-Esteem (Rosenberg, 1965)	–	–	.54*	.56*

[a]Ill persons.
[b]Spouses.
* $p < .05$ or lower.

groups, the reliability of this subscale cannot be inferred. The results are otherwise consistent with those of Hymovich (1983), who reported reliabilities ranging from .93 to .94 on the subscales and on overall reliability of the total scale of .95. The Health Beliefs subscale items relate to views about things that influence a person's life-style. The instrument was developed through interviews of parents of ill children, while in this study subjects included spouse pairs where one member was ill. The Health Beliefs subscale may require revision before it can be reliably used in populations other than the one for which it was developed.

Acceptable internal consistency was demonstrated for the six Coping Scale subscales for spouses. For ill persons, three subscales demonstrated acceptable internal consistency. Low consistency was obtained for Emotional expression and Threat minimization items; very low consistency for Information-seeking items. These results were similar to those reported by Felton and colleagues (1984). In a study of coping in patients faced with one of four chronic illnesses (hypertension, diabetes mellitus, cancer, and rheumatoid arthritis) those authors reported reliability coefficients ranging from .65 to .80; the lowest coefficients for Threat minimization (.65) and Information-seeking (.67); the highest for Cognitive restructuring (.80). It might be thought that the low coefficient for Information-Seeking by ill persons in the present study was due to the fact that this group was a relatively well-informed population and therefore

| Coping Scale (Felton et al., 1984) | | | | | | | | | |
| Wish-fulfilling fantasy | | Self-Blame | | Information seeking | | Threat minimization | | Total | |
I	S	I	S	I	S	I	S	I	S
.40*	.49*	–	.40*	–	–	–.44*	–	–	–
.47*	–	–	–	–	–	–	–.60*	–	–
–	–	–	.58*	–	–	–	–	–	–
–	–	–	.56*	–	–	–	–	–	–
–	–	–	–	–	–	–	.48*	–	.53*
–	–	–	–	–	–	–	–	–	–
–	.42*	–	.51*	–	.65*	–	–	–	.66*
–	–	–	.46*	–	.61*	–	–	–	.50*
.48*	.40*	–	–	–	.43*	–	–	–	.43*
–	.47*	–	.39*	–	.62*	–.41*	.34	–	.70*
–	–.58*	–	–.42*	–	–	–	–	–	–.45*
–	–	.40*	–	–	–	–	–	–	–
–	–	–	.70*	–	–	–	–	–	–
–	–	.43*	.48*	–	.45*	–	–	–	.51*

Table 12.4 Significant Spearman rho Correlations Between the CICI Scores and Scores on the Adjustment Measures: SAS-SR, Acceptance of Illness Scale, ABS, and Self-Esteem Scale

| | CICI (Hymovich, 1981, 1983) | | | | | | | |
| | Concerns | | Health Beliefs | | Help Needs | | Total | |
Scale	I[a]	S[b]	I	S	I	S	I	S
SAS-SR (Weissman & Bothwell, 1976)								
Work Outside Home	–	–	–	–	–	–	–	–
Work at Home	–	–	–	–	–	–	–	–
Spare Time	.39*	–	–	–	–	–	–	–
Family	–	–	–	–	–	.46*	–	–
Children	–	–	.41*	–	–	–	–	–
Total	–	–	–	–	–	–	–	–
Acceptance of Illness (Felton et al., 1984)	–.47*	–	.45*	–	–	–	–.34*	–
ABS (Bradburn, 1969)								
PAS	–	–	–	–	–	–	–	–
NAS	.43*	–	–	–	–	.62*	–	–
Self-Esteem Scale (Rosenberg, 1965)	–	–	–	–	–	–	–	–

[a]Ill persons.
[b]Spouses.
* $p < .5$ or lower.

Table 12.5 Significant Spearman rho Correlations Between the SAS-SR Scores and Scores on the Psychological Adjustment Measures: Acceptance of Illness Scale, ABS, and Self-Esteem Scale

| | Acceptance of Illness (Felton et al., 1984) | | ABS (Bradburn, 1969) | | | | Self-Esteem (Rosenberg, 1965) | |
| | | | PAS | | NAS | | | |
Scale	I[a]	S[b]	I	S	I	S	I	S
SAS-SR (Weissman & Bothwell, 1976)								
Work Outside Home	–	–.55*	.41*	–	–	–	–	–
Work at Home	–	–	–	–	–	–	–	–
Spare Time	–.56*	–	–.51*	–	–	.38*	.42*	.51*
Family	–	–	–	–	–	.59*	–	–
Children	–	–	–	–	–	–	–	.54*
Total	–	–	–	–	–	.34*	–	.59*

[a]Ill persons.
[b]Spouses.
* $p < .05$ or lower.

did not indicate these items as coping behaviors. However, item means and variances were not generally lower for ill persons than for spouses, so this does not account for the difference.

Sociological adjustment (SAS-SR) subscales demonstrated acceptable internal consistency, except for the dimensions of Spare Time and Family for ill persons and Work Outside the Home for spouses. However, in agreement with Edwards and colleagues (1974), we conclude that, while Cronbach's alpha provides an estimate of internal consistency, it is not an appropriate measure of the reliability of the scores because the tool uses branching logic to have subjects skip inappropriate items. Thus, all subjects who were inactive in a particular role did not provide data for items related to that role. This bias was extreme in our study; very small sample sizes were involved in calculations for the subscales of Work Outside Home, Work at Home, and Children; thus, these values cannot be regarded as accurate, even as estimates of internal consistency. Most subjects were included in calculations for Spare Time and Family.

Of the four measures of psychological adjustment, Acceptance of Illness and Self-Esteem demonstrated acceptable internal consistency by both groups. Low consistency was demonstrated for PAS and the NAS. Felton and colleagues (1984), studying chronically ill subjects, estimated the highest reliability on the Acceptance of Illness Scale (alpha = .83), followed by Self Esteem (alpha = .81), and the PAS and NAS (alpha = .64, respectively). Our data from the spouses led to very similar estimates for the PAS and NAS. In this study, ill persons had COPD, a diagnostic group not included in the study by Felton and colleagues (1984). Perhaps symptoms associated with COPD influenced their response to the NAS. Although spouses in this study were not an ill group, living with a chronically ill partner may have influenced their responses to subscale items, particularly PAS.

Validity

It was assumed that specific stressors would be more closely related to certain coping behaviors than to others, and that the pattern of relationships might differ between ill persons and spouses. It was also assumed that while coping and adjustment are usual outcomes of disease-related stressors, they were measures of two distinctly different concepts. Varying levels of correlations between Coping Scale scores and scores on the CICI, SAS-SR, and psychological adjustment scale were therefore expected.

Significant correlations between scores on the Coping Scale and the CICI were unexpectedly few for both groups; those observed were not strong, and some were negative, contrary to expectations. The pattern of relationship differed between ill persons and spouses. These results do not support the idea that increases in stress (in general) lead to increases in coping (in general). The higher correlations in the spouses than in the ill persons may indicate that one or both of these measurement scales is more valid for spouses than for ill persons. On the other hand, they may indicate that the link between stress and coping is stronger among spouses than among ill persons. Spouses differed from the ill persons in that they were not suffering from COPD and they were predominantly female; perhaps such people are less responsive to stress. The failure to find a relationship between total coping and stress, and the existence of some negative correlations between stress and particular coping subscores (Threat Minimization and Cognitive Restructuring), may indicate that some types of coping are a response to stress and so are positively correlated with it, while other types reduce or prevent stress (as measured on the CICI) and so are negatively correlated with it.

Only two correlations between scores on the Coping Scale and the SAS-SR were significant for ill persons (one positive, one negative); many were significant for spouses (all positive). The data from spouses indicates that more coping is done by those with the higher adjustment scores, that is, those who are less well adjusted. The lack of correlation among the ill persons may be due to the subjects' frequently indicated complete absence of certain roles.

Several significant correlations between Coping Scale subscales and psychological scales did emerge for ill persons and spouses, and nearly all were in the predicted direction. Using multiple regression analyses and controlling for medical diagnoses, Felton and colleagues (1984) determined correlations between the Coping Scale subscales and psychological scales used in this study. Although the statistical method used to determine correlations differed, the results do allow for comparison between the two studies. Significant correlations were found between Acceptance of Illness and Emotional Expression, Wish-Fulfilling Fantasy and Self-Blame; between NAS and Self-Blame; and between Self-Esteem and Emotional Expression for spouses in this study and patients in the study by Felton and colleagues (1984). A significant correlation was also found between PAS and Self-Blame for ill persons and patients in the study by Felton and colleagues (1984). The direction of the correlations between coping and adjustment measures implies that the higher the level of adjustment in selected areas, the less selected coping behaviors were utilized. Therefore, the hypothesis was partially supported.

The generally low correlations between CICI stress scores and SAS-SR scores for both groups were in the direction expected. The higher the stress level, the greater the level of impairment for both groups in ability to function in usual social roles. Correlations between stress subscales and psychological adjustment scales for both groups were also generally low. There was an unexpected positive correlation between CICI Health Beliefs and the Acceptance of Illness Scale for ill persons. The low correlations suggest that the scales discriminate between the concepts of stress and adjustment.

Moderate correlations between sociological adjustment subscales and psychological adjustment scales had been predicted and were observed in ill persons and spouses. In addition, nearly all of the correlations for both groups were in the predicted direction. These results support the idea that sociological aspects and psychological aspects are two distinct dimensions of adjustment which are positively related.

High correlations between the three CICI stress subscales had been predicted. The low alpha correlations that were obtained indicated low consistency among subscales for both groups. This indicates that the subscales measure independent aspects of stressors or different types of stressors.

The observed moderate-size, positive correlations among the six Coping Scale subscales had been predicted. Although comparison data were unavailable, this implied that there is a tendency for heavy users of one type of coping strategy to use other types heavily as well. This may be partially due to common causation. On the other hand, subscore intercorrelations were not so high that one would regard the subscores as all measures of the same thing.

The majority of subscale intercorrelations were low for both groups, suggesting that the six coping behaviors represent relatively independent ways of coping.

Moderate-size positive subscale intercorrelations had been predicted for the measure of sociological adjustment (SAS-SR). The majority of correlations for both groups was .35 or below, with ill persons obtaining many negative intercorrelations and generally lower intercorrelations than did spouses. A limitation of this scale is that subjects with any absence of roles are given minimum scores for the corresponding subscales. Minimum scores indicate maximum adjustment. The validity of this scoring method is questionable. Absence of roles occurred more often among ill persons than among spouses. Thus, this problem has its greatest influence in the ill group, but it potentially affects the validity of subscale and total scores in all populations. It may account for the previously mentioned failure of scores on this tool to correlate as strongly as expected with scores on other tools, especially among the ill persons. However, the results among spouses imply that the subscores each assess a separate and relatively independent area of adjustment.

Initially, moderate to high correlations among the four measures of psychological adjustment had been expected. However, the only significant correlations were between scores on the Acceptance of Illness Scale and scores on the PAS and Self-Esteem Scale (both ill and spouses) and, for ill persons only, between the PAS score and the Self-Esteem scale score. All of these correlations were in the predicted direction. The findings of insignificant, moderate-size, or inconsistent (between groups) correlations among the four scales supports the notion that psychological adjustment is multi-dimensional, necessitating the use of a variety of measurements.

IMPLICATIONS

Carmines and Zeller (1979) suggest that although it is difficult to specify a single level of reliability that should apply in all situations, reliabilities should not be below .80 for widely used scales. Only four of the 18 subscales and scales for which internal consistency-reliability was assessed met this standard in both groups; six others met it in one group of subjects. Reliability problems were most severe on the ABS, one of the CICI subscales, three of the Coping Scale subscales, and three of the SAS-SR subscales. The appropriateness of the internal consistency approach to estimating the reliability of the SAS-SR was questioned.

Results of the study suggest that the total scores on the CICI and Coping Scales were invalid and did not correlate with measures with which they were expected to correlate. Subscale scores on the two scales appeared to be more valid than the total scores. Scales used to measure psychological adjustment (Acceptance of Illness, Self-Esteem, and ABS) appeared to be valid. The SAS-SR appeared to be invalid for both groups, particularly for the ill group, where inactivity in roles may be unavoidable. In older well groups, such as the spouse group, inactivity in certain roles – work, children, and family – are generally expected.

Correlations among the subscales and scales related to each of the constructs of stress, coping, and adjustment reached respectable levels: low for stress, moderate for coping, low to moderate for sociological adjustment, and low to moderate for psychological adjustment scales. Failure to reach higher correlations, however, argues for the inclusion of the subscales and scales in further assessments. Relative to coping and adjustment, research should not focus solely on outcome but should study process, for a successful outcome may be arrived at through the use of a number of different behaviors. Further, the data support the notion that the subscale scores of the CICI, Coping Scale, and SAS-SR should be interpreted as measures of different but related concepts.

The significance of this study is its potential contribution to the psychometric evaluation of six existing instruments to assess stress, coping, and adjustment of married couples in which one partner has a chronic illness. These instruments may be useful to nurses in delineating specific difficulties and/or problems in families experiencing a chronic illness. The results may also enable nurses to generate hypotheses to further family response to chronic illness. Specific data can be translated into guidelines in the development of health policy and programs. Results will also provide an initial base for developing and testing interventions for working with families to achieve positive rather than negative outcomes. The end goal is to improve the quality of life for these families and possibly reduce institutionalization of the ill partner due to chronic illness.

REFERENCES

Abram, H. S., Moore, G. L., & Westervelt, F. B. (1971). Suicide behavior in chronic dialysis patients. *American Journal of Psychiatry, 127,* 1199-1207.

Adams, J. E., & Lindemann, E. (1977). Coping with long-term disability. In G. V. Coelho, D. A. Hamburg, & J. E. Adams (Eds.), *Coping and adaptation* (pp. 127-138). New York: Basic Books.

Adsett, C. A., & Bruhn, J. G. (1968). Short-term group psychotherapy for post-myocardial infarction patients and their wives. *Canadian Medical Association Journal, 99,* 557-584.

Agle, D. P., & Baum, G. L. (1977). Psychological aspects of chronic obstructive pulmonary disease. *Medical Clinics of North America, 61,* 749-758.

American Lung Association (1982). *Report of task force on comprehensive and continuing care for patients with COPD.* New York: Author.

Apley, J. (1974). The significance of life events. *Developmental Medicine and Child Neurology, 16,* 218-219.

Barstow, R. E. (1974). Coping with emphysema. *Nursing Clinics of North America, 9,* 137-145.

Bell, J. M. (1977). Stressful life events and coping methods in mental-illness and -wellness behaviors. *Nursing Research, 26,* 136-141.

Ben-Sira, Z. (1983). Loss, stress and readjustment: The structure of coping with bereavement and disability. *Social Science Medicine, 17,* 1619-1632.

Bergner, M., Bobbitt, R. A., Pollard, W. E., Martin, D. P., & Gilson, B. S. (1976). The Sickness Impact Profile: Validation of a health status measure. *Medical Care, 14,* 57-67.

Billings, A. G., & Moos, R. H. (1981). The role of coping responses and social resources in attenuating the stress of life events. *Journal of Behavioral Medicine, 4,* 139-157.

Bilodeau, C. B., & Hackett, T. P. (1971). Issues raised in a group setting by patients recovering from myocardial infarction. *American Journal of Psychiatry, 128,* 73-78.

Binger, C. M., Ablin, A. R., Feuerstein, R. C., Kushner, J. H., Zoger, S., & Mikkelsen, C. (1969). Childhood leukemia. Emotional impact on patient and family. *New England Journal of Medicine, 280,* 414-418.

Bown, O. H. (1961). The development of a self-report inventory and its function in a mental health assessment battery. *American Psychologist, 16,* 402.

Bradburn, N. (1969). *The structure of psychological well-being.* Chicago: Aldine.

Bradford, R. J. (1981). Relationships among marital adjustment, chest pain, and anxiety in myocardial infarction patients. *Issues in Mental Health Nursing, 3,* 381-397.

Braham, S., Houser, H. B., Cline, A., & Posner, M. (1975). Evaluation of the social needs of nonhospitalized chronically ill persons. *Journal of Chronic Disease, 28,* 401-419.

Brooks, N. A., & Matson, R. R. (1982). Social-psychological adjustment to multiple sclerosis. *Social Science Medicine, 16,* 2129-2135.

Brown, J. S., Rawlinson, M. E., & Hilles, N. C. (1981). Life satisfaction and chronic disease: Exploration of a theoretical model. *Medical Care, 19,* 1136-1146.

Bruhn, J. (1977). Effects of chronic illness on the family. *Journal of Family Practice, 4,* 1057-1060.

Bulman, R. J., & Wortman, C. B. (1977). Attributions of blame and coping in the "real world": Severe accident victims react to their lot. *Journal of Personality and Social Psychology, 35,* 351-363.

Canter, A. H. (1951). MMPI Profiles in multiple sclerosis. *Journal of Consulting Psychology, 15,* 253-256.

Cantril, H. (1965). *The pattern of human concern.* New Brunswick, NJ: Rutgers University Press.

Carmines, E. G., & Zeller, R. A. (1979). *Reliability and validity assessment.* Beverly Hills, CA: Sage.

Carter, V. L. (1979). Life change events and myocardial infarction. *Circulation Abstracts, 60,* 11-102.

Chapman, J. M., Reeder, L. G., Massey, F. J., Borum, E. R., Picken, B., Browning, C. G., Coulson, A. H., & Zimmerman, D. H. (1966). Relationship of stress, tranquilizers and serum cholesterol levels in a sample population under stress for coronary heart disease. *American Journal of Epidemiology, 83,* 537-547.

Chodoff, P., Friedman, S., & Hamburg, D. A. (1964). Stress, defenses, and coping behavior: Observations in parents with malignant disease. *American Journal of Psychiatry, 120,* 743-749.

Coelho, G. V., Hamburg, D. A., & Adams, J. E. (Eds.) (1974). *Coping and adaptation.* New York: Basic Books.

Coelho, G. V., Silber, E., & Hamburg, D. A. (1962). Use of the student-TAT to assess coping behavior in hospitalized, normal and exceptionally competent college freshmen. *Perceptual and Motor Skills, 14,* 355-365.

Cohen, F., & Lazarus, R. S. (1979). Coping with stresses of illness. In G. C. Stone, N. E. Adler, & F. Cohen (Eds.), *Health Psychology* (pp. 217-254). San Francisco: Jossey-Bass.

Comty, C. M., Leonard A., & Shapiro F. L. (1974). Psychosocial problems in dialyzed diabetic patients. *Kidney International, 6,* Suppl. 1, 144-153.

Cooper, E. T. (1984). A pilot study on the effects of the diagnosis of lung cancer on family relationships. *Cancer Nursing, 1,* 301-308.

Coopersmith, S. (1967). *The antecedents of self-esteem.* San Francisco: W. H. Freeman.

Costa, P. T., & McCrae, R. R. (1980). Influence of extraversion and neuroticism on subjective well-being: Happy and unhappy people. *Journal of Personality and Social Psychology, 38,* 668-678.

Counte, M. A., Bieliauskas, L. A., & Pavlou, M. (1983). Stress and personal attitudes in chronic illness. *Archives of Physical Medicine and Rehabilitation, 64,* 272-275.

Covino, N. A., Dirks, J. F., Kinsman, R. A., & Siedel, J. V. (1982). Patterns of depression in chronic illness. *Psychotherapeutic Psychosomatics, 37,* 144-153.

Croog, S. H., & Fitzgerald, E. F. (1978). Subjective stress and serious illness of a spouse: Wives of heart patients. *Journal of Health and Social Behavior, 19,* 166-178.

De-Nour, A. K. (1982). Social adjustment of chronic dialysis patients. *American Journal of Psychiatry, 139,* 97-100.

De-Nour, A. K., Shanan, J., & Garty, I. (1977-1978). Coping behavior and intelligence in the prediction of vocational rehabilitation. *International Journal of Psychiatry in Medicine, 8,* 145-158.

Derogatis, L. R., Abeloff, M. D., & Melisaratos, N. (1979). Psychological coping mechanisms and survival time in metastatic breast cancer. *Journal of American Medical Association, 242,* 1504-1508.

DeVon, H. A., & Powers, M. J. (1984). Health beliefs, adjustment to illness and control of hypertension. *Research in Nursing and Health, 7,* 10-16.

Dimond, M. (1979). Social support and adaptation to chronic illness: The case of maintenance hemodialysis. *Research in Nursing and Health, 2,* 101-108.

Dracup, K. (1982). Psychosocial aspects of coronary heart disease. *Implications for Nursing Research, 4,* 257-279.

Dudley, D. L., Glaser, E. M., Jorgensen, B. N., & Logan, D. L. (1980). Psychosocial concomitants to rehabilitation in chronic obstructive pulmonary disease: Part I. Psychosocial and psychological consideration. *Chest, 77-, 413-420.*

Dyk, R. B., & Sutherland, A. M. (1956). Adaptation of the spouse and other family members of the colostomy patient. *Cancer, 9,* 123-138.

Edwards, D. W., Yarvis, R. M., Mueller, D. P., Zingale, H. C., & Wagman, W. J. (1978). Test-taking and the stability of adjustment scales: Can we assess patient deterioration? *Evaluation Review, 2,* 275-292.

Felton, B. J., & Revenson, T. A. (1984). Coping with chronic illness: A study of illness controllability and the influence of coping strategies on psychological adjustment. *Journal of Consulting and Clinical Psychology, 52,* 343-353.

Felton, B. J., Revenson, T. A., & Hinrichsen, G. A. (1984). Stress and coping in the explanation of psychological and adjustment among chronically ill adults. *Social Science Medicine, 18,* 889-898.

Fengler, A. P., & Goodrich, N. (1979). Wives of elderly disabled men: The hidden patients. *The Gerontologist, 19,* 175-183.

Fishman, D. B., & Petty, T. L. (1971). Physical, symptomatic, and psychological improvement in patients receiving comprehensive care for chronic air-way obstruction. *Journal of Chronic Diseases, 24,* 775-785.

Folkman, S., & Lazarus, R. S. (1980). An analysis of coping in a middle-aged community sample. *Journal of Health and Social Behavior, 21,* 219-239.

Fontana, A. F., Marcus, J. L., Noel, B. A., & Rakusin, J. M. (1972). Prehospitalization coping styles of psychiatric patients: The goal-directedness of life events. *The Journal of Nervous and Mental Disease, 155,* 311-321.

Friedman, S. B., Chodoff, P., Mason, J. W., & Hamburg, D. A. (1963). Behavioral observations on patients anticipating the death of a child. *Pediatrics, 32,* 610-625.

Gilberstadt, H., & Farkas, E. (1961). Another look at MMPI profile types in multiple sclerosis. *Journal of Consulting Psychology, 25,* 440-444.

Gilson, B. S., Gilson, J. S., & Bergner, M. (1975). The Sickness Impact Profile: Development of an outcome measure of health care. *American Journal of Public Health, 65,* 1304-1310.

Gorsuch, R. L., & Key, M. K. (1974). Abnormalities of pregnancy as a function of anxiety and life stress. *Psychosomatic Medicine, 36,* 352-362.

Grad, J., & Sainsburg, P. (1968). The effects that patients have on their families in a community care and a control psychiatric service – a two year follow up. *British Journal of Psychiatry, 114,* 265-278.

Graham, S., & Reeder, L. G. (1972). Social factors in the chronic diseases. In H. E. Freeman, S. Levine, and Reeder, L. G. (Eds.), *Handbook of medical sociology* (pp. 63-107). Englewood Cliffs, NJ: Prentice-Hall.

Haan, N. (1977). *Coping and defending.* New York: Academy Press.

Hamburg, D. A. (1974). Coping behavior in life-threatening circumstance. *Psychotherapeutic Psychosomatics, 23,* 13-25.

Hamburg, D. A., & Adams, J. E. (1967). A perspective on coping behavior. *Archives of General Psychiatry, 17,* 277-284.

Hanson, E. I. (1982). Effects of chronic lung disease on life in general and on sexuality: Perceptions of adults patients. *Heart and Lung, 11,* 435-441.

Harris, R. B., Hyman, R. B., & Woog, P. (1982). Survival rates and coping styles of maintenance hemodialysis patients. *Nephrology Nurse, 4,* 30-39.

Holmes, T., & Rahe, R. (1967). The social readjustment rating scale. *Journal of Psychosomatic Research, 2,* 213-218.

Honeyman, M. S., Rappaport, H., Reznikoff, M., Glueck, B. C., & Eisenberg, H. (1968). Psychological impact of heart disease in the family of the patient. *Psychosomatics, 9,* 34-37.

Hymovich, D. P. (1981). Assessing the impact of chronic childhood illness on the family and parent coping. *Image, 13,* 71-73.

Hymovich, D. P. (1983). The chronicity impact and coping instrument: Parent questionnaire. *Nursing Research, 32,* 275-281.

IMS America. (1981, October). *National Disease and Therapeutic Index (NDTI) Monthly Report,* section III.

Jalowiec, A., & Powers, M. J. (1981). Stress and coping in hypertensive and emergency room patients. *Nursing Research, 30,* 10-15.

Janis, I. L. (1958). *Psychological stress.* New York: John Wiley.

Jenkins, C. D. (1971). Psychological and social precursors of coronary disease: Part II. *New England Journal of Medicine, 284,* 244-245, 307-317.

Katz, J. L., Weiner, H., Gallagher, T. F., & Hellman, L. (1970). Stress, distress, and ego defenses. *Archives of General Psychiatry, 23,* 131-142.

Kent, D. L., & Smith, J. K. (1977). Psychological implications of pulmonary disease. *Clinical Notes on Respiratory Disease, 16,* 3-11.

Kerr, W. G., & Thompson, M. A. (1972). Acceptance of disability of sudden onset in paraplegia. *Paraplegia, 10,* 94-102.

Klein, R. F., Dean, A., & Bogdonoff, M. D. (1967). The impact of illness upon the spouse. *Journal of Chronic Disease, 20,* 241-248.

Kobza, L. (1983). Impact of ostomy upon the spouse. *Journal of Enterostomal Therapy, 10,* 54-57.

Krop, H. D., Block, A. J., & Cohen, E. (1973). Neuropsychologic effects of continuous oxygen therapy in chronic obstructive pulmonary disease. *Chest, 64,* 317-322.

Kupst, M. J., Blatterbauer, S., Westman, J., Schulman, J. L., & Pard, M. H. (1977). Helping parents with the diagnosis of congenital heart defect: An experimental study. *Pediatrics, 59,* 266-272.

Laborde, J. M., & Powers, M. J. (1980). Satisfaction with life for patients undergoing hemodialysis and patients suffering from osteoarthritis. *Research in Nursing and Health, 3,* 19-24.

Lazarus, R. S. (1961). *Adjustment and personality.* New York: McGraw-Hill.

Lazarus, R. S. (1966). *Psychological stress and the coping process.* New York: McGraw-Hill.

Lazarus, R. S. (1976). *Patterns of adjustment* (3rd ed.). New York: McGraw-Hill.

Lazarus, R. S. (1981). The stress and coping paradigm. In C. Eisdorfer, D. Cohen, A. Kleinman, & P. Maxim (Eds.), *Models for Clinical Psychopathology* (pp. 177-222). New York: Spectrum.

Lazarus, R. S., & Launier, S. (1978). Stress-related transactions between person and environment. In L. A. Pervin & M. Lewis (Eds.), *Perspectives in international psychology* (pp. 286-327). New York: Plenum.

Leech, J. E. (1982). Psychosocial and physiologic needs of patients with arterial occlusive disease during the preoperative phase of hospitalization. *Heart and Lung, 11,* 442-449.

Lenfant, C., & Moskowitz, J. (1984). National Heart, Lung and Blood Institute: New frontiers in heart, lung, and blood disease. *Circulation, 70,* 1-29.

Lester, D. M. (1973). The psychological impact of chronic obstructive pulmonary disease, In R. F. Johnson (Ed.), *Pulmonary care* (pp. 341-354). New York: Grune & Stratton.

Linkowski, D. C. (1971). A scale to measure acceptance of disability. *Rehabilitation Counseling Bulletin, 14,* 236-244.

Linkowski, D. C., & Dunn, M. A. (1974). Self-concept and acceptance of disability. *Rehabilitation Counseling Journal, 18,* 28-32.

Linn, M. W., Hunter, K. I., & Perry, P. R. (1979). Differences by sex and ethnicity in the psychosocial adjustment of the elderly. *Journal of Health and Social Behavior, 20,* 273-281.

Litman, T. J. (1964). An analysis of the sociological factors affecting the reha-

bilitation of physically handicapped factors. *Archives of Physical Medicine &
Rehabilitation, 8,* 9-16.

Livesley, W. J. (1981). Factors associated with psychiatric symptoms in patients
undergoing chronic hemodialysis. *Canadian Journal of Psychiatry, 27,*
562-566.

Lustig, F. M., Hass, A., & Castillo, D. (1972). Clinical and rehabilitation regime
in patients with COPD. *Archives of Physical Medicine and Rehabilitation, 53,*
315-322.

MacElveen, P. (1977). An observational measure of patient morale. In M. Batey
(Ed.), *Communicating nursing research: The Behavior-Morale Scale* Vol. 9, (pp.
85-92). Boulder, CO: WICHEN Publications.

Matson, R. R., & Brooks, N. A. (1977). Adjusting to multiple sclerosis: An exploratory study. *Social Science and Medicine, 11,* 245-250.

McCubbin, H. I., McCubbin, M. A., Patterson, J. M., Cauble, A. E., Wilson, L.
R., & Warwick, W. (1983). CHIP – Coping Health Inventory for Parents: An
assessment of parental coping patterns in the care of the chronically ill child.
Journal of Marriage and the Family, 45, 359-370.

McSweeny, A. J., Grant, I., Heaton, R. K., Adams, K. M., & Timms, R. M. (1982).
Life quality of patients with chronic obstructive pulmonary disease. *Archives
of Internal Medicine, 142,* 473-478.

Mechanic, D. (1962). *Students under stress: A study in the social psychology of adaptation.* Glencoe IL: The Free Press.

Mechanic, D. (1978). *Students under stress: A study in the social psychology of adaptation.* Madison, WI: University of Wisconsin Press.

Menninger, K., Mayman, M., & Pruyser, P. (1963). *The vital balance.* New York:
Viking Press.

Molumphy, S. D., & Sporawski, M. J. (1984). The family stress of hemodialysis.
Family Relations, 33, 33-39.

Moos, R. H. (Ed.) (1976). *Human adaptation: Coping with life crises.* Lexington, MA:
D. C. Heath.

Moos, R. H. (1977). *Coping with physical illness.* New York: Plenum.

Moos, R. H., & Tsu, V. D. (1977). The crisis of physical illness: An overview. In
R. H. Moos (Ed.), *Coping with physical illness* (pp. 3-21). New York: Plenum.

Morrow, G. R., Chiarello, R. J., & Derogatis, L. R. (1978). A new scale for assessing patients' psychological adjustment to medical illness. *Psychological Medicine, 8,* 605-610.

Neugarten, B., Havighurst, R., & Tobin, S. (1961). The measurement of life satisfaction. *Journal of Gerontology, 16,* 134-143.

Nickerson, E. T. (1971). Some correlates of adjustment by paraplegics. *Perceptual
and Motor Skills, 32,* 11-23.

Ott, C. R., Sivarajan, E. S., Newton, K. M., Almes, M. J., Bruce, R. A., Bergner,
M., & Gilson, B. S. (1983). A controlled randomized study of early cardiac
rehabilitation: The Sickness Impact Profile as an assessment tool. *Heart and
Lung, 12,* 162-170.

Pearlin, L. I., & Schooler, C. (1978). The structure of coping. *Journal of Health
and Social Behavior, 19,* 2-21.

Pfeiffer, E. (1977). Psychopathology and social pathology. In J. E. Birren & K.
Schaie (Eds.), *Handbook of the psychology of aging* (pp. 650-671). New York: Van
Nostrand Reinhold.

Public Services Laboratory, Georgetown University. (1978). Costs of illness, fiscal
year 1975. In *National Heart, Lung and Blood Fact Book* (DHEW Pub. No.
NIH 79-1656). Washington DC.

Rabkin, J. G., & Struening, E. L. (1976). Life events, stress, and illness. *Science,
194,* 1013-1020.

Rahe, R. H. (1977). Epidemiological studies of life change and illness. In Z. J.
Lipowski, D. R. Lipowski & P. C. Whybrow (Eds.), *Psychosomatic medicine:*

Current trends and clinical applications (pp. 421-434). New York: Oxford University Press.

Reeder, L. G., Scharama, P. G. M., & Dirken, J. M. (1973). Stress and cardiovascular health: An international cooperative study: I. *Social Science and Medicine, 7,* 573-584.

Robinson, J. P., & Shaver, P. R. (1973). *Measures of social psychological attitudes (rev. ed.).* Ann Arbor, MI: Institute for Social Research.

Rosenberg, M. I. (1965). *Society and the adolescent self-image.* Princeton, NJ: Princeton University Press.

Russell, R. A. (1981). Concepts of adjustment to disability: An overview. *Rehabilitation Literature, 42,* 330-338.

Sanders, J. B., & Kardinal, C. G. (1977). Adaptive coping mechanisms in adult acute leukemia patients in remission. *Journal of American Medical Association, 238,* 952-954.

Schar, M., Reeder, L. G., & Dirken, J. M. (1973). Stress and cardiovascular health: An international cooperative study: II. The male population of a factory at Zurich. *Social Science and Medicine, 7,* 583-603.

Schoeneman, S. Z., Reznikoff, M., & Bacon, S. J. (1983). Personality variables in coping with the stress of a spouse's chronic illness. *Journal of Clinical Psychology, 39,* 430-436.

Sexton, D. L. (1984). Wives of COPD patients. *Connecticut Medicine, 48,* 37-40.

Sexton, D. L., & Munro, B. H. (1985). Impact of a husband's chronic illness (COPD) on the spouse's life. *Research in Nursing and Health, 8,* 83-90.

Shambaugh, P. W., & Kanter, S. S. (1969). Spouses under stress: Group meetings with spouses of patients on hemodialysis. *American Journal of Psychiatry, 125,* 928-936.

Shantin, L. (1970). The situational attitude schedule: A morale scale for the chronic medical patient. *American Corrective Therapy Journal, 24,* 137-140.

Shontz, F. C. (1955). MMPI responses of patients with multiple sclerosis. *Journal of Consulting Psychology, 19,* 74-76.

Sidle, A., Adams, J., & Cady, P. (1969). Development of a coping scale. *Archives of General Psychiatry, 20,* 226-232.

Skelton, M., & Dominian, J. (1973). Psychological stress in wives of patients with myocardial infarction. *British Medical Journal, 2,* 101-103.

Skipper, J. K., Fink, S. L., & Hallenbeck, P. N. (1968). Physical disability among married women: Problems in the husband-wife relationship. *Journal of Rehabilitation, 34,* 16-19.

Stein, S., & Charles, E. (1971). A study of early life experiences of adolescent diabetes. *American Journal of Psychiatry, 128,* 700-704.

Stein, S., & Charles, E. (1975). Emotional factors in juvenile diabetes mellitus: A study of the early life experiences of eight diabetic children. *Psychosomatic Medicine, 37,* 237-244.

Stern, M. J., Pascale, L., & Ackerman, A. (1977). *Life adjustment post myocardial infarction. Archives of Internal Medicine, 137,* 1680-1685.

Stevenson, J. S. (1977). *Issues and crises during middlescence.* Norwalk, CT: Appleton-Century-Crofts.

Tropauer, A., Franz, M. N., & Dilgard, V. W. (1970). Pscyhological aspects of the care of children with cystic fibrosis. *American Journal of Diseases of Children, 119,* 424-432.

Vaillant, G. (1971). Theoretical hierarchy of adaptive ego mechanisms. *Archives of General Psychiatry, 24,* 107-118.

Vash, C. L. (1975). The psychology of disability. *Rehabilitation Psychology* (Monograph Issue), *22,* 145-162.

Venters, M. (1981). Familial coping with chronic and severe childhood illness: The case of cystic fibrosis. *Social Science and Medicine: Part A, Medical Sociological, 15A,* 289-297.

Videka-Sherman, L. (1982). Coping with the death of a child: A study over time. *American Journal of Orthopsychiatry, 52,* 688-698.

Viney, L. L., & Westbrook, M. T. (1981). Psychological reactions to chronic illness-related disability as a function of its severity and type. *Journal of Psychosomatic Research, 25,* 513-523.

Viney, L. L., & Westbrook, M. T. (1982). Coping with chronic illness: The mediating role of biographic and illness related factors. *Journal of Psychosomatic Research, 26,* 595-605.

von Bertalanffy, L. (1968). *General systems theory.* New York: George Brazillier.

Waltz, C. F., Strickland, O. L., & Lenz, E. R. (1984)., *Measurement in nursing research.* Philadelphia: F. A. Davis.

Weisman, A. D., & Sobel, H. J. (1979). Coping with cancer through self-instruction: A hypothesis. *Journal of Human Stress, 5,* 3-8.

Weisman, A. D., & Worden, J. W. (1976). The existential plight in cancer: Significance of the first 100 days. *International Journal of Psychiatry in Medicine, 7,* 1-15.

Weissman, M. M., & Bothwell, S. (1976). Assessment of social adjustment by patient self-report. *Archives of General Psychiatry, 33,* 1111-1115.

Weissman, M. M., Sholomskas, D., & John, K. (1981). The assessment of social adjustment. *Archives of General Psychiatry, 38,* 1250-1258.

Wender, M., & Dominik, W. (1972). Psychological examination in patients with multiple sclerosis. *Psychiatry, Neurology and Medical Psychology, 24,* 384-392.

White, R. W. (1974). Strategies of adaptation: An attempt at systematic description. In G. V. Coelho, D. A. Hamburg, & J. E. Adams (Eds.), (pp. 47-68), New York: Basic Books.

Wishnie, H. A., Hackett, T. P., & Cassem, N. H. (1971). Psychological hazards of convalescence following myocardial infarction. *Journal of the American Medical Association, 215,* 1292-1296.

Wolf, S., & Goodell, H. (Eds.). (1968). *Harold G. Wolf's stress and disease* (2nd ed.). Springfield, IL: Charles C Thomas.

Wright, B. A. (1960). *Physical disability: A psychological approach.* New York: Harper & Row.

Zeldow, P. B., & Pavlou, M. (1984). Physical disability, life stress, and psychosocial adjustment in multiple sclerosis. *The Journal of Nervous and Mental Disease, 172,* 80-84.

Family Response to Chronic Illness Questionnaire (FRCIQ) Spouse Version

Directions: This questionnaire is to help us learn more about the experiences you have and the things you do to manage these experiences. The information you share will be used to help us plan the appropriate health care for you and your family. Please feel free to ask us about any questions that are not clear.

SECTION A HEALTH INFORMATION*

1. What is your spouse's primary condition or disability?   —
2. How long ago was your spouse's condition first diagnosed?   __(years)   —
3. Does your spouse have any other illnesses or health problems?
   Yes $_2$ No $_1$ —
   If Yes: What are they? (Please specify conditions.)
   1. _____   —
   2. _____   —
   3. _____   —
   4. _____   —
4. How has your spouse's general health been in the *past 6 months?*
   Excellent $_1$ Good $_2$ Fair $_3$ Poor $_4$ —
5. In the *past 6 months*, how many times has your spouse been to the doctor because of illness?
   No Visits $_1$ 1 Time $_2$ 2-3 Times $_3$ 4 or more Times $_4$ —
6. In the *past 6 months*, has your spouse been hospitalized?
   Yes $_2$ No $_1$ —
   If Yes:
   What was your spouse hospitalized for? _____
   How long were the majority of stays?
   Over 2 Weeks $_3$ 1-2 Weeks $_2$ Under 1 Week $_1$ —

Treatment Demand

We're interested in knowing what treatment your spouse is receiving at this time. We'd like to know what your physician has prescribed for your spouse.

7. Is your spouse supposed to be taking medication? Yes $_2$ No $_1$ —
   If Yes: Does your spouse take it orally or receive injections?
   Both $_3$ Injection $_2$ Orally $_1$ —

* Felton, Revenson, & Hinrichsen, 1984.

8. How frequently is your spouse supposed to be taking medication?
   Oral: Injection: (oral) __
   __ __ (times per day)   (injection) __
9. Has your doctor put your spouse on a special diet? Yes 2   No 1   __
   If Yes: What restrictions _____

10. How often has the doctor asked your spouse to come to the clinic for
    check-ups and tests?
    _____ (times per year)   __
11. Is your spouse supposed to be coming to the hospital for special
    treatments? Yes 2   No 1   __
    If Yes: What kind of treatments are they? _____

Adherence

12. How regularly does your spouse keep doctor's appointments for
    checkups and tests?
    Regular 4   Almost always 3   Sometimes miss 2   Almost never 1   __
13. How regularly does your spouse keep appointments for special
    treatments?
    Regular 4   Almost always 3   Sometimes miss 2   Almost never 1   __
14. Are there things that your spouse does – beyond what your doctor
    has prescribed – to keep healthy? Yes 2   No 1   __
    If Yes: What things does your spouse do for his/her health?

Perceived Susceptibility

15. Overall, how vulnerable do you feel your spouse is to illness and disease? __
    Very vulnerable 3   Somewhat vulnerable 2   Not very vulnerable 1
16. What is your assessment of how your spouse's health will be 6
    months from now?
    Refusal 6   Much worse 5   Worse 4   About the same 3   Better 2
    Much better 1   __

Perceived Severity

17. Compared to most other diseases that adults get, how serious do you
    think your spouse's illness is?
    Very serious 3   Somewhat serious 2   Not very serious 1   __
18. How serious do you think the consequences of your spouse's illness are?
    Very serious 3   Somewhat serious 2   Not serious 1   __
19. How important do you think it is for your spouse to take medication
    and follow the doctor's orders?
    Very important 3   Somewhat important 2   Not very important 1
20. How much control do you feel your spouse has over the course of his/
    her illness?
    a.   My spouse has a great influence over what will happen to
         him/her 1
    b.   My spouse has some effect on what will happen to him/her 2

c. My spouse has no effect on what will happen to him/her 3   —
21. Do you know what caused your spouse's illness? Yes 1   No 2   —
If Yes: What was the cause? _____

_____

Limitations

Which of these things is your spouse still healthy enough to do without help?
22. Heavy work, like washing floors and carrying laundry and groceries?
Yes 1   No 2   —
23. Walk eight blocks (half a mile)? Yes 1   No 2   —
24. Walk up and down stairs to the second floor? Yes 1   No 2   —
25. Go out to a movie, to church or a meeting, or to visit friends? Yes 1
No 2   —
Does your spouse's illness interfere with or prevent him/her from doing any of the following things?
26. Eating out at a restaurant?   Yes 2   No 1   —
27. Taking vacations?   Yes 2   No 1   —
28. Concentrating on things?   Yes 2   No 1   —
29. Reading?   Yes 2   No 1   —
30. Are you a member of a support group related to your spouse's chronic illness?   —
Yes 2   No 1
If Yes: How often do you attend meetings?
Frequently 1   Occasionally 2   Never 3   —
If you go to meetings, how helpful have they been?
Do not go 1   Very helpful 2   Somewhat helpful 3   Not very helpful 4   —
If No: Would you be interested in joining a small group of people to discuss medical aspects of the chronic illness and how people personally feel, related to, illness?
Yes 2   No 1   —
If Yes: Would you feel more comfortable in a group of people:
Only about your same age?   Yes 2   No 1   Don't care 0   —
Only the same sex?   Yes 2   No 1   Don't care 0   —

SECTION B CHRONIC IMPACT AND COPING INSTRUMENT (CICI)*

Concerns

All people whose spouses have a chronic health problem have some areas of concern. During the *past 6 months* how much of a concern have the following areas been for you? (Please put an "X" in the appropriate column).

_____

* Hymovich, 1983

Concerns	None/Does not apply (1)	Not sure (2)	A little bit (3)	Quite a bit (4)	A great deal (5)
1. Extra demands on my time					
2. Feeling worn out					
3. Having enough fun and relaxation as I would like					
4. Having enough time alone with my spouse					
5. Talking with or understanding my spouse					
6. Sexual relationship with my spouse					
7. Making my spouse happy					
8. Having enough time or attention from my spouse					
9. Getting out of house with my spouse					
10. Getting out of house alone					
11. Getting to do activities with others					
12. Whether I am taking care of spouse in the best way					
13. Having to travel too far for medical help for my spouse					
14. The weather influencing what my spouse is able to do					
15. Having enough insurance to meet medical expenses of spouse's care					
16. Having accessibility to health care agencies in the community related to my spouse's needs					
17. Wondering about what my spouse's future is likely to be					
18. The responsibility of caring for my spouse worries me					
19. Lack of support from family members					

Health Beliefs

People have different beliefs about many things that influence their life style. Please indicate whether or not you agree with the beliefs stated below.

1. People should take care of their own needs before they can help other family members.
   Agree $_1$ Not Sure $_2$ Disagree $_3$ ___

2. It is necessary to get out of the house often to relieve the strain of caring for another person.
   Agree $_1$ Not Sure $_2$ Disagree $_3$ ___

3. It is usually better not to show or talk about one's feelings to others.
   Agree $_1$ Not Sure $_2$ Disagree $_3$ ___

4. Sometimes just avoiding or trying to forget something makes it easier to handle.
   Agree $_1$ Not Sure $_2$ Disagree $_3$ ___

5. Sometimes just getting away from a situation makes it easier to handle.
   Agree $_1$ Not Sure $_2$ Disagree $_3$ ___

6. I usually have control over things that happen to me or my family.
   Agree $_1$ Not Sure $_2$ Disagree $_3$ ___

7. It is lucky that this is the only condition my spouse has.
   Agree $_1$ Not Sure $_2$ Disagree $_3$ ___

8. My spouse's condition is always going to be there, and there isn't much I can do about it.
   Agree $_1$ Not Sure $_2$ Disagree $_3$ ___

9. Sometimes my spouse's condition is a nuisance.
   Agree $_1$ Not Sure $_2$ Disagree $_3$ ___

10. Things always work out.
    Agree $_1$ Not Sure $_2$ Disagree $_3$ ___

Help Needs

People have asked for help with many aspects of care related to their spouse's health condition including those listed below. Please indicate if you would or would not like to have help with or discuss any of the following.

1. Medical care/needs
   Not sure $_3$ Yes $_2$ No $_1$ ___
2. Diet/nutrition
   Not sure $_3$ Yes $_2$ No $_1$ ___
3. Sleep patterns
   Not sure $_3$ Yes $_2$ No $_1$ ___
4. Recreational/diversional activities
   Not sure $_3$ Yes $_2$ No $_1$ ___
5. Physical support device
   Not sure $_3$ Yes $_2$ No $_1$ ___
6. Information about transportation needs
   Not sure $_3$ Yes $_2$ No $_1$ ___

7. Care of minor illnesses
    Not sure 3   Yes 2   No 1   —
8. Information about your spouse's condition
    Not sure 3   Yes 2   No 1   —

In the past, when you have needed information or help with any of the areas listed above, have you done any of the things listed below? (Check all items that apply.)

9. Written away to others
                Yes 2   No 1   —
10. Asked the clergy
                Yes 2   No 1   —
11. Asked a nurse
                Yes 2   No 1   —
12. Asked a doctor
                Yes 2   No 1   —
13. Asked friends or relatives
                Yes 2   No 1   —
14. Asked spouse
                Yes 2   No 1   —
15. Gone to the library
                Yes 2   No 1   —
16. Ask persons with a similar condition
                Yes 2   No 1   —
17. Nothing
                Yes 2   No 1   —
18. Talked to others   Yes 2   No 1
    Who? Name them _____
                Yes 2   No 1   —
19. Did not know what to do
                Yes 2   No 1   —
20. Other: What?
                Yes 2   No 1   —
21. Have not needed help
                Yes 2   No 1   —

SECTION C COPING SCALE*

1. Being ill often means having to deal with different problems connected with the illness. What are the things that you have to deal with since you learned of your spouse's illness?

   _____

   _____

   _____

2. Sometimes illness brings some positive effects. For you, what are the things that have been positive or beneficial about your spouse being ill?

   _____

   _____

   _____

* Felton, Revenson & Hinrichsen, 1984.

The following is a list of things that people sometimes do in reaction to illness. Please indicate if you have ever done any of these things in reaction to illness and if you have, do you do it seldom, sometimes, often, or most of the time?

I. Cognitive Restructuring

1. Concentrated on something good that could come out of the whole thing.
   Mostly 5   Often 4   Sometimes 3   Seldom 2   Never 1   —
2. Rediscovered what is important in life.
   Mostly 5   Often 4   Sometimes 3   Seldom 2   Never 1   —
3. Felt like you changed or grew as a person in a good way.
   Mostly 5   Often 4   Sometimes 3   Seldom 2   Never 1   —
4. Found new faith or some truth about life.
   Mostly 5   Often 4   Sometimes 3   Seldom 2   Never 1   —
5. Remembered times when your life was more difficult.
   Mostly 5   Often 4   Sometimes 3   Seldom 2   Never 1   —
6. Turned to work or other things to take your mind off the problem.
   Mostly 5   Often 4   Sometimes 3   Seldom 2   Never 1   —
7. Religion became more important.
   Mostly 5   Often 4   Sometimes 3   Seldom 2   Never 1   —
8. Thought about people who were worse off than you.
   Mostly 5   Often 4   Sometimes 3   Seldom 2   Never 1   —
9. Reminded yourself that things could be worse.
   Mostly 5   Often 4   Sometimes 3   Seldom 2   Never 1   —
10. Looked for the silver lining, so to speak; tried to look on the bright side of things.
    Mostly 5   Often 4   Sometimes 3   Seldom 2   Never 1   —
11. Did something totally new that you never would have done if this hadn't happened.
    Mostly 5   Often 4   Sometimes 3   Seldom 2   Never 1   —
12. Changed the way you did things so that the illness was less of a problem.
    Mostly 5   Often 4   Sometimes 3   Seldom 2   Never 1   —
13. Got away from it for a while; tried to rest or take a vacation.
    Mostly 5   Often 4   Sometimes 3   Seldom 2   Never 1   —

II. Emotional Expression

14. Took it out on other people.
    Mostly 5   Often 4   Sometimes 3   Seldom 2   Never 1   —
15. Got help with day-to-day chores or travel.
    Mostly 5   Often 4   Sometimes 3   Seldom 2   Never 1   —
16. Joked about it.
    Mostly 5   Often 4   Sometimes 3   Seldom 2   Never 1   —
17. Let your feelings out somehow.
    Mostly 5   Often 4   Sometimes 3   Seldom 2   Never 1   —
18. Avoided being with people in general.
    Mostly 5   Often 4   Sometimes 3   Seldom 2   Never 1   —
19. Recalled past successes.
    Mostly 5   Often 4   Sometimes 3   Seldom 2   Never 1   —

20. Daydreamed or imagined a better time or place than the one you were in.
    Mostly 5   Often 4   Sometimes 3   Seldom 2   Never 1   —

21. Slept more than usual.
    Mostly 5   Often 4   Sometimes 3   Seldom 2   Never 1   —

III. Wish-Fulfilling Fantasy

22. Wished that you could change what happened.
    Mostly 5   Often 4   Sometimes 3   Seldom 2   Never 1   —

23. Wished that you could change the way you felt.
    Mostly 5   Often 4   Sometimes 3   Seldom 2   Never 1   —

24. Felt bad that you couldn't avoid the problem.
    Mostly 5   Often 4   Sometimes 3   Seldom 2   Never 1   —

25. Wished that the situation would go away or somehow be over with.
    Mostly 5   Often 4   Sometimes 3   Seldom 2   Never 1   —

26. Hoped a miracle would happen.
    Mostly 5   Often 4   Sometimes 3   Seldom 2   Never 1   —

27. Wished you were a stronger person.
    Mostly 5   Often 4   Sometimes 3   Seldom 2   Never 1   —

28. Had fantasies or wishes about how things might turn out.
    Mostly 5   Often 4   Sometimes 3   Seldom 2   Never 1   —

IV. Self-Blame

29. Blamed yourself.
    Mostly 5   Often 4   Sometimes 3   Seldom 2   Never 1   —

30. Thought about fantastic or unreal things that made you feel better.
    Mostly 5   Often 4   Sometimes 3   Seldom 2   Never 1   —

31. Saw the doctor and did what he recommended.
    Mostly 5   Often 4   Sometimes 3   Seldom 2   Never 1   —

32. Got mad at the people or things that caused the problem.
    Mostly 5   Often 4   Sometimes 3   Seldom 2   Never 1   —

33. Criticized or took it out on yourself.
    Mostly 5   Often 4   Sometimes 3   Seldom 2   Never 1   —

34. Realized you brought the problem on yourself.
    Mostly 5   Often 4   Sometimes 3   Seldom 2   Never 1   —

35. Refused to believe that it had happened.
    Mostly 5   Often 4   Sometimes 3   Seldom 2   Never 1   —

V. Information Seeking

36. Looked up medical information.
    Mostly 5   Often 4   Sometimes 3   Seldom 2   Never 1   —

37. Read books/magazine articles (or watched TV) about gout/diabetes/leukemia.
    Mostly 5   Often 4   Sometimes 3   Seldom 2   Never 1   —

38. Came up with a couple of different solutions to the problem.
    Mostly 5   Often 4   Sometimes 3   Seldom 2   Never 1   —

39. Asked someone you respected (other than a doctor) for advice and followed it.

Mostly 5   Often 4   Sometimes 3   Seldom 2   Never 1   —
40. Made a plan of action and followed it.
Mostly 5   Often 4   Sometimes 3   Seldom 2   Never 1   —

VI. Threat Minimization*

41. Kept your feelings to yourself.
Mostly 5   Often 4   Sometimes 3   Seldom 2   Never 1   —
42. Went on as if nothing had happened.
Mostly 5   Often 4   Sometimes 3   Seldom 2   Never 1   —
43. Talked to someone about how you were feeling.
Mostly 5   Often 4   Sometimes 3   Seldom 2   Never 1   —
44. Didn't let it get to you; refused to think too much about it.
Mostly 5   Often 4   Sometimes 3   Seldom 2   Never 1   —
45. Kept others from knowing how bad things were.
Mostly 5   Often 4   Sometimes 3   Seldom 2   Never 1   —
46. Tried to forget the whole thing.
Mostly 5   Often 4   Sometimes 3   Seldom 2   Never 1   —
47. Talked to someone other than a doctor who could do something about the problem for you.
Mostly 5   Often 4   Sometimes 3   Seldom 2   Never 1   —
48. Tried to work it out by yourself.
Mostly 5   Often 4   Sometimes 3   Seldom 2   Never 1   —
49. Accepted sympathy and understanding from someone.
Mostly 5   Often 4   Sometimes 3   Seldom 2   Never 1   —
50. Made light of the situation; refused to get too serious about it.
Mostly 5   Often 4   Sometimes 3   Seldom 2   Never 1   —
51. Went along with fate; sometimes you just have bad luck.
Mostly 5   Often 4   Sometimes 3   Seldom 2   Never 1   —

SECTION D PSYCHOLOGICAL ADJUSTMENT

Acceptance of Illness Scale*

1. I have a hard time adjusting to the limitation of my spouse's illness.
Strongly disagree 5   Disagree 4   Uncertain 3   Agree 2   Strongly agree 1   —
2. Because of my spouse's health, I miss the things I like to do most.
Strongly disagree 5   Disagree 4   Uncertain 3   Agree 2   Strongly agree 1   —
3. My spouse's illness makes me feel useless at times.
Strongly disagree 5   Disagree 4   Uncertain 3   Agree 2   Strongly agree 1   —
4. Health problems make my spouse more dependent on others than I want him/her to be.
Strongly disagree 5   Disagree 4   Uncertain 3   Agree 2   Strongly agree 1   —
5. My spouse's illness makes him/her a burden on our family and friends.

* Felton, Revenson & Hinrichsen, 1984 – adapted from Linkowski, 1971.

Strongly disagree 5   Disagree 4   Uncertain 3   Agree 2   Strongly
agree 1   —
6. My spouse's health does not make me feel inadequate.*
   Strongly disagree 5   Disagree 4   Uncertain 3   Agree 2   Strongly
   agree 1   —
7. My spouse will never be self-sufficient enough to make me happy.
   Strongly disagree 5   Disagree 4   Uncertain 3   Agree 2   Strongly
   agree 1   —
8. I think people are often uncomfortable being around my spouse
   because of his/her illness.
   Strongly disagree 5   Disagree 4   Uncertain 3   Agree 2   Strongly
   agree 1   —

Note: Items marked with an asterisk are revised before scale.

AFFECT-BALANCE SCALE (ABS) (Bradburn, 1969)*

A. During the past few months have you felt:
   1) Bored?   Yes 2   No 1   —
   2) Very unhappy?   Yes 2   No 1   —
   3) Very lonely or remote from other people?   Yes 2   No 1   —
   4) Upset because someone criticized you?   Yes 2   No 1   —
   5) So restless that you couldn't sit in a chair?   Yes 2   No 1   —
B. During the past few months have you felt:
   6) Very happy?   Yes 2   No 1   —
   7) Pleased about having accomplished something?   Yes 2   No 1   —
   8) That things were going your way?   Yes 2   No 1   —
   9) Proud because someone complimented you for
      something you had done?   Yes 2   No 1   —
   10) Enthusiastic about something.   Yes 2   No 1   —
   11) Considering the way your life is going at the
       moment, would you:
       a) Like to continue in much the same sort of
          way?   Continue 1   —
       b) Like to change some parts of it?   Change some 2   —
       c) Like to change many parts of it?   Change many 3   —
   12) How successful have you been at planning your
       life, in your work and with your family? Would
       you say: —
       Very successful 5   A little successful 4
       Undecided 3   Somewhat 2   Very 1
   13) Do you feel you have accomplished most of the
       things you would have liked to, up to this point
       in your life?   Yes 2   No 1   —

Self-Esteem Scale (Rosenberg, 1965)**

1. I feel that I'm a person of worth, at least on an equal plane with
   others.

* Bradburn, 1969.
** Rosenberg, 1965.

Strongly disagree 5   Disagree 4   Uncertain 3   Agree 2   Strongly agree 1

2. I feel that I have a number of good qualifications.   —
Strongly disagree 5   Disagree 4   Uncertain 3   Agree 2   Strongly agree 1

3. All in all, I am inclined to feel that I am a failure.*   —
Strongly disagree 5   Disagree 4   Uncertain 3   Agree 2   Strongly agree 1

4. I am able to do things as well as most other people.   —
Strongly disagree 5   Disagree 4   Uncertain 3   Agree 2   Strongly agree 1

5. I feel I do not have much to be proud of.*   —
Strongly disagree 5   Disagree 4   Uncertain 3   Agree 2   Strongly agree 1

6. I take a positive attitude toward myself.   —
Strongly disagree 5   Disagree 4   Uncertain 3   Agree 2   Strongly agree 1

7. On the whole, I am satisfied with myself.   —
Strongly disagree 5   Disagree 4   Uncertain 3   Agree 2   Strongly agree 1

8. I wish I could have more respect for myself.*   —
Strongly disagree 5   Disagree 4   Uncertain 3   Agree 2   Strongly agree 1

9. I certainly feel useless at times.*   —
Strongly disagree 5   Disagree 4   Uncertain 3   Agree 2   Strongly agree 1

10. At times I think I am no good at all.*   —
Strongly disagree 5   Disagree 4   Uncertain 3   Agree 2   Strongly agree 1

*Note: Items marked with an asterisk are reversed before scale summation.

SECTION E SOCIOLOGICAL ADJUSTMENT SCALE (SAS-SR)*

We are interested in finding out how you have been doing in the last two weeks. We would like you to answer some questions about your work, spare time, and your family life. There are no right or wrong answers to these questions. Please indicate the answers that best describe how you have been in the last two weeks.

Work Outside the Home

Please check the situation that best describes you   —
I am
Worker for pay 1   Housewife 2   Student 3   Retired 4
    Unemployed 5

Do you usually work for pay more than 15 hours per week?   —
    Yes 2   No 1

* Weissman & Bothwell, 1976.

Did you work any hours for pay in the last two weeks?   —
    Yes $_2$ No $_1$

Check the answer that best describes how you have been in the last two weeks.

1. How many days did you miss from work in the last two weeks?   —
   No days missed $_1$
   One day $_2$
   I missed about half the time $_3$
   Missed more than half the time but did make at least one day $_4$
   I did not work any days $_5$
   On vacation all of the last two weeks $_8$

If you have not worked any days in the last two weeks, go on to Question 7.

2. Have you been able to do your work in the last 2 weeks?   —
   I did my work very well $_1$
   I did my work well but had some minor problems $_2$
   I needed help with work and did not do well about half the time $_3$
   I did my work poorly most of the time $_4$
   I did my work poorly all the time $_5$

3. Have you been ashamed of how you do your work in the last 2 weeks?   —
   I never felt ashamed $_1$
   Once or twice I felt a little ashamed $_2$
   About half the time I felt ashamed $_3$
   I felt ashamed most of the time $_4$
   I felt ashamed all the time $_5$

4. Have you had any arguments with people at work in the last 2 weeks? —
   I have had no arguments and got along very well $_1$
   I usually got along well but had minor arguments $_2$
   I had more than one argument $_3$
   I had many arguments $_4$
   I was constantly in arguments $_5$

5. Have you felt upset, worried, or uncomfortable while doing your work during the last 2 weeks?   —
   I never felt upset $_1$
   Once or twice I felt upset $_2$
   Half the time I felt upset $_3$
   I felt upset most of the time $_4$
   I felt upset all of the time $_5$

6. Have you found your work interesting these last 2 weeks?   —
   My work was almost always interesting $_1$
   Once or twice my work was interesting $_2$
   Half the time my work was uninteresting $_3$
   Most of the time my work was uninteresting $_4$
   My work was always uninteresting $_5$

Work at Home: Housewives Answer Questions 7-12 Otherwise, go on to Question 13

7. How many days did you do some housework during the last 2 weeks?   —
   Every day $_1$
   I did the housework almost every day $_2$

I did the housework about half the time 3
I usually did not do the housework 4
I was completely unable to do housework 5
I was away from home all of the last two weeks 8

8. During the last 2 weeks, have you kept up with your housework? This includes cooking, cleaning, laundry, grocery shopping, and errands.   ___
   I did my work very well 1
   I did my work well but had some minor problems 2
   I needed help with my work and did not do it well about half the time 3
   I did my work poorly most of the time 4
   I did my work poorly all of the time 5

9. Have you been ashamed of how you did your housework during the last 2 weeks?   ___
   I never felt ashamed 1
   Once or twice I felt a little ashamed 2
   About half the time I felt ashamed 3
   I felt ashamed most of the time 4
   I felt ashamed all of the time 5

10. Have you had any arguments with salespeople, tradesmen, or neighbors in the last 2 weeks?   ___
    I had no arguments and got along very well 1
    I usually got along well, but had minor arguments 2
    I had more than one argument 3
    I had many arguments 4
    I was constantly in arguments 4

11. Have you felt upset while doing your housework during the last 2 weeks?   ___
    I never felt upset 1
    Once or twice I felt upset 2
    Half the time I felt upset 3
    I felt upset most of the time 4
    I felt upset all of the time 5

12. Have you found your housework interesting in the last 2 weeks?   ___
    My work was almost always interesting 1
    Once or twice my work was not interesting 2
    Half the time my work was uninteresting 3
    Most of the time my work was uninteresting 4
    My work was always uninteresting 5

Spare Time: Everyone Answer Questions 13-21.

Check the answer that best describes how you have been in the last 2 weeks.

13. How many friends have you seen or spoken to on the telephone in the last 2 weeks?   ___
    Nine or more friends 1
    Five to eight friends 2
    Two to four friends 3
    One friend 4
    No friends 5

14. Have you been able to talk about your feelings and problems with at least one friend during the last 2 weeks?   —
    I can always talk about my innermost feelings 1
    I usually can talk about my feelings 2
    About half the time I felt able to talk about my feelings 3
    I usually was not able to talk about my feelings 4
    I was never able to talk about my feelings 5
    Not applicable; I have no friends 8
15. How many times in the last two weeks have you gone out socially with other people? For example visited friends, gone to movies, bowling, church, restaurants, invited friends to your house?   —
    More than 3 times 1
    Three times 2
    Twice 3
    Once 4
    None 5
16. How much time have you spent on hobbies or spare time interests during the last 2 weeks? For example, bowling, sewing, gardening, sports, reading?   —
    I spent most of my spare time on hobbies almost everyday 1
    I spent some spare time on hobbies some of the days 2
    I spent a little spare time on hobbies 3
    I usually did not spend any time on hobbies but did watch TV 4
    I did not spend spare time on hobbies or watching TV 5
17. Have you had open arguments with your friends in the last 2 weeks? —
    I have had no arguments and got along very well 1
    I usually got along well but had minor arguments 2
    I had more than one argument 3
    I had many arguments 4
    I was constantly in arguments 5
    Not applicable; I have no friends 8
18. If your feelings were hurt or offended by a friend during the last 2 weeks, how badly did you take it?   —
    It did not affect me or it did not happen 1
    I got over it in a few hours 2
    I got over it in a few days 3
    I got over it in a week 4
    It will take me months to recover 5
    Not applicable; I have no friends 8
19. Have you felt shy or uncomfortable with people in the last 2 weeks? —
    I always felt comfortable 1
    Sometimes I felt uncomfortable but could relax after a while 2
    About half the time I felt uncomfortable 3
    I usually felt uncomfortable 4
    I always felt uncomfortable 5
    Not applicable; I was never with people 8
20. Have you felt lonely and wished for more friends during the last 2 weeks? —
    I have not felt lonely 1
    I have felt lonely only a few times 2
    About half the time I felt lonely 3

I usually felt lonely 4
I always felt lonely and wished for more friends 5
21. Have you felt bored in your spare time during the last 2 weeks? —
   I never felt bored 1
   I usually did not feel bored 2
   About half the time I felt bored 3
   Most of the time I felt bored 4
   I was constantly bored 5

Family

Answer questions 22-27 about your parents, brothers, sisters, in laws, and children not living at home. Have you been in contact with any of them in the last two weeks.?
Yes 2 – Answer questions 22-27
No 1 – Go to question 28 —

22. Have you had open arguments with your relatives in the last 2 weeks? —
   We always got along very well 1
   We usually got along well but had some minor arguments 2
   I had more than one argument with at least one relative 3
   I had many arguments 4
   I was constantly in arguments 5
23. Have you been able to talk about your feelings and problems with at least one of your relatives in the last 2 weeks? —
   I can always talk about my feelings with at least one relative 1
   I usually can talk about my feelings 2
   About half the time I felt able to talk about my feelings 3
   I usually was not able to talk about my feelings 4
   I was never able to talk about my feelings 5
24. Have you avoided contacts with your relatives these last 2 weeks? —
   I contacted relatives regularly 1
   I have contacted a relative at least once 2
   I have waited for my relatives to contact me 3
   I avoided my relatives, but they contacted me 4
   I have no contacts with my relatives 5
25. Did you depend on your relatives for help, advice, money or friendship during the last 2 weeks? —
   I never need to depend on them 1
   I usually did not need to depend on them 2
   About half the time I needed to depend on them 3
   Most of the time I depend on them 4
   I depend completely on them 5
26. Have you wanted to do the opposite of what your relatives wanted in order to make them angry during the last 2 weeks? —
   I never wanted to oppose them 1
   Once or twice I wanted to oppose them 2
   About half the time I wanted to oppose them 3
   Most of the time I wanted to oppose them 4
   I always wanted to oppose them 5
27. Have you been worried about things happening to your relatives without good reason in the last 2 weeks? —

I have not worried without reason $_1$
Once or twice I worried $_2$
About half the time I worried $_3$
Most of the time I worried $_4$
I have worried the entire time $_5$
Not applicable; my relatives are no longer living $_8$

EVERYONE ANSWERS QUESTIONS 28-33

28. Have you had open arguments with your partner in the last 2 weeks?   —
    We have had no arguments and we get along very well $_1$
    We usually get along well but had minor arguments $_2$
    We had more than one argument $_3$
    We had many arguments $_4$
    We were constantly in argument $_5$
29. Have you been able to talk about your feelings and problems with
    your partner during the last 2 weeks?   —
    I could always talk freely about my feelings $_1$
    I usually could talk about my feelings $_2$
    About half the time I felt able to talk about my feelings $_3$
    I usually was not able to talk about my feelings $_4$
    I was never able to talk about my feelings $_5$
30. Have you been demanding to have your own way at home during the
    last 2 weeks?   —
    I have not insisted on always having my own way $_1$
    I usually have not insisted on having my own way $_2$
    About half the time I insisted on having my own way $_3$
    I usually insisted on having my own way $_4$
    I always insisted on having my own way $_5$
31. Have you been bossed around by your partner these last 2 weeks?   —
    Almost never $_1$
    Once in a while $_2$
    About half the time $_3$
    Most of the time $_4$
    Always $_5$
32. How much have you felt dependent on your partner these last 2 weeks? —
    I was independent $_1$
    I was usually independent $_2$
    I was somewhat dependent $_3$
    I was usually dependent $_4$
    I depended on my partner for everything $_5$
33. How have you felt about your partner during the last 2 weeks?   —
    I always felt affection $_1$
    I usually felt affection $_2$
    About half the time I felt dislike and half the time affection $_3$
    I usually felt dislike $_4$
    I felt dislike $_5$

Children

Have you had unmarried children, stepchildren, or foster children living at
home during the last 2 weeks?   —
Yes $_2$ – Answer questions 34–37

No 1 – Go to question 38

34. Have you been interested in what your children are doing–school, play or hobbies during the last 2 weeks?   —
    I was always interested and actively involved 1
    I usually was interested and involved 2
    About half the time interested and half the time not interested 3
    I usually was disinterested 4
    I was always disinterested 5

35. Have you been able to talk and listen to your children during the last 2 weeks? Include only children over the age of 2.   —
    I always was able to communicate with them 1
    I usually was able to communicate with them 2
    About half the time I could communicate 3
    I usually was not able to communicate 4
    I was completely unable to communicate 5
    Not applicable; no children over the age of 2 8

36. How have you been getting along with the children during the last 2 weeks?   —
    I have had no arguments and got along very well 1
    I usually got along well but had minor arguments 2
    I had more than one argument 3
    I had many arguments 4
    I was constantly in arguments 5

37. How have you felt toward your children these last 2 weeks?   —
    I always felt affection 1
    I mostly felt affection 2
    About half the time I felt affection 3
    Most of the time I did not feel affection 4
    I never felt affection toward them 5

EVERYONE ANSWER QUESTIONS 38-40

38. Have you worried about any of your children without any reason during the last 2 weeks, even if you are not living together now?   —
    I never worried 1
    Once or twice I worried 2
    About half the time I worried 3
    Most of the time I worried 4
    I always worried 5
    Not applicable; children not living 8

39. During the last 2 weeks have you been thinking that you have let down your partner or any of your children at any time?   —
    I did not feel I let them down at all 1
    I usually did not feel that I let them down 2
    About half the time I felt I let them down 3
    Most of the time I felt that I let them down 4
    I let them down completely 5

40. During the last 2 weeks have you been thinking that your partner or any of your children have let you down at any time?   —
    I never felt that they let me down 1
    I felt they usually did not let me down 2
    About half the time I felt they let me down 3
    I usually felt that they let me down 4
    I feel bitter that they have let me down 5

Financial – Everyone Please Answer Question 41

41. Have you had enough money to take care of your own and your family's financial needs during the last 2 weeks?   —
    I had enough money for needs $_1$
    I usually had enough money with minor problems $_2$
    About half the time I did not have enough money but did not have to borrow money $_3$
    I usually did not have enough money and had to borrow from others $_4$
    I had great financial difficulty $_5$

SECTION F DEMOGRAPHICS

We'd like to know a few things about you and your current living situation.

1. How old are you now? _____ (years)
2. What is your sex?
   Female $_2$ Male $_1$ —
3. How would you describe yourself?
   Caucasian $_1$ Asian $_2$ Black $_3$ Spanish-American $_4$
   American Indian $_5$ Other $_6$ _____
                                    Specify   —
4. What is your religion, if any?
   Protestant $_1$ Catholic $_2$ Jewish $_3$ None $_4$ Other $_5$ Specify   —
5. How important would you say religion is to you? Very important, fairly important, fairly unimportant or unimportant?
   Very impt. $_4$ Fairly impt. $_3$ Fairly unimpt. $_2$ Unimpt. $_1$ —
6. How long have you been married to your present spouse?
   _____ (years)   —
7. Do you have children? Yes $_2$ No $_1$ —
   If Yes: How many? _____ (number)   —
           How old is the youngest? _____ (years)
8. Do you live in an apartment or a house?
   Apartment $_2$ House $_1$ —
9. Do you own or rent?
   Own $_2$ Rent $_1$ —
10. How many years have you lived at this address? __ (Years)
11. With whom do you live (in addition to your spouse)?
    Check as many as apply.
    With children   __ (enter no.)   —
    With parents   __ (enter no.)   —
    With other relatives   __ (enter no.)   —
    With unrelated people   __ (enter no.)   —
12. How many people live in your home? __ (enter no.)
13. Which level of education have you completed   —
    Graduate professional training (Graduate degree) $_7$
    Standard college or university graduate $_6$
    Partial college (at least one year or specialized training) $_5$

High school graduate 4
Partial high school (10th or 11th grade) 3
Junior high school (9th grade) 2
Less than 7th grade 1
14. What is your family's annual income?   —
    Over $30,000 5 $21,000 to $30,000 4 $11,000 to $20,000 3
    $5,000 to $10,000 2   Under $5,000 1

PART II
Assessing the Whole Person
– Measuring Wellness

13
Confirmatory Factor Analysis of the Jalowiec Coping Scale

Anne Jalowiec

This chapter discusses the Jalowiec Coping Scale, a measure of coping behavior.

PURPOSE OF STUDY

The purpose of this study was to investigate the construct validity of the Jalowiec Coping Scale (JCS) (Jalowiec, 1979) using a larger sample and more advanced statistical procedures than had been employed in earlier work on the tool. Preliminary examination of the construct validity of the coping scale, using exploratory factor analysis and a small sample, indicated a more complex conceptualization of coping behaviors than the dichotomy originally proposed (Jalowiec, Murphy, & Powers, 1984). The results of that first psychometric study should be considered tentative because the sample size was meager. The present study was therefore indicated in order to test conceptual models for the coping scale suggested by previous work with the instrument, through use of confirmatory factor analysis and an extensive data base.

DESCRIPTION OF PREVIOUS TOOLS

The coping scale was originally developed for the author's thesis study because instrumentation then available (in 1977) either (1) was of the interview type, which was not practical for clinical studies, (2) covered only a limited range of coping behavior, often just defense mechanisms, or (3) pertained only to select populations. The most popular coping tool available during this same time period was Lazarus's Ways of Coping

This dissertation research was partially supported by a grant from the American Nurses' Foundation and by a National Research Service Award Predoctoral Fellowship from the U.S. Public Health Service. The guidance and support of Dr. Marjorie Powers, dissertation advisor, University of Illinois at Chicago, is gratefully acknowledged.

Checklist (Folkman & Lazarus, 1980). This checklist, however, had almost 70 items, and responses were obtained via a yes/no dichotomy. Using such a binary checklist yields less discriminating information on coping behavior than can be obtained from a graded response format. The limited variance in dichotomous responses also attenuates correlations, which serve as the basis for most statistical procedures. Accordingly, Guilford (1954) pointed out that the reliability of a rating scale is a monotonically increasing function of the number of steps used (though leveling off at about seven); therefore, having a greater number of response categories enhances the reliability of a tool by increasing the variance in scores. [It should be noted that Lazarus has since changed to a Likert rating scale and has deleted several items from the checklist (Folkman & Lazarus, 1985)].

Because of the lack of appropriate instrumentation, this author therefore developed the JCS to serve as a fairly generic instrument that would cover a wide range of coping behavior, could be used with diverse populations, would tap the variability in the use of coping methods, and would be practical for clinical settings. In addition, Westlake and Taylor (1985) have recently determined that the JCS has a Fry readability level of sixth grade and hence can be easily understood by most persons.

Conceptual Considerations

Conceptualizations of coping behavior found in the literature have ranged from bidimensional to multidimensional classifications. Some classification schemes apply descriptive labels to the coping behavior (e.g., intrapsychic); whereas other labels are goal-oriented (e.g., maintain self-esteem) or evaluative (e.g., mature v. immature). Although a few themes do recur (e.g., cognitive, active, problem-solving), for the most part, there seems little consensus of opinion on the salient dimensions of coping behavior.

Based on Lazarus and Launier's (1978) bidimensional model of coping behavior, items on the JCS were previously classified by a panel of 20 nursing faculty and graduate students into 15 problem-oriented coping behaviors, which focus on problem resolution, and 25 affective-oriented behaviors, which are aimed at distress mitigation. Overall agreement on the classification was 85%, with more consensus found on problem items (88%) than on affective (83%).

Previous Psychometric Results

Alpha reliability coefficients for total coping scores and for problem and affective subscale scores have ranged from .75 to .86, based on the results of four earlier studies with sample sizes of 135 to 450 (Jalowiec et al., 1984; Murphy, 1982; Murphy, 1984; Powers & Jalowiec, 1986). Retest reliability coefficients, using 2- to 4-week intervals with samples sizes of 9 to 30, have ranged from .78 to .91 (Foster, 1984; Jalowiec, 1979; Langner, 1983). Ample support is thus demonstrated for both homogeneity reliability and stabilily reliability of the JCS.

Principal axis factor analysis was previously done on a sample of 141 subjects to obtain a preliminary assessment of the construct validity of the coping scale (Jalowiec et al., 1984). A two-factor solution failed to support the validity of the dichotomous conceptualization of the coping items as problem-oriented versus affective-oriented. Although 80% of the problem items loaded on the first factor in that solution, only 56% of the affective items loaded on the second factor, thereby suggesting multidimensionality of the coping items rather than bidimensionality. Follow-up analysis indicated, instead, a four-factor pattern for the JCS. These four coping factors were labeled cognitive, tension-modulating, powerlessness, and other-directed (Jalowiec et al., 1984).

Because this preliminary investigation satisfied only minimal sample size requirements (Comrey, 1973; Tabachnick & Fidell, 1983), a large sample validation study was necessary. Therefore, the present study was conducted in an effort to generate more definitive results on the construct validity of the JCS. As used in this study, the coping scale fits loosely into a criterion-referenced framework, with the criteria being the mathematical standards for inclusion of items on a dimension as stipulated by the particular statistical procedure employed.

PROCEDURE FOR DEVELOPMENT

Sample

The coping data used for this study were originally collected by 22 investigators in 10 states and were made available to the author in order to provide a large data base for psychometric analysis of the tool. Data on 1,400 subjects were available and therefore were used as an aggregated sample for this project.

The sample consisted of four types of subjects: patients, 56% ($N = 790$); nurses, 25% ($N = 353$); family members of patients, 10% ($N = 133$); and graduate students, 9% ($N = 124$). Represented in the patient component were hypertensives, dialysis patients, cardiacs, abortion patients, nonserious emergency room (ER) patients, persons on parenteral nutrition at home, epileptic patients, arthritics, patients with chronic obstructuve pulmonary disease (COPD), quadriplegics, cancer patients, and diabetics. Included in the nurse component were ER and intensive care unit (ICU) nurses, other types of hospital staff nurses, and critical care supervisors and faculty. The family group consisted of persons who had family members with chronic or terminal illness, and the student group consisted of graduate students in a health discipline.

So often, nursing studies focus on only one kind of patient or nurse sample, thereby limiting generalizability. However, the diversity of subjects found in this data base enhances the potential for wider applicability of the findings from this study regarding the salient dimensions of coping behavior.

Ages of the subjects ranged from 15 to 95 years, with a mean age of 46. Two-thirds of the sample were female, and half were married. One-fourth of the sample had a college degree, and half were employed. Of the 800 subjects for whom race was reported, almost two-thirds were white.

Scoring the JCS

The JCS lists 40 coping behaviors, gleaned from literature review, which are to be rated on a 1 (never) to 5 (almost always) Likert scale to indicate the extent of use of each strategy. Ratings for items within each subscale are added to obtain a score for each coping scale. Higher scores indicate greater use of that particular coping style. Content validity of the instrument is substantiated by the systematic manner of tool development, the broad literature base from which the items were drawn, the large number of items used to tap the conceptual domain, and the inclusion of diverse coping behaviors.

METHODOLOGY FOR TESTING

Rationale for Methodology

Since the literature and previous work with the JCS had suggested several potential models for the instrument, confirmatory factor analysis was needed to evaluate the differential validity of these models and subsequently to derive a useful conceptual framework for the coping scale. Therefore, confirmatory factor analysis was performed on the coping data from the aggregated sample by using the LISREL VI statistical program (Joreskog & Sorbom, 1983).

LISREL has two statistical models, the measurement model and the structural equation model; the measurement model was used in this study. LISREL was appropriate for this analysis because it would allow both a comparison and a refinement of conceptual models for the coping scale, and would yield both validity and reliability data.

LISREL is currently touted as the state of the art in confirmatory factor analysis (Long, 1983). Previously available factor analytic procedures lacked clear guidelines for evaluating the validity of competing conceptual frameworks. With LISREL, however, the validity of a model can be assessed via significance testing of the maximum likelihood estimates for the parameters in the model (Kroonenberg & Lewis, 1982). LISREL will also identify which parameters for the model do not sufficiently fit the sample data as proposed, so the model can be sequentially modified until a closer fitting framework evolves.

LISREL Procedure

LISREL confirmatory factor analysis involves four major steps: model specification, parameter estimation, assessment of goodness of fit, and modification of the model. Because LISREL is not yet well known to most researchers, an overview of the procedure follows.

Specification

For basic specification of the model in the first step, the investigator indicates the number of factors proposed, which variables are thought to load on which factors, and whether the factors are hypothesized to be correlated or not. Default specifications for additional terms in the model can be changed as needed.

Estimation

Once the model is specified, values for parameters in the model can then be estimated. Parameters to be estimated include factor loadings, factor correlations, and residuals. The purpose of estimation is to find values for these parameters that reproduce as closely as possible the sample covariance matrix (Long, 1983). Five estimation procedures are available; the choice of which to use depends on such considerations as the stage of model development, computer time available, and the type of data being analyzed. The best of the estimates is maximum likelihood (ML) because this procedure maintains consistency and precision as sample size increases (Long, 1983). Maximum likelihood is a technique for generalizing from a sample to a population by deriving parameter estimates for the model being hypothesized for the population so that the estimates converge to the sample data (Gorsuch, 1983).

Assessment of Fit

After parameter estimates are derived, assessment of the goodness of fit (GOF) of the model follows in the third step. Several indicators of the *overall* fit of the model to the data are included in the output, such as chi square, adjusted GOF index, and root mean square residual. Indicators of the *specific* fit of each parameter are also found, such as residuals, standard errors, and modification indices.

A modification index (MI) shows the minimum amount of improvement that will result in the chi square if that parameter were estimated by LISREL. An MI is given for each parameter that has been fixed at zero when the model was specified. Fixing a parameter at zero indicates that an item is not hypothesized to load on a factor; therefore, LISREL will not estimate that factor loading. After the model is estimated, LISREL will then indicate, via the MI, whether the investigator was correct in specifying that parameter as zero. An MI should be nonsignificant and less than 5 to show good fit of the parameter (Joreskog & Sorbom, 1983). Significance of an MI is judged by comparing it to a chi square distribution at 1 degree of freedom.

Regarding the chi square indicator, two things need to be noted. First, when assessing GOF with LISREL confirmatory factor analysis, a *nonsignificant* chi square is needed because this indicates that the parameter estimates for the proposed model closely approximate the sample data (Joreskog & Sorbom, 1983). Second, when the sample size is very large, virtually any model would be rejected because it would be significant based on the regular chi square for the large sample; therefore, *relative* chi square should be used instead because it adjusts for sample size (Carmines & McIver, 1981; Wheaton, Muthen, Alwin, & Summers, 1977). This is the chi square divided by the degrees of freedom. Relative chi square is then assessed for significance by using the chi square table at 1 degree of freedom. Wheaten et al. (1977) suggested that a relative chi square of 5 or less indicates reasonable fit of the model to the data. Table 13.1 summarizes indicators of poor fit and of problems with LISREL models.

Modification

If the GOF indicators do not show *optimal* fit of the model to the data (which is not unusual), then the model can be sequentially modified in the last step to improve the fit. This is accomplished through an iterative

TABLE 13.1 Indicators of Problems with LISREL Models

Relative chi square above 5 or significant
Modification indices above 5 or significant
Small adjusted goodness of fit index
Large root mean square residual
Normalized residuals larger than 2
Large standard errors
Negative variances
Correlations larger than 1
Large correlations between parameter estimates
Small or negative determinant of matrix
Small or negative squared multiple correlations
Small or negative coefficient of determination
Matrices that are not positive definite
Nonidentified parameters
T-values less than 2 or nonsignificant

Source: Compiled from Joreskog & Sorbom (1983).

process whereby at each step the parameter with the highest MI is estimated by LISREL. Two points should be noted about this refining process. First, if it is felt that an item does not fit conceptually with a factor, then that item should be kept fixed at zero even though its MI is high. Second, this refining process is a step-by-step procedure in which only one parameter with a high MI is estimated each time. This is because shifts can result in other estimates from a change in a single parameter; therefore, trying to proceed too quickly with this refining process can lead to a distorted picture of the model (Joreskog & Sorbom, 1983).

The t-value (i.e., parameter estimates divided by their standard errors) also can provide feedback for this modification process. If the t-value is not significant, that parameter can be set to zero to improve the fit (Kroonenberg & Lewis, 1982). This improvement is accomplished not by increasing the chi square itself but by recovering degrees of freedom, which will allow one to judge the significance of the chi square at greater degrees of freedom on the table. This will then result in better approximations of fit (Kroonenberg & Lewis, 1982; Long, 1983).

When the GOF indicators demonstrate adequate concordance between the model and the data, the refining process can be terminated. Overfitting of the model is to be avoided because that can cause problems with improper parameter estimates (i.e., values outside normal boundaries). Overfitting can also capitalize on chance characteristics of the sample and make results harder to replicate with a new group (Kroonenberg & Lewis, 1982).

Models Tested

Seven models for the coping scale were tested with LISREL. The first model was based on the results of the earlier classification study (Jalowiec & Powers, 1981) in which the coping items were labeled by nurses as either problem-oriented or affective-oriented. The second was a two-factor model that had emerged from the previous small-sample analysis (Jalowiec et al., 1984), which explored the validity of this dichotomy. Even though both of these first two models were based on the problem/ affective dichotomy, the composition of problem and affect varied to some degree in each model.

The third model tested was the four-factor structure that had evolved as the best conceptual pattern from the preliminary small-sample investigation (Jalowiec et al., 1984). The other models evaluated were based on frameworks of three, five, six, and seven factors for the coping items; these patterns had been considered in earlier analyses (Jalowiec et al., 1984) but were discarded at that time because they were less than optimal solutions for the data set.

Evaluation of Models

To evaluate the potential utility of each of the seven models under consideration for the coping scale, while at the same time conserving computer resources for subsequent model refinement, each model was subjected to one iteration of LISREL confirmatory factor analysis. Psychometric criteria for all solutions were then compared. Based on the indicators listed in Table 13.2, the three-factor model demonstrated the most potential for a useful model for the coping scale. This trichotomous model was chosen as the most promising framework because it had the following combination of desirable characteristics: a fairly low relative chi square, a high adjusted GOF index, a low root mean square residual, a fairly high coefficient of determination, positive definite matrices, and low factor correlations.

Problems found with the other models included the following. Some matrices were not positive definite in the five-, six-, or seven-factor solutions. A matrix that is not positive definite will be uninvertible (Cattell, 1978); therefore, the model could not be considered identified (Long, 1983). (A model that is identified will have unique and thus meaningful parameter estimates).

Improper parameter estimates were found with some models. For example, the four-factor model had factor loadings larger than 1. Exceedingly high factor correlations (some in the .80s and .90s were found in the four-, five-, six-, and seven-factor models. This designated too much overlap in the content of the factors, thereby implying factor fission. Absence of such negative features and presence of comparatively good fit indicators for a preliminary model suggested that the three-factor structure had the greatest potential for a useful conceptual framework for the JCS.

TABLE 13.2 LISREL Indicators for Seven Coping Scale Models[a]

Model	RCS	AGOFI	RMSR	COD	LEG EST	POS DEF MAT	FAC COR	IDEN
Cl.St.[b]	8.5	.74	.13	−1.29	no	yes	low	yes
2 F	7.8	.75	.12	− .55	no	yes	low	yes
3 F	6.8	.80	.11	.68	yes	yes	low	yes
4 F	6.9	.80	.10	.74	no	yes	high	yes
5 F	6.7	.81	.11	.77	yes	no	high	no
6 F	7.0	.80	.11	.71	yes	no	high	no
7 F	5.4	.85	.09	.98	yes	no	high	no

Abbreviations for indicators are as follows: RCS, relative chi square; AGOFI, adjusted goodness of fit index; RMSR, root mean square residual; COD, coefficient of determination; LEG EST, if estimates were within legal boundaries; POS DEF MAT, if matrices were positive definite; FAC COR, correlations between factors; IDEN, if parameters were identified.
[a]Via confirmatory factor analysis; $N = 1400$.
[b]Cl. St., classification study.

Refinement of Three-Factor Model

Because the GOF indicators showed less than optimal concordance between the parameter estimates for the three-factor model and the sample data, the model was sequentially refined to improve the fit. When the relative chi square did not change except in the third decimal place for four successive iterations, it became obvious that additional refinement would not prove fruitful and moreover, might yield improper estimates and nonidentified parameters due to attempts to overfit the model. Therefore, further modification was not pursued. The refined three-factor model that resulted will be considered both from psychometric and conceptual perspectives.

GOF of Model

Table 13.3 summarizes the psychometric indicators for the refined three-factor model. The relative chi square (RCS) for the refined model was 4.28 and thus was below the .025 level of significance (RCS = 5.02). Therefore, the parameter estimates for the trichotomous model were not appreciably different from the sample data. This RCS satisfies the criterion of less than 5 (Wheaton et al., 1977) for reasonable fit of the model to the data.

The adjusted GOF index (AGOFI) was .87, again indicating close concordance between the model and the data. The root mean square residual (RMSR) was appropriately low (.06). The AGOFI and the RMSR are both indicators of the overall fit of the model. The first is based on the variances and covariances for the parameter estimates whereas the second is based on those for the residuals (Joreskog & Sorbom, 1983). The AGOFI has the advantage of not being sensitive to sample size and also of being robust to departures from normality. If the fit of the model is very good, the AGOFI should be near 1 and the RMSR near 0.

TABLE 13.3 LISREL Indicators for Refined Trichotomous Model

Relative chi square	4.28
Adjusted GOF index	.87
Root mean square residual	.06
Coefficient of determination	.95
Determinant of sample covariance matrix	.81
Largest standard error	.05
Largest first-order derivative	.05
Largest correlation between parameter estimates	.31
Percentage of nonsignificant *t*-values	3.37%
Percentage of normalized residuals over 2	17.07%
Highest modification index	3.49

All modification indices for the final model were below 5, thereby demonstrating sufficient model refinement (Joreskog & Sorbom, 1983). The highest index was 3.49; hence, all MIs were appropriately below the .05 level of significance (MI = 3.84), and thus all parameters fit the data reasonably well.

Although all of the above statistical indicators (RCS, AGOFI, RMSR, MIs) suggested reasonable fit of the model to the data, 17% of the normalized residuals were undesirably above the criterion of 2 cited in the manual. Long (1983) points out, however, that MIs are better determinants of the GOF of the model than residuals because an MI takes into account the change in the fit of all variables *jointly* based on modifying that one parameter, whereas a residual just accounts for the fit of a single parameter. Therefore, the refined trichotomous model did provide a close approximation of the sample data.

Improvement in Fit

The question of whether the final trichotomous model fit the data *significantly* better than the original three-factor model can be answered by the chi square for improvement of fit for nested models, which is calculated on the differences between the chi squares and the degrees of freedom for each model (Long, 1983). In this case, however, the chi square should be significant, so as to indicate that the improvement of the derived model over the original model is meaningful (Carmines & McIver, 1981). The difference in chi squares was 1879 with 6 degrees of freedom ($p < .001$); hence, the refined trichotomous model did fit the data significantly better than the original three-factor model.

Identification

A crucial consideration during the LISREL process is the issue of whether the model is identified. If a model is identified, then unique and meaningful estimates can be derived for the parameters. If estimates were not unique to that model, then other conceptual frameworks might fit the sample data just as well. Identifiability depends on how the model is specified. Therefore, based on model specification, the refined trichotomous model satisfied the following conditions for an identified factor analysis model (Carmines & McIver, 1981; Holzer & Robbins, 1981; Joreskog, 1979; Joreskog & Sorbom, 1983; Long, 1983):

1. The number of independent parameters to be estimated for the model was less than the number of independent covariance equations.
2. The phi matrix (factor correlations) was a symmetric matrix with l's on the diagonal.
3. The theta delta matrix (error terms) was a diagonal matrix with free elements on the diagonal.

4. The lambda matrix (factor loadings) had at least (1 – factors) or 2 fixed zeroes in each column.
5. A metric was established for the latent variables.
6. All matrices were positive definite.

Satisfaction of these conditions therefore indicated that the ML estimates derived from this analysis were unique to the three-factor model; thus, the estimates were meaningful.

REFINED TRICHOTOMOUS MODEL

Table 13.4 shows the item composition for each of the factors in the refined trichotomous model. An item had to have a factor loading of at least .30 to be considered meaningful; this is the minimum noted by Gorsuch (1983), Cattell (1978), Nunnally (1978), Child (1970), Kim and Mueller (1978), and Carmines and Zeller (1979). Explication of the conceptual themes in each factor follows.

Factor I

Loading significantly on the first factor in the trichotomous model (Table 13.4) were 11 items previously classified by the nurses as problem-oriented coping strategies and 2 that were affective-oriented. Based on high squared multiple correlations from the LISREL analysis, the most reliable indicators of Factor I were the following: Try out solutions (SMC = .57), Information-seeking (.53), and Goal-setting (.41). Other coping strategies found here relate to control, objectivity, and discussion of the problem. On the whole, then, the coping methods loading highly on this factor focus on constructive handling of the stressful situation and facing up to the problem. Factor I was therefore labeled as *confrontive* coping behavior. [In agreement with Lazarus and Folkman's (1984) perspective, value-laden labels will be avoided, and so the factor will not be called "constructive."]

The two items with the lowest of the significant loadings on Factor I (seek comfort/help and activity/exercise) were both previously classified as affective coping strategies. Conceptually, it is easier to discern the coping relationship between seeking comfort/help and confronting the problem than between activity and confronting (except for the fact that activity and confronting are both nonpassive behaviors). However, activity and exercise might help relieve some of the distress arising from the situation so that the problem *can* be faced head on, thereby suggesting more of an indirect association between these two elements. Also, exercise may give a person the energy to confront the problem, and activity may generate a sense of control over the situation, thereby facilitating problem management.

TABLE 13.4 Composition of Trichotomous
Model for Coping Scale[a]

No.	Item	Loading
Factor I: Confrontive		
33.	Try out solutions	.92
32.	Information-seeking	.85
36.	Handle problem in steps	.83
38.	Set goals	.81
35.	Make use of past experience	.77
25.	Try to change situation	.73
6.	Think through solutions	.72
20.	Find purpose/meaning	.72
18.	View problem objectively	.67
19.	Maintain control	.58
14.	Discuss problem	.51
30.	Seek comfort/help from others	.43
3.	Activity/exercise	.36
Factor II: Emotive		
22.	Get nervous	.69
1	Worry	.57
26.	Take tensions out on others	.52
15.	Expect the worst	.47
16.	Get mad	.46
27.	Want to be alone	.44
7.	Eat/smoke	.42
24.	Blame others for problem	.37
12.	Daydream	.36
Factor III: Palliative		
37.	Sleep	.71
39.	Don't worry	.65
40.	Compromise	.64
34.	Resignation because it's fate	.64
29.	Do nothing and wait it out	.54
4.	Hope for improvement	.53
10.	Put problem aside	.52
28.	Resignation because it's hopeless	.47
5.	Laugh it off	.46
17.	Accept situation	.42
23.	Withdraw from situation	.42
13.	Try anything	.40
21.	Pray	.36
11.	Let someone else solve problem	.35

[a]Via LISREL confirmatory factor analysis; $N = 1400$.

It was interesting to find that the item "Seek purpose or meaning in the situation" again loaded highly on the first factor, just as it has done in previous work, although the conceptual fit with some of the other items on Factor I may not seem so apparent. This item had previously been classified by the nurses as a problem-oriented coping method. In addition, this item loaded on the problem factor in the initial dichotomous solution and on the cognitive factor in the preliminary four-factor structure. In the present interpretation, finding meaning in the situation can alter the person's perspective so that he/she can then confront the problem in a new light.

Throughout all factor analytic procedures, Factor I has maintained the greatest stability and uniformity. The first 10 items on Factor I loaded significantly on the first factor in all of the different solutions examined in this analysis and in earlier results. The less consistent items were Discuss the problem, Seek comfort/help from others, and Activity/exercise. Similar results were obtained by Murphy (1982) and by Westlake and Taylor (1985). Overall then, Factor I has demonstrated considerable factorial invariance, thereby attesting to the primacy of the confrontive coping style in the adaptive repertoire.

The confrontive coping dimension is similar to Lipowski's (1970) idea of tackling the problem rather than capitulating or avoiding it. In addition, Weisman (1979) labeled as confrontation one of the coping styles he identified in extensive work with cancer patients. The two coping dimensions might not be exactly the same though. The present author's perception is that the word "confrontation" has more of a negative connotation and implies conflictive resistance and counterposing forces; whereas "confrontive" conveys more of a meaning of resolute determination to come to terms with the problem and try to handle it, and therefore has more of a positive focus.

Factor II

All nine items loading significantly on Factor II of the trichotomous model were previously classified by the nurses as affective coping strategies. Examination of the most reliable indicators for this factor provides strong support for labeling Factor II as *emotive* coping behavior. These indicators were as follows: Get nervous (SMC = .32), Take out tensions on others (.29), Worry (.27), and Blame others for your problems (.24). Get mad and Expect the worst also loaded highly here. It's obvious that these coping methods express emotions evoked by the situation and allow for the ventilation of feelings – hence, the emotive label.

All nine items found on the emotive dimension in the present analysis loaded on the affective factor in the earlier dichotomous solution, though some loadings only approached significance. Seven of these nine items loaded on the powerlessness dimension in the previous four-factor results, with the other two items (Take tensions out on others and Daydream) loading on the other-directed factor. Most of the emotive items also proved to be cohesive in Murphy's (1982) and in Westlake and Taylor's (1985) four-factor solutions of JCS data.

The emotive coping style would be akin to Lazarus and Folkman's (1984) emotion-focused dimension, Robbins and Tanck's (1978) dysfunctional behavior, Billings and Moos's (1984) emotional discharge, Kiely's

(1972) affective coping methods, and Kobasa's (Kobasa, Maddi, Donner, Merrick, & White, 1984) regressive coping style. Therefore, many people would feel that the emotive coping behaviors are less desirable ways of handling stress. However, these types of strategies can serve a useful purpose in the coping armamentarium because they allow the person to vent some of the distress generated by the situation so that the person can continue to function. Excessive and inappropriate use of such coping behaviors would of course be the determining factor in how well the emotive strategies serve the person's overall adaptational outcome.

Factor III

Factor III of the trichotomous model consists of many coping behaviors that modulate tension without directly confronting the problem. Ten of the items were previously classified by the nurses as affective coping strategies and four as problem-oriented. The most reliable indicators of this coping dimension were the following: Don't worry (SMC = .41); Resignation due to fate (.33); Resignation due to hopeless (.30); and Sleep (.30). Other items loading here were Compromise, Hope for improvement, Put the problem out of your mind, and Pray. These coping strategies suggest a sense of easing the stress or keeping it under control without directly curing or taking care of the problem. Therefore, Factor III was labeled as *palliative* coping behavior.

Most of the items found on the palliative dimension in the present analysis loaded on the affective factor in the initial dichotomous solution and on the tension-modulating and powerlessness factors in the preliminary four-factor model. Many of these same items also loaded on Westlake and Taylor's (1985) avoidance dimension in their four-factor solution. However, examination of the conceptual composition of the palliative factor suggests more than just avoiding the problem, although an element of evasiveness is present in some of the items. For example, consider the coping strategies having to do with resignation, compromise, and acceptance. These coping behaviors do not imply evasion of the stressful situation but rather of finding some way to alter the perception of the problem so as to be able to still meet the demands of the situation without becoming immobilized by the stress. Therefore, this author feels that a palliative label is more consonant with the tenor of these items than an avoidance label.

The ubiquity and practical utility of this coping approach can be attested to be the recognition of many writers of the existence of a palliative dimension in adaptation. Such a coping style can be identified in the literature in many references (e.g., Ilfeld, 1980; Lazarus & Launier, 1978; Menaghan, 1983; Oskins, 1979; Pearlin & Schooler, 1978; Weisman, 1979).

Nonsignificant Items

Four coping strategies did not load significantly on any of the factors in the trichotomous model. The items and their factor loadings were: Cry (.25 on Factor II); Drink (.18 on Factor II); Take drugs (.07 on Factor II); and Meditate (.22 on Factor III). Since crying is usually such a transitory response, perhaps subjects saw this more as a passing reaction to stress rather than as a coping strategy per se. Further, meager use of such strategies as meditation and biofeedback accounted for the lack of factorial importance of these particular types of coping methods, even though behavioral modification enthusiasts have tried to encourage the use and document the efficacy of such cognitive control strategies.

Drinking and taking drugs have also proved to be problematic items in earlier analyses. It seems that a social desirability bias might be operating here; thus, people just are not admitting to alcohol and drug use for coping. Sidle and his associates (Sidle, Moos, Adams, & Cady, 1969) found, to the contrary, that paper-and-pencil tools were capable of eliciting information on less desirable means of handling stress. Since it is well known that people resort to substance abuse in order to cope, it's hard to find realistic support for deleting these two items from the coping scale based on their nonsignificant factor loadings in JCS results thus far. Instead, a rewording of these items to make them less threatening may help generate more reliable information on the use of these coping methods.

Factor Correlations

Correlations between factors in the trichotomous model were low as would be desired: .02 between Factor I and Factor II; .24 between Factor I and Factor III; and .03 between Factor II and Factor III. These correlations indicate that the factors showed little overlap in content and thus were fairly independent of each other, although significant ($p < .05$) item-total correlations documented that all items do relate in common to the construct of coping. Hence, the confrontive, emotive, and palliative factors represent relatively distinct dimensions of coping behavior.

Reliability

Based on the LISREL analysis, the coefficient of determination for the refined trichotomous model was .95 and thus exceptionally good. This coefficient provides a generalized measure of the reliability for the entire measurement model (Joreskog & Sorbom, 1983) and therefore indicates that the observed variables (coping strategies) are accurately measuring the latent variables (coping dimensions). Cronbach's alpha coefficients were also computed to assess the degree of homogeneity within each factor. Alpha provides a conservative estimate of reliability, thereby establishing a lower boundary for the reliability value (Novick & Lewis, 1967).

For the three factors the alphas were .85, .70, and .75. All coefficients meet or exceed Nunnally's (1978) criterion. The somewhat lower alpha on Factor II reflects both the generally lower SMCs found on items loading here and the smaller number of items on this factor, for alpha is known to be a function of item intercorrelations plus the number of items (Carmines & Zeller, 1979). According to Thorndike (1982), the progressively greater impact of item number on scale reliability occurs because true-score variance increases as a quadratic function of instrument length, whereas error variance increases only as a linear function. Therefore, adding several items should raise the alpha coefficient for the second factor.

Examination of the correlation matrix showed that the highest interitem correlation was .63; therefore, the alphas were not artificially inflated by redundancy of content (Hinshaw & Atwood, 1982). Lack of redundancy is confirmed by the determinant of the sample covariance matrix, which was .81 (out of a possible 1). If the determinant is very small, this would indicate nearly perfect linear relationships between some of the variables - hence, redundancy of items (Joreskog & Sorbom, 1983).

Inspection of the corrected alpha coefficients, which are based on deleting less homogeneous items, showed that the alpha for Factor I would be increased from .85 to .86 by deleting either item 3 (Activity/exercise) or item 30 (Seek comfort/help from others). Similarly, the alpha on Factor III would be increased from .75 to .76 by deleting item 21 (Pray). (The alpha for Factor II would not be enhanced by deletion of any items.) However, these items did have significant item-total correlations and meaningful factor loadings. Therefore, since deleting the indicated items would result in only minimal appreciation of the homogeneity reliability estimates for the first and third factors but would cause the perhaps unnecessary loss of items for the scale, the composition of the factors was retained as generated by LISREL.

SUMMARY

This psychometric study can be summarized as follows:

1. LISREL confirmatory factor analysis was used to compare seven models for the JCS to determine which model had the most potential for a useful conceptual framework for the instrument.
2. Examination of psychometric criteria from LISREL indicated that the three-factor model showed the most potential utility.
3. The trichotomous model was then sequentially refined until GOF criteria indicated optimal concordance between the three-factor model and the sample data.
4. Reliability estimates supported the accurate representation of the

data by the trichotomous model and also the homogeneity of content within each factor.

5. Conceptual examination of the model suggested the labels of confrontive, emotive, and palliative for the three coping dimensions.

CONCLUSION

The strengths of this research rest on (1) the large and diverse data base used to test the models, which enhances the generalizability of the findings on the predominant coping dimensions identified; (2) the foundation laid in earlier work to generate the models for testing; (3) the systematic progression of the psychometric testing of this instrument; and (4) the advanced statistical analysis applied to the models under consideration for the coping scale. The results of the present construct validation study therefore provide strong support for a trichotomous conceptual framework for the JCS.

REFERENCES

Billings, A. G., & Moos, R. H., (1984). Coping, stress, and social resources among adults with unipolar depression. *Journal of Personality and Social Psychology, 46,* 877-891.

Carmines, E. G., & McIver, J. P. (1981). Analyzing models with unobserved variables. In G. W. Bohrnstedt & E. F. Borgatta (Eds.), *Social measurement: Current issues* (pp. 65-115). Beverly Hills, CA: Sage.

Carmines, E. G., & Zeller, R. A. (1979). *Reliability and validity assessment.* Beverly Hills, CA: Sage.

Cattell, R. B. (1978). *The scientific use of factor analysis in the behavioral and life sciences.* New York: Plenum.

Child, D. (1970). *The essentials of factor analysis.* New York: Holt, Rinehart & Winston.

Comrey, A. L. (1973). Common methodological problems in factor analytic studies. *Journal of Consulting and Clinical Psychology, 46,* 648-659.

Folkman, S., & Lazarus, R. S. (1980). An analysis of coping in a middle-aged community sample. *Journal of Health and Social Behavior, 21,* 219-239.

Folkman, S., & Lazarus, R. S. (1985). If it changes it must be a process: Study of emotion and coping during three stages of a college examination. *Journal of Personality and Social Psychology, 48,* 150-170.

Foster, G. M. (1984). *Perceptions of coping in hypertensive men: Comparison by compliance status.* Unpublished master's thesis, University of Colorado, Denver.

Gorsuch, R. L. (1983). *Factor analysis* (2nd ed.). Hillsdale, NJ: Erlbaum.

Guilford, J. P. (1954). *Psychometric methods.* New York: McGraw-Hill.

Hinshaw, A. S., & Atwood, J. R. (1982). A patient satisfaction instrument: Precision by replication. *Nursing Research, 31,* 170-175.

Holzer, C. E., & Robbins, L. (1981). Measurement issues in mental health needs assessment. In D. J. Jackson & E. F. Borgatta (Eds.), *Factor analysis and measurement in sociological research* (pp. 149-176). Beverly Hills, CA: Sage.

Ilfeld, F. W. (1980). Coping styles of Chicago adults: Description. *Journal of Human Stress, 6*, 2-10.

Jalowiec, A. (1979). *Stress and coping in hypertensive and emergency room patients.* Unpublished master's thesis, University of Illinois, Chicago.

Jalowiec, A., Murphy, S. P., & Powers, M. J. (1984). Psychometric assessment of the Jalowiec Coping Scale. *Nursing Research, 33*, 157-161.

Jalowiec, A., & Powers, M. J. (1981). Stress and coping in hypertensive and emergency room patients. *Nursing Research, 30*, 10-15.

Joreskog, K. G. (1979). A general approach to confirmatory maximum likelihood factor analysis. In K. G. Joreskog & D. Sorbom (Eds.), *Advances in factor analysis and structural equation models* (pp. 21-43). Cambridge, MA: Abt Books.

Joreskog, K. G., & Sorbom, D. (1983). *LISREL user's guide: Versions V and VI.* Chicago: International Educational Services.

Kiely, W. F. (1972). Coping with severe illness. In Z. J. Lipowski (Ed.), *Psychosocial aspects of physical illness* (pp. 105-118). Basel: Karger.

Kim, J. O., & Mueller, C. W. (1978). *Factor analysis: Statistical methods and practical issues.* Beverly Hills, CA: Sage.

Kobasa, S. C., Maddi, S. R., Donner, E. J., Merrick, W. A., & White, H. (1984). The personality construct of hardiness. Unpublished manuscript.

Kroonenberg, P. M., & Lewis, C. (1982). Methodological issues in the search for a factor model: Exploration through confirmation. *Journal of Educational Statistics, 7*, 69-89.

Langner, S. (1983). *Reliability of the Jalowiec Coping Scale.* Unpublished manuscript, University of Illinois, Chicago.

Lazarus, R. S., & Folkman, S. (1984). *Stress, appraisal, and coping.* New York: Springer Publishing Co.

Lazarus, R. S., & Launier, R. (1978). Stress-related transactions between person and environment. In L. A. Pervin & M. Lewis (Eds.), *Perspectives in interactional psychology* (pp. 287-327). New York: Plenum.

Lipowski, Z. J. (1970). Physical illness, the individual and the coping process. *International Journal of Psychiatry in Medicine, 1*, 91-102.

Long, J. S. (1983). *Confirmatory factor analysis.* Beverly Hills, CA: Sage.

Menaghan, E. G. (1983). Individual coping efforts: Moderators of the relationship between life stress and mental health outcomes. In H. B. Kaplan (Ed.), *Psychosocial stress: Trends in theory and research* (pp. 157-191). New York: Academic Press.

Murphy, S. (1984). Long-term recovery of bereaved relatives of Mt. St. Helens earthquake victims. Unpublished raw data.

Murphy, S. P. (1982). *Factors influencing adjustment and quality of life of hemodialysis patients: A multivariate approach.* Unpublished doctoral dissertation, University of Illinois, Chicago.

Novick, M., & Lewis, G. (1967). Coefficient alpha and the reliability of composite measurements. *Psychometrika, 32*, 1-13.

Nunnally, J. C. (1978). *Psychometric theory* (2nd ed.). New York: McGraw-Hill.

Oskins, S. L. (1979). Identification of situational stressors and coping methods by intensive care nurses. *Heart and Lung, 8*, 953-960.

Pearlin, L. I., & Schooler, C. (1978). The structure of coping. *Journal of Health and Social Behavior, 19*, 2-21.

Powers, M. J., & Jalowiec, A. (1987). Profile of the well controlled, well adjusted hypertensive patient. *Nursing Research, 36*, 106-110.

Robbins, P. R., & Tanck, R. H. (1978). A factor analysis of coping behaviors. *Journal of Clinical Psychology, 34*, 379-380.

Sidle, A., Moos, R. H., Adams, J., & Cady, P. (1969). Development of a coping scale. *Archives of General Psychiatry, 20*, 225-232.

Tabachnick, B. G., & Fidell, L. S. (1983). *Using multivariate statistics.* New York: Harper & Row.

Thorndike, R. L. (1982). *Applied psychometrics.* Boston: Houghton Mifflin.

Weisman, A. (1979). *Coping with cancer.* New York: McGraw-Hill.

Westlake, S. K., & Taylor, L. L. (1985, April). *Psychometric properties of the Jalowiec Coping Scale.* Poster presented at the Ninth Annual Midwest Nursing Research Society Conference, Chicago.

Wheaton, B., Muthen, B., Alwin, D. F., & Summers, G. F. (1977). Assessing the reliability and stability in panel models. In D. R. Heise (Ed.) *Sociological methodology 1977* (pp. 84-136). San Francisco: Jossey-Bass.

COPING SCALE

People react in many ways to stress and tension. Some people use one way to handle stress; others use many coping methods. I am interested in finding out what things people do when faced with stressful situations. Please estimate *how often* you use the following ways to cope with stress by picking one number for *each item*.

Coping Method	Never	Occasionally	About half the time	Often	Almost Always
1. Worry (A)[1]	1	2	3	4	5
2. Cry (A)	1	2	3	4	5
3. Work off tension with physical activity or exercise (A)	1	2	3	4	5
4. Hope that things will get better (A)	1	2	3	4	5
5. Laugh it off, figuring that things could be worse (A)	1	2	3	4	5
6. Think through different ways to solve the problem or handle the situation (P)[2]	1	2	3	4	5
7. Eat; smoke; chew gum (A)	1	2	3	4	5
8. Drink alcoholic beverages (A)	1	2	3	4	5
9. Take drugs (A)	1	2	3	4	5
10. Try to put the problem out of your mind and think of something else (A)	1	2	3	4	5
11. Let someone else solve the problem or handle the situation (P)	1	2	3	4	5
12. Daydream; fantasize (A)	1	2	3	4	5
13. Do anything just to do something, even if you're not sure it will work (P)	1	2	3	4	5
14. Talk the problem over with someone who has been in the same type of situation (P)	1	2	3	4	5
15. Get prepared to expect the worst (A)	1	2	3	4	5

16. Get mad; curse; swear (A)	1	2	3	4	5
17. Accept the situation as it is (P)	1	2	3	4	5
18. Try to look at the problem objectively and see all sides (P)	1	2	3	4	5
19. Try to maintain some control over the situation (P)	1	2	3	4	5
20. Try to find purpose or meaning in the situation (P)	1	2	3	4	5
21. Pray; put your trust in God (A)	1	2	3	4	5
22. Get nervous (A)	1	2	3	4	5
23. Withdraw from the situation (A)	1	2	3	4	5
24. Blame someone else for your problems or the situation you're in (A)	1	2	3	4	5
25. Actively try to change the situation (P)	1	2	3	4	5
26. Take out your tensions on someone else or something else (A)	1	2	3	4	5
27. Take off by yourself; want to be alone (A)	1	2	3	4	5
28. Resign yourself to the situation because things look hopeless (A)	1	2	3	4	5
29. Do nothing in the hope that the situation will improve or that the problem will take care of itself (A)	1	2	3	4	5
30. Seek comfort or help from family or friends (A)	1	2	3	4	5
31. Meditate; use yoga, biofeedback, or "mind over matter" (A)	1	2	3	4	5
32. Try to find out more about the situation so you can handle it better (P)	1	2	3	4	5
33. Try out different ways of solving the problem to see which works the best (P)	1	2	3	4	5
34. Resign yourself to the situation because it's your fate, so there's no sense trying to do anything about it (A)	1	2	3	4	5
35. Try to draw on past experience to help you handle the situation (P)	1	2	3	4	5

36. Try to break the problem down into "smaller pieces" so you can handle it better (P)	1	2	3	4	5
37. Go to sleep, figuring things will look better in the morning (A)	1	2	3	4	5
38. Set specific goals to help you solve the problem (P)	1	2	3	4	5
39. "Don't worry about it, everything will probably work out fine" (A)	1	2	3	4	5
40. Settled for the next best thing to what you really wanted (P)	1	2	3	4	5

[1]A = affective-oriented coping method.
[2]p = problem-oriented coping method.

14
Measuring Social Support: Revision and Further Development of The Personal Resource Questionnaire

Clarann Weinert

This chapter discusses the Personal Resource Questionnair (PRQ) a measure of social support.

A current focus of attention in the health-related and social science disciplines is the study of social forces in the environment that contribute to the maintenance and promotion of people's health. Wortman (1984) noted in her comprehensive review of the concept and measurement of social support that although the nature, meaning, and measurement of this concept are still debated, social support has been claimed to have positive effects on a wide variety of outcomes, including physical health, mental well-being, and social functioning. Although the concept has been around for a long time in the guise of caring, friendship, community cohesion, or unconditional positive regard (Tilden, 1985) it was Caplan's work in 1974 that had a strong influence on viewing social support as various forms of aid or assistance supplied by family members, friends, neighbors, and others. In the last decade hundreds of studies and numerous review articles and books have appeared dealing with social support (Wortman, 1984). Despite impressive research efforts, the empirically substantiated body of knowledge regarding social support has some major limitations. Norbeck, Lindsey, & Carrieri (1981) stated that there is a lack of conceptual agreement on what social support is and how it functions to protect health or buffer the effects of stressors. There are wide discrepancies among the approaches that researchers have taken to measure the support construct (Gottlieb, 1983; Tilden, 1985; Wortman, 1984), and

Prepared for the Measurement of Clinical and Educational Nursing Outcomes Project, University of Maryland, School of Nursing, Wealtha McGurn, Ph.D., R.N., consultant.

social support continues to be measured differently from study to study, usually by instruments that have not been tested for reliability and validity (Norbeck et al., 1981; Rock, Green, Wise, & Rock, 1984). The purpose of this study was to further develop and test a social support instrument that has been used in nursing, the Personal Resource Questionnaire (PRQ) (Brandt & Weinert, 1981).

CONCEPTUAL BASIS OF THE PRQ

Definition of Social Support

To begin to address the issues of measuring social support, Brandt and Weinert (1981) designed the PRQ. This measure of social support was developed through a synthesis of ideas, with principal reliance on Weiss's (1969, 1974) model of relational functions. Social support is defined in a comprehensive fashion as composed of the following dimensions: (a) provision for attachment/intimacy, (b) social integration – being an integral part of a group, (c) opportunity for nurturant behavior, (d) reassurance of worth as an individual and in role accomplishments, and (e) the availability of informational, emotional, and material help.

Description

As one of the first-generation social support instruments the PRQ begins to address the issues of definition and measurement of social support, as well as providing a way to compare results across studies. The PRQ, a norm-referenced instrument, is a two-part measure of social support. Part 1 consists of 10 life situations in which one might be expected to need some assistance; it provides descriptive information concerning the person's resources and their satisfaction with the help they received from their resources. Part 2 is a 25-item Likert scale developed according to Weiss's (1969, 1974) relational dimensions; it measures the respondent's *perceived level* of social support.

Development

Before the initial utilization of the PRQ in empirical investigations, content and face validity were established, and the tool was pilot-tested to evaluate the format and wording of the questions. The original version of the PRQ was initially used in the dissertation research of the authors (Brandt, 1982; Weinert, 1982) of the tool. The initial use and psychometric evaluation of the PRQ provided reasonable evidence that the instrument may be an effective way to assess the social environment. Some slight modifications in the wording were made following the first two studies. Since that time Brandt and Weinert have conducted several studies designed to evaluate specific aspects of the PRQ. Results of psychometric testing are published elsewhere (Brandt, 1984; Brandt & Weinert, 1981; Weinert, 1984; Weinert & Brandt, 1987), and are reviewed in subsequent sections of this chapter.

The PRQ has received considerable attention from nurse researchers and researchers in other health-related fields and is currently being used in approximately 75 studies. Continued use and evaluation of the PRQ had identified some issues that required further study. The Measurement of Clinical and Educational Nursing Outcomes Project provides an excellent opportunity to address these issues.

PURPOSE OF STUDY

The specific aims of the study included the following:

1. Content analysis of the open-ended question in Part 1 to assess the adequacy of the content domain of the eight life situations.
2. Consideration of rewording of the items in the nurturance subscale.
3. Assessment of the multidimensionality of the subscales in Part 2.

This chapter consists of three distinct sections, one section for each of the aims of the study. In each section there is a discussion of an aim, the methodology used for the analysis, the results of the analysis, and suggestions for revision and further evaluation of the PRQ.

ADMINISTRATION AND SCORING

The PRQ is designed to be a self-administered tool that requires the respondent to circle a response for each item. Part 1 provides descriptive information and is not scored in the strict sense. The number and types of resources may be identified across each situation. Overall satisfaction can be obtained by summing the level of satisfaction for each of the situations that were experienced in the past six months. The second part of the PRQ has a seven-point Likert format, composed of 25 items, rated from "strongly agree" (7) to "strongly disagree" (1). Five of the items are written in the negative and must be recoded, resulting in a scale in which higher scores indicate higher levels of perceived social support. The items are then summed for a total score ranging from 25 to 175.

INSTRUMENT DEVELOPMENT PROCESS AND METHODOLOGY FOR TESTING

PRQ Part 1: Open-ended Questions

Problem

In Part 1 of the PRQ there were eight life situations developed to represent the domains of events for which one might need assistance. The domains were derived from a review of the literature and from evaluation of existing social support and social network instruments. The eight situations included the domains of (a) immediate help, (b) extended help with an ill family member, (c) help in the event of short-term illness, (d) problems regarding family/friend, (e) problems with spouse/partners, (f) loneliness, (g) financial problems, and (h) global concerns with life. Content validity was initially established by the use of teams of experts to evaluate these domains.

To further validate the adequacy of these domains a ninth question was included in 1982 as a part of the modification of the original PRQ. This question reads: "What has been the greatest concern or problem for you in the past six months?" The respondent described the problem and then indicated to whom they had turned for assistance and their level of satisfaction with the help they received.

Method

An available data set from a study conducted in 1982 by Weinert and Brandt (1987) was used to analyze the responses to the open-ended question. The sample consisted of 120 adults, aged 30 to 37 years, who had graduated from the same university. The majority of the respondents were Caucasian, married, employed full-time, with an average family income of $20,000 to $30,000. Three-fourths of the sample were men, the mean number of years of education was 17.4, and all respondents lived in the greater Seattle area.

One hundred twelve written responses to the open-ended question were provided by the 120 participants. These responses were typed and the eight domains operationalized. Two judges, nurse researchers who were not familiar with the development of the PRQ, were instructed to indicate the domain into which each open-ended response belonged. They were also to indicate those responses that could not be assigned to a domain. Both of the tool developers also served as judges.

Results

Thirty-seven of the 112 responses were rated by at least one of the four judges as not fitting into any of the eight domains. These 37 items were content-analyzed to identify common elements. Fourteen of the responses clearly represented a domain of problems in the work setting. Sixteen responses formed a domain of issues related to concerns about health or decisions such as going back to school. The remaining seven responses could be categorized in one of the original eight domains. The content analysis procedure and the resulting categories were validated by a nurse researcher who is an expert in analytic techniques.

Discussion

Further revision and evaluation of Part 1 of the PRQ were indicated by this analysis. Items to tap the domains of job problems and personal concerns were designed. Slight modification of the wording of some of the original eight situations was carried out with the expectation that more explicit wording would facilitate the respondents' identification with the situation.

A new segment was added to each question in Part 1, asking respondents to describe the situation to which they are responding; this was done to provide information as to how the respondents interpret each question and to further validate each of the domains. This version of the PRQ, with the additional segment for validation of domains, is being used only in a major project conducted by the author and is not included in the new PRQ-85, which is available to other researchers.

The frequency of selection of the various resource persons was also evaluated. It was found that the option "former spouse" was never selected and thus was eliminated as an option. Feedback from researchers who had used the PRQ and the information written in by respondents under the "other" category indicated difficulty with some of the categories of resource persons the respondents would turn to for help in the situation, and thus several items were slightly modified. An example of such a modification was to separate the category "friend, co-worker, or neighbor" into two separate categories of "friend" and "neighbor or co-worker."

Rewording of the Nurturance Items

Problem

The items for Part 2 were developed using Weiss's (1969, 1974) dimensions of social relationships. Weiss noted that the "opportunity for nurturance is provided by relationships in which an adult takes responsibility for the well-being of a child and thus can develop a sense of being needed." When the PRQ was developed, the concept of nurturance was broadened by adding "or younger persons" to the nurturance items. An example of a nurturance item is "I have a sense of being needed by a child or younger person."

A common concern repeatedly expressed by respondents and researchers using the PRQ was the restriction of nurturant behaviors to only children or younger people. *The American Heritage Dictionary* (Morris, 1976) defines nurture as "the act of promoting development or growth." By this definition it is reasonable to contend that one can nurture – that is, promote development or growth of – a person, regardless of age relationship.

Method

The issue of broadening the concept of nurturance beyond age relationships was presented to a panel of judges. The six judges were nurse researchers known for their work and expertise in the area of social support. The original nurturance items and the proposed revised items were sent to each judge. They were asked to examine the items and to indicate if the revised items were an acceptable substitution for the original items and if the integrity of the concept of nurturance was threatened by these revisions. All six experts agreed that the revisions were appropriate and that they did not appear to alter the concept of nurturance as it relates to the construct of social support.

　　Dr. Ann Muhlenkamp, Arizona State University, used the revised items in a study conducted with a sample of older persons living in a trailer/mobile home setting in the Tempe area. She reported (A. Muhlenkamp, personal communication, April 1985) an estimate of the internal consistency, Cronbach alpha, of .89 for the total scale and .66 for the Nurturance subscale. When her results were compared with other available samples of older adults (Iverson, 1981; Muhlenkamp, 1983b; Weinert, 1982), it was found that the revised wording did not essentially effect the total alpha nor the Nurturance subscale alpha. That the internal consistency estimate remained consistent with other estimates for similar groups indicated that the subscale was not weakened by these revisions (see Table 14.1).

　　The revised nurturance items are used in the PRQ-85. For example, the nurturance item "I have a sense of being needed by a child or younger person" now reads "I have a sense of being needed by another person."

TABLE 14.1 Internal Consistency for PRQ-Part 2 (Reliability Coefficients) with Older Adults

Scales	Iverson (1981)[a]	Muhlenkamp (1983b)[b]	Weinert (1983)[c]	Muhlenkamp (new wording) (1985)[d]
Total PRQ	.90	.85	.87	.89
Subscales				
Intimacy	.67	.71	.71	.76
Social				
Integration	.59	.54	.55	.62
Nurturance	.80	.68	.63	.66
Worth	.66	.61	.62	.60
Assistance/				
Guidance	.70	.65	.71	.66

[a]N, 120; [b]N, 97; [c]N, 177; [d]N, 132.

Discussion

Muhlenkamp (personal communication, April 1985) reported that the mean score for the Nurturance subscale was 28.4. One of Dr. Muhlenkamp's students used the original wording for the nurturance items in a study of a similar group of older persons at a senior center in Tempe (Hubbard, Muhlenkamp & Brown, 1984). A mean score of 24.8 was obtained. Perhaps the broadening of the concept to include nurturant behaviors toward people of all ages allowed the respondents in Muhlenkamp's study to identify more strongly with nurturant behaviors, which may have resulted in the higher mean score.

The PRQ-85, which contains the revised nurturance items, will be evaluated using various age groups of respondents. The mean scores, internal reliability estimates, intersubscale correlations, subscale to total scale correlations, and the factor structure will be compared with existing samples to evaluate the impact of the revisions on the perceived social support scale.

Multidimensionality of Part 2

Problem

Social support is defined in this chapter as a construct composed of five underlying dimensions: intimacy, social integration, nurturance, worth, and assistance. Items on the perceived social support portion of the PRQ were written to reflect these five dimensions.

Evaluation across various studies indicated moderate intercorrelations among the subscales. The intercorrelation among subscales for the Seattle sample ($N = 120$) described earlier in this chapter range from .37 to .82. Across studies (Iverson, 1981; Lobo, 1982; Murtaugh, 1982) the intercorrelations among the subscales Intimacy, Social Integration, Worth, and Assistance/Guidance have ranged from .52 to .73. However, lower correlations have consistently been obtained between the Nurturance subscale and the other four subscales, ranging from .27 to .59. Estimates of internal consistency for the Nurturance subscale have been acceptable with alphas between .58 and .88. These results indicated that nurturance may be an independent scale. Theoretically, nurturance is distinct from the other four dimensions. The Nurturance subscale items were designed to measure the support a person provides *to* younger people; whereas the Intimacy, Social Integration, Worth, and Assistance/Guidance subscales measure support *received from* others. In this study, factor analysis was conducted as a means of examining the substructure of the perceived social support scale.

Method/Results

The sample utilized for this aspect of the project was the one described earlier consisting of 120 men and women in their mid-thirties living in the greater Seattle area (Weinert & Brandt, 1987). Cronbach's alpha was used to assess the internal consistency of the instrument. For this sample an alpha of .93 was obtained for the full 25-item scale. The alpha coefficients for each subscale ranged from .63 to .70. The pattern and range of coefficients has been consistent across multiple studies.

In the current analysis the individual items demonstrated an item-total correlation of .50 or above except for two items that were between .42 and .50. Thus, all items were above the .30 criterion of acceptability as stated by Kerlinger (1973) and were retained in the factor analysis.

A preliminary factor analysis was undertaken to see if the statistical pattern of relationships underlying the data resembled the multidimensional theoretical pattern of five subscales. Although the sample size of 120 is marginal for factor analysis on a 25-item tool, it was felt that an exploratory factor analysis could provide preliminary information about the consistency between the hypothesized factors and empirical data. Rao's canonical factoring (RAO) was selected as it is designed to find a factor solution in which the correlation between the set of hypothesized factors and the set of data variables is maximized (Nie, Hull, Jenkins, Steinbrenner, & Bent, 1975). Oblique rotation was utilized because the initial factor axes are allowed to rotate to best summarize any clustering of variables. With oblique rotation the factors are allowed to be correlated if such correlations exist in the data (Nie et al., 1975).

An unrestricted Rao's canonical factoring extraction identified five factors. All factors met the Kaiser criterion of eigenvalues of greater than 1 to determine factors meaningful to extract and rotate (Kim & Mueller, 1978). Inspection of the magnitude of the eigenvalues of the factors, the point of discontinuity of the percentage of explained variance, and the loading of items does not substantiate the five hypothesized factors. A three-factor Rao's canonical oblique factor rotation was then conducted.

The loading of items clearly indicates that Factor II is a nurturance subscale composed of four of the five original nurturance items. One item, "I have the opportunity to encourage others to grow and develop their interests and skills," loaded on Factor I. This may be a function of the wording of the item as it is the only Nurturance subscale item that does not specifically identify a child or younger person.

Factor III is composed of all five of the original Intimacy subscale items and one Worth item. While the eigenvalue and percentage of variance explained is diminished, it appears that Intimacy is a separate subscale. A separate subscale for intimacy is logical and is a major component of nearly all of the currently held definitions of social support (see Table 14.2).

All other items loaded on Factor I, which seems to represent a subscale that could be labeled Affirmation/Assistance. Two of the factors in this three-factor solution correspond closely to the original items for the Intimacy and Nurturance subscales, with Social Integration, Worth, and Assistance/Guidance items forming a single factor.

The intercorrelations among the three factors were −.36 between Factors I and II, .55 between Factors I and III, and −.30 between Factors II

TABLE 14.2 Factor Structure and Factor Loadings for the PRQ-Part 2

Items	I	II	III
		Factors	
Affirmation/Assitance			
SI	.75		
W	.67		
A	.39		
SI	.65		
W	.83		
A	.66		
SI	.81		
N	.61		
A	.68		
SI	.53		
W	.86		
SI	.82		
A	.66		
W	.46		
A	.64		
Nurturance			
N		−.80	
N		−.72	
N		−.96	
N		−.96	
Intimacy			
I			.77
I			.72
I			.58
I			.69
W			.59
I			.76
Eigenvalue	33.13	15.62	4.22
% Total variance	62.5	29.5	8.0
Cumulative %	62.5	92.0	100.0

A, Assistance subscale item; I, Intimacy subscale item; N, Nurturance subscale item; SI, Social Integration subscale item; W, Worth subscale item.

and III. Low to moderate correlations would be expected if factors contribute uniquely to the total construct. High correlations would indicate lack of distinctiveness of factors and redundancy in measurement. It appears that the Nurturance subscale is a separate subscale and that Factors I and III may be overlapping. This finding was further substantiated by the fact that six of the items loaded nearly equally on Factors I and III, indicating that these items contributed to both factors and were not clearly distinguishable.

The items that loaded on each of the three factors were examined for their internal consistency. The alpha for Factor I (Affirmation/

Assistance) was .91; for Factor II (Nurturance), .91; and for Factor III (Intimacy), .82. Table 14.3 shows the alpha coefficients from several previous studies (Eyers & Ellison, 1982; Lobo, 1982; Muhlenkamp, 1983a; Murtaugh, 1982; Weinert, 1982; Weinert & Brandt, in press) using the original item clusters to represent the five hypothesized dimensions of social support. The alpha coefficient of .91 for the factored subscale of Nurturance was substantially higher than previous reliability estimates for the original five Nurturance subscale items.

Discussion

This factor analysis was exploratory and should be considered as a preliminary evaluation because of the small sample size in relation to the number of items on the PRQ. Because the adequacy of the sample is marginal, analysis using a larger sample is desirable. Hence, results must be interpreted with caution. Additional data sets are available at this time, but they must be inspected relative to the homogeneity of samples before combining them for further factor analysis. The alternate wording of the Nurturance subscale items may result in changes in the factor structure, and thus further analysis will be conducted. Further factor analysis with larger and more adequate samples will allow for decisions to retain or eliminate items that have overlapping loadings. Nunnally (1978) indicated that removing overlapping items can change the factor structure and cautioned against ignoring the correlations among items used to define a factor. The correlations among the variables for each of the three factors were at an acceptable level. However, two variables in Factor I correlated with some of the other variables in that factor at the .20 to .30 level and should be investigated further before being considered as appropriate items for Factor I.

TABLE 14.3 Internal Consistency for PRQ-Part 2 (Reliability Coefficients)

| | Youth Adults | | Middlescent Adults | | | |
Scales	Murtaugh (1982)[a]	Lobo (1982)[b]	Weinert (1982)[c]	Eyers & Ellison (1982)[d]	Muhlenkamp (1983b)[e]	Weinert & Brandt (in press)[f]
Total PRQ	.90	.88	.89	.93	.88	.93
Subscales						
Intimacy	.66	.70	.75	.77	.74	.83
Social Integration	.76	.70	.61	.80	.63	.83
Nurturance	.79	.68	.77	.58	.73	.88
Worth	.90	.73	.70	.71	.61	.78
Assistance	.69	.69	.75	.66	.72	.79

[a]*N*, 77; [b]*N*, 188; [c]*N*, 149; [d]*N*, 45; [e]*N*, 133; [f]*N*, 120.

SUMMARY

The aims of this project addressed three distinct aspects of the PRQ. The aims were to validate the content domains of Part 1, to consider the rewording of the nurturance items in Part 2, and to assess the multidimensionality of the subscales in Part 2. For each of these aims I have discussed the method of analysis and the results of the analysis and have presented specific areas of further study. The outcomes of this project have resulted in the development of a new version of the PRQ, the PRQ-85, which is currently being used in several studies. Data from these studies will be used for further psychometric evaluation. It is anticipated that the contributions of the findings from this project and the continued work on this first-generation measure will result in a valid and reliable measure of social support.

REFERENCES

Brandt, P. (1982). Relationship of mothers' negative life exposures and social support to the restrictive discipline and environmental stimulation of her developmentally disabled child. (Doctoral dissertation, University of Washington, 1981). *Dissertation Abstracts International, 42*(12). DA8212498A.

Brandt, P. (1984). The stress buffering effects of social support on maternal discipline. *Nursing Research, 33*(5), 277-280.

Caplan, G. (1974). *Social systems and community mental health.* New York: Behavioral Publications.

Eyers, S., & Ellison, E. (1982). (Social support: Mothers and children study). Unpublished raw data.

Gottlieb, B. (1983). *Social support strategies.* Beverly Hills, CA: Sage.

Hubbard, R., Muhlenkamp, A., & Brown, N. (1984). The relationship between social support and self-care practices. *Nursing Research, 33*(5), 266-270.

Iverson, C. (1981). *An exploratory study of the relationship among presence and perception of life change, social support and illness in an aging population.* Unpublished master's thesis, University of Washington, Seattle, WA.

Kerlinger, J. (1973). *Foundations of behavioral research.* New York: Holt, Rinehart, and Winston.

Kim, J., & Mueller, C. (1978). *Factor analysis: statistical methods and practical issues.* Beverly Hills, CA: Sage.

Lobo, M. (1982). Mother's and father's perceptions of family resources and marital adjustment and their adaptation to parenthood. (Doctoral dissertation, University of Washington, 1982). *Dissertation Abstracts International, 43*(3), DA9219243.

Morris, W. (Ed.). (1976). *The American Heritage dictionary of the English language.* Boston: Houghton Mifflin.

Muhlenkamp, A. (1983a). Assessment of social support in a health fair population. Unpublished raw data.

Muhlenkamp, A. (1983b). Social support: Elderly participants in a senior center. Unpublished raw data.

Muhlenkamp, A. (1985). Social support and elderly persons living in trailer and mobile home settings. Unpublished raw data.

Murtaugh, J. (1982). *A descriptive study of social support and depression in low income women*. Unpublished master's thesis, University of Washington, Seattle, WA.

Nie, N., Hull, C., Jenkins, J., Steinbrenner, K., & Bent, D. (1975). *Statistical package for the social sciences*. New York: McGraw-Hill.

Norbeck, J., Lindsey, A., & Carrieri, V. (1981). The development of an instrument to measure social support. *Nursing Research, 30*(5), 264-269.

Nunnally, J. C. (1978). *Psychometric theory*. New York: McGraw-Hill.

Rock, D., Green, K., Wise, B., & Rock, R. (1984). Social support and social network scales: A psychometric review. *Research in Nursing and Health, 7*, 325-332.

Tilden, V. (1985). Issues of conceptualization and measurement of social support in the construction of nursing theory. *Research in Nursing and Health, 8*(2), 199-206.

Weinert, C. (1982). Long-term illness, social support, and family functioning. (Doctoral dissertation, University of Washington, 1981). *Dissertation Abstracts International, 42*(12), DA821647A.

Weinert, C. (1983). (Social support: Rural people in their new middle years.) Unpublished raw data.

Weinert, C. (1984). Evaluation of the PRQ: A social support measure. In K. Baynard, P. Brandt, & B. Raff (Eds.), *Social support and families of vulnerable infants, 3*(5), (pp. 59-97). White Plains, New York: March of Dimes Defects Foundation.

Weinert, C., & Brandt, P. (1987). Measuring social support with the PRQ. *Western Journal of Nursing Research*.

Weiss, R. (1969). The fund of sociability. *Trans-Action, 6*(9). 36-43.

Weiss, R. (1974). The provisions of social relationships. In D. Rubin (Ed.), *Doing unto others* (pp. 17-26). Englewood Cliffs, NJ: Prentice-Hall.

Wortman, C. (1984). Social support and the cancer patient. *Cancer, 53* (May 15 Supplement), 2339-2360.

Personal Resource Questionnaire (PRQ-85)*

Developed by Patricia Brandt and Clarann Weinert, S.C.

In our everyday lives ther are personal and family situations or problems that we must deal with. Some of these are listed below. Please consider each statement in light of your own situation. Circle the number before the person(s) that you *could count on* in each situation that is described. You may circle more than one number if there is more than one source of help that you *count on*. In addition, we would like to know if you have had this situation or a similar one in the past six months and how satisfied you are with the help you received.

Q-1a. If you were to experience urgent needs, who would you turn to for help?
1 Parent
2 Child or children
3 Spouse or partner or significant other
4 Relative or family member
5 Friend
6 Neighbor or co-worker
7 Spiritual advisor (minister, priest, etc.)
8 Professional (nurse, counselor, etc.)
9 Agency
10 Self-help group
11 No one (no one available)
12 No one (prefer to handle it alone)
13 Other (explain) _____

b. Have you had urgent needs in the past six months?
1 Yes
2 No

c. If you have experienced urgent needs in the past six months, to what extent do you feel satisfied with the help you received?
1 Very satisfied
2 Fairly satisfied
3 A little satisfied
4 A little dissatisfied
5 Fairly dissatisfied
6 Very dissatisfied

Q-2a. If you needed help for an extended period of time in caring for a family member who is sick or handicapped, who would you turn to for help?
1 Parent
2 Child or children

* © Weinert, 1987.

    3 Spouse or partner or significant other
    4 Relative or family member
    5 Friend
    6 Neighbor or co-worker
    7 Spiritual advisor (minister, priest, etc.)
    8 Professional (nurse, counselor, etc.)
    9 Agency
   10 Self-help group
   11 No one (no one available)
   12 No one (prefer to handle it alone)
   13 Other (explain) _____

b. Have you needed help in caring for a sick or handicapped family member in the past six months?
    1 Yes
    2 No

c. If you have needed help in caring for a sick or handicapped family member in the past six months, to what extent do you feel satisfied with the help you received?
    1 Very satisfied
    2 Fairly satisfied
    3 A little satisfied
    4 A little dissatisfied
    5 Fairly dissatisfied
    6 Very dissatisfied

Q-3a. If you were concerned about your relationship with your spouse, partner, or intimate other, who would you turn to for help?
    1 Parent
    2 Child or children
    3 Spouse or partner or significant other
    4 Relative or family member
    5 Friend
    6 Neighbor or co-worker
    7 Spiritual advisor (minister, priest, etc.)
    8 Professional (nurse, counselor, etc.)
    9 Agency
   10 Self-help group
   11 No one (no one available)
   12 No one (prefer to handle it alone)
   13 Other (explain) _____

b. Have you had concerns about your relationship with your spouse, partner, or intimate other in the past six months?
    1 Yes
    2 No

c. If you have had concerns about your relationship with your spouse, partner, or intimate other in the past six months, to what extent do you feel satisfied with the help you received?
    1 Very satisfied
    2 Fairly satisfied
    3 A little satisfied
    4 A little dissatisfied

      5 Fairly dissatisfied
      6 Very dissatisfied

Q-4a. If you needed help or advice for a problem with a family member or friend who would you turn to for help?

      1 Parent
      2 Child or children
      3 Spouse or partner or significant other
      4 Relative or family member
      5 Friend
      6 Neighbor or co-worker
      7 Spiritual advisor (minister, priest, etc.)
      8 Professional (nurse, counselor, etc.)
      9 Agency
    10 Self-help group
    11 No one (no one available)
    12 No one (prefer to handle it alone)
    13 Other (explain) _____

   b. Have you needed help or advice regarding a problem with a family member or friend in the past six months?

      1 Yes
      2 No

   c. If you were have needed help or advice in the past six months regarding a problem with a family member or friend, to what extent do you feel satisfied with the help you received?

      1 Very satisfied
      2 Fairly satisfied
      3 A little satisfied
      4 A little dissatisfied
      5 Fairly dissatisfied
      6 Very dissatisfied

Q-5a. If you were having financial problems, who would you turn to for help?

      1 Parent
      2 Child or children
      3 Spouse or partner or significant other
      4 Relative or family member
      5 Friend
      6 Neighbor or co-worker
      7 Spiritual advisor (minister, priest, etc.)
      8 Professional (nurse, counselor, etc.)
      9 Agency
    10 Self help group
    11 No one (no one available)
    12 No one (prefer to handle it alone)
    13 Other (explain) _____

   b. Have you had financial problems in the past six months?

      1 Yes
      2 No

   c. If you have had financial problems in the past six months to what extent do you feel satisfied with the help you received?

      1 Very satisfied

    2 Fairly satisfied
    3 A little satisfied
    4 A little dissatisfied
    5 Fairly dissatisfied
    6 Very dissatisfied

Q-6a. If you felt lonely, who would you turn to?
    1 Parent
    2 Child or children
    3 Spouse or partner or significant other
    4 Relative or family member
    5 Friend
    6 Neighbor or co-worker
    7 Spiritual advisor (minister, priest, etc.)
    8 Professional (nurse, counselor, etc.)
    9 Agency
   10 Self-help group
   11 No one (no one available)
   12 No one (prefer to handle it alone)
   13 Other (explain) _____

  b. Have you felt lonely in the past six months?
    1 Yes
    2 No

  c. If you have felt lonely in the past six months to what extent do you feel satisfied with the help you have received?
    1 Very satisfied
    2 Fairly satisfied
    3 A little satisfied
    4 A little dissatisfied
    5 Fairly dissatisfied
    6 Very dissatisfied

Q-7a. If you were sick and not able to carry out your usual activities for a week or so, who would you turn to for help?
    1 Parent
    2 Child or children
    3 Spouse or partner or significant other
    4 Relative or family member
    5 Friend
    6 Neighbor or co-worker
    7 Spiritual advisor (minister, priest, etc.)
    8 Professional (nurse, counselor, etc.)
    9 Agency
   10 Self-help group
   11 No one (no one available)
   12 No one (prefer to handle it alone)
   13 Other (explain) _____

  b. During the past six months, have you been sick for a week and not able to carry out your usual activities?
    1 Yes
    2 No

  c. If you have been sick for a week during the past six months to what

extent do you feel satisfied with the help you received?
1 Very satisfied
2 Fairly satisfied
3 A little satisfied
4 A little dissatisfied
5 Fairly dissatisfied
6 Very dissatisfied
Q-8a. If you were upset and frustrated with the conditions of your life, who would you turn to for help?
1 Parent
2 Child or children
3 Spouse or partner or significant other
4 Relative or family member
5 Friend
6 Neighbor or co-worker
7 Spiritual advisor (minister, priest, etc.)
8 Professional (nurse, counselor, etc.)
9 Agency
10 Self-help group
11 No one (no one available)
12 No one (prefer to handle it alone)
13 Other (explain) _____
b. Have you been upset and frustrated with the conditions of your life in the past six months?
1 Yes
2 No
c. If you have been upset and frustrated with the conditions of your life in the past six months to what extent do you feel satisfied with the help you received?
1 Very satisfied
2 Fairly satisfied
3 A little satisfied
4 A little dissatisfied
5 Fairly dissatisfied
6 Very dissatisfied
Q-9a. If you were having problems with your work at home or at your place of employment who would you turn to for help?
1 Parent
2 Child or children
3 Spouse or partner or significant other
4 Relative or family member
5 Friend
6 Neighbor or co-worker
7 Spiritual advisor (minister, priest, etc.)
8 Professional (nurse, counselor, etc.)
9 Agency
10 Self-help group
11 No one (no one available)
12 No one (prefer to handle it alone)
13 Other (explain) _____

b. Have you had problems related to your work in the past six months?
    1 Yes
    2 No

c. If you have had problems with your work situation in the past six months, to what extent do you feel satisfied with the help you received?
    1 Very satisfied
    2 Fairly satisfied
    3 A little satisfied
    4 A little dissatisfied
    5 Fairly dissatisfied
    6 Very dissatisfied

Q-10a. If you needed someone to talk to about your day-to-day personal concerns, who would you turn to for help?
    1 Parent
    2 Child or children
    3 Spouse or partner or significant other
    4 Relative or family member
    5 Friend
    6 Neighbor or co-worker
    7 Spiritual advisor (minister, priest, etc.)
    8 Professional (nurse, counselor, etc.)
    9 Agency
    10 Self-help group
    11 No one (no one available)
    12 No one (prefer to handle it alone)
    13 Other (explain) _____

b. Have you needed someone to talk to about day-to-day personal concerns in the past six months?
    1 Yes
    2 No

c. If you have needed someone to talk to about day-to-day personal concerns in the past six months, to what extent do you feel satisfied with the help you received?
    1 Very satisfied
    2 Fairly satisfied
    3 A little satisfied
    4 A little dissatisfied
    5 Fairly dissatisfied
    6 Very dissatisfied

Q-11 Below are some statements with which some people agree and others disagree. Please read each statement and *circle* the response most appropriate for you. There is no *right* or *wrong* answer.
    1 Strongly disagree
    2 Disagree
    3 Somewhat disagree
    4 Neutral
    5 Somewhat agree
    6 Agree
    7 Strongly agree

STATEMENTS

a.	There is someone I feel close to who makes me feel secure	7	6	5	4	3	2	1
b.	I belong to a group in which I feel important	7	6	5	4	3	2	1
c.	People let me know that I do well at my work (job, homemaking)	7	6	5	4	3	2	1
d.	I can't count on my relatives and friends to help me with problems	7	6	5	4	3	2	1
e.	I have enough contact with the person who makes me feel special	7	6	5	4	3	2	1
f.	I spend time with others who have the same interests that I do	7	6	5	4	3	2	1
g.	There is little opportunity in my life to be giving and caring to another person	7	6	5	4	3	2	1
h.	Others let me know that they enjoy working with me (job, committees, projects)	7	6	5	4	3	2	1
i.	There are people who are available if I needed help over an extended period of time	7	6	5	4	3	2	1
j.	There is no one to talk to about how I am feeling	7	6	5	4	3	2	1
k.	Among my group of friends we do favors for each other	7	6	5	4	3	2	1
l.	I have the opportunity to encourage others to develop their interests and skills	7	6	5	4	3	2	1
m.	My family lets me know that I am important for keeping the family running	7	6	5	4	3	2	1
n.	I have relatives or friends who will help me out even if I can't pay them back	7	6	5	4	3	2	1
o.	When I am upset, there is someone I can be with who lets me be myself	7	6	5	4	3	2	1
p.	I feel no one has the same problems as I	7	6	5	4	3	2	1
q.	I enjoy doing little "extra" things that make another person's life more pleasant	7	6	5	4	3	2	1
r.	I know that others appreciate me as a person	7	6	5	4	3	2	1
s.	There is someone who loves and cares about me	7	6	5	4	3	2	1
t.	I have people to share social events and fun activities with	7	6	5	4	3	2	1
u.	I am responsible for helping provide for another person's needs	7	6	5	4	3	2	1
v.	If I need advice there is someone who would assist me to work out a plan for dealing with the situation	7	6	5	4	3	2	1
w.	I have a sense of being needed by another person	7	6	5	4	3	2	1
x.	People think that I'm not as good a friend as I should be	7	6	5	4	3	2	1
y.	If I got sick there is someone to give me advice about caring for myself	7	6	5	4	3	2	1

15

Functional Assessment of the Elderly: The Iowa Self-Assessment Inventory

Woodrow W. Morris and Kathleen C. Buckwalter

This chapter discusses the Iowa Self Assessment Inventory, a measure of functional capabilities of the elderly.

Multidimensional functional assessment of older persons is gradually becoming a regular part of overall planning for the provision of services to those who come to the attention of providers. The best-known methodology for such assessment is the Multidimensional Functional Assessment Questionnaire (MFAQ) (Duke University, 1978). It is also referred to as the OARS Methodology, the acronym being taken from Duke's Older American's Resources and Services program. Lawton, Moss, Fulcome, and Kleban (1982) have pointed out that every later assessment system bears an immense debt to the OARS designers for providing the first integrated system for evaluating the older person and thereby a model against which purported improvements can be compared.

The OARS methodology was initiated in 1972 on the request of the U.S. Administration on Aging "to structure and conceptualize an approach to understanding a persistent issue of special relevance to an aging society – alternatives to institutionalization, or better, institutionalization as an alternative in a continuum of health and welfare services" (Duke University, 1978, p. 3).

The Duke efforts led to the conceptualization of a basic model that would be useful not only for approaching the specific question of options in long-term care but also would have general applicability to program evaluation and to resource allocation decisions. The element of the model with which we are most concerned is that of providing a procedure for measuring the functional status of individuals and a related scheme for classifying individuals with similar status (equivalence classes).

As Fillenbaum & Smyer (1981) have pointed out, the effort was focused on being able to measure functional status of elderly clients. Surveys of the literature and clinical experiences indicated that information was necessary on five dimensions – social resources, economic resources, mental health, physical health, and activities of daily living (ADL) – to obtain a comprehensive overview of individual functioning.

In developing the OARS methodology certain constraints were imposed and certain standards were desired. First, the questionnaire had not only to be valid and reliable, but it also had to be sufficiently detailed to be clinically useful; the entire range of functioning from excellent to totally impaired had to be covered; and it had to be sufficiently brief to permit rapid data gathering. The questionnaire also had to be readily understood by those for whom it was intended and sufficiently straightforward that it would be easy to administer. Finally, the information obtained for each of the five dimensions covered by the questionnaire had to be readily summarizable on a brief scale, with the meanings of the points of the scale being uniform across the dimensions. In addition, in each dimension, certain information was considered basic to a determination of level of functioning:

Social Resources – quantity and quality of relationships with friends and family; availability of care in time of need.

Economic resources – adequacy of income and resources.

Mental health – extent of psychiatric well-being, presence of organicity.

Physical health – presence of physical disorders, participation in physical activities.

ADL – capacity to perform various instrumental and physical (bodily care) tasks that permit individuals to live independently.

Lawton and his colleagues (1982) described the Philadelphia Geriatric Center Multilevel Assessment Instrument (MAI), an assessment approach built on a conceptual model of the well-being of older people (Lawton, 1972, Lawton et al., 1982) and designed explicitly to deal with some deficiencies and gaps in existing assessment systems. It very explicitly incorporates much earlier work from the OARS, from many other investigators, and from the authors and their colleagues at the Philadelphia Geriatric Center.

According to these authors, assessment ideally should be based on a conceptual scheme and lead to the refinement of a functional taxonomy and the generation of hypotheses on theoretical and applied issues with relevance far beyond the assessment task itself. To this end, Lawton (1977) suggested that any conception of the "good life" for the aged had to include four major sectors, each with multiple domains: behavioral competence, psychological well-being, perceived quality of life, and environmental quality. Each of these sectors implies a structure for assessment that defines the qualities to be assessed and the relationships among them.

Lawton et al. (1982) points out three limitations in existing assessment devices that led to the development of the MAI: their failure to represent all domains, their incomplete psychometric development, and their restricted versatility.

Under the first point, it is noted that a weakness in the OARS is its failure to deal with most aspects of the environment. Further, in the conceptual scheme of behavioral competence, it is essential to separate such activities as leisuretime pursuits, solitary time use, and organizational participation from informal social behavior with family, friends, and acquaintances; the OARS combines these in the social domain. In addition, the OARS combines cognitive ability and psychological well-being into the single domain of mental health. This curious decision mixes two aspects of the individual that not only have totally different implications for treatment but also, in the terms of our present approach, make it impossible to separate an essential aspect of competence (cognition) from an outcome (psychological well-being).

With respect to the second limitation, incomplete psychometric development, Lawton et al. (1982) points out that every instrument could stand improvement in these technical aspects. As a model in the environmental area, however, the set of assessment instruments produced by Moos and his colleagues (Moos, 1974; Moos, 1978; Moos, Gauwain, Lemke, Max, & Mehren, 1979) are exemplary in their painstaking establishment of reliability, validity, and guides for the user that are clear and still use the full range of the data produced. In the behavioral competence sector the OARS has been similarly treated so as to yield extremely detailed information on the psychometric properties of a 6-point summary rating scale completed by the user on the basis of interview items designated as relevant to each of the five domains. These ratings, rather than the interview items themselves, are the basis of much of the use of the OARS as reported to date. Optimum use of the OARS thus relies heavily on the training and clinical perspicacity of the user in translating overall item content into the summary rating scales. Considering the richness of the primary data and the psychometric superiority of longer item sets, it seems highly desirable to offer the user the alternative of using either summary ratings or the richer psychometrically derived item indices.

The third limitation discussed by Lawton et al. (1982) concerned the lack in most instruments of structural versatility. Although arguments persist over the hazards of creating "short forms" of standard instruments, the fact is that the length of many of the best instruments is a deterrent to their use. In gerontology this is an especially critical problem because of the large volume of assessments that must be made in settings where time is at a premium, where paraprofessional staff make assessments, and where the endurance of the older person may be limited. To some extent the OARS meets this need by allowing summary ratings to be made on the basis of partial information if necessary. These ratings nonetheless suffer from the psychometric deficiency inherent in the scales' limited 6-point range. Thus, a need is seen for a nest of assessment instruments of different lengths, whose psychometric properties are provided so that the user may know exactly what kinds of trade-offs characterize the choice of longer or shorter versions.

Another major obstacle in the more universal assessment of relatively independent, well elderly adults using the Duke University (1978) instrument is that the required interview may take from 45 min to more than 1 hour to complete. Thus, if it were desirable to assess 100 persons, it would require at least 100 hr of interview time alone. This would take a single interviewer some 25 days at the rate of four subjects per day; or 5 interviewers seeing four persons each day would complete the job in five days.

If consideration is limited to independent, well elderly, it would seem appropriate to assume that they themselves should be capable of providing the essential information for assessment, using a self-administered format of the assessment instrument. Such an approach would require a carefully worded set of instructions, the self-administered form and, at most, a brief (e.g., 5-10 minutes) visit with each subject to clarify any unclear responses and/or to obtain replies to unanswered items.

This study was conducted in two phases. The purpose of phase 1 was to examine the feasibility of obtaining multitudinal functional assessment information using a self-administered mode in contrast with the usual internal mode, with the intent of simplifying the process. Phase II was undertaken to develop a psychiatric inventory to assess social resources; economic resources; mental health, physical health, and cognitive states; and the ability to carry out the usual ADL among relatively well-elderly persons.

PHASE I STUDY

Purpose

Phase I of this study (Morris & Boutelle, 1985) examined four research questions about this kind of self-assessment.

1. With what reliability will four judges be able to rate assessment protocols from a sample of relatively independent, well elderly persons?
2. To what degree will the ratings of the judges based on interview protocols agree with those based on self-administered protocols?
3. Will the sequence with which the two modes are administered be reflected in any systematic differences in ratings?
4. Can a system of objective scores be devised that will agree with the ratings of the judges?

Participants

A sample of 24 residents of a housing project for low-income elderly and handicapped persons was invited and agreed to participate in the study designed to seek answers to the research questions. Halfway through data collection, two males withdrew, leaving a sample of 12 female and 10 male subjects. The ages of the participants ranged from 63 to 89 years; 45% were widowed and 32% were married. Of those 36% who had some post-high school education, three had completed collegiate graduate or professional school programs. All were low-income persons, with annual income ranging from $3,700 to $15,000, equally divided above and below $7,000.

Design of the Phase I Study

Two forms of the Duke University *Multidimensional Functional Assessment: The OARS Methodology* were used. In addition to the questionnaire described in the manual (Duke University, 1978), which we shall refer to as the *interview mode*, a *self-administered mode* was developed by converting the wording of the original items used in the interview to direct questions addressed to the respondent, followed by multiple-choice answers. Care was taken to maintain similar wording and response choices as in the original instrument.

The interview instrument is a 21-page form, not including the five rating scales. Its component parts, in the order in which they occur, are as follows:

A *preliminary questionna*ire, which is essentially a mental status examination comprising 10 items covering orientation for time and place, general information, and serial subtractions of 3s, beginning with 20. The score is the total number of errors.

Five items seeking information regarding the respondent's sociodemographic background precede the section dealing with social resources.

The *social resources* section comprises 9 items, ranging from marital status, current living arrangements, and questions directly focused on contacts with other persons to the extent to which care would be available in case of illness or injury.

The *economic resources* section comprises 16 items, concerned first with income and assets, then with attitudes toward the adequacy of financial needs and resources, and ending with four items focused on comparisons with the individual's financial status compared with others and extent to which needs are being met now and in the future.

The *mental health* section comprises 6 items, one of which, however, is a 15-item "psychiatric evaluation," which purports to assess the presence and degree of psychiatric problems. The section ends with another comparison of self with others and present versus recent past.

The *physical health* section is made up of 19 items that include surveys of common medications being taken and present illnesses and the degree to which they interfere with activities, as well as specific questions about vision, hearing, use of supportive devices and prostheses, extent to which each respondent has been a patient in hospital, nursing home, or rehabilitation center, has been seen by a physician, has felt need for health care, and has participated in vigorous physical activities. Finally, three items ask for an overall health rating, comparison of present health status with recent past, and degree of interference with activities.

The final section, *activities of daily living*, consists of 15 items divided more or less equally between instrumental activities of daily living and physical activities of daily living.

To make the self-administered format as easy to read as possible, a larger 10-point type style was used with double-spacing between items and with $1^1/_2$ spaces between lines within items. This resulted in a 15-page booklet using only one side of each page. The self-administered format assumes reading ability as well as sufficient visual acuity in the elderly participant to complete the questionnaire.

Procedures

The respondents were divided into two groups, each with 11 subjects (5 men and 6 women). One group was first assessed by interview over a span of 3 days by the same interviewer. Two weeks later the self-administered form of the instrument was distributed to the same persons for completion. At that time the self-administered format was also distributed to the members of the second group. Two weeks later the members of the second group were assessed by the same interviewer.

Four judges assigned ratings based on both interview and self-report protocols, using written sets of rating criteria based on those used at Duke University. Two of the judges were university staff members who had completed training in the assessment methodology. The authors of the study were the other two judges.

All of the protocols were coded, and no names or other identifying information were made available to the judges, although it should be noted that all knew that the subjects were low-income persons qualifying as residents of the Housing and Urban Development Project (HUD) in which they were living.

Rating criteria and other instructions were provided to the judges. The rating criteria deviated somewhat from that used in the OARS methodology since we have always believed that rating scheme to be biased toward impairment (with four of the six rating categories suggesting impairment and only two for excellent or good functioning). In this study, the rating of 3, which was defined as "Mildly impaired" in the original instrument was changed to "Moderate," and 4 became "Mildly impaired"; 5 was used to indicate "Moderately impaired," and 6 signified "Severe impairment."

Thus, ratings of 1 to 3 were used to signify positive status, and ratings of 4 to 6 were used to reflect a negative status.

The meaning of the ratings may be made more specific by describing the significance of high (i.e., 1 and 2) ratings. For example, in the category of social resources, such ratings suggest an individual who has numerous and consistent contacts with other persons both as individuals and in group settings. More often than not they have family members who are accessible and with whom they have frequent and satisfying contacts. People high in social resources tend to belong to and participate in social groups as well as religious groups. Finally, such persons report that their social resources are as plentiful now as in the past and that they are both satisfying and supportive.

The more the ratings of individuals deviate from this high profile, the more their resources, statuses, and abilities are deemed less than ideal or that they are impaired.

With these factors in mind, the judges made their ratings privately and independently, with no other information than that contained in the protocols. The judges made their ratings on each group of protocols in the order in which they had been administered.

Scoring

Finally, in order to study the feasibility of objectifying the assessment process, a scoring system was devised separately for the interview and self-report modes. Each item was scored by assigning numerical weightings to the various responses in keeping with the rating criteria – that is, positive, healthy, favorable responses were scored 1 with higher numbers assigned to responses that indicated deviations toward impairment. The potential score ranges for the interview and the self-report formats were as follows for each of the sections:

	Interview	Self-administered
Social resources	7-23	14-45
Economic resources	11-29	14-38
Mental health	7-25+	20-36+
Physical health	18-50+	16-51+
ADL	14-42	17-50

The maximum scores for the interview and self-report formats were as follows for each of the sections:

	Interview	Self-report
Social resources	13	14
Economic resources	20	20
Mental health	33	34
Physical Health	93	93
ADL	21	22

Precise ceilings cannot be stated for the mental health and physical health sections because the scores are somewhat indeterminate, being dependent in part on such elements as the number of symptoms noted, the number of illnesses reported and their effects on daily activities, and the number of medications being taken.

Data Analysis

Analyses of variance and kappa statistics of the ratings among the four judges were calculated for ratings based on both interview and self-administered protocols, taking into account the sequence with which the protocols were obtained. Finally, objective scores were derived as described earlier and were correlated with the ratings of the judges separately for the two data sources.

Reliability of Ratings

The data in Table 15.1 were obtained by calculating the kappa statistics to measure the extent of agreement among the four judges for each mode of data collection. The statistical analyses followed the procedures outlined by Fleiss (1971) and Light (1971). In addition, analysis of variance of the ratings was calculated, from which intraclass correlation coefficients were obtained.

The correlation coefficients among the several pairs of judges were high, and no significant differences were found among the several pairs of judges on any of the five variables (Table 15.1). The agreement among the four judges, as estimated by kappa, shows that in all instances, agreement among them was greater than what would have been expected by chance ($p < .001$). The intraclass correlation coefficients, all statistically

TABLE 15.1 Overall Reliability of Ratings of Judges for Interview and Self-Administered Modes

Variables	Interview mode			Self-administered mode		
	Kappa	Standard error	z	Kappa	Standard error	z
Social resources	.5410	.0435	12.44*	.5958	.0439	13.57*
Economic resources	.3219	.0338	9.52*	.3020	.0390	7.75*
Mental health status	.3436	.0354	9.70*	.2654	.0361	7.35*
Physical health status	.4259	.0453	9.40*	.2120	.0524	4.05*
ADL	.3352	.0400	8.38*	.5905	.0410	14.41*

Agreement among four judges on ratings based on interview and self-administered protocols ($N = 22$).
*$p < .001$.

significant at an alpha level of .01, were as follows for the interview-based ratings: social resources, .92; economic resources, .90; mental health, .90; physical health, .95; and ADL, .93. Analogous results for the self-administered ratings were social resources, .86; economic resources, .94; mental health, .84; physical health, .82; and ADL, .95. It is clear from both the kappa analysis and the intraclass correlations that there was significant agreement among the four judges.

Agreement among Judges and the Sequence of Administration

The ratings of the judges were submitted to analysis of variance, and since there were no significant variances, the ratings were averaged. The average ratings based on interview protocols were compared with the average ratings based on self-administered protocols, with findings that suggest no significant differences between these two modes of data collection. Analysis of the sequence with which the protocols were administered (i.e., interview first or self-report first) indicates that sequence did not result in any meaningful differences, as shown in Table 15.2.

Objective Scores

Objective scores derived from interview protocols were correlated with the ratings of the judge for each of the five areas, with resulting correlations ranging from 0.69 to 0.86. Similarily, when self-report scores were correlated with the judges' ratings, the resulting coefficients ranged from 0.71 to 0.95. All of the correlations were significant at the .01 level of probability.

Table 15.3 presents the alpha coefficients of reliability based on objective scores derived from both interview and self-report protocols.

TABLE 15.2 Combined Ratings by Sequence

Variables	Interview first		Self-report second		F_a value[a]	Interview first		Self-report second		F_a value[a]
	M	SD	M	SD		M	SD	M	SD	
Social resources	1.68	0.88	1.93	1.02	1.51	2.23	1.20	1.86	0.88	2.64
Economic resources	2.18	0.79	2.41	0.84	1.71	2.39	0.97	2.48	1.11	0.17
Mental Health status	2.16	1.12	2.11	1.13	0.04	2.20	0.93	2.11	0.95	0.21
Physical health status	3.20	0.98	3.16	1.03	0.04	3.11	1.38	3.30	0.98	0.51
ADL	2.16	1.22	1.59	1.30	0.26	2.11	1.15	2.05	0.96	0.09

The effective range of ratings in all cases was from 1 to 4: less than 3% of the 880 ratings were 5, most of which were in the physical health category.
[a]Number of degrees of freedom in each comparison was 86 and 1: F value required at the .01 level = 7.20.

TABLE 15.3 Means, Standard Deviation, and Alpha Coefficients of Reliability of Objective Scores Derived from Interview and Self-Report Protocols

Variables	Interview $(N = 22)$		Self-Report $(N = 22)$		t^a	Alphas	
	M	SD	M	SD		Interview	Self-report
Social resources	9.91	2.01	10.23	2.65	0.44	0.49	0.69
Economic resources	15.10	2.87	15.05	2.83	0.06	0.79	0.82
Mental health status	25.32	4.89	25.59	4.91	0.18	0.86	0.85
Physical health status	79.87	8.66	80.96	7.86	0.43	0.78	0.73
ADL	17.05	2.74	17.23	2.90	0.21	0.81	0.77

[a]With $df = 42$, $t = 2.704$ is required at the .01 level of probability.

Comparison of Findings with Duke University Experience

Fundamentally, responses obtained either from interviews or self-administered assessment are sought in order to secure accurate information regarding the functional status of respondents in terms of the five dimensions comprising the methodology. Fillenbaum and Smyer (1981) reported on an assessment of the interrater reliability of the OARS methodology. They utilized a sample of 11 users of the methodology, each of whom rated the protocols of 30 participants in a validity study. Each rater assigned ratings on each of the five dimensions for all 30 participants.

Interrater reliability was assessed using the intraclass correlation coefficient derived from an analysis of variance performed on each of the five scales. The obtained results, all significant at an alpha level of .001, were as follows: social, .823; economic, .783; mental health, .803; physical health, .662; and self-care capacity, .865. The authors concluded that it was evident that substantial rating agreement existed among the group of raters. Our experience presented here found equally high intraclass correlations among the judges for both the interview-based and the self-administered ratings.

Fillenbaum and Smyer (1981) noted that the raters in their study were in complete agreement on 74% of the ratings. In the present study, identical ratings among the four judges occurred over half of the time; agreement within a one-point spread in the interview mode occurred as follows: social, 95%; economic, 86%; mental health, 77%; physical health, 77%; and ADL, 86%. For the self-administered protocols, agreements within a 1-point spread were social, 82%; economic, 91%; mental health, 68%; physical health, 73%; and ADL, 86%. Overall disagreement on placement in an impaired or unimpaired rating category (in this study ratings of 1-3 compared to ratings of 4-6) occurred only about 9% of the time. These findings support the reliability with which ratings based on both interviews and self-administered approaches may be made by trained raters.

Although these results are encouraging in that they demonstrate that skilled judges agree on their ratings, whether based on interview or self-administered protocols, it appears that it would be feasible to dispense with the use of judges altogether by devising and refining objective scores that might be used in lieu of ratings. Correlations between objective scores and ratings are high enough to suggest confidence in such scores.

Conclusions and Recommendations for Phase I

The purpose of the Phase I study was to examine the feasibility of obtaining multidimensional functional assessment information using a self-administered mode in contrast with the usual interview mode, with the idea in mind of simplifying the assessment process. Objective scoring was a second step in the same direction. The evidence suggests that both are viable processes and make the process more readily available and economical. The only caveat that must be asserted is that these findings pertain to well elderly persons still living relatively independently, with good visual acuity and an ability to read and respond to written items. Whether and to what extent self-assessment may be useful among ill elderly or elderly persons requiring accommodations in long-term care institutions is yet to be determined.

This kind of a study would be worth doing. Perhaps a more worthwhile and logical next step is the development of a psychometrically constructed inventory that could be easily and quickly scored and would provide information basic to understanding the needs and status of individuals for survey purposes, and of members of large groups of elderly persons. The Phase II study attempts the development of such an instrument.

PHASE II STUDY

Purpose

Because of the developmental and exploratory nature of Phase II, the following research questions will be examined in lieu of specific hypotheses.

1. With what reliability will subjects be able to report their resources, status, and abilities using such an inventory?
2. What relationships are there between inventory scale scores and sociodemographic characteristics of the subjects?
3. In institutional settings, what are the correlations between inventory scale scores and staff evaluations of the functional status of the subjects?
4. What intercorrelations are there among the several scale scores?

We are now launching a program of data collection from a variety of sources such as the following:

1. Residents of retirement homes.
2. Residents of HUD-sponsored 202 housing projects.
3. Respondents from the several Area Agencies on Aging across Iowa.
4. Respondents from outpatient programs of health care facilities, including the University of Iowa Geriatric Clinic at university hospitals, a specialty clinic at the College of Dentistry, and Veterans Administration Medical Centers at Iowa City and Knoxville.

In addition to seeking answers to the four research questions noted earlier, the data obtained will be submitted to detailed item analyses and to factor analysis to confirm the existence of the six scales comprising the inventory. With this information in hand, the inventory will be revised again to provide the most efficient and effective instrument possible.

The purpose of the Phase II study was to develop a psychometric inventory to assess social resources; economic resources; mental health, physical health, and cognitive status; and the ability to carry out the usual ADL among relatively well elderly persons.

Conceptual Basis

The conceptual basis for the Iowa Self Assessment Inventory is similar to that of the OARS methodology with some of the improvements suggested by Lawton et al. (1982). Thus, the entire instrument was designed to include as many domains as possible; it includes those noted by Lawton with the exception of the environment. To at least a modest degree the inventory includes items related to behavioral competence, sampling activities in the area of leisure time pursuits, interests, and organizational participation embedded in the area of social behavior with family, friends, and acquaintances. Finally, a separate cognitive status scale was included in the inventory. Furthermore, as we have noted above, the inventory is designed as a psychometric instrument to which older persons find it easy to respond, since all of the items are answered using the same format. Also, the inventory does not depend on the clinical acumen of the user but can be reviewed for completeness by a clerk and scored by hand, mechanically, or conceivably, by machine.

Review of the Self-Report Literature

Others have studied self-report assessment procedures. Slavonic (1983) studied self-administered assessment by obtaining responses from about 30 male geriatric veterans to the OARS questionnaire, which had been mailed to them and returned by mail to the author. Responses were scored by means of a computer-based program developed by George, Landermann, & Fillenbaum (1982). Using interview-based protocols as criteria, Slavonic correlated self-administered (mail) scores and found highly significant moderate-size correlations between the five health dimension scores and the same five health dimension scores on the interview. She concluded that the mail-out approach is a highly promising method for conducting health status surveys of the elderly.

Linn and Linn (1984) describe the development of a Self-Evaluation of Life Function (SELF) scale for elderly adults that is brief but comprehensive. SELF is a 54-item, multidimensional self-report scale that appears to measure the following dimensions: physical disability, symptoms of aging, self-esteem, social satisfaction, depression, and personal control. The scale was derived from studies of 826 persons aged 60 years and older. The item structure was based on factor analysis.

Test-retest reliability was based on intraclass correlations between ratings at baseline and 3 to 5 days later for 101 subjects. Scale reliabilities were as follows: physical disability, .96; symptoms of aging, .93; self-esteem, .59; social satisfaction, .81; depression, .84; and personal control, .79. Some of the scales were modestly intercorrelated. As might be expected, depression was related both to symptoms of aging and to self-esteem.

Linn and Linn (1984) also report that the SELF scale discriminated among known groups of institutionalized patients, those living independently, and patients attending mental health clinics. All scales discriminated among groups at a highly significant level statistically in the expected direction, both with and without age covaried. The best discriminator was physical disability, and the least sensitive was personal control.

Description of Instrument and Scoring

The preliminary form of the Iowa Self Assessment Inventory includes six scales of 20 items each. Each item is followed by a four-point rating scale in which 4 is to be selected if the respondent believes the item is completely true about him/her; 3 is to be selected if the item is more often true than not; 2 is to be selected if the item is more often false than not; and 1 is to be selected if the item is completely false about him/her. Thus, the maximum score on each scale would be 80 and the minimum 20. The scoring orientation is such that the higher the score, the healthier or better the individual would appear to be functioning. The preliminary items were reviewed by a panel of 20 of our colleagues across the country representing the disciplines of geriatrics, geriatric nursing, anthropology, psychology, education, social work, and public health. The items were then rewritten based on the panel's critical comments and suggestions to constitute the present form of the inventory.

The Phase II study plans call for the administration of the inventory to diverse samples of elderly persons in a variety of living arrangements in various degrees of health and relative independence.

Instrument Development Process

The inventory was administered to 87 older persons; 64 were participants in a congregate meals program, and 23 were homebound persons receiving home-delivered meals.

Since all of those attending the congregate meals program were relatively independent and well, but the members of the home-delivered-meals group were by definition physically ill, relatively frail, and dependent, we drew the following hypotheses concerning expected scale scores:

1. It was expected that the homebound persons would have significantly lower scores on the social resources, physical health, and ADL scales.
2. It was expected that there would be no significant differences between the two groups on the economic resources, mental health, and cognitive status scales.

Data Analysis and Findings

Before presenting findings that bear directly on these two hypotheses, it is worth commenting on the findings in more general terms. For example, the ranges of scores among the congregate-meals group were from 38 to 77, (mean, 62) on the social resources scale, from 22 to 77, (mean, 61) on the mental health scale, from 39 to 79, (mean, 61) on the physical health scale, from 49 to 77, (mean, 68) on the ADL scale, and from 45 to 78, (mean, 61) on the cognitive status scale. Comparable ranges and means for the homebound group were from 39 to 74 (mean, 57) on the social resources scale, from 41 to 77 (mean, 61) on the economic resources scale, from 38 to 76 (mean, 56) on the physical health status scale, from 38 to 77 (mean, 62) on the ADL scale, and from 36 to 80 (mean, 63) on the cognitive status scale. Such a spread of scores on each of the scales for both groups is an encouraging finding.

The results of comparisons between the two groups on each of the scales are presented in Table 15.4. These results generally support the retention of the hypotheses noted earlier. The only scale for which findings were different from those hypothesized was the economic resources scale. Homebound elderly had significantly ($p < .01$) lower scores on the economic scale than did the well elderly.

The intercorrelations among the six scales for the well elderly group ranged from .05 to .63. Correlations significant at $p < .01$ were found between social resources and mental health status (.55), social resources and physical health status (.57), economic resources and mental health status (.50), mental health status and physical health status (.63), and physical health status and ADL (.54). None of the scales was significantly correlated with cognitive status. The role of physical health in this group of

TABLE 15.4 Means, Standard Deviations, *t*-test Comparisons, and Alpha Coefficients for Inventory Scale Scores Derived from the Well Elderly and Homebound Elderly Respondents

Scales	Well Elderly (N = 64)		Homebound Elderly (N = 23)			Alphas	
	M	SD	M	SD	*t*-Value	Well elderly	Homebound elderly
Social resources	62.04	9.10	56.54	11.84	2.29*	.71	.80
Economic resources	66.10	10.02	61.42	9.71	1.94*	.82	.75
Mental health status	60.79	9.93	60.45	11.99	0.13	.80	.87
Physical health status	68.12	10.17	55.95	9.94	2.12**	.79	.74
ADL	68.12	7.70	62.17	12.25	2.69*	.70	.85
Cognitive status	61.09	9.53	62.95	13.77	1.86	.80	.92

*p < .01; **p < .05.

aged persons pervades all of the other scales and to a significant degree on three scales: social resources, mental health, and ADL. This finding deserves further investigation. The mental health status scale correlated significantly with three other scales: social resources, economic resources, and physical health. This also should be investigated further.

The intercorrelations among the scale scores of the homebound group ranged from .13 to .70. Correlations significant at *p* < .01 were found between mental health status and physical health status (.57), mental health status and cognitive status (.71), physical status and ADL (.70), physical status and cognitive status (.66), and ADL and cognitive status (.55). In this instance, the cognitive status scale scores were significantly correlated with three other scales: mental health, physical health, and ADL. Mental health status also was significantly correlated with physical health, and physical health also was significantly correlated with ADL. Otherwise, there was less overlap among the scale scores of this group than was the case with the well elderly.

Analysis of sociodemographic characteristics of respondents demonstrated no significant differences between female and male subjects in the well elderly group. The *t*-values for the well elderly ranged from 0.30 to 1.38, below the *t* = 2.58 required at the .01 level of probability, with df = 61. In the homebound group the only significant difference was in ADL (*t* = 3.08, *df* = 20). For the homebound group *t*-values ranged from 0.16 to 3.08, with *df* = 20, *t* = 2.58 as required at the .01 level of probability.

Pearson correlations of scale scores with age and level of education were similarly nonsignificant for both groups. Correlations of scale scores with age for the well elderly ranged from −0.32 to 0.02 and for the homebound elderly from −0.27 to 0.02. Correlations of scale scores with level of education ranged from (0.03 to 0.27) for the well elderly and from (0.31 to 0.02) for the homebound elderly.

Finally, analysis of variance among the three types of living arrangements of respondents (alone, with spouse, or with others) revealed no significant differences in the various scale scores, as shown in Table 15.5.

Thus, according to these preliminary Phase II findings, gender, age, educational level, and type of living arrangement failed to significantly affect scale scores for either the well elderly or the homebound group.

Practical Applications

There are many situations in which assessment of the functioning of older persons would have been of value had costs, time factors, and person-power been available for the implementation of assessment procedures. With the demonstration of the feasibility of self-assessment, at least among well elderly, relatively independent persons, it should be possible for agencies concerned with needs assessment, holistic health assessment, case management, evaluation of functioning over time, and admission to various living arrangements for the elderly to consider making functional assessments. Self-assessment also should be a useful tool in large-scale community surveys in which information is sought concerning the service needs of elderly citizens for planning service programs, new housing units, or simply to understand better the demographics of the elderly segment of the population.

Clinical Applications

Multidimensional functional assessment is essential to good case management. It can be a valued tool for making wise, informed decisions regarding those who apply for a variety of special living arrangements for older adults, including retirement homes, housing for low-income elderly and handicapped persons, congregate living arrangements for frail elderly individuals, residential care, and possible intermediate care facilities.

TABLE 15.5 Analysis of Variance among Three Types of Living Arrangements

Scales	Alone (N = 29)		With spouse (N = 22)		With others (N = 12)		F-value[a]
	M	SD	M	SD	M	SD	
Social resources	61.03	8.56	64.18	9.47	61.25	9.76	0.82
Economic resources	63.45	11.55	69.32	5.29	68.42	9.79	2.73
Mental health status	58.86	10.46	61.82	8.69	63.77	8.33	1.37
Physical health status	58.69	10.63	64.27	9.29	61.17	9.36	1.97
ADL	67.21	8.36	70.82	5.44	65.42	8.96	1.97
Cognitive status	62.00	9.98	61.14	8.84	59.67	10.18	0.25

[a]With $df = 2$ and 60, $F = 4.98$ is required at the .01 level of probability.

Long-term care providers need systematic information about the functional levels of their residents as they relate to the services their facilities are prepared to supply. They need to know that important behaviors can be measured and how such functions change over time. Thus, the functional assessment of applicants and residents can provide important information regarding the extent to which the individual's functioning fits the pattern of services offered. If assessment is conducted over time – say, once a year – changes in any of the five areas assessed may be monitored, behavioral modification efforts instituted, and their effects measured.

Multidimensional functional assessment could be a useful addition to the usual intake procedures in a wide variety of health care settings, including medical and dental outpatient clinics, hospitals, adult day health care programs, and community and home health care service agencies.

The geriatric patient needs to be seen and treated as a whole person rather than simply on the basis of presenting symptoms. Such a person will surely benefit if his/her conditions are seen against the background of an assessment of the five broad areas of functioning. Physicians, dentists, nurses, pharmacists, and other health care professional personnel need to be cognizant of, for example, the implications to a person's physical health of that individual's social and economic resources, mental health status, and ability to carry on ADL. Furthermore, these same factors are of value in considering alternative sources of health care, such as whether care can be provided at home, elsewhere in the community, or in a long-term care facility.

Community Surveys

Studies conducted by the Comptroller General of the United States (Laurie, 1977; U.S. General Accounting Office, 1980) are models of investigations that yield valuable data using multidimensional functional assessment methods. These studies sampled 1,609 older persons in Cleveland, Ohio, who were interviewed over a span of six months and reinterviewed a year later. Already available data based on interviews of 868 persons in Oregon and 128 persons in northeastern Kentucky were also analyzed. The reports do not specify the number of interviewers who were used to conduct these studies, but they must have entailed great costs in time, money, and energy. The studies were valuable because they shed light on differences between rural and urban elderly, differences by region of the country, and relative conditions with respect to health, security, loneliness, outlook on life, extent of impairment, need for services, unmet needs, and the predominant sources of help for other persons. Such large-scale surveys form the basis for helping to develop a national policy to better provide for the elderly.

From our initial findings regarding self-administered assessment, future large-scale surveys might be carried out at a fraction of the cost of studies using interviewers. This should encourage those who are concerned with policy studies or community-wide assessment for particular purposes, who might otherwise be unable to do so because of cost and personal needs, to proceed with a smaller budget and fewer staff than that required with interviews.

An example of the latter may be seen in an Iowa City, Iowa, study (Munson, 1983) designed to estimate the interest of the elderly population of Johnson County in congregate living facilities. A random sample of 600 persons, 55 years of age and older, was drawn from available population lists. A response rate just under 50% was obtained, and the 284 (95%) usable responses formed the basis of the study. In addition to specific items relating to available services and attitudes toward congregate housing, the bulk of the self-administered questionnaire comprised items taken from the OARS methodology. No follow-up was required because a comparison of the sample obtained with the population sought showed an adequate fit.

The original intent of the Iowa City study was to measure the demand or need for congregate housing in Johnson County. On completion and analysis of the survey, it was clear that the city knew more about its senior citizens and their needs than before, but in addition, based on the self-administered assessment of the elderly themselves, Iowa City committed itself eventually to development of a congregate facility for the elderly. In view of the constraints under which the study was conducted, any approach other than self-report would have been impossible (the cost constraint was $4,000 and the time constraint allowed four months for the formulation, distribution, statistical analysis, and preparation of the written report).

Conclusions and Recommendations for Phase II

The initial findings based on the Iowa Self Assessment Inventory are encouraging. It is clear that the scales are sensitive to such differences as gross frailty and physical illness, social deprivation due to physical health status, and the consequent inability to carry out the usual ADL. Furthermore, in those instances in which no differences were expected, only one was found. This preliminary evidence suggests that an objectively scored inventory promises to make multidimensional functional assessment readily available and economical of both time and money. Again, the caveat must be expressed that the use of such an inventory depends completely on the respondent's ability to read, understand, and make the responses required. As suggested in the overall research and development design described earlier, it is the author's intent to carry out further necessary data collection so that the inventory can be available as a psychometrically sound assessment tool.

Also, to date the inventory has been developed using Iowans as respondents. A necessary future step will be the extension of the sample to older persons in other parts of the country so that sociodemographic variables such as urban-rural locus, ethnicity, and regional cultural differences may be examined. Readers who might be interested in participating in such additional data collection may contact the authors expressing their interest.

REFERENCES

Duke University, Center for the Study of Aging and Human Development. (1978). *Multidimensional functional assessment: The OARS methodology* (2nd ed.). Durham, NC: Author.

Fillenbaum, G. G., & Smyer, M. A. (1981). The development, validity and reliability of the OARS Multidimensional Functional Assessment Questionnaire. *Journal of Gerontology, 36,* 428-434.

Fleiss, J. L. (1971). Measuring nominal scale agreement among many raters. *Psychological Bulletin, 76,* 378-382.

George, L. K., Landermann, R., & Fillenbaum, G. G. (1982). *Developing measures of functional status and service utilization: Refining and extending the OARS methodology.* Durham, NC: Duke University, Center for Aging and Human Development.

Laurie, W. F. (1977). *Report to the Congress on the well-being of older people in Cleveland, Ohio* (Publication No. HRD 77-70). Washington DC: U.S. General Accounting Office.

Lawton, M. P. (1972). Assessing the competence of older people. In D. Kent, R. Kastenbaum, & S. Sherwood (Eds.), *Research, planning and action for the elderly* (pp. 122-143). New York: Behavioral Publications.

Lawton, P. L., Moss, M. S., Fulcomer, M., & Kleban, M. H. (1982). A research and service oriented multilevel assessment instrument. *Journal of Gerontology, 37,* 91-99.

Light, R. J. (1971). Measures of response agreement for qualitative data: Some generalizations and alternatives. *Psychological Bulletin, 76,* 365-377.

Linn, M. W., & Linn, B. S. (1984). Self-Evaluation of Life Function (Self) Scale: A short, comprehensive self-report of health for elderly adults. *Journal of Gerontology, 39,* 603-612.

Moos, R. H. (1974). *Evaluating treatment environments: A social ecological approach.* New York: John Wiley.

Moos, R. H. (1978). *Evaluating educational environments.* San Francisco: Jossey-Bass.

Moos, R. H., Gauwain, M., Lemke, S., Max, W., & Mehren, B. (1979). Assessing the social environments of sheltered care settings. *The Gerontologist, 19,* 74-82.

Morris, W. W., & Boutelle, S. (1985). Multidimensional functional assessment in two modes. *The Gerontologist, 25,* 638-643.

Munson, D. E. (1983). *Congregate housing: A study of local elderly needs.* Iowa City, IA: Iowa City, Iowa, Housing Commission.

Slavonic, M. J. (1983). *Assessment of the functional health status of the male geriatric veteran: Criterion validity of a mail-out questionnaire.* Unpublished master's thesis, University of Nevada, Reno.

U.S. General Accounting Office (1980). *Comparisons of the well-being of older people in three rural and urban locations* (Publication No. HRD 80-41). Washington, DC: U.S. General Accounting Office.

Iowa Self Assessment Inventory

Directions: The statements on the following pages are about things that can affect our lives in one way or another. We are asking you and a number of other older people to describe your own situations using these statements. In this way, we hope to understand some of the problems and needs of older people living in your community.

Please use the following key in rating each statement:

                4 – True
                3 – More often true than not
                2 – More often false than not
                1 – False

Please read each statement carefully and then circle the number corresponding to the answer that *best* applies to you. We realize that some of the statements may not apply directly to you all of the time, but please try to do the best you can. Do not worry about giving exactly the right answer; your answer may simply mean that the statement is true (or false) to some degree.

Please do not omit any statements. Thank you for your help.

Background Information

Name _____ Date _____

Sex   Male __ Female __   Age on last birthday _____

How far did you go in school?
__ Through the 8th grade
__ Some high school
__ Graduated from high school
__ Some business or trade school
__ Completed business or trade school
__ 1-3 years of college
__ Completed 4-year college
__ Some graduate or professional college
__ Completed graduate or professional college

Who lives in your household with you?
__ No one, I live alone
__ My spouse
__ A child (or children)
__ A friend
__ Other, please specify _____

		Rating (Circle one number for each statement)			
1.	I know at least 4 people whom I can go to visit where they live.	4	3	2	1
2.	Days go by when I do not talk with anyone on the telephone.	4	3	2	1
3.	I have no one who would take care of me if I were sick or disabled for more than a year.	4	3	2	1
4.	I could stay with someone if I were sick for a month.	4	3	2	1
5.	I visit friends in their homes.	4	3	2	1
6.	Friends, other than relatives, seldom visit me.	4	3	2	1
7.	I sometimes meet a friend somewhere other than our homes.	4	3	2	1
8.	I do not see relatives as often as I want too.	4	3	2	1
9.	I see friends as often as I want too.	4	3	2	1
10.	I have someone nearby in whom I trust and confide.	4	3	2	1
11.	At least once a month I attend a meeting of a club, fraternal organization, or other social group.	4	3	2	1
12.	I feel uncomfortable whenever I am in a group of people.	4	3	2	1
13.	At least once a month I attend religious services.	4	3	2	1
14.	I have fewer contacts with other people than most older people I know.	4	3	2	1
15.	I wish my contacts with family, friends, and others were more satisfying.	4	3	2	1
16.	My contacts with other people are more satisfying now than they were 5 years ago.	4	3	2	1
17.	I enjoy getting together with others to play cards, bingo, or other games.	4	3	2	1
18.	I can visit a friend or relative who lives out of town for overnight or longer.	4	3	2	1
19.	I enjoy doing volunteer work that brings me in contact with others.	4	3	2	1
20.	I never write letters to friends or relatives.	4	3	2	1
21.	I have enough money to meet my regular daily expenses.	4	3	2	1
22.	I have enough money to meet unexpected emergencies.	4	3	2	1
23.	My monthly expenses are so high I cannot always pay my bills.	4	3	2	1
24.	I need financial help.	4	3	2	1
25.	I get help from family or friends for the cost of food or meals.	4	3	2	1

26.	I go to the lunch program.	4	3	2	1
27.	I use food stamps.	4	3	2	1
28.	I use special senior citizens' discounts when available.	4	3	2	1
29.	I have health or medical insurance in addition to Medicare.	4	3	2	1
30.	I am doing better financially than most older people I know.	4	3	2	1
31.	I have enough money to buy those little "extras."	4	3	2	1
32.	The cost of transportation is a problem for me.	4	3	2	1
33.	My finances at the present time are excellent.	4	3	2	1
34.	My financial resources are better now than 5 years ago.	4	3	2	1
35.	I have had to cut back on desired activities since retirement.	4	3	2	1
36.	I have some savings and/or investments.	4	3	2	1
37.	I receive Supplemental Security Income (SSI).	4	3	2	1
38.	I receive income from a pension.	4	3	2	1
39.	I live in low-rent housing.	4	3	2	1
40.	I depend on my family for financial help.	4	3	2	1
41.	I seldom worry about things.	4	3	2	1
42.	I feel like life is well worth living.	4	3	2	1
43.	After a year or more, I am still grieving over the loss of someone with whom I was very close.	4	3	2	1
44.	I wake up fresh and rested most mornings.	4	3	2	1
45.	My life is full of things that keep me interested.	4	3	2	1
46.	I am a happy person.	4	3	2	1
47.	I am aware of my heart pounding.	4	3	2	1
48.	I feel lonely even when I am with people.	4	3	2	1
49.	People treat me like I am "different."	4	3	2	1
50.	People are trying to take advantage of me.	4	3	2	1
51.	I would rate my emotional health as excellent.	4	3	2	1
52.	My outlook on life is better now than 5 years ago.	4	3	2	1
53.	I feel good about myself.	4	3	2	1
54.	I am frustrated by changes in my ability to participate in sexual activities.	4	3	2	1
55.	I enjoy sexual activities.	4	3	2	1
56.	I sleep just as well as I ever did.	4	3	2	1
57.	Food tastes as good to me as it ever did.	4	3	2	1
58.	I am satisfied with my sexual life.	4	3	2	1
59.	Thoughts of dying are frequently on my mind.	4	3	2	1
60.	I worry about whether I will be able to care for myself in the future.	4	3	2	1
61.	During the past year I have been to a doctor fewer than 4 times.	4	3	2	1
62.	During the past year I have been so sick I was unable to carry on my usual activities.	4	3	2	1
63.	During the past year I have not been a patient in a hospital.	4	3	2	1
64.	I need more health care than I am now receiving.	4	3	2	1
65.	I fall frequently.	4	3	2	1

66.	My eyesight is good.	4	3	2	1
67.	My hearing is good.	4	3	2	1
68.	I have no physical disabilities or illnesses at this time.	4	3	2	1
69.	I take 3 or more medicines each day.	4	3	2	1
70.	I take laxatives to avoid constipation.	4	3	2	1
71.	I have fewer health problems than most older people I know.	4	3	2	1
72.	I need a cane, crutches, walker, or wheelchair to get around.	4	3	2	1
73.	My doctor has recommended that I cut down on drinking alcohol.	4	3	2	1
74.	I participate in vigorous physical activities.	4	3	2	1
75.	My overall health is excellent.	4	3	2	1
76.	My health is better than it was 5 years ago.	4	3	2	1
77.	I smoke.	4	3	2	1
78.	I have a dry cough.	4	3	2	1
79.	I have stiffness in some of my joints.	4	3	2	1
80.	I have a heart condition that interferes with my activities.	4	3	2	1
81.	I use the telephone without help from others.	4	3	2	1
82.	Whenever I go places beyond walking distance, I need help.	4	3	2	1
83.	I do my own shopping without help.	4	3	2	1
84.	I am not able to prepare my own meals.	4	3	2	1
85.	I need some help with my housework.	4	3	2	1
86.	I am not able to take my own medicine.	4	3	2	1
87.	I eat without assistance from others.	4	3	2	1
88.	I handle my own finances without help.	4	3	2	1
89.	I dress and undress without help.	4	3	2	1
90.	I need help in caring for my appearance (for example, combing my hair and, for men, shaving).	4	3	2	1
91.	I walk without help.	4	3	2	1
92.	I am unable to get in and out of bed without help.	4	3	2	1
93.	I am unable to take a bath or shower without help.	4	3	2	1
94.	I have trouble getting to the bathroom in time.	4	3	2	1
95.	I use public transportation by myself.	4	3	2	1
96.	I do my own laundry.	4	3	2	1
97.	Getting around town is a problem for me.	4	3	2	1
98.	My ability to carry on my daily activities is excellent.	4	3	2	1
99.	My ability to carry on my daily activities is worse than it was 5 years ago.	4	3	2	1
100.	My ability to carry on my daily activities is as good as other older people I know.	4	3	2	1
101.	I have trouble remembering the names of people I know.	4	3	2	1
102.	I have more trouble keeping track of my money than I used to.	4	3	2	1
103.	I forget appointments.	4	3	2	1
104.	Learning new things is harder for me than it used to be.	4	3	2	1
105.	I forget where I put things.	4	3	2	1

106.	I lose my train of thought in the middle of a conversation.	4	3	2	1
107.	My thinking is as good as it ever was.	4	3	2	1
108.	I forget to take medicine when I am supposed to.	4	3	2	1
109.	I am not always sure of the date.	4	3	2	1
110.	I can do arithmetic as well as ever.	4	3	2	1
111.	I feel lost in places I used to know well.	4	3	2	1
112.	I have trouble remembering things that happened very recently.	4	3	2	1
113.	I remember things that happend 10 or more years ago.	4	3	2	1
114.	After watching a movie I don't understand what it was about.	4	3	2	1
115.	My mind is just as sharp as ever.	4	3	2	1
116.	My mind is sharper than most older people I know.	4	3	2	1
117.	I can recall past events when I want to.	4	3	2	1
118.	I enjoy activities that stimulate my mind.	4	3	2	1
119.	I welcome opportunities to learn new things.	4	3	2	1
120.	I have no trouble remembering things like my address and zip code.	4	3	2	1

16
Reliability and Validity of the Lifestyle Assessment Questionnaire

Judith M. Richter

This chapter discusses the Wellness Inventory Section of the Lifestyle Assessment Questionnaire, a measure of wellness behaviors.

The purpose of this study was to provide an analysis of the psychometric properties of the Wellness Inventory section of the Lifestyle Assessment Questionnaire (LAQ), which was developed in 1976 by Dr. William Hettler of the University of Wisconsin. The LAQ has undergone several revisions since its development and is currently recommended to students at the University of Wisconsin as their entrance health assessment. "The LAQ consists of four sections: (1) wellness inventory, (2) personal growth, (3) risk of death (health hazard appraisal), and (4) medical alert sections" (Hettler, 1982, p. 212).

The wellness section of the instrument is designed to encourage students to recognize strengths in each of the wellness dimensions and also to encourage students to identify areas where they might improve. Another purpose of this section is to educate the student about wellness behaviors. "Wellness" refers to the promotion of health by reducing risk of illness and increasing life satisfaction. Health can be considered a result of a "wellness life-style." The wellness component of the LAQ makes the tool particularly desirable for use by nurses if we are to consider health to be the result of a wellness life-style. Doerr and Hutchins (1981) in their review of 12 health hazard appraisal tools described the LAQ as a tool developed with a broad construct of health as a conceptual base. Health concepts incorporated in the LAQ include mental health, knowledge and values, coping abilities, and environmental, occupational, and spiritual factors.

SCORING AND ADMINISTRATION

The tool is a paper-and-pencil test that is self-administered. It takes about 45 min to complete the questionnaire. It would take about 20 minutes to complete the wellness section of the tool, which has 173 items. The results are mailed to the University of Wisconsin-Stevens Point Foundation for scoring.

The Wellness Inventory section of the LAQ is designed to help the individual assess his/her current level of wellness. The score for each of the 11 subsections is the percentage of possible points on the wellness statements. The higher the score, the higher the level of wellness. The subject receives a printout with a percentage of possible points achieved for each life-style dimension of wellness, in addition to the average score for people taking the questionnaire in the group and the total average of all people who ever used the questionnaire. The wellness dimensions included in the tool can be found in Table 16.1.

TABLE 16.1 Wellness Inventory – LAQ

Physical exercise – measures one's commitment to maintaining physical fitness.

Physical nutritional – measures the degree to which one chooses foods that are consistent with the dietary goals of the United States as published by the Senate Select Committee on Nutrition and Human Needs.

Physical, self-care – measures the behaviors that help one prevent or detect early illnesses.

Physical, vehicle safety – measures one's ability to minimize chances of injury or death in a vehicle accident.

Physical, drug usage – measures the degree to which one is able to function without the unnecessary use of chemicals.

Social-environmental – measures the degree to which one contributes to the common welfare of the community. This emphasizes the interdependence with others and nature.

Emotional awareness and acceptance – measures the degree to which one has an awareness and acceptance of one's feelings and related behaviors, including the realistic assessment of one's limitations.

Intellectual – measures the degree that one engages her/his mind in creative, stimulating mental activities, expanding knowledge and improving skills.

Occupational – measures the satisfaction gained from one's work and the degree to which one is enriched by that work.

Spiritual – measures one's ongoing involvement in seeking meaning and purpose in human existence. It includes an appreciation for the depth and expanse of life and natural forces that exist in the universe.

Institute for Lifestyle Improvement UN-SP Foundation, University of Wisconsin-Stevens Point, Stevens Point, WI 54481.

The test has been widely used by people in the age range of 18 to 70 years. Reliability and validity estimates of the tool have been limited, however (Hettler, Janty, & Moffat, 1977). It was decided that additional reliability and validity estimates would enable nurses to make some decisions about the merit of the tool with young female college students.

The wellness component is especially important for consideration by educators. As the profession of nursing is trying to incorporate more health promotion content in nursing practice, it is important that we find effective ways of assessing and teaching health promotion content.

PRETEST: INSTRUMENT DEVELOPMENT PROCESS

The sample for the study consisted of 88 junior-year female college students who were enrolled in an introductory course in nursing. The project was approved by the Human Subjects Review Committee at the University of Northern Colorado. The students were asked to participate in the study and signed consent forms indicating their agreement to be part of the project. Only one student refused to participate in the study, and there were incomplete data on two students. Data were collected from the remaining 85 nursing students. The mean age of the students who participated was 21 years, 5 months.

PRETEST: METHODOLOGY FOR TESTING

Stability

Reliability was established by using 15 subjects who had been randomly selected from the larger group and retesting the subjects after two weeks. Reliability of the subscales ranged from .81 to .97; thus, the stability of the wellness inventory was supported with test-retest analysis using Pearson R.

Homogeneity

Cronbach's coefficient alpha was computed on the wellness scale data to estimate internal consistency reliability. The purpose of evaluating internal consistency is to determine whether something in common is being measured. According to Nunnally (1978), a coefficient of .70 is sufficient as a reliability measure when the researcher is conducting basic research or is working with a new scale. Reliability results obtained with the wellness subscales met these criteria except in the Exercise and Vehicle Safety subscales (Table 16.2).

TABLE 16.2 Reliability of Lifestyle Assessment Questionnaire, Internal Consistency (*N* = 85)

Wellness subscale	Alpha	No. of variables
Exercise	.67	12
Nutrition	.81	13
Self-care	.72	14
Vehicle safety	.69	9
Drug use	.82	13
Social/environment	.81	17
Emotional awareness	.94	30
Emotional management	.89	22
Intellectual	.83	14
Occupational	.85	15
Spiritual	.91	14

Content Assessment

Content Validity

Content validity refers to the extent to which an instrument achieves the purpose for which it was intended (Waltz, Strickland, & Lenz, 1984). To determine content validity, two experts were independently given a copy of the LAQ and were asked to "(1) assess the relevancy of the items to the content addressed by the objectives, and (2) judge if they believed the items of the tool adequately represented the content or behaviors in the domain of interest" (Waltz et al., 1984, p. 142). The Index of Content Validity (CVI) was used to quantify the extent of agreement between the two judges. "To compute the CVI, two content specialists are given the objectives and items and are asked to independently rate the relevance of each item to the objectives, using a four-point rating scale: (1) not relevant, (2) somewhat relevant, (3) quite relevant, and (4) very relevant. The CVI is defined as the proportion of items given a rating of quite/very relevant by both raters involved" (Waltz et al., 1984, p. 142).

Two experts, who were specialists in measurement and the study of health promotion, independently evaluated the wellness section of the LAQ. The CVI was .98. Both raters stated that each wellness subsection adequately represented the behaviors in the domain of interest and added some relevant remarks.

For example, an item from the Physical Self-care subscale ("I select foods that keep my cholesterol level, high density lipids, and triglycerides in a range that minimize my chances of the disease") was believed by one rater to have terminology not easily understood by a layperson. It was also questioned whether this item was more appropriate for the Physical/ Nutritional subsection. Another comment was that the Physical/Vehicle

Safety subsection should have included an item about seat belt use. One rater made the comment that the Social/Environmental subsection actually includes two types of questions: how I contribute to the community and how I choose the environment for myself.

Another useful comment was that questions in the Emotional Management subscale that relate to expression of feelings should include the term "appropriate." For example, there is no way of knowing that if a respondent indicates that he/she expresses feelings of anger that he/she does so in an appropriate manner. Both raters questioned whether the section relating to intellectual behaviors was realistic or understandable by subjects. For example, one item asked whether the respondent read 12 or more books a year. Another item asked if the respondent visited museums three or more times a year.

Another issue addressed by one rater was that there was clearly a socially acceptable "correct" answer for each item. In an effort to avoid the potential of subjects answering items in a socially acceptable manner, they were assured that their responses were held confidential and that data would be analyzed in a manner that did not evaluate individual responses. After the study was completed, students were asked to complete a questionnaire anonymously that asked if they answered the LAQ as honestly as they could or whether they hesitated to answer honestly because of concern about anonymity. Only two students indicated that they did not answer as honestly as they could.

Predictive Validity

Hypothesis testing was conducted to determine if the LAQ did what it was intended to do, that is, change health behaviors in subjects over the course of 6 months. In their review of 12 health risk appraisal instruments, Doerr and Hutchins (1981) indicated that a major issue was "how effective is the instrument in motivating behavioral change?" (p. 301).

One of the first studies attempting to evaluate the impact of a health hazard appraisal (HHA) tool on behavioral change was published by LaDou, Sherwood, and Hughes (1975). One hundred seven employees of a research center were randomly selected from a group of 488 and given the HHA. They were counseled once, 2 weeks after the test, and told what changes needed to take place and how risk age could be reduced. The employees were retested 1 year later, and the risk age was significantly reduced (1.4 years lower) after adjusting for age difference. A problem with this study was that there was no control group. Characteristics of the participants, other than age and areas in which change took place, were not discussed.

The ability of HHA to stimulate appropriate risk reduction behavior was evaluated by Lauzon (1978). Three hundred forty-six volunteers were randomly assigned to one of three groups: one given HHA with counseling, another given HHA with written feedback only, and a control group given neither. It was hypothesized that the group given HHA with counseling would have more behavioral change than the group given HHA without counseling, and the group without counseling would display more behavior change than the control group. Analysis included percentage of positive behavior change between pre-and post-test. Results supported the researcher's hypothesis except in the 30-to-40-year-old group, where there was no demonstrated change between the group who was given HHA only and the control. One major limitation of the study was that 12 weeks was too short a time to properly evaluate behavior change.

Leppink and DeGrassi (1978) evaluated results of HHA scores of 366 participants who were randomly selected from a health risk appraisal program. Subjects' responses were compared to determine differences that occurred at entry, at 6 months, and at 18 months. Data were analyzed to compare percentages of changed behavior in a positive direction, a negative direction, and no change in behavior. Seventy-one percent of the participants had made one or more positive changes in risk behavior. Most of the positive behavioral change was made during the first 6 months. There was very little increase in these percentages 18 months later.

The review of literature reveals limited information about the impact of HHA on behavior change at 6 months. Health risk appraisal has been found to be more effective when accompanied by an educational process (Doerr & Hutchins, 1981), yet there were no studies that examined differences in outcome in subjects who were given HHA alone, HHA with counseling, and HHA with an educational process. There were no studies that evaluated the effectiveness of a wellness assessment tool on behavior change.

POSTTEST: INSTRUMENT DEVELOPMENT PROCESS

A quasi-experimental study was designed to determine the impact of the LAQ on changes in behavior after 6 months. The purpose was also to compare a change in health behaviors in three different groups of nursing students after 6 months.

The sample for the study consisted of 78 female junior-year nursing students. Group 1 ($N = 21$) was enrolled in a 10-week, two-credit course entitled Health Promoting Behaviors. Group 2 ($N = 30$) participated in a personal health assessment program in a multidisciplinary health clinic. Group 3 ($N = 27$) received no treatment other than the LAQ, and they served as the control group.

Although a random assignment would have been the ideal way of completing the study, it was not possible given the philosophy of the School of Nursing. Students were allowed to select the class rotation plan that fit with their work schedules and personal life needs.

The nursing students took the LAQ in July during the summer quarter. Class time was alloted for the students to complete the test. Written results with an interpretation were given to the students 3 weeks later.

At the end of 6 months, after Group 1 and Group 2 had been exposed to didactic information or interventions related to wellness, all three groups again took the LAQ. It was hypothesized that there would be no significant difference in LAQ wellness subscales after 6 months, between students in Group 1 versus Group 2 versus Group 3. MANOVA was used to compare the independent variable (3 groups of nursing students) with the dependent variables (11 wellness subscales). The level of significance for accepting statistical tests was at the .05 level.

POSTTEST: FINDINGS

The results indicated a significant difference on only 1 of the 11 subscales, the Exercise subscale ($F = 5.24$, $p < .01$) (see Table 16.3). Using the Scheffe Multiple Comparison test, it was found that the difference existed between Group 2 (clinic assessment/health promotion) and Group 1 (health promotion course) and between Group 3 (control group) and Group 1. Subjects in Group 2 (clinic assessment/health promotion) and Group 3 (control group) had a decrease in mean scores for exercise. Subjects who had taken the health promotion course (Group 1) were the only subjects who reported an improvement in exercise behaviors after 6 months.

Although wellness content and experiences were introduced to students, there was a trend for health behaviors to change in an adverse direction over the course of 6 months (Table 16.4). this was an unexpected finding of the study.

TABLE 16.3 Wellness Subscales Compared by MANOVA

Subscale	df	Sum of squares	Mean square	F-value	p
Exercise	2	344.913	172.456	5.24	.01*
Nutrition	2	29.014	14.507	.86	.43
Self-care	2	166.916	83.457	2.29	.11
Vehicle safety	2	36.786	18.393	1.22	.30
Drug use	2	6.209	3.104	.15	.86
Environment	2	40.335	20.168	.56	.57
Emotional awareness	2	162.491	81.246	.82	.44
Emotional management	2	58.857	29.428	.49	.61
Intellectual awareness	2	30.627	15.314	.38	.68
Occupation	2	46.737	23.368	.69	.51
Spiritual	2	135.275	67.638	1.30	.28

TABLE 16.4 Mean Score Differences by Group

LAQ Subscales	Group 1 Health promotion course			Group 2 Clinic assessment			Group 3 Control		
	Pre	Post	Difference	Pre	Post	Difference	Pre	Post	Difference
Physical Exercise	30.22	30.76	0.38	31.97	27.53	4.63	31.65	27.5	3.96
Nutritional	29.57	29.24	1.04	28.39	25.63	2.57	27.94	26.74	2.11
Self-care	34.52	29.42	5.52	30.48	26.63	3.67	30.09	28	1.78
Vehicle safety	17.89	17.04	1.05	16.77	13.83	2.77	16.61	13.74	2.19
Drug use	19.61	17.57	2.43	17.71	15.63	2.03	17.35	15.81	1.70
Social-environmental	36.48	33.43	2.67	36.61	31.70	4.47	34.32	31.11	3.60
Emotional:									
Awareness and acceptance	47.04	42.67	3.95	48.87	42.37	5.57	46.29	43.44	2.19
management	40.17	37.71	2.09	39.71	35.27	3.83	41.10	36.93	4.22
Intellectual	39.61	34.71	4.48	36.90	33.57	2.97	37.22	33.33	3.96
Occupational	25.83	25.00	.57	24.97	22.80	1.80	24.06	21.41	2.56
Spiritual	27.04	26.90	.43	25.77	22.46	2.70	27.94	25.14	3.78

Significant univariate F-values: $F = 5.24$, $p = < .01$.

There are a number of possible reasons for the deterioration in wellness behaviors. The LAQ was given prior to enrollment in the upper division in nursing. The students expressed anxiety and concern about their performance in the clinical courses during the junior year of nursing school. It may be that the wellness content and experiences were introduced at a time when students were more interested in learning about pathology. Some students expressed frustration at knowing what they should do to be healthy yet being unable to attain health goals because of heavy school schedules. Further research is necessary to evaluate the positive and negative effects associated with self-awareness of health behaviors. Results of this study suggest that self-awareness of health behaviors is not necessarily a motivator for improving health behaviors.

SUMMARY OF PSYCHOMETRIC SUPPORT

In summary, stability and homogeneity coefficients for the wellness subscales achieved satisfactory standards for reliability. Content validity of the tool was established (.98 CVI) with the evaluation by two experts in measurement and health promotion. Predictive validity was not established with the quasi-experimental design described in this chapter. Health behaviors did not improve as a result of taking the LAQ. The addition of content and experiences in health promotion did not positively affect health-promoting behaviors. In fact, there was a trend for health behaviors in nursing students to deteriorate generally over the course of 6 months.

CONCLUSIONS AND IMPLICATIONS

The research presented here provides an important step in the assessment of a wellness scale designed for use by college students. It is suggested that future research focus on a larger sample and also a sample of older adults and males.

It is further suggested that research be conducted to evaluate the impact of self-awareness on change in health behaviors. The timing of introduction of health promotion content must also be evaluated.

Information about wellness behaviors can provide direction to nurse clinicians in the design of health-promoting nursing interventions. The development of reliable and valid tools that will measure the many domains of wellness is the first phase in the assessment process of health-promoting behaviors.

REFERENCES

Doerr, B. J., & Hutchins, E. B. (1981). Health risk appraisal: Process, problems and prospects for nursing practice and research. *Nursing Research, 30,* 299-306.

Hettler, B. (1982). Wellness promotion and risk reduction on a university campus. In M. Faber and A. Reinhardt (Eds.), *Promoting health through risk reduction.* New York: Macmillan.

Hettler, D., Janty, C., & Moffat, C. (1978). A comparison of seven methods of health hazard appraisal. In *Proceedings of the Thirteenth Meeting of the Society of Prospective Medicine* (pp. 36-44). MD: Society of Prospective Medicine.

LaDou, J., Sherwood, J. N., & Hughes, L. (1975). Health hazard appraisal in patient counseling. *Western Journal of Medicine, 122*(2), 177-180.

Lauzon, R. R. J. (1978). A randomized controlled trial of the ability of HHA to stimulate appropriate risk reduction behavior. In *Proceedings of the Thirteenth Meeting of the Society of Prospective Medicine* (pp. 102-103). Bethesda, MD: Health and Education Resources.

Nunnally, J. C. (1978). *Psychometric theory* (2nd ed.). New York: McGraw-Hill.

Waltz, C., Strickland, O., & Lenz, E. (1984). *Measurement in nursing research.* Philadelphia: F. A. Davis.

Lifestyle Assessment Questionnaire

PURPOSE

The Lifestyle Assessment Questionnaire is designed to help you assess your current level of wellness and the potential risks or hazards you choose to face at this point in your life. The LAQ is organized into four sections: (1) Wellness Inventory; (2) Topics for Personal Growth; (3) Risk of Death Section; and (4) Alert Section: Medical/Behavioral/Emotional. The results that you will receive from completing the questionnaire will reflect your strengths and the possible consequences of risks that you choose to take. The questionnaire results will also assess your interest in improving the quality of your life. You will also receive sources of information that will help you learn more about gaining higher levels of wellness. Your results will be provided in the Lifestyle Assessment Questionnaire Interpretation Guide, which will explain the scoring and the meaning of your results for each of the four sections of this instrument.

CONFIDENTIALITY

The Institute for Lifestyle Improvement will maintain the confidentiality of your answers. The Institute will not permit any individually identified information from your questionnaire to be released to any person or organization other than the source from whom the LAQ was received.

GENERAL INSTRUCTIONS

The attached answer sheet is to be used for recoiding your answers for the Lifestyle Assessment Questionnaire. Please make certain that you complete all of the information at the top of the answer sheet, requesting your name, occupation, age, weight, height, and Social Security number. Results cannot be obtained for Section 3, Risk of Death, if you fail to provide this information. Use a No. 2 pencil for making your responses. Only your answer sheet need be returned for scoring. You may retain the questionnaire.

WELLNESS INVENTORY SECTION

Instructions: This section will help determine the current level of wellness that you are experiencing. We hope that it will also give you ideas for areas in which you might improve. If you are uncomfortable in answering any item in this section or following sections, you may leave that item blank. Please respond to these statements using the following choices marking your responses on the attached answer sheet using a #2 pencil only.

A – Almost always this is true (90% or more of the time)
B – Very frequently this is true (approximately 75% of the time)
C – Frequently this is true (approximately 50% of the time)
D – Occasionally this is true (approximately 25% of the time)
E – Almost never this is true (less than 10% of the time)
    If item does not apply to you do not mark item

Physical Exercise –

Measures one's commitment to maintaining physical fitness.
1. I exercise vigorously for at least 20 minutes three or more times per week.
2. I determine my activity level by monitoring my heart rate.
3. I stop exercising before I feel exhausted.
4. I approach exercise in a relaxed manner.
5. I stretch before exercising.
6. I stretch after exercising.
7. I walk or bike whenever possible.
8. When feeling tired, I arrange for sufficient sleep.
9. I participate in a strenuous sport (tennis, running, swimming, handball, basketball, etc.)
10. I use foot gear of good quality, designed for the activity in which I participate.
11. If I am not in shape, I avoid sporadic (once a week or less often) strenuous exercise.
12. After vigorous exercise, I "cool down" (very light exercise such as walking) for at least five minutes before sitting or lying down.

Physical/Nutritional –

Measures the degree to which one chooses foods that are consistent with the dietary goals of the United States as published by the Senate Select Committee on Nutrition and Human Needs.
13. When choosing non-vegetable protein, I select lean cuts of meat, poultry, and fish.
14. I maintain an appropriate weight for my height and frame.
15. I minimize salt intake.
16. I eat fruits and vegetables fresh and uncooked.
17. I eat breakfast.
18. I intentionally include fiber in my diet on a daily basis.
19. I drink enough fluid to keep my urine light yellow.
20. I plan my diet to ensure an adequate amount of vitamins and minerals.
21. I minimize foods in my diet that contain large amounts of refined flour (bleached white flour, typical store bread, cakes, etc.)
22. I minimize my intake of fats and oils including margarine and animal fats.
23. I include items from all four basic food groups in my diet each day (fruits

and vegetabes; milk group; breads and cereals; meat, fowl, fish or vegetable proteins).

24. To avoid unnecessary calories, I choose water as one of the beverages I drink.
25. I avoid adding sugar to my food and I minimize my intake of pre-sweetend foods such as sugar-coated cereals, syrups, chocolate milk, and most processed and fast foods.

Physical/Self-Care –

Measures the behaviors that help one prevent or detect early illnesses.
26. I record immunizations to maintain up-to-date immunization records.
27. I examine my breasts or testes on a monthly basis.
28. I have my breasts or testes examined yearly by a physician.
29. I have a Pap test annually (Males – do not mark).
30. I take action to minimize my exposure to tobacco smoke.
31. When I'm experiencing illness or injury, I take necessary steps to correct the problem.
32. I brush my teeth after eating.
33. I floss my teeth after eating.
34. My resting pulse is 60 or less.
35. I get an adequate amount of sleep.
36. I engage in activities that keep my blood pressure in a range that minimizes my chances of disease (e.g., stroke, heart attack, and kidney disease).
37. I select foods that keep my cholesterol level, high-density lipids, and triglycerides in a range that minimizes my chances of disease.
38. If I were to engage in sex and didn't want children at that time, I would use a contraceptive method.
39. I take action to prevent contracting and/or transmitting verereal disease.

Physical/Vehicle Safety –

Measures one's ability to minimize chances of injury or death in a vehicle accident.
40. I do not operate vehicles under the influence of alcohol or other drugs.
41. I do not ride with vehicle operators who are under the influence of alcohol or other drugs.
42. I stay within the speed limit.
43. I use the information I learned in a driver education or defensive driving course.
44. When traffic lights change from green to yellow, I prepare to stop.
45. I maintain a safe driving distance between cars based on speed and road conditions.
46. Vehicles which I drive are maintained to assure safety.
47. Because they are safer, I use radial tires on cars that I drive.
48. I use caution when riding bicycles or motorcycles (e.g., helmets, adequate lights, etc.)

Physical/Drug Usage –

Measures the degree to which one is able to function without the unnecessary use of chemicals.
49. I use drugs only when necessary.

50. I avoid the use of tobacco.
51. I consume two alcoholic drinks per day or less.
52. Because of the potentially harmful effects of caffeine (e.g., coffee, tea, colas, etc.), I limit my consumption.
53. I avoid using marijuana.
54. I avoid the use of hallucinogens (LSD, PCP, MDA, etc.).
55. I avoid the use of stimulants ("uppers" – e.g., cocaine, amphetamines, "pep pills," etc.)
56. I avoid the use of depressants ("downers" – e.g., barbiturates, minor tranquilizers, etc.).
57. I avoid using a combination of drugs unless under medical supervision.
58. I follow the instructions provided with any drug I take.
59. I avoid using drugs obtained from unlicensed sources.
60. I understand the expected effect of drugs I take.
61. I consider alternatives to drugs.

Social/Environmental –

Measures the degree to which one contributes to the common welfare of the community. This emphasizes the interdependence with others and nature.
62. I take steps to conserve energy in my place of residence.
63. I consider energy conservation when choosing a mode of transportation.
64. I offer support to members of my family when appropriate.
65. I contribute to the feeling of acceptance within my family.
66. I do my part to promote clean air.
67. When I see a safety hazard, I take action (warn others or correct the problem).
68. I avoid unnecessary radiation.
69. I report criminal acts I observe.
70. I contribute time and/or money to community projects.
71. I actively seek to become acquainted with individuals in my community.
72. I use my creativity in constructive ways.
73. My behavior reflects fairness and justice.
74. When possible, I choose an environment which is free of noise pollution.
75. When possible, I choose an environment which is free of air pollution.
76. I participate in volunteer activities benefiting others.
77. I go out of my way to help others.
78. I beautify those parts of my environment under my control.

Emotional Awareness and Acceptance –

Measures the degree to which one has an awareness and acceptance of one's feelings. This includes the degree to which one feels positive and enthusiastic about oneself and life.
79. I have a good sense of humor.
80. I feel positive about myself.
81. I feel there is a satisfying amount of excitement in my life.
82. My emotional life is stable.
83. I am aware of my needs.
84. I trust and value my own judgment.

85. When I make mistakes, I learn from them.
86. I feel comfortable when complimented for jobs well done.
87. It is okay for me to cry.
88. I have feelings of sensitivity for others.
89. I feel enthusiastic about life.
90. I find it easy to laugh.
91. I am able to give love.
92. I am able to receive love.
93. I enjoy my life.
94. I have plenty of energy.
95. My sleep is restful.
96. I trust others.
97. I feel others trust me.
98. I accept my sexual desires.
99. I understand how I create my feelings.
100. At times I can be both strong and sensitive.
101. I am aware when I feel anger.
102. I can accept my anger.
103. I am aware when I feel sad.
104. I can accept my sadness.
105. I am aware when I feel happy.
106. I can accept my happiness.
107. I am aware when I feel frightened.
108. I can accept my feelings of fear.

Emotional Management –

Measures the capacity to appropriately control one's feelings and related behaviors including the realistic assessment of one's limitations.
109. I am able to be open with those with whom I am close.
110. I can express my feelings of anger.
111. I can express my feelings of sadness.
112. I can express my feelings of happiness.
113. I can express my feelings of fear.
114. I can compliment myself for a job well done.
115. I accept constructive criticism without reacting defensively.
116. I recognize that I can have wide variations of feelings about the same person (such as loving someone even though you are angry with her/him at the moment).
117. I am able to develop close, intimate relationships.
118. I make conscious decisions about my sexual activity based on personal/spiritual values.
119. I stick to the limits I set for myself.
120. I can say "no" without feeling guilty.
121. I would feel comfortable seeking professional help to better understand and cope with my feelings.
122. I set realistic objectives for myself.
123. I can relax my body and mind (without using drugs).
124. I can be alone without feeling lonely.
125. I am able to be spontaneous in expressing my feelings.

126. I accept responsibility for my actions.
127. I am willing to take the risks that come with making changes.
128. I manage my feelings to avoid unnecessary suffering.
129. I make decisions with a minimum of stress and worry.
130. I accept the responsibility for creating my own feelings.

Intellectual –

Measures the degree that one engages her/his mind creatively, stimulating mental activities, expanding knowledge, and improving skills.
131. I read a newspaper daily.
132. I read twelve books or more yearly.
133. I read on the average one or more national magazines weekly.
134. When I watch TV, I choose educational programs.
135. I visit a museum or art show at least three times yearly.
136. I attend lectures, workshops, and demonstrations at least three times yearly.
137. I regularly use some of my time participating in hobbies such as photography, gardening, woodworking, sewing, painting, baking, art, music, writing, pottery, etc.
138. I read about local, state, national, and international political/public issues.
139. I make an effort to learn the meaning of new words.
140. I engage in some type of writing activity such as a regular journal, letter writing, preparation of papers or manuscripts.
141. I am interested in understanding the views of others.
142. I devote time to sharing ideas, concepts, thoughts, or procedures to advance the knowledge of others.
143. I gather information to enable me to make independent decisions.
144. I regularly listen to radio and/or TV news.

Occupational –

Measures the satisfaction gained from one's work and the degree to which one is enriched by that work.
   Please answer these items from your primary frame of reference, (e.g., your job, student, homemaker, etc.). If you are unemployed or retired, do not mark this section.
145. I enjoy my work.
146. My work contributes to my personal needs.
147. I feel that my job in some way contributes to others and/or society.
148. I interact cooperatively with others in my work.
149. I take advantage of opportunities to learn new skills in my work.
150. My work is challenging.
151. I feel my job responsibilities are consistent with my values.
152. I find satisfaction from the work I do.
153. I find healthy ways of reducing excessive stress when it occurs in my job.
154. I use recommended health and safety precautions.
155. I make recommendations for improving occupational health and safety.
156. I am satisfied with the degree of freedom to exercise independent judgments in my job.

157.   I am satisfied with the amount of variety in my work.
158.   I believe I am competent in my job.
159.   My co-workers and supervisors respect me as a competent individual.

Spiritual –

Measures one's ongoing involvement in seeking meaning and purpose in human existence. It includes an appreciation for the depth and expanse of life and natural forces that exist in the universe.

160   I feel good about my spiritual life.
161.   Prayer, meditation, and/or quiet personal reflection is/are important part(s) of my life.
162.   I contemplate my purpose in life.
163.   I reflect on the meaning of events in my life.
164.   My values guide my daily life.
165.   My values and beliefs help me to meet daily challenges.
166.   I recognize that my spiritual growth is a lifelong process.
167.   I am concerned about humanitarian issues.
168.   I enjoy participating in discussions about spiritual values.
169.   I feel a sense of compassion to others need.
170.   I seek spiritual knowledge.
171   My spiritual awareness occurs other than at times of crises.
172.   I believe in something greater or that I am part of something greater than myself.
173.   I share my spiritual values.

TOPICS FOR PERSONAL GROWTH SECTION

Instructions: This section is intended to help you identify areas in which you would like more information for continued learning assistance. In response to your selection from the following topics we will provide you with resources or services to meet your requests.

With regard to the following list, I would like information on the following topics:
1. Responsible alcohol use
2. Stop smoking programs
3. Sexual dysfunction
4. Contraception
5. Venereal disease
6. Depression
7. Loneliness
8. Exercise programs
9. Weight reduction
10. Self-breast exam
11. Medical emergencies
12. Vegetarian diets
13. Relaxation, stress reduction
14. Mate selection
15. Parenting skills

16. Marital (or couples) problems
17. Assertiveness training (how to say no without feeling guilty)
18. Biofeedback for tension headache
19. Overcoming phobias (e.g., high places, crowded rooms, etc.)
20. Educational/career goal setting/planning
21. Spiritual or philosophical values
22. Interpersonal communication skills
23. Automobile safety
24. Suicide thoughts or attempts
25. Drug abuse
26. Anxiety associated with public speaking, tests, writing, etc.
27. Enhancing relationships
28. Time management skills
29. Nutrition
30. Death and dying
31. Learning skills (speed reading, comprehension, etc.)

RISK OF DEATH SECTION

Instructions: This section is intended to help you identify the problems most likely to interfere with the quality of your life. This will give you a statistical assessment of the most likely causes of death facing you for the next ten (10) years. This section will also indicate what impact various personal behavioral choices have on that risk of death. Although this section will give you a printout indicating a statistical measurement of your risk based on national morbidity and mortality data, the printout will be no guarantee. We do feel, however, that it is a fairly accurate assessment of your current state of risk and offers suggestions for improving the quality of life and useful longevity.

Preexisting disease or chance occurrence can completely negate the recommendations or suggestions made on the printout of this section.

Please make certain that you complete all of the information at the top of the answer sheet requesting your name, occupation, age, weight, height, and Social Security number.

Record all of your answers for Section 3 on the attached answer sheet, marking your responses in the appropriate boxes using a #2 pencil only.

1. Sex:
   1. Male
   2. Female
2. Race:
   1. White
   2. Black
   3. Other
3. How would you describe you body build?
   1. Small
   2. Medium
   3. Large

4. What is your systolic (top number) blood pressure?
   1. 190 or more
   2. 170-189
   3. 150-169
   4. 130-149
   5. Less than 130
   Note: If you don't know your blood pressure, we will use the average for your age, race, and sex.
5. What is your diastolic (lower number) blood pressure?
   1. 103 or more
   2. 97-102
   3. 91-96
   4. 85-90
   5. Less than 85
6. What is your blood cholesterol level?
   1. 270 or more
   2. 230-269
   3. 210-229
   4. 190-209
   5. Less than 190
   Note: If you don't know your cholesterol level, we will use the average for your age, race, and sex.
7. Are you:
   1. An uncontrolled diabetic
   2. A controlled diabetic
   3. Not a diabetic
8. Which of the following best describes how much physical activity you get per week including work?
   1. Climb less than 5 flights of stairs or walk less than $1/2$ mile 4 times per week (or equivalent activity)
   2. Climb 5-15 flights of stairs or walk $1/2$-$1^1/2$ miles 4 times per week (or equivalent activity)
   3. Climb 15-20 flights of stairs or walk $1^1/2$-2 miles 4 times per week (or equivalent activity)
9. Family history of heart disease:
   1. Both parents died before age 60 of heart disease
   2. One parent died before age 60 of heart disease
   3. Neither parent died before age 60 of heart disease
10. Do you smoke tobacco?
    1. Yes
    2. No
11. If item 10 is yes, how much do you smoke per day?
    1. 2 packs of cigarettes or more
    2. $1^1/2$-2 packs of cigarettes
    3. 1-$1^1/2$ packs of cigarettes
    4. $1/2$-1 pack of cigarettes or heavy pipe or cigar
    5. Less than $1/2$ pack of cigarettes or light pipe or cigar
12. If item 10 is yes, how many years have you been smoking?
    1. Less than 2
    2. 2-5

    3. 5-10
    4. 11-15
    5. 16 or more
13. Are you a former smoker?
    1. Yes
    2. No
14. If item 13 is yes, how much did you smoke per day?
    1. 2 packs of cigarettes or more
    2. $1^1/_2$-2 packs of cigarettes
    3. 1-$1^1/_2$ packs of cigarettes
    4. $^1/_2$-1 pack of cigarettes or heavy pipe or cigar
    5. Less than pack of cigarettes or light pipe or cigar
15. If item 13 is yes, how many years ago did you quit?
    1. 0-2 years
    2. 3-4
    3. 5-6
    4. 7-8
    5. 9 or more
16. Do you drink alcoholic beverages?
    1. Yes
    2. No
17. If item 16 is yes, how many drinks per week?
    1. More than 40 drinks
    2. 25-40
    3. 8-24
    4. 3-7
    5. 1-2
18. When consuming alcohol, I consume not more than one drink per hour.
    1. Yes
    2. No
19. How many miles a year do you travel in a motor vehicle as a driver or passenger?
    1. Under 10,000
    2. 10,000-20,000
    3. 20,000-30,000
    4. 30,000-40,000
    5. Over 40,000
20. While traveling in a motor vehicle how often do you use seat belts?
    1. 20% or less of the time
    2. 20%-40%
    3. 40%-60%
    4. 60%-80%
    5. 80%-100%
21. How often do you find you are experiencing depression?
    1. Frequently
    2. Seldom
    3. Never
22. Has anyone in your immediate family (parents, brothers, sisters) committed suicide?
    1. Yes

2. No

23. In regard to your heart, have you had:
    1. A murmur without preventive antibiotics
    2. A murmur with preventive antibiotics
    3. No murmur
24. In regard to your heart, have you had:
    1. Rheumatic fever without preventive antibiotics
    2. Rheumatic fever with preventive antibiotics
    3. No rheumatic fever
25. To the best of your knowledge, do you have any signs or symptoms of rheumatic heart disease?
    1. Yes
    2. No
27. Do you carry a weapon with you?
    1. Yes
    2. No
28. Have you ever had bacterial pneumonia?
    1. Yes
    2. No
29. Have you ever had emphysema?
    1. Yes
    2. No
30. Has anyone in your family (parents, brothers, sisters) had diabetes?
    1. Yes
    2. No
31. Have you ever had polyps (growth in the intestines?)
    1. Yes
    2. No
32. Have you ever had undiagnosed rectal bleeding?
    1. Yes
    2. No
33. Have you ever had ulcerative colitis?
    1. Yes, 10 or more years ago
    2. Yes, less than 10 years ago
    3. No
34. Have you had a rectal examination with a lighted instrument within the last year?
    1. Yes
    2. No

If female, answer the following questions:

35. Do you perform a regular monthly self-breast examination?
    1. Yes
    2. No
36. Do you have a yearly exam by your physician?
    1. Yes
    2. No
37. How many of your blood relatives (mother, sisters, aunts) have had breast cancer?

    1. 2 or more
    2. 1
    3. None
38. Have you ever had fibrocystic breast disease or other noncancerous disease?
    1. Yes
    2. No
39. Are you Jewish? (Cancer of the cervix is very rare in Jewish women.)
    1. Yes
    2. No
40. Age of first intercourse. (Cancer of the cervix is more common in females who have first intercourse in teens and/or have multiple partners.)
    1. Under 20 years old
    2. 20-25 years old
    3. Over 25 years old or never
41. Pertaining to a Pap smear, mark the response most accurate for you. The following responses are irrelevant if you have had an abnormal Pap test ever. Abnormal Pap tests deserve regular follow-up.
    1. Haven't had one in last five (5) years
    2. Had 1 normal within the last five (5) years
    3. Had 1 normal within last year
    4. Had 3 normal within the last five (5) years
    5. Had one normal each of the last five (5) years
42. Have you experienced undiagnosed vaginal bleeding?
    1. Yes
    2. No
43. Do you now take birth control pills?
    1. Yes
    2. No

ALERT SECTION MEDICAL/BEHAVIORAL/EMOTIONAL

Instructions: This section is intended to be used to identify high-risk problems or past medical problems that we feel are important in establishing one's medical records. This can be used for a personal record by the individual or can be used by professionals as a problem list to be incorporated with the remainder of the individual's medical records. Please mark the number that is most correct in answering each question. Any question that you do not feel comfortable answering or you think is not pertinent please leave blank.

Mark your answers on the attached answer sheet using a #2 pencil only.

Medical

1. Do you have diabetes?   1. Yes 2. No
2. Do you have a seizure disorder (epilepsy)?   1. Yes 2. No
3. Do you have known heart trouble(acquired or congenital)? 1. Yes 2. No
4. Did any of your blood relatives die of heart disease under the age of 50?   1. Yes 2. No

 5. Have you had major heart surgery?   1. Yes 2. No
 6. Do you have a physical disability that interferes with rou-
    tine activities including physical fitness programs?   1. Yes 2. No
 7. Have you had a skin test for TB in the past two (2) years?   1. Yes 2. No
 8. If item 7 is yes, which result did you have?   1. Reaction
                                                                  2. No Reaction
 9. Do you take any medication regularly such as daily or sev-
    eral times per week?   1. Yes 2. No
10. Do you have allergies to drugs?   1. Yes 2. No
11. Are you allergic to penicillin?   1. Yes 2. No
12. Are you allergic to sulfa?   1. Yes 2. No
13. Are you allergic to aspirin?   1. Yes 2. No
14. Do you have additional drug allergies not listed above?   1. Yes 2. No
15. Do you have asthma?   1. Yes 2. No

Immunizations

16. Did you have baby shots for DPT (diphtheria whooping
    cough, and tetanus)/ Ask your parents or doctor.   1. Yes 2. No
17. Have you had a booster for tetanus in the last five (5)
    years? (Recommended interval is 5-10 years.).   1. Yes 2. No
18. Have you had a form of polio vaccine?   1. Yes 2. No
19. With regard to German measles:
    1. Have had a blood test showing immunity or received
        rubella immunization
    2. Never had a blood test or the blood test showed no
        immunity to rubella (German measles).
20. Have you had a Pap test in the last year?   1. Yes 2. No
21. Have you ever had an abnormal Pap test?   1. Yes 2. No
22. Were you exposed to DES (diethylstilbesterol) while your
    mother was pregnant with you? (Ask you mother to check
    with her doctor if you are not sure.)   1. Yes 2. No

Behavioral/Emotional

Note: The leading cause of death among young adults is auto accidents.
23. Do you drive a car, motorcycle, or bike after drinking alcohol? 1. Yes 2. No
24. Do you ride with "drinking" drivers?   1. Yes 2. No
Note: The second leading cause of death among young adults is suicide.
25. Have you seriously considered killing yourself within the
    past year?   1. Yes 2. No
26. Have you ever attempted suicide?   1. Yes 2. No
27. Have any of your relatives committed suicide?   1. Yes 2. No
28. Do you frequently feel that life is not worth living?   1. Yes 2. No
29. Does each day look so dull that you would rather not wake
    up in the morning?   1. Yes 2. No
30. Do you feel overly tired and without motivation much of the
    time?   1. Yes 2. No
31. Do you feel you have a serious emotional problem?   1. Yes 2. No
32. Do you have a history of/or have you recently experienced
    hallucinations (hearing or seeing things others don't)?   1. Yes 2. No

33. Do you have difficulty feeling close to people? 1. Yes 2. No
34. Do you worry excessively? 1. Yes 2. No
35. Do you feel you've had an excessive number of illnesses in
    the past year? 1. Yes 2. No
36. Do impulsive behaviors cause you serious problems? 1. Yes 2. No
37. Are you unhappy too much of the time? 1. Yes 2. No
38. Do you cry too often? 1. Yes 2. No
39. Do you have difficulty controlling your temper? 1. Yes 2. No

THE MAJOR DETERMINANT FOR JOYFUL LIVING IS YOU AND YOUR LIFESTYLE

The circle graph below indicates the factors that contribute to increasing your enjoyment and quality of life. While it is true that doctors and hospitals have a significant role to play in the quality of our lives, this graph clearly indicates that it is individuals, through the choices that they make each day, that contribute the greatest percentage toward maximizing the quality of life and health. We believe this instrument can be a useful adjunct in helping individuals identify the most likely causes of death and disability, but more important, identify the areas of self-improvement that will lead to higher levels of joy and wellness. This instrument can be used to begin a positive, wellness approach toward living. It is our belief that this instrument can help people realize that they are the most important provider of health or "illth" care. Many of the common killers in America are the direct result of individual behaviors. We all know that our behaviors can improve our chances for leading a long, useful life. Collectively, all of our behaviors can be described as our lifestyle.

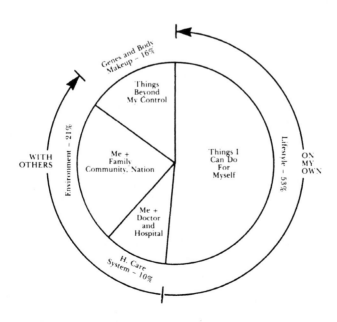

WORDS FROM THE PAST

"To ward off disease or recover health, men as a rule find it easier to depend on the healers than to attempt the more difficult task of living wisely."

— Rene Dubois

"It's what you do hour by hour, day by day, that largely determines the state of your health; whether you get sick, what you get sick with, and perhaps when you die."

— Lester Breslow, M.D.

"For many years, while engaged in the practice of medicine, the author of this volume has been more and more impressed with the idea that the causes of the suffering, diseases, and premature deathes, which we witness around us on every hand, lie nearer our own doors . . . and that the men and women of today, are, at least, equally as responsible for existing suffering, as those who have gone before them, and often much more so. In fact, he feels satisfied that by far the greatest portion of all the suffering, disease, deformity, and premature deaths which occur, are the direct result of either the violation of, or the want of compliance with the laws of our being; calamities, which, were the requisite knowledge possessed by the community, can and should be avoided."

— Taken from the Preface to *Avoidable Causes of Disease* by John Ellis, 1859

17
Validity and Reliability of a Measure of Women's Health Beliefs

Carol Ann Gramse

This chapter discusses the Health Beliefs Instrument, a measure of women's attitudes toward breast cancer and breast self-examination.

Women's health beliefs, more specifically women's health beliefs regarding breast cancer and breast self-examination were identified as the specific outcome variable to be measured. This instrument was designed and reported by Stillman (1977).

REVIEW OF LITERATURE ON HEALTH BELIEFS

Several authors have developed general theories of health behavior in an effort to establish a foundation for prediction of whether health practices will be undertaken. The health beliefs model proposed by Rosenstock (1974) forms the theoretical foundation for assessment of the variable related to women's health beliefs regarding breast cancer and breast self-examination.

The way individuals perceive the world around them determines their behavior in any given situation. Rosenstock's model of health beliefs identifies two variables believed to influence the taking of a preventive action. Specifically, two sets of perceptions are important: (1) psychological state of readiness to take action and (2) the extent to which a specific course of action is seen as beneficial in reducing threat (Rosenstock, 1974).

Psychological readiness is composed of perceived susceptibility (or vulnerability) and perceived seriousness. Optimal conditions for taking action are thought to depend on several factors. The individual must perceive that he/she is susceptible to a health threat. Cancer of the breast is a condition that many women consider a personal threat (Gramse, 1982; Hallal, 1982; Stillman, 1977).

Readiness for action also includes the perceived serious consequences for the individual should the health threat materialize. Breast cancer certainly connotes serious consequences for most women. Although there is an 85% 5-year survival rate when diagnosis and treatment occur early, by the time most women discover a lump, 60% have lymph node involvement, reducing the survival rate to 40 to 45% (American Cancer Society, 1985a, b).

Finally, the course of action being recommended would be effective in reducing or eliminating the threat. Since widespread mammography screening is not feasible, nor is it indicated for all age groups, monthly breast self-examination supplemented by yearly physical examinations remains the most viable health activity for early detection of cancer of the breast. Breast self-examination does not prevent breast cancer, but it does limit the progress of the disease (American Cancer Society, 1985b; Edwards, 1980; Foster et al., 1978; Thiessin, 1971; Turnball, 1978).

Individuals must also perceive that there is a relative absence of barriers to taking action. Breast self-examination meets this criteria in that it is painless, cost-free, and can be performed in the privacy of one's home when it is convenient for the woman. Since a woman must also perceive cues or triggers to action, breast self-examination is widely publicized.

Chapion's (1985, p. 376) convenience sample ($N = 301$) revealed that barriers accounted for the largest portion of variance (23%) on the dependent variable of frequency of breast self-examination. Health motivation accounted for 2% of the variance and perceived benefits; seriousness and susceptibility did not add significantly to this health behavior.

EXISTING TOOLS AND PROCEDURES FOR MEASURING WOMEN'S HEALTH BELIEFS

Several investigators have examined women's attitudes toward breast cancer and breast self-examination and other factors influencing whether or not a woman will practice breast self-examination (Cortrell, 1973; Edwards, 1980; Gallup Organization, 1974; Howe, 1981; Rose, 1978; Scilken, 1977; Thiessen, 1971; Turnball, 1978). These investigators' examinations of generalized health beliefs have limitations because such beliefs represent only one of the variables that enter into the prediction of behavior. In other words, a low level of prediction follows use of a broad measure of generalized health beliefs. The narrower the definition of generalized women's health beliefs, the higher the prediction that results. Therefore, a more specific measure of women's health beliefs should allow for greater prediction in a specific situation. The instrument in this study measures the specific outcome of women's health beliefs about breast cancer and breast self-examination.

Several nursing studies utilize the health beliefs model and report data collected about women's health beliefs about breast cancer and breast self-examination (Gramse, 1982; Hallal, 1982; Stillman, 1977). Invariably, these nurse investigators, along with the researchers cited above, do not describe methodologies used to construct the tools, nor do they report estimates of validity or reliability. This chapter reports refinement of a tool designed in the general framework of the health beliefs model, with the intention of measuring a specific outcome, women's health beliefs about breast cancer and breast self-examination. Before continued investigations can utilize this instrument and build on previously reported significant findings, supporting evidence of validity and reliability must be estimated.

The multitrait multimethod (MTMM) approach was selected to provide the necessary documentation. Prior to elaboration of the MTMM approach, a discussion of the initial conceptual basis for items included to measure women's health beliefs about breast cancer and breast self-examination is presented.

VALIDITY OF WOMEN'S HEALTH BELIEFS

Conceptual Basis of Women's Health Beliefs about Breast Cancer and Breast Self-Examination

The concept of health beliefs is theoretically defined as a set of perceptions an individual holds about his/her susceptibility to any illness, the seriousness of that illness on his/her life, and the benefits of taking action that would enhance the early detection of that illness, or if that disease occurred, would reduce its severity. The applied definition of such a concept to this study is women's health beliefs about breast cancer and breast self-examination. These beliefs are a set of perceptions a woman holds about her susceptibility to breast cancer, the seriousness of the effect of that illness on her life, and the benefits of breast self-examination in enhancing early detection of breast cancer, or if breast cancer occurred, reducing its severity.

Purpose of Women's Health Beliefs

Operationally, the instrument developed by Stillman (1977) measured the perceived susceptibility and the benefits of breast self-examination. Perceived seriousness of breast cancer was not measured, as cancer has been documented in previous research to be perceived as serious (Haefner & Kirscht, 1970; Kegeles, 1965). The even-numbered items are intended to reflect a women's perceived susceptibility to breast cancer, and the odd-numbered items are intended to reflect a woman's perceived benefits of breast self-examination in reducing the threat of breast cancer.

Content Validity

Stillman (1977) related the estimation of content validity to the conceptual basis for the items included in the instrument. The questionnaire was submitted to a panel of five nursing experts. Their areas of expertise were not identified. The objectives for evaluation of the questionnaire were presented to these judges, who were then asked to determine whether the 10 items represented women's health beliefs for perceived susceptibility to breast cancer and perceived benefits of breast self-examination. No method of rating the ways judges were to indicate their agreement is discussed. Stillman reported that on all items the panel agreed 100% that the items represented the domain of women's health beliefs, and more specifically, perceived susceptibility and perceived benefits.

Refinement of Content Validity

To refine this approach to establishing content validity, measurement of the Content Validity Index (CVI) was performed as discussed by Waltz, Strickland, & Lenz (1984, p. 142). Two content/measurement nursing experts were selected. One, a nurse educator with clinical experience and classroom expertise in oncology nursing, had taught specifically the content area of breast cancer. The other expert is an active nurse investigator and recent author on research in qualitative theories and methodologies in nursing.

A written explanation of the instructions to assess content validity was given to them. These instructions provided theoretical definitions of health beliefs and operational definitions of women's health beliefs about breast cancer and breast self-examination. The content experts were asked to link the relevance of the odd-numbered items to perceived susceptibility to breast cancer and the even-numbered items to perceived benefits of breast self-examination in enhancing early detection of breast cancer. They were asked to rate the relevancy of each item to the operational definition using a 4-point scale: (1) not relevant, (2) somewhat relevant, (3) relevant, and (4) quite relevant. In reviewing the instrument items, the experts were directed to be alert for the presence of ambiguous wording, unclear or imprecise statements, and the unlikelihood of yielding the desired response(s), perceived susceptibility or perceived benefits. The CVI is defined as the proportion of items given a rating of 3 or 4 by both experts. Fifteen items were rated quite/very relevant (3 or 4) on a scale of 1 to 4, giving a CVI of 0.75, which is a mildly acceptable level of content validity (Waltz et al., 1984).

Construct Validity

Construct validity is one of several ways to derive validity – the extent to which an instrument measures what it was intended to measure. Estimation of construct validity can provide stronger theoretical support to findings and strengthen conclusions that may be drawn. It is an important procedure for estimating validity of measures when the intent is to infer the degree to which the individual possesses some hypothetical trait or quality presumed to be reflected in the test score. Its greatest utility is for affective types of measures, measures that seek to quantify interests, values, and attitudes. Individual differences in test scores are intended to reflect individual differences in the trait (interest, value, or attitude) about which the inference is being made.

The MTMM approach to estimate construct validity was selected because it produces more data with more efficiency than other approaches used to estimate construct validity, such as contrasted-groups or known-groups approaches. The MTMM approach is based on two premises: (1) that different measures of the same construct should correlate highly with each other (convergent validity principle) and (2) that measures of different constructs should have low correlations with each other (discriminant validity principle).

Several criteria must be met in order to use this particular strategy. Specifically, (1) one must measure at least two traits to assess discriminant validity; (2) one must employ at least two different methods of measuring a trait to assess convergent validity; (3) one must be able to administer all instruments to every subject at the same time.

To carry out this strategy, constructs must be selected that can be measured using several methods. Then instruments are developed that can employ these similar measurement methods, such as the Likert rating scale, Q-sort, semantic differential, and so on. For example, one construct might employ a semantic differential and an adjective checklist, thus meeting the criteria of employing at least two measurement methods. The next step involves meeting the criteria of utilizing at least two traits. The second construct in this example must be capable of being measured by the semantic differential and the adjective checklist techniques. Thus, similar methods and dissimilar traits gives this approach its name.

When this MTMM technique is employed, attention is focused not only on the size of the correlations but on the pattern of relationships between correlations as well. It is assumed that performance on each instrument employed is independent and not influenced by performance on any other instrument. The size of a correlation between two measures is a function of both trait and method variance. Trait variance is the variability in a set of scores resulting from individual differences in the trait being measured. Method variance is variance resulting from individual differences in a subject's ability to respond appropriately to the type of method used.

Validity techniques that focus only on the size of the correlation between two measures are not able to account for the extent to which each of these types of variances (trait variance and method variance) are represented in their results. When validity is evident, the correlation between two measures of the same construct will be more a function of trait than method variance. In order to assess that this is so, it is therefore necessary to focus not only on the size of the correlations but also on the patterns of the relationships between correlations of measures of the same and different constructs, using common and different methods as well. The MTMM approach can provide evidence of (1)convergent validity (that is, different measures of the same construct, which should correlate highly with each other); (2) discriminant validity (that is, measures of different constructs, which should have low correlations with each other); (3) construct validity; and (4) estimates of reliability using the internal consistency coefficient alpha.

Multitrait Selection

Women's health beliefs have been identified as one trait to be measured and are described above in detail. To represent a measure of a different construct, value of health was selected. It is defined as the individual's perception of how important health is to that individual.

Multimethod Selection

Having selected one trait employing a Likert type of method, value of health was measured by a modification of the Value Survey, developed by Wallston, Wallston, Kaplan, & Maides (1976). Using an alphabetical listing of 10 values, including health, individuals are asked to rate the relative degrees of importance of each item for themselves. A Likert scale of 1 to 3 with important, next important, and most important, was selected.

A new method using a visual analog approach was selected. This method was identified because in using scaling techniques, subjects sometimes fall in between arbitrary scale divisions. The visual analog approach helps individuals to set the boundary, rather than the researcher, who arbitrarily sets the scale range 1 to 4, 1 to 7, and so on. The subject simply rates himself/herself within the field of the visual scale shown.

Modification Procedures

Information about structure, design, and scoring is important in tool development. Each tool must be modified in construction and scoring to reflect each method of measurement. Modifying the Likert scale to the visual analog construction was done simply by drawing a line for the continuum from "strongly agree" to "strongly disagree," and similarly for the continuum of degree of importance.

Scoring

Scoring for the women's health beliefs instrument consists of an overall women's beliefs score or two subscores on beliefs of perceived susceptibility to breast cancer (even-numbered items) and beliefs of perceived benefits of breast self-examination (odd-numbered items). In the Likert format, one simply sums the numbers circled. Items 1, 4, 5, and 8 are rated four if "agree strongly" is chosen; items 2, 3, 6, 7, and 9 are reversed scored. The 10th item is rated 1 if "below average" is chosen; a response of "above average" receives a score of 3. Using the visual-analog method, one measures from left to right, using a centimeter ruler. The score is the absolute value, to one decimal point, for the mark placed on the line next to each item, a length of 3 cm. Values obtained for items 1, 4, 5, and 8 were subtracted from 3 to maintain consistency with the Likert scoring procedure. For the Likert format, the range of scores for beliefs of perceived susceptibility is 5 to 19; the range of scores for beliefs of perceived benefits is 5 to 20. In the visual analog format, the range was scores of 0 to 30, in absolute terms, for each subscale of perceived benefits and perceived susceptibility, and a range of 0 to 60 for an overall measure of women's health beliefs.

The score for the value of health is simply the absolute value of the number circled in the Likert format or the value obtained when measuring the mark placed on the visual analog field. It was defined that an individual's perception of the value of health is the value of item F on the list of value items. The range of scores for this item was 1 to 3 (Likert format) and 0 to 6 (visual analog format). If one sums all items, the range of scores for all items valued by the individual is 10 to 30 and 0 to 60 on each scale, respectively.

MTMM Matrix

I have identified two constructs, women's health beliefs and value of health, each being measured by a Likert and a visual-analog scale method. A 2×2 matrix results (2 methods and 2 traits). However, perceived benefits and perceived susceptibility are conceptualized to reflect two dimensions of health beliefs and hence are shown as two scores. The resulting matrix is thus 3 traits $\times$ 2 methods: (1) perceived benefits/Likert, (2) perceived benefits/visual analog, (3) perceived susceptibility/Likert, (4) perceived susceptibility/visual analog, (5)health value/Likert, and (6) health value/visual analog.

Sampling Procedure

The next step in the MTMM procedure is to select a sample to which each of the instruments will be administered at the same time. A simple probability sampling technique was utilized to minimize bias in selecting 250 potential women subjects from a large college within a metropolitan university. A list of 350 nine-digit random numbers was generated from a table of random numbers. These numbers represented social security numerical identification, from which 250 individuals with first names indicating they were women were selected. No other demographic information was collected.

A cover letter was mailed to these potential subjects inviting them to participate in nursing research that involved developing questionnaires to find out more about women and their health-related activities. They were told how they were selected and that their participation was voluntary, anonymous, and confidential and would consist of 15 min to complete four questionnaires. Stamped, addressed envelopes were provided along with this researcher's name, address, and work telephone number should they have any questions.

A final sample size of 148 women responded to the invitation to participate in the tool development research project. Table 17.1 provides summary statistics for subject responses to the different constructs using the Likert and visual analog methods. Stillman (1977) reported mean scores of 16.70 and 18.43, respectively, for perceived susceptibility and perceived benefits. Standard deviation and variance were not reported by her. Gramse (1982) reported mean scores of 15.58 and 17.55 for these two variables, with standard deviation of 2.36 and variance of 2.24. Table 17.1 shows values close to those reported by both of these investigators.

MTMM STATISTICAL ANALYSIS

Procedure and Results

Analysis of the MTMM approach involves construction of a matrix from the calculation of the reliability of each instrument, using an index of internal consistency (alpha) and the correlation (r) between each pair of forms. These figures have been entered in the 3 trait × 2 method matrix as shown in Table 17.2. Several steps are used to evaluate the size, as well as the pattern of relation between correlations so entered into the matrix.

Step 1

Initially entered were the reliability estimates for each form to create the reliability diagonal (correlation coefficients are in parentheses). These values should be sufficiently high for the procedure to continue, since reliability is a prerequisite for validity. The values of the reliability diagonal range from .62 to .88, indicating mild to moderate evidence for reliability.

Step 2

Convergent validity was examined by entering in the lower left block of the matrix the correlation between the two measures of each trait assessed, using the two different methods (Likert and visual analog) to create the validity diagonal (correlation coefficients are circled). These values should be lower than the coefficient in the reliability diagonal yet

TABLE 17.1 Summary Statistics for MTMM (*N* = 148)

Method	Mean	Variance	Standard deviation	No. of variables
Likert				
Total health beliefs, range 10-39	32.42	15.87	3.98	10
Perceived susceptibility, range 5-19	14.79	5.45	2.33	5
Perceived benefits, range 5-20	17.63	7.56	2.75	5
Health value (all items), range 10-30	22.35	13.94	3.73	10
Health value (item F only), range 1-3	2.69	–	.66	48
Visual analog				
Total health beliefs, range 0-60	41.77	47.20	6.87	10
Perceived susceptibility, range 0-30	19.05	20.08	4.48	5
Perceived benefits, range 0-30	22.72	10.92	3.31	5
Health value (all items), range 0-60	43.35	13.72	8.59	10
Health value (item F only), range 0-6	5.42	–	.94	48

high enough to provide evidence of convergent validity (different methods measuring the same construct should correlate highly with each other). The values obtained were mildly high yet were less than those figures obtained in the reliability diagonal (.35-.61).

The correlation for value of health was computed using scores for item F only (not total test scores). This item operationalizes the theoretical definition for value of health and raises an issue regarding the number of items that may be needed for indexing a health value. One-item scales

TABLE 17.2 Intercorrelations between Likert and Visual Analog Rating Measures of Health Beliefs and Value of Health ($N = 148$)

Trait	Likert			Visual analog		
	PS	PB	VH	PS	PB	VH
Likert						
Perceived susceptibility	(.74)					
Perceived benefits	.22	(.62)				
Value of health	.16	.15	(.83)			
Visual analog						
Perceived susceptibility	.56	.03	.19	(.69)		
Perceived benefits	.12	.61	.14	.31	(.88)	
Value of health	−.25	−.09	.35	.24	−.01	(.78)

are notoriously difficult to obtain reliability on; that is, an individual responding to one item tends to vary a great deal. Nunnally (1967) suggests that in indexing any construct or concept one needs approximately 7 items in a completed instrument. The correlation obtained (.35) adds credence to this suggestion.

Step 3

The correlation between measures of the three different constructs employing the Likert rating scale is entered in the upper left of the matrix (upper left solid triangle). The correlation between measures of the three different constructs employing the visual-analog scale is entered in the lower right block of the matrix (lower right solid triangle). These are also called the heterotrait monomethod triangles.

These coefficients indicate the relationship between measures of different constructs that use the same method of measurement (visual analog and Likert) and thus are a function of the relationship existing between the three constructs and the use of a common method. The size of these coefficients will be lower than the values on the validity diagonal, and on the reliability diagonal as well if variability is more a function of trait than of method variance. This would provide evidence of construct validity. As shown in Table 17.2, the values in the Likert triangle (.22, .15, .16) and the values in the visual-analog triangle (−.01, .24, .31) follow this pattern, thus suggesting some evidence of construct validity.

Step 4

The remaining correlations between measures of different constructs measured by different methods are entered in the lower left block in the matrix (lower left broken triangles). These are also called heteromethod triangles. The values for these coefficients should be lower than the values in the validity diagonal (circled values) and the corresponding values of the heterotrait monomethod triangles (solid line). This would provide evidence of discriminant validity. One can suggest that there is some evidence of discriminant validity since these correlations coefficients (−.09, −.25, .12, and .03, .14, .19) follow this pattern except for one value (.19). This might possibly be explained again by having used only one item (F) for the value of health and not the total test scores.

RELIABILITY

Procedures and Results

Reliability estimates were not reported by Stillman (1977), nor was an attempt made to compare data from the study sample ($N = 122$) to the pilot results. Reliability is necessary but not a sufficient condition for validity. Using the sampling procedure described above, 100 women were identified. A cover letter was mailed to these potential subjects, inviting them to participate in nursing research that involved developing a questionnaire to find out more about women and their health-related activities. They were told how they were selected and that their participation was voluntary, anonymous, and confidential and would consist of 10 min to complete a questionnaire. They were also told that tool development required that in 2 weeks they would have to again complete the same questionnaire.

Coefficient of Stability

The test-retest procedure was utilized to estimate reliability since the nursing outcome variable, women's health beliefs, is an affective measure. Although women can change their beliefs over time, since there is not a long period between testing, such beliefs are expected to remain stable. Therefore, the coefficient of stability is an appropriate estimate of reliability.

To estimate the test-retest reliability for this instrument, potential subjects were sent the questionnaire through the mail. Initially, 48 women responded to the invitation to participate in establishing stability of the tool. Table 17.3 provides summary statistics for subject responses in terms of total test score and subscores for respective beliefs of perceived susceptibility and perceived benefits. The same test was readministered to the same subjects approximately 2 weeks later. Of these subjects, 27 women responded to the retest follow-up letter, and 21 women required a second letter to remind them to participate in the test-retest procedure.

In determining the extent to which the two sets of scores were correlated, the Pearson product-moment correlation coefficient (r) was taken as the estimate of reliability. The test-retest correlation for perceived susceptibility was .69 and for perceived benefits, .61. Although both values

TABLE 17.3 Summary Statistics for Women's Health Beliefs (*N* = 48)

Scale	Mean	Variance	Standard deviation	No. of variables
Initial testing				
Total health beliefs (range 10-39)	32.37	22.09	4.70	10
Perceived susceptibility (range 5-19)	14.78	10.33	3.21	5
Perceived benefits (range 5-20)	17.59	4.10	2.02	5
Retest testing				
Total health beliefs (range 10-39)	32.95	17.60	4.19	10
Perceived susceptibility (range 5-20)	15.32	9.07	3.01	5
Perceived benefits (range 5-20)	17.63	3.39	1.84	5

[a]Stillman (1977) *N* = 122	Perceived susceptibility Perceived benefits	16.70 18.43
[b]Gramse (1982) *N* = 212	Perceived susceptibility Perceived benefits	15.58 17.55

are low, they were significant at better than .05 probability levels. These low values may in part be explained by the small sample of items from the domain(s) in perceived susceptibility and perceived benefits, as well as the small sample size (*N* = 48). Increasing the size of the sample and the number of items can improve reliability estimates.

Internal Consistency

Internal consistency reliability was also estimated as an indication of performance of the subjects across all items on the questionnaire. The alpha coefficient was selected as the preferred index of internal consistency reliability because it measures the extent to which performance on any one item on a questionnaire is a good indicator of performance on any other item in the same instrument. As such, alpha was determined to see how any one perceived susceptibility item was consistent with all other perceived susceptibility items and similarly how any one perceived bene-

TABLE 17.4 Internal Consistency, Alpha Coefficients ($N = 48$)

Scale	Number of items	Alpha	Total test variance	Alpha if deleted
Initial testing				
Perceived susceptibility	5	.73	10.33	.78 (#8)
Perceived benefits	5	.65	4.10	.68(#7)
Total health beliefs	10	.75	22.09	.80(#7)
Retest testing				
Perceived susceptibility	5	.75	9.07	.78(#2)
Perceived benefits	5	.51	3.39	.63(#5)
Total health beliefs	10	.78	17.60	.80(#3)

fits item was consistent with all other perceived benefits items. Table 17.4 depicts the alpha coefficients for each subscale, as well as for the test as a whole for each administration of the test.

The resulting low alpha values for perceived benefits (.65 and .51) indicate that this subscale has a very low degree of internal consistency reliability; that is, since the item intercorrelations are low, performance on any one item is not a good predictor of performance on any other perceived benefits item. This may in part be explained by the small sample of items from the domain "beliefs in perceived benefits." This subscale also had a marginally significant coefficient of stability (.61, $p = .043$).

The high alpha values for the perceived susceptibility (.73 and .75) indicated that this subscale as a whole is measuring one attribute, perceived susceptibility to breast cancer. Note, too, that although the coefficient of stability was again marginally significant (.69, $p = .006$), the r value had a much stronger significance level for this sample.

INTERPRETATIONS AND RECOMMENDATIONS

Implications for Measurement of Women's Health Beliefs

Before one can test the relationships between a specific trait and other traits, one must have some confidence of one's measure of that trait. Such confidence can be supported by evidence of convergent and discriminant validation and estimates of reliability. Campbell and Fiske (1959) state this in different words. Any conceptual formulation of trait will usually include implicitly the proposition that this trait is a response tendency that can be observed under more than one experimental condition and that this trait can be meaningfully differentiated from other traits.

The evaluation of the reliability data and the MTMM correlation matrix formed by intercorrelating several trait method units must take into consideration the many factors that are known to affect the magnitude of correlations. The whole approach assumes adequate sampling of individuals. Results produced in this tool development study raise several points regarding reliability and validity to be considered in further development of this tool.

Reliability Issues

Although probability sampling was utilized, the fact that the initial reliability coefficients entered into the MTMM matrix were mildly to moderately high might be explained by the final sample size of 148. Since reliability can be increased by raising the sample size, this would be strongly recommended for future studies.

Random errors of measurement affect reliability. The test-retest procedure yielded small but significant r values. Sources of random error might have been individual differences at measurement time and temporal factors (since approximately 40% of the subjects had to be reminded to complete the retest procedure and the time period between initial and retest responses was 3-8 weeks). Of course, imprecision in the tool itself may be operating.

A number of sampling factors may affect the alpha coefficient obtained. The domain-sampling model suggests that the reliability of scores obtained on a sample of items increased with the number of items sampled. The domain of women's health beliefs reflects beliefs in perceived susceptibility and perceived benefits. The alpha values obtained for the questionnaire as a whole are higher values, reflecting alpha as a function of test length. Increasing the number of items for both scales is recommended.

Similarly, from the formula for alpha, it is apparent that alpha is dependent on the total test variance. Table 17.4 shows that the higher the value of the total test variance, the greater the alpha value obtained.

The reliability analyses for each scale were examined further to determine the change in alpha values if individual test items are deleted. The subsequent changes in alpha warranted further examination of five items, especially item 7 from the perceived benefits subscale. Alpha would be strengthened if this item were reworded or deleted in further administrations of the instruments.

In examining the distribution of scores, it was noted that value of health (item F) was severely restricted in range as the scores clustered together in one end of the scale. Since variables that are restricted in range cannot correlate highly with other variables, the value of the health correlation coefficient was indeed low (standard deviation of .66 and intercorrelation of .24). It should be noted that the value of health alpha coefficients of .83 and .78 in Table 17.2 were reflective of all items in the value survey, not just item F. By definition one-item scales cannot be used to calculate an internal consistency coefficient. Since reliability can be increased by raising the number of items, this again would be strongly recommended in future validity studies, especially for measurement of value of health as depicted in this study.

Validity Issues

The validity coefficients obtained indicate where further effort is needed in refining conceptual developments for both health beliefs and value of health, rather than abandoning development of these two tests. Since the heterotrait monomethod triangle for the visual analog method shows a value of .31 (lower right solid triangle), which was not extremely lower than the value .35 in the validity diagonal, variability is suggested as a function of method variance (Campbell & Fiske, 1959; Waltz et al., 1984). This value (.31) suggests examining methods used to measure perceived benefits, in particular the visual analog method.

Wherever possible, the several methods in one matrix should be completely independent of each other; there should be no prior reason for believing that they share method variance (Campbell & Fiske, 1959). This requirement is necessary to permit the values in the heterotrait, heteromethod triangles (broken lines) to approach zero. That three of these values (.14, .19, and .12) were this high suggests that this requirement of independence was not entirely met. One can conclude that one of the methods does not really measure the trait "perceived benefits" since the values (.12 and .14) should have been closer to zero.

If the nature of the traits rules out such independence, efforts should be made to obtain as much diversity as possible from data sources. It is noted that data was collected randomly from 148 subjects.

Several aspects of the MTMM matrix have additional bearing on the construct validity question. The most direct evidence (convergence) comes from the correlations between two different methods for measuring the same trait. In the validity diagonal, the correlation of .61 for perceived benefits is reasonably substantial. This entry should also be higher (in terms of absolute magnitude) than those correlations between measures that have neither method nor trait (broken triangles) in common. Similarly, the correlation of .56 for perceived susceptibility is higher (in terms of absolute value) than correlations between measures in heterotrait heteromethod (broken-line triangles). Thus, some evidence exists for construct validity for perceived benefits and perceived susceptibility, yet, as mentioned previously, method of measurement of perceived benefits is suspect.

SUMMARY

Using the MTMM approach, as well as various estimates of reliability, has suggested some evidence of validity and reliability for women's health beliefs about breast cancer and breast self-examination. The analyses suggested an increase in sample size, increase in number of items for each scale, and a reexamination of the methods used to measure these constructs. The instruments are undergoing further testing for reliability and validity estimation. This is a necessary prerequisite if use of these instruments in studying health – in particular, women's health beliefs as defined in this study – is to contribute to the science of nursing in a meaningful way.

REFERENCES

American Cancer Society. (1985a). *Cancer facts and figures.* New York: Author.
American Cancer Society. (1985b). *Cancer statistics 1985.* New York: Author.
Campbell, S., & Fiske, S. (1959). Convergent and discriminant validity by multitrait-multimethod matrix. *Psychological Bulletin, 56,* 81.
Chapion, V. (1985). Use of the health belief model in determining frequency of breast self-examination. *Research in Nursing and Health, 8,* 373-379.
Cortrell, R. (1973). Breast cancer detection in an employee health clinic. *Journal of Occupational Medicine, 15,* 114-117.
Edwards, V. (1980). Changing breast self-examination behavior. *Nursing Research, 29,* 301-307.
Foster, R. S., Lang, S. P., Costanza, M. C., Morden, J. K., Haines, C. R., & Yates, J. W. (1978). Breast self-examination – practices and breast cancer stage. *New England Journal of Medicine, 299,* 265-270.
Gallup Organization. (1974). Women's attitudes regarding breast cancer. *Occupational Health News, 22,* 20-23.
Gramse, C. A. (1982). The relationship of internal-external health expectancies, value of health, health beliefs, and health behavior regarding breast self-examination in women. (Doctoral dissertation, New York University, 1982). *Dissertation Abstracts International, 43*(2), 385-388.
Haefner, D. P., & Kirscht, J. P. (1970). Motivational and behavioral effects of modifying health beliefs. *Public Health Report, 85,* 478-483.
Hallal, J. (1982). Health beliefs, health locus of control and self concept regarding breast self-examination in adult women. *Nursing Research, 31,* 137-142.
Howe, H. L. (1981). Social factors associated with breast self-examination among high risk women. *American Journal of Public Health, 71,* 251-255.
Kegeles, S. S. (1965). Survey of beliefs about cancer detection and taking Papanicolau tests. *Public Health Reports, 80,* 815-823.
Nunnally, J. C. (1967). *Psychometric theory.* New York: McGraw-Hill.
Rose, R. (1978). Surveys reveal women's attitudes to breast self-examination. *New Zealand Nursing Journal, 7*(3), 24-26.
Rosenstock, I. M. (1974). The health belief model and preventive health behavior. In M. Becker (Ed.), *The health belief model and personal health behavior* (pp. 27-59). Thorofare, N J: Charles B. Slack.
Scilken, M. P. (1977). *The relationship between locus of control, body cathesix, perception of disability, and the practice of breast self-examination.* Unpublished doctoral dissertation, New York University, New York.
Stillman, M. (1977). Women's health beliefs about breast cancer and breast self-examination. *Nursing Research, 26,* 121-127.
Thiessen, E. U. (1971). Breast self-examination in proper perspective. *Cancer, 28,* 1537-1543.

Turnball, E. (1978). Effect of basic preventive health practices and mass media on the practice of breast self-examination. *Nursing Research, 27,* 98-102.

Wallston, B. S., Wallston, K. A., Kaplan, G. D., & Maides, S. A. (1976). Development and validation of the health locus of control (HLC) scale. *Journal of Consulting and Clinical Psychology, 44,* 580-585.

Waltz, C., Strickland, O., & Lenz, E. (1984). *Measurement in nursing research.* Philadelphia: F. A. Davis.

VALUE SURVEY

Instructions : Read the items below carefully. Next to the items, circle the number as follows that reflects the degree of importance to you.

1 - important
2 - next important
3 - most important

A.	A comfortable life (a prosperous life)	1	2	3
B.	An exciting life (a stimulating, active life)	1	2	3
C.	A sense of accomplishment (lasting contribution)	1	2	3
D.	Freedom (independence, free choice)	1	2	3
E.	Happiness (contentedness)	1	2	3
F.	Health (physical and mental well-being)	1	2	3
G.	Inner harmony (freedom from inner conflict)	1	2	3
H.	Pleasure (an enjoyable, leisurely life)	1	2	3
I.	Self-respect (self-esteem)	1	2	3
J.	Social recognition (respect, admiration)	1	2	3

HEALTH BELIEFS INSTRUMENT

Please read each statement and indicate how you agree with each statement by circling the number next to each item. Remember, there is no right or wrong answer.

1 = Strongly Agree
2 = Agree Little
3 = Disagree Little
4 = Disagree Strongly

1. If more women examined their breasts regularly, there would be fewer deaths from breast cancer.   1 2 3 4
2. My health is too good at present to even consider thinking that I might get breast cancer.   1 2 3 4
3. Whether I find a lump in my breast myself doesn't really matter because by then it's too late anyway.   1 2 3 4
4. Whenever I hear of a friend or relative (or public figure) getting cancer, it makes me realize that I could get it too.   1 2 3 4
5. If I examine my own breasts regularly, I might find a lump sooner than if I just went to the doctor for a checkup.   1 2 3 4
6. There are so many things that could happen to me that it's pointless to think about any one thing like breast cancer.   1 2 3 4
7. Even though it's a good idea, I find examining/having to examine my breasts an embarrassing thing to do.   1 2 3 4
8. The older I get, the more I think about the possibility of getting breast cancer someday.   1 2 3 4
9. Examining my breasts often makes/would make me worry unnecessarily about breast cancer.   1 2 3 4
10. If I had to think about the possibility that I might someday get breast cancer, I rate my chances as compared with other woman as:
    1. below average (less likely I would get it)
    2. average
    3. above average (likely I would get it)

18

Measuring Family Well-Being; Conceptual Model, Reliability, Validity, and Use

Shirley Metz Caldwell

This chapter discusses the Family Well-Being Assessment Tool, a measure of various aspects of family life on a continuum from well-being to stress.

The Family Well-Being Assessment (FWA) is an instrument designed to measure various aspects of family life on a continuum from well-being to stress. An earlier version of this instrument was called Family Stress Assessment and was used in an investigative study in 1983 (Caldwell, 1983). The present version has been refined through work done for the University of Maryland's Measurement of Clinical and Educational Nursing Outcomes Project. The instrument uses a 6-point Likert scale, with low scores demonstrating less stress or a greater perception of well-being.

The conceptual model for the FWA was begun by Thomas (1981), whose beginning theory of family stress I have adapted and expanded with his permission, since it was generally consistent with my concept of family stress/well-being. Thomas proposed that family stress research should be conceptualized by assessing family structural components, by assessing the family function or roles, and by assessing individual and family vulnerability. In the past, family stress research focused on isolated aspects of the total picture. Although selected traits of the relationship of parents and children have been investigated extensively, such relationships are almost always dealt with out of context, as if the family as a whole did not exist. It is my belief that a family is an interactional system of two or more members in the process of, or at the level of, defining the nature of their kinship or intimate relationship, which is in agreement with Watzlawick, Beavin, & Jackson (1967). The FWA attempts to assess family as an interactional system based on Thomas's work and on my conception of family stress/well-being.

REVIEW AND ANALYSIS OF EXISTING TOOLS

In 1980-1981, when searching for a tool to measure family stress/well-being, Straus and Brown's (1978) review of abstracts of published instruments, *Family Measurement Techniques*, and Buros's *Mental Measurement Yearbooks* (1972, 1978) were reviewed. One of the most promising tests identified was Moos's (1975) Family Environment Scale (FES). The 90 items on Form R (Real Form) are all true-false statements regarding relationships, personal growth, and system maintenance. Although reviewers identified good face validity, overall validity was disappointing (Buros, 1972). I concluded that there was little empirical evidence that the FES adequately assessed the important features of family environment, particularly in regard to my conceptualized model of family interaction and relationships.

An instrument by Pratt (1976) from *Family structure and effective health behavior: The energized family*, was also reviewed. Components of this measure, such as interaction pattern, freedom constraint, coping effort, and role structure, appeared to have relevance for my conceptual ideas; however, the instrument did not seem appropriate for all members of the family. I was searching for an instrument that would test each individual's perception of his family, concerning, for example, how it coped with stress. Few researchers have used perceptions of each family member (Masters, Cerreto & Mendlowitz, 1983). The approach of seeking to understand how different individuals in the same family perceive stress is a newer direction for family research (McCubbin et al., 1980).

Another instrument that was considered was Pless and Satterwhite's *Family Functioning Index*. This instrument was developed because the authors recognized the need to understand that the family unit "is of pervasive importance in many aspects of child health. Nevertheless the knowledge a doctor has of a family is often fragmentary" (p. 613). The instrument had been tested for 5 years and had established reliability; however, the subscales of this test also did not adequately fit my conceptual model of stress or well-being.

My attention then was directed to stress research done at Vanderbilt University by Pettegrew and associates (Pettegrew et al., 1980). Pettegrew's measure was developed from his background in communication and social psychology. He also worked with Thomas. Pettegrew worked with me in shortening the earlier version of the Family Stress Assessment (FSA) instrument for use with children. It was believed that the adult version took too much time. Wording changes were also needed for children, such as, "My job as a parent is extremely important in comparison to other interests in my life." The result was the development of a shorter version, basically three items per subscale, suitable for use with children aged 9 years and older. It was pilot-tested for reading comprehension with 10 children, 9 to 12 years old.

THEORETICAL BASIS

The theoretical basis of the FWA instrument incorporates viewing the family as a social system (Katz & Kahn, 1966; Miller, 1971). The family is believed to be the primary influence on the behavior and experience of each individual member. What affects one member of the family has an impact on the other family members (Sabbeth, 1984). Thus, members must adapt to stressors from other parts of the system as well as to stress that is self-generated. Conversely, the sense of well-being of one member has an effect on other members.

Thomas's (1981) conceptual model defines the family system as (1) the relationship of structure, the units of which the family is composed; (2) the interrelationship of function or roles in the way the family tasks are done; and (3) the vulnerability to other influences such as those of genetic, physiological, sociological, or psychological origin. This basic idea was used and expanded on to produce the following components that describe the FWA Instrument. The Likert scale responses range from STRONG agreement through Moderate agreement, slight agreement, slight disagreement, and Moderate disagreement to STRONG disagreement.

Family Structure

Family structure provides each member with a sense of identity. This structure is believed to develop from family interaction. Mehrabian (1970) declared that over 90% of the message in personal relationships comes through nonverbal cues (facial expression, posture, and tone of voice), rather than what is said (verbal). The "how" qualifies the "what." If the two do not match, confusion, mistrust, anxiety, and doubt result (Bandler, Grinder, & Satir, 1976).

A family atmosphere that allows members to express themselves freely, congruently, and clearly about problematic relational issues and fosters their resolution through mutual participation in decision making will enable family members to have a sense of family well-being. Such an atmosphere will promote productive coping with the stresses of family life (Caldwell, 1983; Eiser, 1985; Haley, 1980; Nuckolls, 1975). For the FWA instrument, family structure is operationalized by subscales that measure family stress, satisfaction, support, cohesion, and adaptation.

Family Stress

Family stress is defined by using the systems perspective. It measures the individual's perception of strain, frustration, and tension present in the home. When unclear messages are used among family members, family relationships are affected. Family coalitions and boundaries arise as these interactions result in regularly recurring patterns (Minuchin, 1974). Such interactions do not promote positive growth and health; in fact, they may be an inducement to illness (Eiduson, 1983; Leahey & Wright, 1985). Bard (1970) found that 37% of the patients in his study believed that interpersonal relationships were stressful enough to have caused an illness. Marital discord has been reported to correlate with child deviance, low self-esteem, and physical and psychological disorders (Benoliel, 1970; Matteson, 1974; Minuchin et al., 1975; Satir, 1972).

Other researchers have found that sibling rivalry and illness play a significant role in psychopathology, physical violence, and low self-esteem (Bank & Kahn, 1976; Crain, Sussman & Weil, 1966; Steinmetz, 1978). The degree of well-being within the family unit is thus closely related to the quality of interaction between family numbers.

Examples of items that measure family stress include (1) "There is a lot of strain on the members of our family"; (2) "I would definitely say that my home is a stressful place for family members to live."

Family Satisfaction

This aspect measures the individual's perception of family well-being, satisfaction, and happiness in the family as a whole and is closely related to the quality of interaction. Well-functioning families in which conflicts were few, stress between subsystems was low, chronic disease was well controlled, and finances were not a major problem rated higher on family satisfaction (Novak & Van der Veen, 1970; Swift, Seidman & Stein, 1967). Pratt (1976) stated that a family that fostered personal health practices of the members was characterized by frequent, meaningful, and varied forms of interaction among the members. This includes how messages are communicated as well as the specific responses that are emitted later.

Sample items from the instrument that measure family satisfaction are (1) "Being a member in this family is extremely satisfying to me compared with other interests in my life"; (2) "In general, my family is the kind of family I want to be a member of."

Family Support

Family support is defined as information leading the family member to believe that he/she is cared for, loved, and valued (Cobb, 1976). Studies from various contexts have reported findings that indicate that failure to provide or receive adequate social support tends to jeopardize well-being (Kaplan & Cassel, 1975; Kiritz & Moss, 1974; Minuchin, Rosman, & Baker, 1978). Stress was found to be induced by pressures from significant others or by a lack of support from others during trying times (Lazarus, 1966).

Family support also appears to protect people in crisis from a wide range of health problems: arthritis, tuberculosis, cancer, depression, alcoholism, and the social breakdown syndrome (Cobb, 1976; Nuckolls, 1975). In addition, family support may reduce the amount of medication required, accelerate recovery, and facilitate compliance with prescribed medical regimens (Cerreto & Travis, 1984; de Araujo, van Arsdel, Holmes, & Dudley, 1973; Egbert, Battit, Welch, & Bartlett, 1964; Simpson & Smith, 1979). Other studies have reported that the loss of supportive family relationships increases the risk of mortality and morbidity (Berkman, 1969; Koski, Ahlas, & Kumento, 1976). It therefore seems reasonable to believe that the giving and acceptance of support in the family network is a central factor in individual and family health.

Two examples of items that measure family support include the following: (1) "Your family pays attention to what you are saying"; (2) "Your family members stand up for each other to outsiders."

Family Cohesion

The items included here measure the balance between separateness and belonging that exists for each family member (Minuchin, 1974) and is one of the new subscales. Family cohesion is defined as "the emotional bonding that family members have toward one another and the degree of individual autonomy they experience" (Olson & McCubbin, 1982, p. 49). In each family, this will be perceived differently by each individual and should change across time (Carter & McGoldrick, 1980). The construct of cohesion appears to be an important aspect of family life (Olson & McCubbin, 1982; Olson, Russell, & Sprenkle, 1980).

A lack of family or social cohesiveness has been linked to such health outcomes as arthritis, mental disorders, hypertension, coronary heart disease, and tuberculosis (Berkman & Syme, 1979; Cassel, 1974; Wirsching & Stierlin, 1985). Van der Veen (1979) found that emotionally healthy families could be distinguished from disturbed families in the amount of perceived family integration identified. Cohesiveness reduces family members' susceptibility to stress within the group but may increase individual stress for those members who try to change from the family norm (Costell & Leiderman, 1968). Cohesion should therefore be a changing, adapting element in the family, depending on the ages of the children and the parents (Carter & McGoldrick, 1980).

Sample items that measure cohesion are (1) "My family rarely does anything together for fun"; (2) "Even when I am away from my family, I know they are interested in what I am doing."

Family Adaptation

This new subscale is designed to measure "the ability of a marital or family system to change its power structure, role relationships and rules in response to situational and developmental stress" (Olson & McCubbin, 1982, p. 51). Adaptability is concerned with the degree that a family is rigid, structured, flexible, or chaotic as stress develops. It is believed that the middle categories of adaptability, which range from structured to flexible, are the healthiest. Functional families may be distinguished by their ability to change appropriately to meet arising needs (Beavers, 1976). Minuchin et al. (1978) and Lewis, Beavers, Gossett, and Phillips (1976) have also found a high amount of rigidity in psychosomatic families.

The family structural system, of which adaptation is a component, is constantly exposed to internal and external changes (Toffler, 1970). Consequently, this system must be able to adapt when circumstances warrant the need for alternative patterns of interaction and division of tasks. Various studies have demonstrated a positive relationship between an increased number of life-changing events and the onset of illness (Holmes & Rahe, 1966, 1967). Events requiring considerable behavioral adaptation produce stress and frequently will be detrimental to an individual's health.

Family well-being is also dependent on the family unit's ability to evolve and adapt to the various stages in the family's life cycle – birth, growth, illness, marriage, old age, and finally death (Carter & McGoldrick, 1980). According to Erikson and others, there are psychological crises that confront individuals at each stage of family development. The extent to which these tasks will be successfully negotiated will depend, to a considerable degree. on the adaptability of the family (Carter & McGoldrick, 1980; Duvall, 1964; McCubbin et al., 1980).

Sample items from the FWA that measure adaptation include (1) "I adapt quickly to changing situations in my family"; (2) "If someone in our family is sick, our home is really upset and disorganized." Items for this subscale were found to have the lowest reliability so are currently deleted for further refinement.

Family Role Processes

Role has been a basic concept in family theory and research (Ackerman, 1958; Rossi, 1968). A role is defined as a goal-directed pattern or sequence of acts, tailored by the cultural process for the transactions a person may carry out in a social group or family (Spiegel, 1960, p. 363). The term "family role" designates individual behavior and expectations within the family setting. Thus, family roles are a network of duties and expectations that support family functioning. In the FWA conceptual model, the subscales to operationalize family role processes include (a) role conflict, (b) role overload, (c) role ambiguity, (d) role nonparticipation, and (e) role preparedness (parents only).

Role processes are believed to be vital conductors of well-being and/or stress within the family system. They are believed to be a gauge of the family climate; however, the degree to which role processes affect family stress needs further investigation. Role processes have been researched in specific organizational settings and were found to be correlated with health outcomes (Caplan, Cobb, French, Harrison, & Pinneau, 1975; Pettegrew et al., 1980).

Role Conflict

This is believed to arise when there are disagreements concerning roles, or mismatched role expectations. Pratt (1976) viewed family conflict as the blocking or impeding of efforts of family members to cope, function, and work toward personal objectives and fulfillment. Pathology is associated with the inability to resolve such dilemmas and break cycles of conflict which tend to perpetuate themselves.

Conflict and tension have been shown to be consistently correlated to illness in the family (Croog, 1970; Meissner, 1966; Minuchin et al., 1978; Pratt, 1976). Conflict appears to play an important part in the types and levels of illness within the family. Van der Veen (1979) found emotionally healthy families could be distinguished from disturbed families by the amount of perceived conflict. Perceived high conflict was also related to less cohesion, less intellectual-cultural orientation, and less meaningful organization.

Some sample items from the FWA used to measure role conflict are (1) "I am asked to do things around my home without enough time or help to do them"; (2) "I have a hard time satisfying the conflicting demands of the members of my family."

Role Overload

The definition for this subscale is the discrepancy between a set of obligations and an individual's resources to meet these diversified demands (Thomas, 1981). It appears to be a significant source of stress in families with a chronically ill child (Benoliel, 1970; Koski, 1969; Simpson & Smith, 1979) but has received little attention in family research. In addition, the dual career family places a greater burden on women because they continue to assume "female role" responsibilities for the home and children as well as the additional responsibilities of work outside the home (Caldwell, 1983; Cooper & Payne, 1978). When analyses were conducted for dual career families with regard to involvement in household responsibilities, it was determined that family members cooperated little in household activities; they remained the mother's responsibility (Davey & Paolucci, 1980; Walker & Woods, 1976).

Other writers argue that the family may be viewed as a direct source of stress and role overload for men because of the competition for the father's time and resources (McKeever, 1981; Renshaw, 1976). Thus, the strains of modern-day living appear to be potentially burdensome for both husbands and wives.

Role overload items from the FWA include (1) "My family expects me to do more at home than I am able to do"; (2) "I have too many responsibilities at home."

Role Ambiguity

This is believed to occur when members have inadequate knowledge or unclear role expectations of what their family expects or thinks of them. Feelings of security among family members appear to be related to clearly defined family structural and role systems. Various psychological problems within the family have been associated with vague boundaries (Minuchin, 1974) and unclear communication patterns (Haley, 1980; Satir, Stackowiak, & Taschman, 1975). However, family researchers are just beginning to operationally define "role ambiguity" so that the concept can be tested within the family context.

Sample items used include (1) "I am not sure what my family expects of me"; (2) "In my family, I don't really know what my family thinks of me."

Role Nonparticipation

Role nonparticipation is perceived to be different from role overload. It results when there is little or no participation in the family decision-making process, little sense of belonging, poor communication, and a lack of influence. These factors have been found to be consistent and significant indicators of job-related stress (Margolis, Kroes, & Quinn, 1974). They also appear to be applicable to the family system since freedom to participate in decisions that affect life is highly valued in American culture. However, studies done by Backman (1970) found that over half of the teenagers sampled reported they had little input into the home rules affecting their lives. Backman also noted a tendency for husbands to exercise the most authority in the family. Pratt (1976) concluded that a significant segment of American families believe in greater authority for men than for women. Others (Haley, 1970; Simpson & Smith, 1979; Taylor, 1980) found that families who share responsibility and are permitted to express themselves on relevant family matters cope better with the stress of family living.

Sample items for role nonparticipation include (1) "My family regularly takes time to discuss family issues"; (2) "I feel that it is useless to make suggestions regarding family issues because decisions are made regardless of my opinion."

Role Preparedness

These items are only included in the parents' form and measure parental perception of how previous experience and learning has equipped them to be parents. Parenting is learned primarily from the role models in the family from which each parent comes, and sometimes from experience that may be obtained while caring for younger siblings (Elder, 1977; Rossi, 1968). However, since families have become smaller, older siblings do not care for younger siblings so frequently as in previous generations. Rossi believes parenting is the role that most people feel the least prepared for, but it is one that lasts a lifetime.

Examples of items used for this subscale include (1) "I feel I am unprepared to do my job as a parent"; (2) "My training to be a parent was inadequate in preparing me for the daily demands of the role."

Vulnerability

It is recognized that other influences, such as those of genetic, physiological, sociological, psychological, or spiritual origin are also involved in family stress. In addition, extrafamilial support variables have an influence on family stress. Two subscales to measure family vulnerability are included. They are Psychosomatic Symptoms and Life Satisfaction.

Psychosomatic Symptoms

These items measure possible predispositions toward such disorders as headaches, insomnia, stomach disorders, and nervousness. Although somewhat elusive, the impact of psychosomatic problems must be addressed. It is possible that certain predispositions to pathology may be transferred within families from one generation to succeeding generations, as well as symptoms that may have developed as a response to stress in the family. Some researchers have found that siblings of chronically ill children have increased physical problems, possibly to get attention. In other words, certain family members may have predispositions toward such disorders as headaches, enuresis, stomach disorders, phobias, insomnia, constipation, and primary affective disorders (Crain et al., 1966; Lavigne & Ryan, 1979; Masters et al., 1983; Minuchin et al., 1978). In fact, the close relationship between depressive trends and psychosomatic/hypochondrical symptoms is considered a clinical axiom. Meissner (1966) believed that stressors that disrupted the emotional balance of the family were more readily internalized by the psychosomatic-prone individual. Pratt (1976) suggested that the family structure and family health climate account for about one-third of the total variance in health problems of the members. Vulnerability thus appears to be influenced by the type and amount of stress imposed on the individual by the family structural and functional components and mediated by genetic, physiological, sociological, psychological, and spiritual resources.

Sample items from the FWA that measure psychosomatic symptoms include (1) "I am bothered by nervousness, feeling fidgety or tense"; (2) "I am troubled by headaches."

Life Satisfaction

Life satisfaction is defined as the individual's perception of life in general. Research previously done by Holmes and Rahe (1967) found that circumstantial aspects of living can create stress in the individual that is felt in the family and influences the family environment. Pettegrew et al. (1980) attempted to use a life satisfaction variable as a control for stress due to nonwork factors. They concluded that life satisfaction is a factor independent from job stress, a finding corroborated by Caldwell (1983). However it would seem that more research is needed before such a conclusion can be made.

Sample items of life satisfaction include (1) "I currently find my life quite lonely"; (2) "I currently find my life very enjoyable."

FAMILY WELL-BEING: A CONCEPTUAL MODEL

If the concept of multiple, interactional factors is valid, then it is essential to develop a model identifying the component parts and their dynamic relationship to family stress/well-being. Using this model, the FAW instrument can measure these component parts and lead us to a greater understanding of the influence of these components on the individual member and the family as a whole. From this knowledge, we can then make more appropriate family interventions to decrease stress and increase family health.

The central claim of this model is that the family is responsible for creating and maintaining a physical, emotional, social, and spiritual environment that will preserve and enhance the well-being of its members. Family pathology is predicted on the assumption that family structure, functional role processes, and vulnerability are significant factors in the predisposition, inception, and maintenance of many diseases and overall family stress.

In essence, family structure, role process, and vulnerability and the disease processes are elements of an open system (Miller, 1971; von Bertalanffy, 1968). Biochemical, physiological, psychological, social, and spiritual systems interact to transmit stress throughout the system. Family well-being is threatened. However, an existing dysfunctional system of family structure, role process, and vulnerability has a strong independent influence on the development and maintenance of illness within family members. Pratt's (1976) findings suggest that it is not simply a number of separate factors that affect health, but it is the family's overall pattern of arrangements for relating to, and working with, each other that is important.

Family structure, functional role process, and vulnerability are by no means novel concepts in the study of family systems and health. Their novelty and uniqueness are attributable to their placement in a dynamic, multidimensional model (see Figure 18.1) that posits an interaction between the components as necessary (versus exclusive) dimensions in the analysis of family well-being. It should be emphasized that the combination of stressors, family structure, functional role processes, and vulnerability are not the sole cause of any specific disease state. Nuckolls (1975) believed that instead of searching for a specific relationship, it is perhaps more useful to view factors as *detractors or enhancers* of the overall health or as interacting contributors to both the susceptibility to and prognosis of disease in general. The factors may account for a sizable proportion of the etiology and pathology, but they do not by themselves account for a particular health outcome. Perhaps they are best conceptualized as predictors of increased risk.

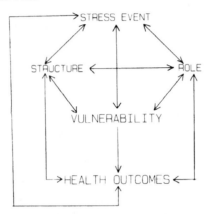

FIGURE 18.1 Model for family well-being.

The FWA has thus been developed on the basis of a conceptual framework of interrelated and interdependent concepts applicable to family well-being. This instrument appears capable of assessing family well-being using these concepts (Caldwell, 1983; Caldwell & Pickert, 1985; Pettegrew et al., 1980). What remains to be demonstrated is the configuration and strength of the relationship between family structural components and functional role process, vulnerability, and state of family health.

The conceptual framework that has been developed provides a mapping sentence. A mapping sentence serves two functions in relation to theory building. It allows the researcher to articulate visually the elements of the construct under investigation. It also provides a means of identifying specific facets of the construct, the components of which can be expanded or modified to extend and enrich the theory and improve the measuring instrument (Elizur, 1970; McCubbin et al., 1980). Embedded within this framework is a mandate for research scholars to turn their attention to the entire family as an important unit of study. The following mapping sentence of family well-being is offered to demonstrate the hypothesized relationship of stress, family structure, functional role processes, and vulnerability to family well-being.

Mapping Sentence

The FWA is the cognitive assessment by members of a nuclear family of their perceptions of the extent to which the following are present in family life: (1) family structural components – family stress, family satisfaction, family support, family cohesion, and family adaptation; (2) family functional role processes – role conflict, role overload, role ambiguity, role nonparticipation, and role preparedness; and (3) family vulnerability – psychosomatic and life satisfaction.

The components of the mapping sentence are indicators of family stress or well-being, ranging from very strong to very weak manifestations on each item. If these measures of family stress can identify families at high risk, then intervention and treatment strategies can be developed to decrease or control those factors causing family stress (adapted from Thomas, 1981).

PROCEDURES FOR REVISION AND FURTHER DEVELOPMENT

The Family Adaptation subscale items need further wording refinement, then retesting for internal consistency so that the scale will strengthen the instrument. In addition, factor analysis would help confirm the appropriateness of the subscale. Some items appear to overlap, and if so, the appropriate times should be counted in more than one subscale. An answer sheet that would facilitate hand scoring would aid individual use of the instrument.

ADMINISTRATION AND SCORING

FWA provides a norm-referenced affective assessment of family members' perceptions of the extent to which the following are present in family life: family structural components of family (a) stress, (b) satisfaction, (c) support, (d) cohesion, and (e) adaptation; role process of (a) conflict, (b) overload, (c) ambiguity, (d) nonparticipation, and (e) preparedness; and family vulnerability as measured by (a) psychosomatic and (b) life satisfaction. Individual family members rate each item of family well-being on a 6-point Likert scale ranging from STRONG agreement through Moderate agreement, slight agreement, slight disagreement, and Moderate disagreement to STRONG disagreement.

There are two versions of the test: a shorter 45-item test for children 9 to 18 years of age (10 subscales) and a longer 54-item test for parents (11 subscales). The time required to complete the test is 15 to 20 min. All items are measured on a 6-point Likert-type scale, scored from 1 to 6, with 1 being most desirable. The number of items in each subscale varies from three to eight. Some items require reverse coding. A total Well-Being score is obtained by summing the average score of each subscale. The total possible range is 11 to 66. Low score indicates well-being or low stress. Item numbers on the children's version of the instrument are not consecutive but match similar items on the parent's version so that differences can be more easily identified for individual families. An SPSS computer program is available for computer scoring.

Using data from my studies of families plus data from student research, Table 18.1 provides the means and standard deviations for each subscale and total score. The children and parents of families with chronically ill children are separated from children and parents of families without chronically ill children because there are significant differences between these families. Further reference to these studies are described in the discussion of reliability and validity.

TABLE 18.1 Means and Standard Deviations of FWA Testing Results (1986)

Subscales	Children from families with		Parents from families with	
	Chronically ill children ($N = 110$) $\bar{x}$ (SD)	No chronically ill children ($N = 98$) $\bar{x}$ (SD)	Chronically ill children ($N = 96$) $\bar{x}$ (SD)	No chronically ill children ($N = 91$) $\bar{x}$ (SD)
Family Stress	2.58* (1.31)	2.30 (1.08)	3.05*** (1.06)	2.55 (1.01)
Family Satisfaction	1.97* (1.20)	1.72 (0.88)	1.93* (0.83)	1.75 (0.75)
Family Support	2.33 (1.05)	2.22 (0.89)	2.18* (0.83)	1.95 (0.87)
Family Cohesion	2.43 (0.95)	2.28 (0.73)	2.43** (0.63)	2.23 (0.61)
Family Adaptation	3.52 (1.01)	3.24 (0.91)	2.65 (0.94)	2.58 (0.71)
Role Conflict	3.25 (1.23)	3.23 (1.17)	3.64 (1.01)	3.40 (1.03)
Role Overload	2.70 (1.36)	2.60 (1.10)	2.73 (1.14)	2.63 (1.00)
Role Ambiquity	2.45 (0.95)	2.28 (0.94)	2.28** (0.79)	2.00 (0.74)
Role Nonparticipation	3.08** (1.18)	2.70 (0.95)	2.17** (0.74)	1.84 (0.67)
Role Preparedness	–	–	2.34 (0.88)	2.39 (0.84)
Psychosomatic Symptoms	2.93** (1.10)	2.58 (0.89)	2.72*** (0.98)	2.30 (0.75)
Life Satisfaction	1.98 (1.10)	1.98 (0.94)	2.06*** (0.89)	1.66 (0.69)
Total scale	2.58* (0.80)	2.38 (0.70)	2.50** (0.63)	2.25 (0.59)

Low scores = more well-being and less stress.
Note significant differences all favor families with no chronically ill children.
*$p < .05$; **$p < .01$; ***$p < .001$.

RELIABILITY AND VALIDITY METHODOLOGY

Reliability

Reliability, the consistency with which an instrument assesses a domain and the measurements are repeatable (Waltz, Strickland, & Lenz, 1984), was assessed in four ways:

1. Item analysis, an aspect of Cronbach's alpha was performed. Items were deleted if they detracted from the subscale alpha by more than 4. None of the deleted items is included in the current instrument.
2. A correlational matrix was run. Items with extremely high (>.88) or low (primarily negative) correlations were deleted.
3. Internal consistency, using Cronbach's alpha, has been done twice, once in 1985 using original data (Caldwell, 1983). Inappropriate terms (i.e., items that had two ideas) were deleted so that alpha values ranged from .37 to .86 for the subscales. Cronbach's alpha were recomputed in 1986 using the revised instrument and the data from the increased sample size of 204 children and 185 parents. Results are shown in Table 18.2. The number of items per subscale varies from 3 to 8, so the subscales were considered worthwhile for this stage of instrument development. Overall instrument reliability was .89 for the children's version and .90 for the parents. Tables 18.3 and 18.4 provide subscale correlations for all children and all parents.
4. Test-retest, also called a coefficient of stability and recommended for determining the reliability of affective measures, was administered to 11 families ($N = 82$). utilizing a retest time of 1 to 3 weeks, as recommended for determining the reliability of affective measures. It was found to be .88.

Validity

The validity of the instrument or extent to which the measure achieves the purposes for which it was intended (Waltz et al., 1984) was assessed three ways:

1. Face validity is not a stringent method of assessing validity. However, because the instrument was developed from a conceptual framework, each of the items for the subscales was developed from the definition.
2. Content validity relates to how well the content matches the objective to be measured and was assessed by two specialists, Ora Strickland, RN, Ph.D., FAAN, Doctoral Program Evaluator, University of Maryland, and Linda Cronenwett, RN, Ph.D., Director of Nursing Research, Dartmouth Hitchcock Medical Center, Hanover, NH, each with a special interest in family research. Their interrater

TABLE 18.2 Cronbach's Alpha Reliability of Subscales of the FWA (1986a)

Subscale	No. of items	Alpha level
Family Stress (FSt)		
Children	3	.64
Parents	3	.80
Family Satisfaction (FSat)		
Children	3	.72
Parents	3	.70
Family Support (FS)		
Children	8	.81
Parents	6	.86
Family Cohesion (FC)		
Children	7	.63
Parents	7	.67
Family Adaptation (FA)		
Children	4	.22
Parents	4	.38
Role Conflict (RC)		
Children	3	.49
Parents	4	.68
Role Overload (RO)		
Children	3	.64
Parents	5	.79
Role Ambiguity (RA)		
Children	4	.48
Parents	6	.74
Role Nonparticipation (RNp)		
Children	3	.37
Parents	5	.71
Role Preparedness (RP)		
Parents (only)	4	.55
Psychosomatic Symptoms (PS)		
Children	6	.62
Parents	6	.74
Life Satisfaction (LS)		
Children	5	.79
Parents	5	.84
Total scale		
Children	45	.89
Parents	54	.90

Sample size: Children, 204; parents, 185.

agreement or Content Validity Index for each of the subscales ranged from .9 to 1. Items were rated from 1 (not relevant) to 4 (very relevant). Items rated 3 or 4 were retained. Those rated 1 or 2 were deleted.

3. Construct validity is of greatest importance when testing the affective domain. Previous research using contrasting groups found the instrument was able to separate high-stress persons from low-stress

persons (Pettegrew et al., 1980) and high-stress families from low-stress families (Caldwell & Pichert, 1985).

Construct validity was further supported when data from families without a chronically ill child, (Keys, 1986; Yeagley, 1985), hypothesized to have lower stress, were compared to data from families with a chronically ill child (Caldwell, 1985; Chandler, 1985). Parents showed a greater difference than the children.

Data from parents of chronically ill children were compared to data from parents of children not chronically ill ($N = 91$). The t-tests for individual subscale differences and the total overall instrument scores demonstrated less stress or a greater perception of well-being for parents of the children not chronically ill. The findings were statistically significant at $p < .01$ for six of the subscales, at $p < .05$ for two more, and not statistically significant for Family Adaptation, Role Overload, and Role Preparedness. Role Conflict difference is reported at $p < .06$. The level of significance

TABLE 18.3 Subscale Correlational Matrix for Children ($N = 204$)

	FST	FSat	FS	FC	FA	RC	RO	RA	RNp	PS	LS
FST	–	.51	.50	.42	.26	.46	.51	.45	.42	.45	.51
FSat		–	.60	.62	.12	.40	.36	.36	.43	.22	.55
FS			–	.64	.22	.52	.54	.43	.56	.36	.56
FC				–	.11	.40	.37	.40	.54	.21	.51
FA					–	.25	.20	.19	.26	.34	.23
RC						–	.65	.46	.39	.36	.39
RO							–	.40	.42	.35	.45
RA								–	.43	.39	.48
RNp									–	.21	.43
PS										–	.33
LS											–

TABLE 18.4 Subscale Correlational Matrix for Parents ($N = 185$)

	FST	FSat	FS	FC	FA	RC	RO	RA	RNp	RP	PS	LS
FST	–	.63	.48	.44	.40	.54	.51	.51	.36	.45	.43	.55
FSat		–	.62	.60	.41	.49	.50	.66	.56	.49	.35	.65
FS			–	.61	.46	.56	.47	.56	.62	.39	.26	.54
FC				–	.53	.51	.51	.56	.54	.42	.31	.48
FA					–	.46	.49	.47	.39	.32	.27	.38
RC						–	.65	.52	.36	.35	.32	.47
RO							–	.64	.34	.52	.21	.48
RA								–	.59	.60	.29	.51
RNp									–	.35	.19	.46
RP										–	.14	.30
PS											–	.44
LS												–

for differences between the two groups using the total instrument was $p < .01$ (see Table 18.4).

Children's perceptions were found to be less different. For each subscale, and the total score, children from families without a chronically ill child ($N = 98$) perceived less stress than did children from families that included a chronically ill child ($N = 110$). The t-test for difference was statistically significant)($p < .05$) for three subscales – Family Adaptation, Family Stress, and Family Satisfaction – and $p < .01$ for Psychosomatic Symptoms and Role Nonparticipation. The level of significance for difference between the two groups using the total instrument was $p < .05$) (see Table 17.1).

RESULTS AND IMPLICATIONS

The FWA instrument was used in a two-year follow-up study of families previously studied by Caldwell (1986b) and was found to be a sensitive instrument for measuring individual and family stress. By using the subscales, researchers are able to better understand how the major sources of perceived stress vary for individual family members. Two major grants have been written that will include further use of the instrument in assessing individual and family well-being or stress.

Three graduate students also used the FWA instrument. Yeagley (1985) looked at stress differences between families who used the birthing room experience versus families who used the traditional labor and delivery experience. No significant differences were found between the two groups of families. Chandler (1985) measured stress in families with a child with cancer and compared results to the children with diabetes studies by Caldwell (1985). No significant differences in total stress were found between the two groups; however, family stress (FSt) was perceived as higher by children having cancer than by children with diabetes. In addition, both children with cancer and their siblings experienced more psychosomatic symptoms (PS) such as headaches and stomach upsets than did children in the diabetes group. Keys (1986) measured stress in families that have no chronically ill children. These measures are being compared to the measures obtained for children from families with diabetic children. These analyses have not been completed. The FWA instrument has also been found to be sensitive to individual differences in the same family (Caldwell, 1983).

Currently, the author and a co-therapist are using results from the instrument to provide direction for family counseling in families that have a child newly diagnosed with insulin-dependent diabetes. The use of this instrument can provide health care providers and family counselors with increased information about the family that will aid them in identifying areas at risk so that appropriate interventions can be implemented. The anticipated result would be a healthier family system requiring fewer health care provider visits or family counseling sessions.

REFERENCES

Ackerman, N. W. (1958). *Psychodynamics of family life, diagnosis and treatment in family relationships.* New York: Basic Books.

Backman, J. G. (1970). *Youth in transition: Vol. 2. The impact of family background and intelligence on tenth-grade boys.* Ann Arbor, MI: University of Michigan Press.

Bandler, R., Grinder, J., & Satir, V. (1976). *Changing with families.* Palo Alto, CA: Science and Behavior Books.

Bank, S., & Kahn, M. D. (1976). Sisterhood-brotherhood is powerful. In S. Chess & A. Thomas (Eds.), *Annual progress in child psychiatry and development* (pp. 311-337). New York: Brunner/Mazel.

Bard, M. (1970). The price of survival for cancer victims. In A. Strauss (Ed.), *Where medicine fails* (pp. 99-110). Chicago: Aldine.

Beavers, W. R. (1976). A theoretical basis for family evaluation. In J. M. Lewis, W. R. Beavers, J. T. Gassett, & V. A. Phillips (Eds.), *No single thread: Psychological health in family system* (pp. 46-98). New York: Brunner/Mazel.

Benoliel, J. Q. (1970). The developing diabetic identity: A study of family influence. In M. J. Batey (Ed.), *Communicating nursing research: Methodological issues in research* (pp. 14-32). Boulder, CO: Western Interstate Commission on Higher Education.

Berkman, L. F., & Syme, S. L. (1979). Social networks, host resistance, and mortality: A nine-year follow-up study of Alameda County residents. *American Journal of Epidemiology, 2,* 186-204.

Berkman, P. L. (1969). Spouseless motherhood, psychological stress, and physical morbidity. *Journal of Health and Social Behavior, 10,* 323-334.

Buros, O. K. (Ed.). (1972). *Mental measurements yearbook* (7th ed.). Highland Park, NJ: Gryphon Press.

Buros, O. K. (Ed.). (1978). *Mental measurements yearbook* (8th ed.). Highland Park, NJ: Gryphon Press.

Caldwell, S. M. (1983). *Family communication patterns, siblings, and insulin-dependent diabetic children.* Unpublished doctoral dissertation, Vanderbilt University, Nashville, TN.

Caldwell, S. M. (1986a, June). *Family well-being assessment.* Paper presented at the 21st annual conference of the association of the Care of Children's Health, San Francisco.

Caldwell, S. M. (1986b). Systems theory applied to families with insulin-dependent diabetic children. In S. Stinson, J. C. Kerr, P. Giovannetti, P. Field, & J. MacPhail (Eds.), *Proceedings: International Nursing Research Conference* (p. 85). Edmonton, Alberta: University of Alberta Press.

Caldwell, S. M., & Pichert, J. W. (1985). Systems theory applied to families with a diabetic child. *Family Systems Medicine, 3*(1), 34-44.

Caplin, R., Cobb, S., French, J. R. P., Harrison, R. V., & Pinneau, S. R. (1975). *Job demands and worker health* (DHEW Publication No. (NIOSH), 75-160). Washington, DC: U.S. Government Printing Office.

Carter, E. A., & McGoldrick, M. (1980). *The family life cycle: A framework for family therapy.* New York: Gardner Press.

Cassel, J. (1974). An epidemiological perspective of behavior factors in disease etiology. *American Journal of Public Health, 64,* 1040-1043.

Cerreto, M. C., & Travis, L. B. (1984). Implications of psychological and family factors in the treatment of diabetes. *Pediatric Clinics of North America, 31*(3), 689-710.

Chandler, D. L. (1985). *Stress and self-concepts of chronically-ill children and their healthy siblings.* Unpublished master's thesis, Vanderbilt University, Nashville, TN.

Cobb, S. (1976). Social support as a moderator of life stress. *Psychosomatic Medicine, 38*, 300-315.

Cooper, C. L., & Payne, R. (Eds.). (1978). *Stress at work*. New York: John Wiley.

Costell, R. M., & Leiderman, H. (1968). Physiological concomitants of social stress: The effects of conformity to pressure. *Psychosomatic Medicine, 30*, 298-310.

Crain, A. J., Sussman, M. B., & Weil, W. B. (1966). Effects of a diabetic child on marital integration and related measures of family functioning. *Journal of Health and Human Behavior, 7*, 122-127.

Croog, S. (1970). The family as a source of stress. In S. Levine & N. Scotch (Eds.), *Social stress* (pp. 19-53). Chicago: Aldine Press.

Davey, A., & Paolucci, T. (1980). Family interaction: A study of shared time and activities. *Family Relations, 29*, 43-49.

de Araujo, G., von Aradel, P. P., Holmes, T. H., & Dudley, D. L. (1973). Life change, coping ability and chronic intrinsic asthma. *Journal of Psychosomatic Research, 17*, 359-363.

Duvall, E. (1964). *Family development*. Philadelphia: J. B. Lippincott.

Egbert, L. D., Battit, G. E., Welch, C. E., & Bartlett, M. K. (1964). Reduction of past operative pain by encouragement and instruction of patients. *New England Journal of Medicine, 270*, 825-827.

Eiduson, B. T. (1983). Conflict and stress in nontraditional families: Impact on children. *American Journal of Orthopsychiatry, 53*(3), 426-435.

Eiser, C. (1985). *The psychology of childhood illness*. New York: Springer-Verlag.

Elder, G. H., Jr. (1977). Family history and the life course. *Journal of Family History, 2*, 279-304.

Elizur, D. (1970). *Adapting to innovation*. Jerusalem: Jerusalem Academic Press.

Haley, J. (1970). Approaches to family therapy. *International Journal of Psychiatry, 9*, 233-242.

Haley, J. (1980). *Leaving home: The therapy of disturbed young people*. New York: McGraw-Hill.

Holmes, R., & Rahe, R. (1966). Life crisis and disease onset; parts I, II, III. Unpublished research reports, Department of Psychiatry, University of Washington School of Medicine, Seattle WA.

Holmes, R. H., & Rahe, R. (1967). Social readjustment rating scale. *Journal of Psychomatic Research, 11*, 213-218.

Kaplan, B. H., & Cassel, J. C. (1975). *Family and health: An epidemiological approach*. Chapel Hill Inc: University of North Carolina.

Katz, D., & Kahn, R. L. (1966). *The social psychology of organizations*. New York: John Wiley.

Keys, J. E. (1986). A comparison of perceived stress and self-concept measures for children from families with and without chronically-ill children. Unpublished raw data.

Kiritz, S., & Moos, R. H. (1974). Physiological effects of social environments. *Psychosomatic Medicine, 36*, 96-114.

Koski, M. L. (1969). The coping process in childhood diabetes. *Acta Paediatrica Scandinavica, 198* (Suppl.), 1-56.

Koski, M. L., Ahlas, A., & Kumento, A. (1976). A psychosomatic follow-up study of childhood diabetics. *Acta Paedopsychiatrica, 42*, 12-26.

Lavigne, J. V., & Ryan, M. (1979). Psychologic adjustment of siblings of children with chronic illness. *Pediatrics, 63*, 616-627.

Lazarus, R. D. (1966). *Psychological stress and the coping process*. New York: McGraw-Hill.

Leahey, M., & Wright, L. M. (1985). Intervening with families with chronic illness. *Family Systems Medicine, 3*(1), 60-69.

Lewis, J. M., Beavers, W. R., Gossett, J. T., & Phillips, V. A. (1976). *No single thread: Psychological health in family systems.* New York: Brunner/Mazel.

Margolis, B. L., Kroes, W. H., & Quinn, R. P. (1974). Job stress: An unlisted occupational hazard. *Journal of Occupational Medicine, 16,* 654-661.

Masters, J. C., Cerreto, M. C., & Mendlowitz, D. R. (1983). The role of the family in coping with childhood illness. In T. Purish & L. A. Bradley (Eds.), *Coping with chronic diseases: Research and applications* (pp. 381-407). New York: Academic Press.

Matteson, R. (1974). Adolescent self-esteem, family communication, and marital satisfaction. *Journal of Psychology, 86,* 35-47.

McCubbin, H., Joy, C., Cauble, E., Corneau, J., Patterson, J., & Needle, R. (1980). Family stress and coping: A decade review. *Journal of Marriage and the Family, 42*(4), 125-141.

McKeever, P. T. (1981). Fathering the chronically ill child. *Maternal Child Nursing, 6,* 124-128.

Mehrabrian, A. (1970). *Tactics of social influence.* Englewood Cliffs, NJ: Prentice-Hall.

Meissner, W. W. (1966). Family dynamics and psychosomatic processes. *Family Process, 5,* 142-146.

Miller, J. C. (1971). Systems theory and family psychotherapy. *Nursing Clinics of North America, 6*(3), 395-406.

Minuchin, S. (1974). *Families and family therapy.* Cambridge, MA: Harvard University Press.

Minuchin, S., Baker, L., Rosman, B. L., Liebman, R., Milmon, L., & Todd, T. C. (1975). A conceptual model of psychosomatic illness in children: Family organization and family therapy. *Archives of General Psychiatry, 32,* 1031-1038.

Minuchin, S., Rosman, B. L., & Baker, L. (1978). *Psychosomatic families: Anorexia nervosa in context.* Cambridge, MA: Harvard University Press.

Moos, R. H. (1975). Assessment and impact of social climate. In P. McReynolds (Ed.), *Advances in psychological assessment* (Vol. 3, pp. 8-41). San Francisco: Jossey-Bass.

Novak, A., & Van der Veen, F. (1970). Family concepts and emotional disturbances in the families of disturbed adolescents with normal siblings. *Family Process, 9,* 157-171.

Nuckolls, K. B. (1975). Life crisis and psychosocial assets: Some clinical applications. In B. H. Kaplan & J. Cassel (Eds.), *Family and health: An epidemiological approach.* Chapel Hill, NC: University of North Carolina, Institute for Social Science Research.

Olson, D. H., & McCubbin, H. I. (1982). Circumplex model of marital and family systems: V. Application to family stress and crisis intervention. In H. I. McCubbin, A. E. Gauble, & J. M. Patterson (Eds.), *Family stress, coping, and social support* (pp. 48-72). Springfield, IL: Charles C. Thomas.

Olson, D. H., Russell, C. S., & Sprenkle, D. H. (1980). Circumplex model of marital and family systems: II. Empirical studies and clinical intervention. *Advances in Family Intervention, 1,* 129-176.

Pettegrew, L., Thomas, R. C., Costello, D. E., Wolf, G. E., Lennox, L., & Thomas, S. L. (1980). Job related stress in a medical center organization: Management of communication issues. In D. Nimmo (Ed.), *Communication yearbook 4* (pp. 625-653). New Brunswick, NJ: Transaction.

Pless, I. B., & Satterwhite, B. (1973). A measure of family functioning and its application. *Social Science & Medicine, 7,* 613-621.

Pratt, L. (1976). An exploration of the dynamics of the overlapping worlds of work and family. *Family Process, 15,* 143-165.

Rossi, A. (1968, February). Transition to parenthood. *Journal of Marriage and the Family,* pp. 26-39.

Sabbeth, B. (1984). Understanding the impact of chronic childhood illness on families. *The Pediatric Clinics of North America, 31*(1), 47-57.

Satir, V. (1972). *Peoplemaking.* Palo Alto, CA: Science and Behavior Books.

Satir, V., Stackowiak, J. S., & Taschman, H. A. (1975). *Helping families to change.* New York: Jason Aronson.

Simpson, O. W., & Smith, M. A. (1979). Lightening the load for parents of children with diabetes. *Maternal Child Nursing, 4,* 293-296.

Spiegel, J. P. (1960). The resolution of conflict within the family. In N. W. Bell & E. F. Vogel (Eds.), *A modern introduction to the family.* Glencoe, IL: The Free Press.

Steinmetz, S. K. (1978). Violence between family members. *Marriage and Family Review, 1,* 1-16.

Straus, M. A., & Brown, B. W. (1978). *Family measurement techniques: abstracts of published instruments, 1935-1974* (Rev. ed.). Minneapolis: University of Minnesota Press.

Swift, C. F., Seidman, F., & Stein, H. (1967). Adjustment problems in juvenile diabetes. *Psychosomatic Medicine, 29,* 555-576.

Taylor, S. C. (1980). The effects of chronic childhood illnesses upon well siblings. *Maternal-Child Nursing Journal, 9,* 109-116.

Thomas, R. C. (1981, May). Conceptual foundation for a theoretical model of family well-being. Paper presented at the convention of the Health Communications Division of the International Communication Association, Minneapolis.

Toffler, A. (1970). *Future shock.* New York: Random House.

Van der Veen, F. (1979). Dimensions of the family concept and their relation to gender, generation, and disturbance. In J. G. Howells (Ed.), *Advances in family psychiatry* (Vol. 1) (pp. 171-190). New York: International Universities Press.

von Bertalanffy, L. (1968). *General systems theory.* New York: George Braziller.

Walker, K., & Woods, M. (1976). *Time use: A measure of household production of family goods and services.* Washington, DC: Center for the Family of the American Home Economics Association.

Waltz, C., Strickland, O., & Lenz, E. (1984). *Measurement in nursing research.* Philadelphia: F. A. Davis.

Watzlawick, P., Beavin, J., & Jackson, D. (1967). *Pragmatics of human communication.* New York: W. W. Norton.

Wirsching, M., & Stierlin, H. (1985). Psychosomatics: I. Psychosocial characteristics of psychosomatic patients and their families. *Family Systems Medicine, 3*(1), 6-16.

Yeagley, S. C. (1985). *Siblings at birth: Long term stress effects.* Unpublished master's thesis, Vanderbilt University, Nashville, TN.

Family Well-Being Assessment

There is much about how families work together and support each other that researchers don't understand. The following questions concern what it is like to be a member of your family. Please answer each question as honestly as possible but don't spend too much time on any one question. All questions pertain to *your role as a parent. All of your answers will remain anonymous.*

There are two sections in this questionnaire. Each section will have slightly different answer categories. Before beginning each section, please read the answer categories for that section very carefully, and then proceed by *circling* the answer that best represents your particular feelings.

In this section the following scale is used for all questions. Circle the answer that best suits your agreement or disagreement with the statement.

YES = STRONG Agreement
Yes = Moderate agreement
yes = slight agreement
no = slight disagreement
No = Moderate disagreement
NO = STRONG Disagreement

1. At times I cannot get my work done without doing things that my spouse disagrees with.	YES	Yes	yes	no	No	NO
2. I know what my family expects of me as a parent from one day to the next.	YES	Yes	yes	no	No	NO
3. Most of the time other family members expect me to be a better parent.	YES	Yes	yes	no	No	NO
4. My family regularly takes time to discuss family issues.	YES	Yes	yes	no	No	NO
5. There is a lot of strain on the members of our family.	YES	Yes	yes	no	No	NO
6. In general, my family is the kind of family I want to be a member of.	YES	Yes	yes	no	No	NO
7. My life is currently very rewarding.	YES	Yes	yes	no	No	NO
8. I have a hard time satisfying the conflicting demands of the members of my family.	YES	Yes	yes	no	No	NO
9. I am sure what my family expects of me.	YES	Yes	yes	no	No	NO
11. My family expects me to do more at home than I am able to do.	YES	Yes	yes	no	No	NO
12. I have influence over what happens in my family.	YES	Yes	yes	no	No	NO

14. My spouse understands that I need to have time alone with my friends.	YES	Yes	yes	no	No	NO
15. I currently find my life very hopeful.	YES	Yes	yes	no	No	NO
16. I would definitely say that my home is a stressful place for family members to live.	YES	Yes	yes	no	No	NO
17. I am extremely satisfied with my role as a parent.	YES	Yes	yes	no	No	NO
18. I currently find my life quite lonely.	YES	Yes	yes	no	No	NO
19. There is a difference between the way my spouse thinks things should be done and the way I think they should be done.	YES	Yes	yes	no	No	NO
21. I receive enough information to effectively carry out my duties as a parent.	YES	Yes	yes	no	No	NO
22. Even when we are not together as a family, I have a sense of family support.	YES	Yes	yes	no	No	NO
26. My life is currently quite empty.	YES	Yes	yes	no	No	NO
27. My job as a parent is extremely fulfilling in comparison to other interests in my life.	YES	Yes	yes	no	No	NO
30. Other family members feel I am a very capable parent.	YES	Yes	yes	no	No	NO
31. I ask other family members questions, and I often do what they suggest.	YES	Yes	yes	no	No	NO
32. In my family I don't really know what my family thinks of me.	YES	Yes	yes	no	No	NO
33. I would describe my home as a tightly wound spring ready to explode.	YES	Yes	yes	no	No	NO

The following section contains questions which describe your and your family's reactions related to situations at home. Please indicate the extent to which each question applies to your family situation by *circling* the most appropriate point on the scale.

YES	= Almost always
Yes	= Very often
yes	= Frequently
no	= Occasionally
No	= Not very often
NO	= Almost never

54. I experience stomach upsets.	YES	Yes	yes	no	No	NO
55. Your spouse supports you and your decisions in front of other family members and friends.	YES	Yes	yes	no	No	NO
56. I have trouble getting to sleep or staying asleep.	YES	Yes	yes	no	No	NO
57. Your family pays attention to what you are saying.	YES	Yes	yes	no	No	NO
59. I am troubled by headaches.	YES	Yes	yes	no	No	NO

60. I worry a great deal about my family.	<u>YES</u>	Yes	yes	no	No	<u>NO</u>
62. Your family members stand up for each other to outsiders.	<u>YES</u>	Yes	yes	no	No	<u>NO</u>
63. I am bothered by nervousness, feeling fidgety or tense.	<u>YES</u>	Yes	yes	no	No	<u>NO</u>
65. I have had a recent loss or gain of weight.	<u>YES</u>	Yes	yes	no	No	<u>NO</u>
66. When you really need to talk with someone, the children in your family are willing to listen.	<u>YES</u>	Yes	yes	no	No	<u>NO</u>
67. Your spouse pays attention to what you are saying.	<u>YES</u>	Yes	yes	no	No	<u>NO</u>
68. When you really need to talk to your spouse s/he is willing to listen.	<u>YES</u>	Yes	yes	no	No	<u>NO</u>
69. If I choose to do things differently than family custom, this would create a lot of family tension.	<u>YES</u>	Yes	yes	no	No	<u>NO</u>
71. My family asks my opinion on important matters.	<u>YES</u>	Yes	yes	no	No	<u>NO</u>
72. I feel I am unprepared to do my job as a parent.	<u>YES</u>	Yes	yes	no	No	<u>NO</u>
73. I am told about important things that are happening with my family.	<u>YES</u>	Yes	yes	no	No	<u>NO</u>
74. I am unsure of what all my responsibilities are as a parent.	<u>YES</u>	Yes	yes	no	No	<u>NO</u>

Family Well-Being Assessment

There is much about how families work together and support each other that researchers don't understand. The following questions concern what it is like to be a member of your family. Please answer each question as honestly as possible but don't spend too much time on any one question. All questions pertain to *you as a child*. *All of your answers will remain anonymous.*

There are two sections in this questionnaire. Each section will have slightly different answer categories. Before beginning each section, please read the answer categories for that section very carefully, and then proceed by *circling* the answer that best represents your particular feelings.

In this section the following scale is used for all questions. Circle the answer that best suits your agreement or disagreement with the statement.

YES	= STRONG Agreement
Yes	= Moderate agreement
yes	= slight agreement
no	= slight disagreement
No	= Moderate disagreement
NO	= STRONG Disagreement

1. I am asked to do things around my home without enough time or help to do them. YES Yes yes no No NO
2. I know what my family expects of me as a child from one day to the next. YES Yes yes no No NO
3. Most of the time other family members expect me to be a better child. YES Yes yes no No NO
4. My family regularly takes time to discuss family matters. YES Yes yes no No NO
5. There is a lot of tenseness, pressure on the members of our family. YES Yes yes no No NO
6. My family is the kind of family I want to be a member of. YES Yes yes no No NO
7. My life right now is very happy. YES Yes yes no No NO
8. I have a hard time pleasing my parents because they each expect different things from me. YES Yes yes no No NO
9. I am sure what my family expects of me. YES Yes yes no No NO
11. My family expects me to do more at home than I am able to do. YES Yes yes no No NO
12. What I think can change what happens in my family. YES Yes yes no No NO
13. I am allowed to make more personal YES Yes yes no No NO

420

decisions now than a year ago.

14.	My family recognizes the value of private time for each member.	YES	Yes	yes	no	No	NO
15.	I look forward to living my life.	YES	Yes	yes	no	No	NO
16.	I would definitely say that my home is a stressful place for family members to live.	YES	Yes	yes	no	No	NO
17.	All in all, I would say I am extremely satisfied with being a member in this family.	YES	Yes	yes	no	No	NO
18.	I currently find my life quite lonely.	YES	Yes	yes	no	No	NO
19.	There is a difference between the way my parents think things should be done.	YES	Yes	yes	no	No	NO
21.	I get enough direction to know what is expected of me as a child in our family.	YES	Yes	yes	no	No	NO
22.	Even when I am away from my family, I know they are interested in what I am doing.	YES	Yes	yes	no	No	NO
26.	My life is really quite empty.	YES	Yes	yes	no	No	NO
27.	Being a member in this family is very important to me compared with friendships outside of my home.	YES	Yes	yes	no	No	NO
31.	I ask other family members questions and I often do what they suggest.	YES	Yes	yes	no	No	NO
32.	I don't really know what my family thinks of me.	YES	Yes	yes	no	No	NO
33.	I would describe my home as a stressful place to live.	YES	Yes	yes	no	No	NO
35.	Most of my friends are friends of the entire family.	YES	Yes	yes	no	No	NO
36.	My family rarely does anything together for fun.	YES	Yes	yes	no	No	NO
38.	I listen very carefully to my parents so they know I am listening to them.	YES	Yes	yes	no	No	NO
39.	I have too many responsibilities at home.	YES	Yes	yes	no	No	NO
41.	My life right now is very enjoyable.	YES	Yes	yes	no	No	NO
42.	In my home, I feel that it is useless for me to make suggestions regarding family issues.	YES	Yes	yes	no	No	NO

The following section contains questions that describe your and your family's reactions related to situations at home. Please indicate the extent to which each question applies to your family situation by *circling* the most appropriate point on the scale.

YES	=	Almost always
Yes	=	Very often
yes	=	Frequently
no	=	Occasionally
No	=	Not very often
NO	=	Almost never

53. When you really need to talk to your mother, she is willing to listen.   YES Yes yes no No NO

54. I have stomach upsets.   YES Yes yes no No NO

55. Your parents support you and your decisions in front of other family members and friends.   YES Yes yes no No NO

56. I have trouble getting to sleep or staying asleep.   YES Yes yes no No NO

57. Your brother/sister pays attention to what you are saying.   YES Yes yes no No NO

58. When you really need to talk with your father, he is willing to listen.   YES Yes yes no No NO

59. I am troubled by headaches.   YES Yes yes no No NO

60. I worry a great deal about my family.   YES Yes yes no No NO

61. Your mother pays attention to what you are saying.   YES Yes yes no No NO

62. Your family members stand up for each others to outsiders.   YES Yes yes no No NO

63. I am bothered by nervousness, feeling fidgety or tense.   YES Yes yes no No NO

64. Your father pays attention to what you are saying.   YES Yes yes no No NO

65. I have recently lost or gained weight.   YES Yes yes no No NO

66. When you really need to talk with your brother/sister, s/he is willing to listen.   YES Yes yes no No NO

19

Identifying Social and Intellectual Stimulation Available to Young Children in The Home

Helen Lerner

This chapter discusses the Home Screening Questionnaire, a measure of stimulation available in the home environment for young children.

It is generally recognized that young children's home environment greatly affects their growth and development and general health. To understand fully the child's pattern of development, it is essential for those involved in providing health care to the child to have a good knowledge of the child's home environment. With this knowledge, it is possible to identify children who are at risk for developmental delay.

The Home Screening Questionnaire (HSQ) is an instrument for evaluating the home environment of children from birth to three years of age; it was developed by Coons, Gay, Fandal, Ker, and Frankenburg (1981) in Denver, Colorado, for use by health care workers and educators in evaluating environmental factors in the home that are related to a child's growth and development. This measure is based on the Home Observattion for Measurement of the Environment (HOME) developed by Dr. Bettye Caldwell (1967) to measure the home environment of young children. The HOME is a 45-item instrument divided into six subscales: (1) emotional and verbal responsivity of the mother, (2) avoidance of restriction and punishment, (3) organization of physical and temporal environment, (4) provision of appropriate play materials, (5) maternal involvement with the child, and (6) opportunities for variety in daily stimulation. A home visit with a trained observer is required to score this instrument. The visit takes approximately 1 hour. Using a questionnaire

The author gratefully acknowledges the support and cooperation of the staff and patients at the Bronx Lebanon Hospital Center – Concourse and Fulton Division.

in an outpatient setting to help identify chidren at risk for developmental delay because of inadequate stimulation in their home environment is more practical than a time-consuming home visit. In certain urban areas, such as New York City, it is very difficult to make home visits because of disorganized family life and poor housing conditions that require families to make many moves or live illegally with relatives. Also, false addresses are often given on a chart so that the family will be eligible for service at a particular hospital.

In addition to its use in screening, this tool can enable nurses and other professionals to evaluate the effects of parent education programs and the provision of guidance and counseling by looking at whether the families that participated in programs of parent education or special counseling programs were less likely to score in the "at risk" category on the HSQ than were families in the general population.

The HSQ has 33 short-answer items and a 50-item toy checklist. There is one instrument for children 0 to 3 and another for children 3 to 5 years. Studies were undertaken to determine the reliability and validity of the HSQ in Denver. The ethnic breakdown of the standardization sample was as follows: Anglo, 62%; Black, 4%, Spanish, 25%, other, 9%. In order for the researcher to use this instrument in New York City where the majority of families were Black and Hispanic rather than Anglo, a study of the instrument's reliability and validity had to be conducted.

STATEMENT OF THE PROBLEM

Environment stimulation is an important component of health in young children, because it is essential for the promotion of growth and development. Stimulation available to the young child in the home includes the caretaker and the physical enviroment that the caretaker provides. This physical environment includes such things as toys and books. Stimulation outside the home, such as going to the grocery store or playground, is also important. The environment of young children facilitates the intake and processing of information or it can hinder that process. Such factors are crucial in affecting the young child's growth and development and consequently the child's state of health.

Parental activities are also important to the family's well-being. These activities include school or college attendance, interest in books and reading, and financial decision making.

It is very important to obtain such information in low-income families because of the high incidence of developmental disabilities in this group. Since it is difficult and time-consuming to make home visits to obtain this information, it would be very useful to have a form that can be filled out by a parent or caretaker when the child comes to clinic. It is essential to have a measure that is reliable and valid.

An instrument to assess the child's environment can provide information on which to plan nursing intervention. Barnard (1982) states that the assessment can provide data that the nurse or other professional can use to decide which of the famly's ongoing behaviors should be supported. Therapeutic plans for change can be implemented when appropriate.

REVIEW AND ANALYSIS OF SELECTED LITERATURE

The following review of the literature includes environmental effects on young children, use and testing of the HSQ, and use and testing of a questionnaire developed by the Nursing Child Assessment Staff at th University of Washington. This instrument was also used to evaluate the stimulation offered to young children in the home environment and is based on the HOME Inventory.

There has been extensive literature on environmental stimulation. Much of this research began in the 1960s and continues in the present. Yarrow, Rubinstein & Pederson (1975) noted that awareness of the infant state was very important. stated that awareness of the infant state led mothers to a better understanding of infant behavior. They describe how the infant's character and changing states mediate or buffer the impact of stimuli. Yarrow et al. found that a sensitive mother is aware of infant states and responds to a variety of signals from the baby. An alert and vigorous infant elicits more and different responses than does a lethargic one. Thus, a cyclical pattern is set up. The response to maternal stimulation encourages more maternal stimulation. Yarrow concludes that an infant who is healthy encourages maternal stimulation, and one who is in poor health may lack the responses to encourage maternal stimulation.

Bee, Van Ergen, Streissguth, Nyman, & Leckie (1969) and Clarke-Stewart (1973), reporting on the behavior of lower-income and middle-income mothers, noted that middle-income mothers were more helpful and gave less negative feedback than did lower-income mothers. Lower-income mothers were more controlling and disapproving. They interacted less frequently with the child, and the interaction was seldom playful.

Marcus and Corsini (1978) looked at parental expectations related to socioeconomic class. It was found that low-socioeconomic-status parents have relatively low expectations of their children with respect to tasks. A group of low-income parents, as compared with middle-income parents had significantly lower expectations of their preschoolers on prescribed tasks.

Lewis and Wilson (1972) observed interaction between 32 infants and their caregivers of five different socioeconomic statuses. They found that lower-class infants receive stimulation but that the stimulation was less directed toward specific purposes than was the stimulation given to middle-income infants. It was found that lower-income mothers responded less often to an infant's vocalization with a vocalization than did middle-income mothers.

Caldwell (1967) reports the development of a preschool inventory for Head Start in 1965. This was later adapted to become the HOME Inventory. She stated that no description of the child's development was complete without a description of the environment in which it occurred. The inventory was administered by a person going to the child's home when the child was awake and could be observed. Two-thirds of the items relied on observation and one-third on information obtained during an interview. The interobserver agreement on coding items was 94.6% for the total scale. The agreement within subscales ranged from 91.8% to 100%. It was felt that the high reliability was due to the fact that all items were scored in a yes/no manner.

Caldwell (1971) noted that the performance of children from the lowest socioeconomic levels begins to drop betwen 18 months and 2 years. Scores are significantly lower on measures of ability and achievement.

Elardo, Bradley, and Caldwell (1975) found that after 12 months of age the most enriching environment experienced by children was that in which the mother or other primary caretaker provided the infant with a variety of materials and positively responded to the child.

Bradley and Caldwell (1976) also see parents as having the greatest impact on mental development during the first 3 years of life. Early home stimulation, as measured by the HOME inventory, is related to increases and decreases in mental test performance over 6 to 36 months of age. There is a correlation of .54 between the HOME at 6 months and 36-month IQ scores measured by the Stanford-Binet test.

Hollenbeck (1978) found that scores on the HOME inventory associated with social class in a positive way. He found that middle-class parents provided relatively large numbers of play materials.

Bradley (1985) reports the results of the Longitudinal Observation and Intervention Study designed to explore the question of when the decline in development so often observed in children reared in economically disadvantaged circumstances occurs. The HOME inventory was used to assess the child's environment. One form of the HOME inventory was used for children aged 0 to 3 years, and the other form was used for children aged 3 to 6 years. In all subgroups of the sample, the association between play materials and intelligence was significant. For boys and girls the 12-month play material scores were efficient predictors of 3-year-old IQ. The score for the Maternal Involvement subscale at 12 months was also related to the score on the Bayley Scales of Infant Development at 24 months.

Pouissant (1976) sees a child's image of himself/herself and the future as a reflection of socioeconomic and ethnic background. Several factors influence the development of the young child. First, children's ideas of themselves depend on the response of others. The child must feel that "I am a good person." Second, the parents must display respect for the child. Third, parents provide a positive self-concept that is linked with feelings of competence.

Egbuonu and Starfield (1982) report that children from low-income famlies have many more health problems and disabilities than do non-poor children. Low-income families, in particular, have a more difficult time providing health care and a stimulating environment for their toddlers. Since case finding is an important nursing function, it is important for nurses to monitor the child's environmental status, as well as undertaking the more traditional role of monitoring the child's physical health, to provide early diagnosis of problems and the basis for early intervention to correct these problem areas.

In summary, the literature on environment and children indicates that the environment contributes to the child's health and development. Low-income children are at higher risk for a poor environment and thus for delays in development.

Presently, the most frequent way to measure the stimulation offered to the young child at home is by a home visit and scoring of the HOME inventory designed by Caldwell (1967). Since requiring a home visit may be difficult and costly, the administration of the questionnaire form of this instrument, designed to be used in a clinic, school, or physician's office, can be quite helpful. The only two instruments that have been developed at this time in a questionnaire format are the HSQ for children of 0 to 3 years and 0 to 6 years and the questionnaire developed by the Nursing Child Assessment staff at the University of Washington, both of which measure the environment of the young child. Reliability and validity have been obtained with these instruments. These data have been collected from populations that are different from those served by hospitals and clinics in the Bronx. Low-income families served by health care facilities in the Bronx are largely either Black or Hispanic, with very few low-income Anglo famlies. Also, the Hispanic families in the Bronx are most often from Puerto Rico or Central America. Many Hispanic families in Denver are Mexican.

A questionnaire was developed by the Nursing Child Assessment program (NCAP) staff at the University of Washington. Hammond and Snyder (1978) report that 27 out of the 45 items on the HOME were revised into a multiple-choice and open-ended question form that was filled out by the mother prior to the clinic visit. Sixteen of the remaining 18 items were completed by the clinic staff during the observation portion of the clinic session. There are 23 items on the questionnaire; 22 of them can be scored.

Hammond and Snyder (1978) state that reliability studies on the questionnaire method versus the interviewing method were not performed because it would have been necessary to obtain data on the same items by both of the methods at the same time on the same subjects. This was not possible with 2-year-old subjects.

They further state that the validity of the data collected by questionnaire, interview in the home, or by a combined method of the two was examined in relation to the scores on the Stanford-Binet received by the children at 48 months. This was the same measure as the one used in the Bradley and Caldwell study (1976), where the full interview was used. Bradley and Caldwell administered the Stanford-Binet at 54 months to 49 children, and the NCAP sample of 133 children received the Stanford-Binet at 48 months.

The Pearson correlation coefficients obtained for each method with the scores on the Stanford-Binet were as follows: .57 for the full interview method, .42 for the questionnaire form, and .60 for the combined method of questionnaire and interview. These correlations were all statistically significant at the .01 level. Analyses showed that all forms were as valid as the interview form for predicting 4-year-old IQ. The difference between the correlations was also statistically significant. The combined form of the HOME had a statistically significant higher correlation with 4-year-old IQ than did the questionnaire form. It was suggested by Hammond and Snyder (1978) that whenever possible the questionnaire should be supplemented by having an interviewer score the remaining HOME items during an observation of the mother and infant.

This form of the HOME questionnaire is recommended for use only by those persons already trained in the traditional use of the HOME. The questionnaire form should be used only in conjunction with direct observation of the mother and child for more valid data. The total score only is used for interpretation, and the questionnaire was used only with 2-year-olds, so use with other age groups needs further study.

CONCEPTUAL BASIS OF THE HSQ

When Coons and others (1981) developed the HSQ, they noted that environmental factors and their effect on the young child's growth and development has been documented by the literature search. Many children growing up in economically and educationally disadvantaged homes later have problems learning in school. Children who have difficulty learning in school are also less likely to be able to compete in the job market as adults.

Since there are many children from poor homes who develop well and do not need referral and assistance, it is not necessary or economically feasible to refer all poor children for intervention. As previously discussed, the measure of the home environment that can identify children who are at risk for the development of low IQ or who do poorly on standardized tests of development is the HOME inventory.

Administering the HOME inventory requires that a person trained in the administration of the HOME visit the child's home and spend an hour there. This is not feasible for determining if large numbers of children are at risk. Therefore, the HSQ was developed, using the HOME inventory as a guide for the selection, writing, and scoring of items. The goal was to identify quickly, easily, and economically those children whose home environments did not provide adequate stimulation as defined by low scores on the HOME inventory.

To facilitate parent response to the questionnaire, it is written at a third- or fourth-grade reading level (Coons et al., 1981). Depending on the parent's reading ability, it should take 15 to 20 min to complete. The HSQ consists of multiple-choice items, fill-in-the-blank items, and yes/no questions. There is also a 50-item toy checklist. The parent checks those toys that are available to the child in the home.

SCORING THE HSQ ITEMS

Each HSQ item that positively contributes to the child's development is printed on the form contained in the HSQ manual, with the appropriate scoring shown next to it. Scoring of the toy checklist is based on categories of the toys. These categories were derived from the HOME inventory. A total of 11 points can be scored from the toy checklist on the HSQ for 0 to 3 years. On the HSQ for 3 to 6 years, 14 points can be scored from the toy checklist. Some toys can receive credit in more than one category.

STUDIES OF RELIABILITY AND VALIDITY

The HSQ was developed by selecting items from the HOME inventory and writing them in questionnaire form. The reliability and validity of this instrument in relation to the HOME had to be established.

Coons et al. (1981) reported that a three-phase pilot study was undertaken to establish agreement between the HSQ and the HOME inventory. During each phase of the pilot study, approximately 50 parents completed the questionnaire. A follow-up interview was conducted with the same 50 parents using the HOME inventory 2 to 4 weeks later. HSQ items were then revised to improve agreement with the HOME items. Two types of disagreements occurred between the items on th HSQ and the items on the HOME: underestimates that constituted a fail on the HSQ and a pass on the HOME and overestimates that were a pass on the HSQ and a fail on the HOME. Since the HSQ was designed as a screening instrument, a low rate of overestimates was desirable. Items were revised until they met the criteria of an overestimate rate of less than 10%, which meant they would pass the HSQ and fail the HOME, and an underestimate rate of less than 30% for each item, which meant they would fail the HSQ and pass the HOME. The correlations for the HSQ and HOME inventory were .71 and .81 for 0 to 3 years (0-3 group) and 3 to 6 years (3-6 group) respectively.

Coons et al. (1981) report a second study that was done to investigate aspects of the HSQ. The samples in this group were larger, 911 in the

0-3 group and 590 in the 3-6 group Of these, 505 in the 0-3 group and 294 in the 3-6 group were followed with the HOME tool 2 to 4 weeks later.

The sample reported for the second study indicated a group with a higher number of parents who attended or completed college. Fifteen percent of the mothers in the 0-3 group had reported attending or completing college, and 14% of the mothers in the 3-6 group had reported attending or completing college.

To calculate reliability in this study, a Kuder Richardson Formula 20 (Waltz, Strickland, & Lenz, 1984) analysis was done. The internal consistency coefficients were .74 for the 0-3 HSQ and .80 for the 3-6 HSQ. To calculate test-retest reliability, a second HSQ was given to 30 parents of the 0-3 group and 24 parents of 3-6 group 1 to 4 months following the first. The test-retest reliability coefficient was considerably lower (.62) for the 0-3 group than for the 3-6 group (.86). When calculations were done only on children of 1-3 years, the test-retest reliability coefficient was .82. This may have to do with the considerable developmental changes in the first year of life, making changes in the parent's reponse probable. However, this does suggest that the HSQ is less reliable for children under the age of 1 year.

The ability of the HSQ to identify low HOME scores is quite high (81%) in the 0-3 group and (86%) in the 3-6 group. The accuracy of identifying high HOME scores is only moderate: 66% in the 0-3 group and 55% in the 3-6 group. Overreferral appears to be high particularly in the 3-6 group. Since the HSQ can be used as a screening instrument, it is more desirable that the instrument be accurate in determining low scores than in keeping overreferrals to a minimum. False referrals can be screened out by further diagnostic procedures. The families found by this study to need referral were 62% and 66% for the 0-3 and 3-6 groups, respectivey. The study group felt that these were reasonable percentages considering the high rates of school problems in a group of children who come from poor families.

The authors cautioned about the use of the HSQ with groups in other countries because values and customs differ. This may limit its use in the New York area, where there is a small and growing population of immigrants from countries in South and Central America and the Caribbean Islands. But is is essential to assess these children. Even though methods of child rearing may be different, if the famlies are choosing to live in the United States, their children will be competing cognitively with children from other cultures when they enter school and will need to have the same kind of skills.

Additional reliability and validity data needed to be obtained on both instruments if they were to be used in clinics in the New York City area, where a different population of ethnic groups is involved.

It is hoped that testing the HSQ with an urban population in New York City will extend its use to populations other than those represented in

Denver and form the basis for wider use of the questionnaire to determine the child's home environment.

Rosenbaum, Chua-Lim, Wilhite, & Mankad (1983) describe a Denver prescreening questionnaire for use in a low-income population. The results of their study showed that such a prescreening questionnaire was applicable to assess early child development (birth to 12 months) beyond the Denver population, thereby increasing its appropriateness for general use on a widespread basis in pediatric settings.

In summary, previous testing on the questionnaires has proved them reliable and valid and useful for certain populations.

MEHODOLOGY FOR TESTING THE RELIABILITY AND VALIDITY OF THE HSQ ON THE DESIGNATED POPULATION

Hypothesis 1: Both the questionnaire and the inteview form of the HSQ will be reliable.

Hypothesis 2: The scores on both the questionnaire and the interview form of the HSQ will show a statistically significant correlation ($p<.05$) with the Bayley Scales of Infant Development, the Mental Scale Record Form.

Definition of Terms

A Black family in this study refers to a family in which the mother identifies herself as Black and has at least one parent who was born in a country in the Western Hemisphere. The mother must be able to speak, read, and write English.

A Hispanic family in this study refers to a family in which the mother identifies herself as Hispanic and has at least one parent who came from a country in the Western Hemisphere where Spanish is the language spoken. The mother must be able to speak, read, and write English.

Sample

The study was conducted at pediatric clinics in two different hospitals in the South Bronx. All parents of children from 12 to 30 months who came to the clinic on the day the researcher was there were asked to participate in the study. Parents who agreed to participate had their participation in the research explained to them, and a consent form was read and signed. All but three of the mothers who were approached agreed to participate in the study. The sample obtained consisted of 41 children who ranged in age from 12 to 30 months. The mean age was 20.8 months. Eighteen of the sample were Hispanic, and 23 were Black. The mothers' ages ranged from 18 to 42 years with a mean age of 26.4 years. Twenty-three of the mothers were 25 years of age or below. Nineteen of the children were first-born; nine, second-born; nine, third-born; and three, fourth-born; data were missing on one child. Of the population sampled, four were low-birth-weight infants; 12 mothers reported other complications during labor and deliver, and 25 mothers reported no complications. Thirty-two mothers reported the child's health as good, and nine reported problems with the child's health.

The mothers' educational levels ranged from third grade to 1 year of college. Nineteen mothers reported being at least high school graduates.

The households were composed as follows: 12 mothers living alone, 20 living with the child's father, and 8 living with extended family; one mother lived with a friend.

Thirty-two mothers did not work. Nine mothers reported being employed.

PROCEDURES FOR ADMINISTRATION AND SCORING

Two content validity experts were asked to rate the questionnaire. Both content validity experts were nurses. One was a pediatric nurse practitioner who worked with low-income families in the Bronx. The other was director of an outpatient department that served only low-income families. Both had extensive knowledge of child development, and both also had a knowledge of the community where their facilities were located. The target population consisted of Black and Hispanic children. One of the nurses was Black, and one was Hispanic. Criterion validity was assessed by means of the Bayley Scales of Infant Development, the Mental Scale Record Form, as the criterion.

The Mental Scale Record Form of the Bayley Scales of Infant Development is designed to assess early abilities such as "object constancy," memory and learning, problem-solving ability, the beginnings of verbal communication, and early evidence of the ability to form generalizations. The Bayley was standardized on a sample of children from 2 to 30 months. The sample was controlled for sex and color within each age group and was chosen to reflect accurately selected strata of the U.S. population (Bayley, 1969). This instrument is recommended for use both clinically and for research. The split-half reliability of the Mental Scale on 14 age groups from 2 to 30 months ranged from .83 to .95. Coefficient correlation of the Mental Scale score with the Stanford-Binet score was .57, which indicates that there was a substantial degree of agreement.

Mothers who came to the pediatric clinic or to the Women's, Infants', and Children's (WIC) program with their children had the study described to them; they were then asked if they would like to participate. All but three persons approached agreed to participate in the study. Once the mothers agreed to participate, they were asked to come to a quiet room with their children. They read the consent form or had it read to them and then signed it. The Bayley Scales of Infant Development, the Mental Scale Record Form, was administered. Then the mother was given the questionnaire to fill out. After the questionnaire was filled out, the researcher or an assistant gave the mother the same questions in an interview format. The mother was then asked to wait outside.

The Bayley Scales of Infant Development, the Mental Scale Record Form, was then scored to obtain a mental development index (MDI). The results were explained to the mother. Each item on the Bayley was reviewed with the mother. The numbers on the left side, which gave the age range at which the child would perform the items, was explained to the mother in relation to how her child reacted to the item. The actual numbers of the total score were not used in the explanation because of concern with identifying the child with a low or high score that would not be predictive. Children with exceptionally low scores (below 80) were discussed with the mother. The researcher stated that the child might need some special support in a particular area such as language. The mother's permission was then obtained for reporting this to the pediatrician, and a referral was made. This happened with only two children, and in both cases the mother was aware of the problem and was anxious for a referral.

The MDI was scored only after the questionnaire and interview were obtained, to minimize bias in an unfunded study, since the researcher or an assistant had to perform both tasks.

The questionnaire and the interview were scored at a later time by the researcher or one of her assistants, using the suggested scoring procedure in the HSQ manual. This was also done to minimize bias, even though the scoring was objective, so that the researcher or assistant did not relate the score to the one obtained on the Mental Scale Record Form of the Bayley.

RESULTS AND STATISTICAL ANALYSIS

The scoring procedure from the manual by Coons et al. (1981) was utilized. A total score of 43 was the highest possible score that could be achieved on the HSQ. This total score was obtained by adding the score on the short answer items and the score on the toy checklist. A score of 33 or above was regarded by the authors of the HSQ as a "nonsuspect" result. A score of 32 or below was regarded as "suspect." The mean score on the questionnaire in this study was 25.8, with a standard deviation of 5.376. Of the 38 persons filling out the questionnaire, 4 scored above 33. The scores ranged from 16 to 37. The other three people in the group were unable to read.

The mean score on the HSQ when it was administered by the interview method was 28.829, with a standard deviation of 4.711. When the questionnaire was administered by the interview method, 12 persons scored

33 or above. The scores ranged from 17 to 37.

Internal consistency reliability was used to measure the reliability of the instrument. When internal consistency was calculated for the questionnaire form, the alpha was .87. The reliabiilty for the HSQ when administered by the interview method was .56.

To assess the validity of the instrument, content validity procedures, and criterion validity, assessment using the MDI as the criterion was done. Assessment of the content validity index (CVI) by the two content specialists had previously resulted in a CVI of .95.

To assess criterion-related validity, Pearson product-moment correlations were done for the total scores of the HSQ when administered by both the questionnaire method and the interview method and the separate toy list scores for each HSQ with the MDI (see Table 19.1). The correlation for the HSQ administered by questionnaire and the toy checklist for that HSQ were not significant. The correlation for the total score on the HSQ administered by the interview form was significant at the .03 level. If you separate out the score on the toy list from the total score, the correlation is even higher and is significant at the .02 level. This finding agrees with Bradley (1985), who reports path analyses on Bayley scores and the Play Materials subscale on the Home Inventory. He reports significant paths running from 12-month scores on the Play Materials subscale to Bayley scores at 12 and 24 months.

There were problems with the administration of the questionnaire. It took the mothers a long time to complete the instrument. The average time was about 20 to 25 min, which made administration in a busy pediatric clinic difficult.

Some questions caused particular difficulty. One question asked, "About how many times do you have to spank or slap your child to get him to mind?" The word *mind* is not a familiar word to most urban New Yorkers that we saw, and it frequently had to be explained. The toy checklist consisted of 50 items. When the mothers saw this, they frequently became extremely anxious. They were reassured by the researcher or assistant that they were not expected by any means to have all of those toys. The mothers frequently stated that even so there was "so much to read."

When the questionnaire was administered as an interview, another problem arose. Some questions had four or five possible answers, and the mother was to choose only one or two. Often by the time the last choice was read, the mother had forgotten what the first choice was and the question had to be read again.

Hypothesis I – both the questionnaire and the interview form of the HSQ will be reliable – demonstrated reliability. This hypothesis was partially supported. The questionnaire form achieved a reliability of .87, which is acceptable. However, the interview form achieved a reliability of .56, which is not acceptable.

TABLE 19.1 Pearson Product-Moment Correlation of Mental Development Index (MDI) Scores with Home Screening Scores by Questionnaire (HSQ) and Interview (HSI) Methods and with Toy List Scores from Each Screening (TLSQ and TLSI)

Scores	MDI
HSQ	$r = 0.1457$
	$p = .198$
HSI	$r = 0.2967*$
	$p = .3$
TLSQ	$r = 0.1895$
	$p = .118$
TLSI	$r = 0.3156$
	$p = .022$

* >.05 significance level

Hypothesis 2 – the scores on both the questionnaire and the interview form of the HSQ will show a statistically significant correlation (<.05) with the Bayley Scales of Infant Development, the Mental Scale Record Form – was also found to be only partly supported. The scores on the questionnaire form of the HSQ did not show a statistically significant correlation with the MDI score of the Bayley Scales of Infant Development, the Mental Scale Record Form. However, the score on the interview form showed a statistically significant correlation with the MDI. Criterion-related validity studies tend to overestimate the strength of the predictor criterion relationship Waltz et al. (1984).

DISCUSSION

There were several things that compounded what seemed like an essentially simple study. First, there were extensive problems in the population being studied regarding literacy. The questionnaire was difficult for all but a handful of mothers to read. It took a great deal of time and effort to fill out the questionnaire and a great deal of clarification was needed. Of the 13 mothers who scored 30 or above on the questionnaire, five left out at least one item. Of the 25 mothers who scored 29 or below, 14 left out at least one item. Three mothers were unable to read the questionnaire at all.

Second, the Bayley Scales of Infant Development, the Mental Scale Record Form, was difficut to administer to many of the children. Compared to a middle-income group of children that the researcher had evaluated in a prior study, their attention span was very short. Many times the performance on the second or third trial of an item seemed less effective than on the first trial. This resulted in a great deal of frustration.

Also, parents often interfered and tried to do the item for the child or help the child with the item and had to be cautioned not to interfere. Most of the children did particularly poorly on language items. Many of the parents commented that they thought the languge items were too advanced for the children and that children of the age of their child were not ready to use language. Yarrow (1984) found a relationship between the child's ability to persist at tasks and the MDI scored at 13 months. The 6-month environment scores were related to persistence and competence in the tasks at 20 months.

There is also the concern that children would obtain a lower MDI score when the Bayley Scales of Infant Development, the Mental Scale Record Form, was administered in the clinic than would be achieved by the child if the test was administered in the child's own home. Horner (1980) tested 9- and 15-month-old infants in a home and a clinic setting. The test results of the majority of infants fluctuated very little between the two settings.

Third, there was concern about possible contamination of the study by having the same person giving the Bayley Scales of Infant Development, the Mental Scale Record Form, and administering the questionnaire and interview, even though the Bayley was not scored until after the questionnaire and interview were done. In this unfunded study this was the only procedure feasible. In view of this concern, six questionnaires and interviews were administered to parents who had not been previously involved in the study. The questionnaire was not looked at until after the interview was administered. Then both instruments were scored. The scores on six questionnaires and interviews revealed the same pattern: The scores on the questionnaires were consistently lower than those on the interviews. Parents tended to leave out items on the questionnaire, as with the other sample. The range of scores was similar, from 22 to 35. Scores were consistently higher on the interview form of the HSQ. A larger sample of independently adminstered questionnaires needs to be obtained.

Fourth, the low reliability index for the interview form of the questionnaire is of concern. The low value obtained may be due to several factors. A high alpha is obtained when the test as a whole measures one attribute. It may be that for very poor urban families the test is measuring more than just one attribute – that is, their financial status, their interest in stimulating their child, and their mental health. It may be that the reliability would be higher if the HSQ were divided into subscales. There are also a large number of HSQ scores, from both the questionnaire and the interview method, at the lower end of the scale. This means a lesser variance, which would give a lower alpha. The group studied may also be homogeneous in the particular attribute measured. The group seen at this particular hospital may not be typical of the larger population in New York City. Sixty-two percent of the Denver population had low HSQ scores. Approximately 90% of the New York City population had low HSQ scores when the HSQ was administered by questionnaire. Seventy-one percent had low scores when the HSQ was administered by the interview method.

Regarding the validity, there is a small but statistically significant correlation between the total score on the HSQ when administered by interview and the MDI. In her study using the HOME, on which this instrument was based, Caldwell (1967) had a low positive correlation on the Bayley at 12 months and a much higher correlation at 36 and 54 months when other instruments were used. It may be that the predictive validity of the HSQ, like that of the HOME, is stronger than the concurrent validity.

There must be some adjustment of the HSQ as it presently stands to make it more reliable and valid for the population of New York City. The difficulties in administration can be addressed by changing the wording in the question that was unclear to parents because the word *mind* was used. This word should be changed to *behave*. The toy list can also be shortened to facilitate reading. Only certain items on the toy list are scored for points. Other items listed receive no points on the score whether or not the parent checks them. Eliminating some of the items that receive no points toward the score would shorten the toy list and facilitate reading but would not disrupt the scoring of the instrument. The number of options for several questions can also be reduced without interfering with the scoring. For example, one question asks: "How often does someone read stories or show pictures to your child?" The choices are "hardly ever," "once or twice a month," "at least once a week" "at least three times a week" and "at least five times a week." The answers "at least three times a week" and "at least five times a week" each received 1 point. None of the other answers receives credit. Therefore, the choices were reduced to "hardly ever," "less than three times a week," and "three times a week or more." This would reduce the amount of reading that the parents must do.

IMPLICATIONS FOR THE NURSING PROFESSION

There are several implications in this study for the provision of nursing care. Because of the great problem of reading and reading comprehension for persons in lower socioeconomic groups, one must be very careful about forms and educational materials that are prepared for them, and we should never rely on their reading a pamphlet or instruction sheet for information. Most people are too embarassed to say that they cannot read or understand something that is given to them. Information needs to be read and explained to parents very carefully, using a vocabulary that they can understand.

It is possible also that the problems in reliability and validity and the low scores the parents receive do reflect reality. If it were possible to obtain a score on the HOME inventory for the same persons, they might achieve a correspondingly low score. This should alert nurses again to the great problem of the risk of developmental delay for children whose parents may be poor. Differences in development may be occurring earlier than thought, although there is increasing recognition of this fact by those who work with very young children.

In view of the risk of developmental delay, it should be of concern to nurses that parents with financial problems have considerably less money to spend on toys, particularly the kinds of toys that children need to play with to develop the skills to function in a very technological society. For example, fewer than half of the children had the opportunity to play with puzzles. Means must be found to provide children with these experiences. Bradley and Caldwell (1982) reported that intellectual competency for Black children was first associated with organization of the home. The next most important factors were emphasis on enriching materials and experiences.

Developing an appropriate instrument to measure home environment in a clinic setting for families in New York City appears to be a difficult task but an essential one. The HSQ needs further testing and possible modification to refine it into an effective tool fo this population.

The HSQ is available from DDM Inc., P.O. Box 20037, Denver, CO 80220; (303) 335-4729. the cost is $6.00 for a packet of 25.

REFERENCES

Bayley, N. (1969). *Manual for the Bayley Scales of Infant Development*. Berkeley, CA: University of California Institute of Human Development.

Bee, H., Van Ergen, L. F., Streissguth, A. P., Nyman, B. A., & Leckie, M. S. (1969). Social class differences in maternal teaching strategies and speech patterns. *Develomental Psychology, 1*, 726-734.

Bradley, R. (1985). Play maternals and intellectual development. In C. C. Brown & A. W. Gottfried (Eds.), *Play interactions: The role of toys and parental involvement in children's development (pp. 129-142)*. Skillman NJ; Johnson and Johnson Baby Products. (Pediatric Round Table Series. H)

Bradley, R., & Caldwell, B. M. (1976). Early home environment and changes in mental test performance in chidren from 6 to 36 months. *Developmental Psychology, 12*, 93-97.

Bradley, R., & Caldwell, B. (1982). The consistency of home environment and its relation to child development. *International Journal of Behavior Development, 5*, 445-465.

Caldwell, B. (1967). Descriptive evaluation of child development and of developmental settings. *Pediatrics, 40*, 46-54.

Caldwell, B. (1971). The effects of early experiences on a child's development. In J. Segal (Ed.), *The mental health of the child* (pp. 179-192). (Public Health Services Publication No. 2168). Washington, DC: U.S. Government Printing Office.

Clarke-Steward, K. A. (1973). Interactions between mothers and their young children: Characteristics and consequences. *Monographs of the Society for Research in Child Development, 38*, 1-109.

Coons, C., Gay, E., Fandal, A. W., Ker, C., & Frankenburg W. K. (1981). *The Home Screening Questionnaire reference manual*. Denver: University of Colorado Health Sciences Center.

Egbuonu, L., & Starfield, B. (1982). Child health and social status. *Pediatrics, 69,* 550-557.

Elardo, R., Bradley, R., & Caldwell, B. M. (1975). The relation of infants' home environment to mental test performances from six to thirty-six months: A longitudinal analysis. *Child Development, 46,* 71-76.

Hammond, M. A., & Snyder, C. (1978). The validity of obtaining the Home Observation for Measurement of the Environment by Mother Questionnaire. In K. E. Barnard (Ed.), *Nursing child assessment satellite training project: Instructor's learning resource manual* (pp. 119-127). Seattle: University of Washington School of Nursing.

Hollenbeck, A. R. (1978). Early home environment: Validation of the Home Observation for Measurement of the Environment Inventory. *Developmental Psychology, 14,* 416-418.

Horner, T. M. (1980). Test-retest reliability and home clinic characteristics of the Bayley scales of infant development in nine and fifteen month old infants. *Child Development, 51,* 751-758.

Lewis, M., & Wilson, C. D. (1972). Infant development in lower class American families. *Human Development, 15,* 112-127.

Marcus. T. L., & Corsini, D. A. (1978). Parental expectations of preschool children related to gender and socioeconomic status. *Child Development, 49,* 234-246.

Poussiant, A. F. (1976). Building a strong image in the black child. In S. White & B. Walsh (Eds.) *Human development – Today's world* (pp. 96-102). Boston: Little, Brown.

Rosenbaum, M. S., Chua-Lim, C., Wilhite, H., & Mankad, V. N. (1983). Applicability of the Denver prescreening developmental questionnaire in a low-income population. *Pediatrics, 71,* 359-363.

Waltz, C. F., Strickland, O. L., & Lenz, E. R. (1984). *Measurement in nursing research.* Philadelphia; F. A. Davis.

Yarrow, L. J. (1984). Infantile persistence at tasks: Relationship to cognitive function and early experience. *Annual Progress in Child Psychology and Child Development.* 217-229.

Yarrow, L. J., Rubinstein, J. L., & Pedersen, F. A. (1975). *Infant and environment.* Washington, DC: Hemisphere.

PART III
Measuring Factors in Community-Based Care

20

Specific Outcomes of Nurse-Directed Colorectal Cancer Screening

Roberta L. Messner and Sylvia S. Gardner

This chapter discusses the results of a nurse-run screening program for colorectal cancer. The Hemoccult® test (filter paper impregnated with guaiac) was used as a screening tool.

There has been virtually no improvement in the survival rate for colorectal cancer in the past 50 years (DeVita, Hellman, & Rosenberg, 1982). It is estimated that 140,000 new cases of colorectal cancer will be diagnosed in 1986 in the United States alone, claiming the lives of 60,000 individuals (American Cancer Society, 1986).

At present, more than one-half of all cases of colorectal cancer are discovered when metastases become evident. At this point, the 5-year survival rate is reduced to 51% for colon cancer and 38% for rectal cancer (American Cancer Society, 1986). When colorectal cancer is detected in an early stage, however, the 5-year survival rate is 90% for colon cancer and 80% for rectal cancer (American Cancer Society, 1986), underscoring the importance of early detection (Johnson, 1985).

Only breast and colorectal cancer have randomized controlled trials with an end point of mortality (RCTM) proving that early detection significantly decreases mortality (Eddy, 1983). The early detection of cancer is dependent on two conditions: the existence of a premalignant or detectable preclinical phase and the availability of appropriate tests for detection (Johnson, 1985).

* At the time this study was conducted, Ms. Messner was the Gastroenterology Nurse Clinician at the Veterans Administration Medical Center, Huntington, West Virginia.

The authors express appreciation to the West Virginia State Medical Association for allowing the representation of data previously published in *The West Virginia Medical Journal*.

Colorectal cancer originates with the development of a benign adenomatous polyp or lesion in the large bowel or rectum, (Mitchell & Silman, 1983). A polyp is described as a lesion protruding into the lumen of the bowel wall; it is referred to as sessile if it has no stalk and as pedunculated if a stalk is present (Williams, 1983). The typically prolonged premalignant state of 5 to 10 years or longer for adenomatous polyps enhances the opportunity for early detection and cure (Memorial Sloan-Kettering Cancer Center, 1982). Because there are no early warning signs, individuals often remain asymptomatic for colorectal cancer until the disease has progressed. Therefore, preventive programs for the early detection of colorectal cancer should be targeted toward asymptomatic individuals.

The potential for malignant degeneration varies according to the anatomical location of the polyp and increases with the presence of one or more adenomas, as time elapses, in polyps with a villous component and as the size of the polyp surpasses 0.5 cm (Sherlock & Winawer, 1984). For adenomas greater than 3 to 5 cm in size, carcinoma in the polyp has been reported with a 55% frequency (Winawer, Miller, & Sherlock, 1984).

While screening tests are not designed to be diagnostic, they are important in identifying individuals with a particular characteristic (Larson, 1986). Studies on the role of nursing in screening and case finding for colorectal cancer are virtually nonexistent. Nurses, however, have many opportunities to assess clients at risk for colorectal cancer in an asymptomatic stage, to institute serial fecal occult blood screening, and to initiate referrals and follow-up care for clients with positive findings (Messner, Gardner, & Webb, 1986).

In the year preceding this study, 27 cases of colorectal cancer were diagnosed at the study medical center, providing the stimulus for this multidisciplinary research (Gardner, Messner, & Webb, 1985). The research objectives were as follows:

1. To what extent does serial fecal occult blood testing as a primary screening modality detect premalignant and malignant colorectal lesions in men over age 40 who are at standard risk for developing colorectal cancer and are asymptomatic for gastrointestinal disease?
2. To what degree does the provision of education and counseling by nursing pre-and postscreening affect the rate of returning the stool specimens and consenting to diagnostic investigations?

REVIEW OF THE LITERATURE

Colorectal cancer affects individuals of both sexes and all racial and ethnic groups, although significant international differences do exist (DeVita et al., 1982). These disparities appear to be primarily related to dietary factors, although a number of other risk factors also contribute to the development of colorectal cancer in varying degrees. The most easily determinable risk factor for colorectal cancer is age; 98% of colorectal cancers occurs in persons over age 40 (Memorial Sloan-Kettering Cancer Center, 1982). The incidence of colorectal cancer increases at age 40 and doubles at age 50 and each consecutive decade until it levels off at age 80 (Young et al., 1981). Individuals age 40 and over with no additional risk factors are considered to be at standard risk for the development of colorectal cancer. These are additional subgroups in the population who because of certain personal and/or familial factors, such as familial polyposis coli, Gardner's syndrome, and Peutz-Jeghers syndrome, are at high risk for developing colorectal cancer (Sherlock & Winawer, 1984). These situations necessitate earlier and more intense screening (Winawer et al., 1984).

Screening refers to an approach for a large population, whereas case finding is an approach for individual clients and small groups within the health care system. In utilizing the fecal occult blood test for screening and early case finding, outcomes are evaluated in terms of the early detection of colorectal cancer as well as the detection of premalignant colorectal lesions (Winawer et al., 1984).

The ability of hemoglobin to catalyze the oxidation of guaiac resin by hydrogen peroxide has been used for over a century to demonstrate the presence of fecal occult blood (Frommer & Logue, 1981). Greegor (1967, 1971) showed that early colorectal cancer could be detected by the use of guaiac-impregnated slides prepared by individuals at home following a prescribed dietary regimen. He reported no missed colorectal cancers in clients on a high-roughage, meat-free diet when testing them by using two slides each day for 3 consecutive days. In individuals with colorectal cancer, the pathological staging was such that they could be expected to have a more favorable outcome. Recent data suggest that detecting colorectal cancer prior to the onset of symptoms prolongs survival (Winawer et al., 1984). Removal of polypoid colonic lesions, which may be premalignant, is usually achievable through a colonoscopy/polypectomy procedure.

A study on public attitudes toward colorectal cancer (Shapiro, 1982) revealed that screening for colorectal cancer is not a routine component of the physical examination for individuals at risk for the disease. This can be attributed to a number of factors. Colorectal cancer has often been referred to as "the cancer nobody talks about" ("Cancer Nursing News", 1984). As a result of embarrassment, cultural taboos, or fear of death or the need for a colostomy, asymptomatic individuals are frequently hesitant to approach the practitioner about screening modalities for the early detection of colorectal cancer. According to the American Cancer Society (1983), individuals tend to assign greater significance in their self-definition to heart, lungs, and stomach. By contrast, the possibility of exerting control over conditions of colon and rectum appear relatively limited; therefore, dismissal of the colon and rectum tends to remove these areas from the perceived possible sites of cancer. In addition, symptoms of colorectal cancer may be inappropriately attributed to the aging process (Messner & Gardner, 1985).

According to Hoffman, Young, and Bright-Asare (1983), educational efforts in regard to colorectal cancer screening are tedious and time-consuming and may not fit within the practitioner's time constraints. However, Winchester (1983) and Johnson (1985) assert that early detection for specified individuals at risk for cancer are best accomplished in outpatient settings where a one-to-one relationship between the practitioner and client is enhanced. This atmosphere is conducive to comprehensive testing as the benefits and risks can be more carefully explained than in mass screening programs. In addition, it is less time-consuming to obtain informed consent from individuals with whom the practitioner has a long-standing relationship than from individuals the practitioner has just met.

While colorectal cancer is amenable to public screening programs, data are inconclusive concerning the mortality benefit, cost-effectiveness, and precise mechanisms for facilitating compliance. Poor compliance has been observed in screening of individuals with inadequate orientation and education (Winawer et al., 1984; Winchester, 1983). In a 1978 American Cancer Society screening of 54,000 individuals in Chicago, the compliance rate for returning the specimen kits was 26%. Eighty-six percent of individuals with positive fecal guaiac tests consented to further diagnostic evaluation (Winchester, Sylvester, & Maher, 1983). A compilation of many studies revealed that compliance with fecal occult blood testing was 15% for "unmotivated" client populations as compared to 80% for "motivated" groups (Winawer et al., 1984). At present, the American Cancer Society and the International Work Group recommend that fecal occult blood testing be instituted only when clients have already gained entrance into the health care system (Winawer et al., 1984).

POPULATION AND SAMPLE

The study sample was 300 Caucasian male veteran subjects of predominantly lower socioeconomic status who came to one nurse practitioner in the ambulatory care walk-in clinic between November 1982 and March 1983. All subjects were at standard risk for colorectal cancer by virtue of their age and were asymptomatic for gastrointestinal disease. Subjects at increased risk for colorectal cancer or who were symptomatic for gastrointestinal disease were treated appropriately but not included in the study. Subjects included in the study had already entered the health care system; all aspects of the study were incorporated into the investigators' daily clinical practice.

BIOLOGICAL INSTRUMENTATION

Selection of the biological instrument for use in the early case finding of colorectal cancer was based on the diagnostic accuracy of the instrument as defined by its sensitivity, specificity, predictive value, and accuracy, as well as ability to achieve reasonable client compliance (Hoffman, 1984). Ostrow, Mulvaney, & Hansell (1972) have demonstrated that normal adults lose approximately 1.5 ± 0.5 ml of blood per 100 g of feces daily. The biological instrument needed to be sensitive enough to detect fecal occult blood loss above the normal range without giving false-positive tests, that is, positive readings in the absence of gastrointestinal pathology.

The Hemoccult® test (Smith Kline Diagnostics, Sunnyvale, California) consists of filter paper impregnated with guaiac, which undergoes phenolic oxidation when exposed to hemoglobin in the stool and hydrogen peroxide in the test reagent (Fleisher, Schwartz, & Winawer, 1980). The positive reaction produced by hemoglobin is the result of the pseudoperoxidase activity that interacts with the hydrogen peroxide, causing the guaiac paper to turn blue (Winawer et al., 1984). The Hemoccult test was selected as the most promising biological instrument for the study on the merits of the balance between specificity and sensitivity, predictive value (both of which influence instrument validity), ease of use and interpretation, and the ability to achieve acceptable levels of subject compliance (Frommer & Logue, 1981).

The level of sensitivity (the degree to which a true characteristic is correctly measured) for fecal occult blood testing is a compromise between too many false-positive results in normal subjects and an unacceptable number of false negatives in subjects with increased gastrointestinal blood loss (Frommer & Logue, 1981). Sensitivity and specificity are inversely correlated; hence, increasing an instrument's sensitivity decreases its specificity, and vice versa (Larson, 1986).

Although a number of similar products are currently available, there is a paucity of information concerning other competitive products (Frommer & Logue, 1981). The sensitivity of the Hemoccult® test has been compared to other commercial products by the use of visual performance tests to measure "working" test sensitivities, by instrument-based performance tests to measure "inherent" test sensitivites, and by slide composition tests to analyze the content of the guaiac filter paper. The components of the Hemoccult test have been carefully selected and engineered to produce a positive test only when fecal occult blood loss exceeds clinically defined limits (Smith-Kline, 1980). Frommer and Logue (1981) compared four competitive products with the Hemoccult test in in vitro testing. Two of the products were found to be too sensitive and could be expected to produce an increased number of false positives, while another competitive product was found to be grossly insensitive. The Hemoccult fecal occult blood test has been shown to be one-fourth as sensitive as comparable products; however, the lesser sensitivity has been accompanied by a reduction in false-positive tests (Ostrow, Mulvaney, Hansell, & Rhodes, 1973). An inappropriate increase in instrument sensitivity results in a greater number of unnecessary invasive procedures for the client and increased health care costs.

According to Hoffman (1984), fecal guaiac screening is 99% specific for blood in the stool, not colorectal cancer. Sufficient quantities of blood anywhere in the gastrointestinal tract can result in a positive test. Medications such as anti-inflammatory drugs, iron, or preparations containing aspirin are gastric irritants that may cause the normal gastrointestinal mucosa to bleed (Winawer, Fleisher, Baldwin, and Sherlock, 1982). Nonhuman hemoglobin present in food such as red meat and the peroxidase activity of some fresh fruits and some uncooked vegetables, such as turnips and radishes, may also result in a false-positive test (Fink, 1983; Winawer et al., 1982). Although false negativity with the Hemoccult method appears to be low, there are various possible explanations for false-negative results. These include sampling errors in slide preparation, conversion of initially positive slides to negative, or a lesion that did not bleed at the time of sampling (Winawer, Miller, & Schottenfeld, 1977). Ascorbic acid as an oxidation inhibitor may produce a false-negative test, even in the presence of blood in the stool (Winawer et al., 1982).

The predictive value of a positive test is the likelihood that the characteristic under study is truly present. The predictive value of a negative test is the likelihood that the characteristic under study is truly absent (Larson, 1986). Screening individuals at increased risk for colorectal cancer, as opposed to indiscriminate mass public screening, increases the predictive value of positive test results (Hoffman, 1984).

The ability to achieve reasonable client compliance with an instrument is influenced by such factors as convenience, aesthetics, and the risk imposed to clients. In studies of fecal occult blood testing with the Hemoccult method, client compliance with the preparation of slides has been shown to be feasible (Winawer et al., 1977).

METHODOLOGY

In a one-to-one educational session with one nurse investigator, subjects were provided with information about colorectal cancer in lay terminology. Subjects were informed that the fecal occult blood test was not specific for cancer but would detect microscopic or "hidden" blood in the stool, and if present, further investigation to discover the cause of the bleeding would be necessary. They were assured that blood in the stool could result from a number of gastrointestinal conditions and that the likelihood of having colorectal cancer was small but not too small to ignore. It was stressed that if they should have colorectal cancer, discovering it early would make cure very likely. In Appalachian West Virginia, many clients view "the bowel issue" as too personal for discussion and are crisis-oriented as opposed to prevention-oriented (Gardner et al., 1985). Therefore, cultural variables specific to the Appalachian people were given careful consideration.

Written and verbal instructions for specimen collection were provided to ensure proper procedure for specimen collection, preservation, and storage (Waltz, Strickland, & Lenz, 1984). For 48 hr before the first stool sample was to be taken, as well as throughout the test, subjects were advised to eat a diet that was high in fiber (fruits, vegetables, bran, etc.) but not to eat any turnips or horseradish. Subjects were instructed that red meats should be deleted from the diet but that fish and poultry were acceptable. Subjects were instructed not to injest any iron preparations, vitamin C, or any medications containing aspirin, since these may interfere with test results.

Subjects were instructed to take two *tiny* samples of the stool each day for 3 days in a row and smear them on the enclosed slides with the wooden applicator, for a total of six specimens. They were told to place the slides in the enclosed "ziplock" plastic bag after obtaining the final specimen, store the specimens at room temperature, sign and date the kits, and mail them immediately in the preaddressed, stamped envelope. The importance of obtaining a *series* of stool specimens was emphasized. Because almost all colorectal lesions bleed on an intermittent basis and a given lesion may have a daily variation in the rate of bleeding, random testing may yield many false-negative results (Morris, Hansell, Ostrow, & Lee, 1976). A high-fiber diet encourages colorectal lesions to bleed sufficiently to produce a positive test.

Hemoccult stool screening kits were dispensed between November 1982 and March 1983 by one nurse investigator. The timing of specimen collection coincided with the winter season, as it has been suggested that hot weather may decrease specimen positivity (Frommer & Logue, 1981). A screening kit consisted of six "windows" of guaiac-impregnated filter paper. Pertinent data regarding the date of kit distribution, the client's age, and significant medical and family history were recorded in a master log book. On receipt of the specimens, one nurse investigator tested all of the specimens, verifying that they were received within 2 days of obtaining the last stool sample. Prolonged storage of fecal occult blood tests (for longer than 5 days after specimen application) can convert a weakly positive reaction to a negative one (Winawer et al., 1982).

To ensure accuracy of test results, prior to reading the slides, the built-in Hemoccult Performance Monitor was tested for validity, or that the instrument indeed measured occult blood. The reagent (Hemoccult Developer®), which was stored at room temperature, protected from heat, sunlight, fluorescent light, and ultraviolet light, and kept tightly capped to prevent evaporation (Smith Kline Diagnostics, 1980b), was checked to ascertain that it was not outdated. Hands, gloves, and working area were cleaned and free of blood prior to testing of specimens. As indicated in the product instructions, one drop of the Hemoccult Developer was applied between the positive and negative portions of the performance monitor and read within 30 sec. Validity was established if the negative portion of the performance monitor did not change in color and the positive portion of the performance monitor turned blue.

A major strength of the Hemoccult instrument is its objectivity, or the degree of agreement between the reading of positive or negative assigned by two independent observers; that is, two practitioners interpreting the same specimen are likely to read the same result. The Hemoccult provides measurement of the occult blood with relative precision (reliability) and sensitivity and with minimal likelihood of product malfunction. Interrater reliability was established prior to the study in the following manner: Two raters independently recorded readings (positive or negative) of the same stool specimen using the same measurement instrument on the same measurement occasion (Waltz et al., 1984). Full agreement as to a positive or negative test result was obtained in 100% of specimens ($N = 120$).

Specimens were not rehydrated on the basis of the manufacturer's recommendation and studies that suggest that rehydration increases the percentage of false-positive results (Frame & Kowulich, 1982; Frommer & Logue, 1981). Hemoglobin, as well as other interfering compounds such as peroxidases present in certain foods and bacteria, is reactivated during the rehydration process, thereby increasing false-positive results (Winawer et al., 1984). To read the Hemoccult slides, the perforated windows in back of the slides were opened. Two drops of the Hemoccult Developer were applied to the back of each stool specimen and read within 60 sec. In the presence of occult blood, a positive result (defined as any trace of blue) was observed. In the absence of any detectable blue color, the test was read as negative.

Test results were recorded in the master log book by one nurse investigator to lessen the likelihood of transcription errors (which would affect validity of results) and to account for unreturned specimens. After interviewing subjects with positive slides to ascertain compliance with the prescribed testing procedures, the subjects were counseled regarding the process for recommended diagnostic workup. The possible risks of invasive procedures were explained and appropriate informed consents were obtained. For consistency, diagnostic evaluation of subjects with positive findings was made in the outpatient gastroenterology clinic by one gastroenterologist. One nurse investigator assisted the gastroenterologist with all endoscopic procedures. Subjects underwent complete history and physical examinations, digital rectal examinations, and flexible sigmoidoscopies to 60 cm from the anal ring. Subjects with polyps, as well as those without demonstrable lesions on sigmoidoscopy, then underwent full colonoscopy. Subjects still demonstrating no gastrointestinal pathology underwent upper gastrointestinal barium and endoscopy studies.

TABLE 20.1 Clinical Data in 300 Patients[a] Provided With Serial Hemoccult Stool Screening Kits

	No.	%
Patient compliance for returning specimens	240	80
Usable specimens returned	235	98
Patients with usable slides who had one or more positive slides (unrehydrated)	22	9
Patients with one or more positive slides who completed the diagnostic workup[b]	22	100
Patients with positive slides who demonstrated some gastrointestinal pathology on diagnostic workup	22	100
Patients completing diagnostic workup who had polypoid colonic lesions	5	23
Premalignant	2	9
Non-premalignant	3	14
Patients with one or more positive slides who had colorectal cancer	0	0
False-positive slides	0	0

[a]Average age, 59.4 years; range, 44-77 years.
[b]Two of these 22 patients completed the diagnostic workup at another hospital.

ANALYSIS OF DATA

Two hundred forty subjects (80%) of the study sample returned the fecal occult blood kits, of which 235 (98%) were usable specimens (see Table 20.1). Twenty-two subjects had one or more guaiac-positive slides. One hundred percent compliance with the recommended procedure for specimen collection was reported by all subjects with positive guaiac slides. Following one-to-one education and counseling by nursing, all subjects with one or more positive slides consented to and received a complete diagnostic workup. Two subjects who relocated during the study were referred to another facility, where they received a diagnostic evaluation.

The excellent subject compliance was attributed to the one-to-one relationship the nurse investigators had established with the subjects and their families. This was considered to be especially significant in view of the characteristic attitudes and behaviors of the Appalachian people and the exclusively male sample. The American Cancer Society (1983) noted that women report a greater awareness of their colon and rectum and an increased interest in checking these sites for cancer.

Table 20.2 shows the clinical diagnoses among subjects in whom occult bleeding was detected by serial Hemoccult stool screening. While only one subject had six of six slides positive, diagnostic procedures revealed an explanation for fecal occult blood in 100% of subjects. The seriousness of the lesions did not correlate with the percentage of positive slides. This

TABLE 20.2 Clinical Diagnoses of the 20 Patients with Positive Hemoccult Tests Who Underwent a Diagnostic Workup at the Study Medical Center

Diagnosis	No.
Duodenal ulcer	4
Diverticular disease	3
Pedunculated colonic polyps	3
Alcohol gastritis	2
Inflammatory bowel disease	2
Sessile colonic polyps	2
Billroth II anastomatic ulcer	1
Duodenitis	1
Esophagitis	1
Hemorrhoids	1

was consistent with the findings of Hoffman and associates (1983), who distributed approximately 11,888 Hemoccult kits in an urban public hospital setting. Diagnostic workup revealed colonic pathology in 100% of subjects. The significance of examining a *series* of stool specimens was confirmed, as only one subject had all six slides positive.

Five subjects had polypoid lesions demonstrated on colonoscopy. The three subjects with pedunculated polyps, two of which were premalignant villous adenomas, had complete removal of their lesions by cautery snare during full colonoscopy. Because of the potential dangers in removing sessile polyps by cautery snare, the two subjects with sessile polyps (which were not premalignant) underwent biopsy of the lesions. All subjects with polypoid lesions were entered into a long-range polyp surveillance program. Although no malignant lesions were identified, the polypoid lesions discovered resulted in a protocol for comprehensive surveillance for five subjects, the eradication of polypoid lesions in three subjects (two of which were premalignant), and education regarding the prevention and early detection of colorectal cancer for 300 subjects and their families.

According to Hoffman and colleagues (1983), in colorectal cancer screening and case finding, determining risk and benefit for a population requires large numbers of subjects. Therefore, individual investigators are at a disadvantage for validating the results reached through personal experience.

DISCUSSION AND CONCLUSIONS

Physiologic indicators are of increasing importance to nurse researchers in the quantification of physiologic variables and in the measurement of outcomes of nursing interventions and to nurse clinicians in making decisions about health promotion, maintenance, and restoration (Waltz et al., 1984). Larson (1986) asserts that screening tests are useful when there is an important health problem that can be detected in an early stage; when the screening test is simple, convenient, reliable, and cost-effective; and when an effective treatment or intervention is available. Screening for colorectal cancer by use of the Hemoccult instrument meets all of these criteria when specific procedures are followed.

To exert a reduction in mortality from colorectal cancer, screening programs must reach and be accepted by the target population. The prevention and early detection of colorectal cancer represents a compelling multidisciplinary responsibility. Although the number of subjects tested was somewhat limited, this study demonstrated an effective modality for the early detection of premalignant and malignant colonic lesions; however, the number of subjects with false-negative results is not known because subjects with negative results were not followed longitudinally.

This research approach is congruent with Orem's (1980) self-care nursing model, which could be adapted by nurses in a variety of settings. Self-care agency does not occur in a vacuum but represents a collaborative process between the nurse and client. In this study, self-care agency of the subjects was fostered by nursing through one-to-one education and counseling. Because the current research was multidisciplinary, it was not framed in the authentic locus of nursing. Additional nursing research in this area could extend the conceptualization of Orem's model.

The feasibility of designing and performing research-related activities as a part of daily nursing practice was demonstrated by this study. This is dependent on the motivation of nurses to recognize opportunities for clinical investigation, the willingness of nurses to collaborate with other members of the multidisciplinary team, and the provision of administrative support. If the nurse selects as a research site a familiar environment, such as the institution of employment, the obstacles of gaining entry into a new system can be avoided, thereby facilitating the research process. Lack of funding, a frequently cited deterrent to nursing research, may be more easily managed if researchers and administrators can collaborate to utilize the existing budget. Therefore, many of the barriers described by nurse investigators can be overcome in the clinical practice setting.

Whitehead (1929) described science as a river with two sources, the theoretical and the practical. Theory and clinical practice have widely demonstrated the profound benefits of early case finding of colorectal cancer in asymptomatic individuals at risk for developing the disease. Until primary prevention of colorectal cancer is possible, efforts must be geared toward secondary prevention or early detection as a means of reducing morbidity and mortality from the disease (Winchester, 1983).

The American Cancer Society (1985) estimates that if only 10% of the over-age-50 target population who are not presently receiving regular examination for colorectal cancer would receive examination during each of the next three years, 10,000 lives could be saved and 170,000 person-years could be added to the lives of individuals who are discovered to have colorectal cancer. This would result in a savings of more than $160 million in treatment costs and more than $190 million in otherwise lost earnings (American Cancer Society, 1985).

Serial Hemoccult stool screening provides an excellent opportunity for nursing measurement and recording of physiological functioning to explore ways in which nursing interventions can be improved (Polit & Hungler, 1983). Research that examines the effect of nursing intervention on the prevention and early detection of colorectal cancer is important for the improvement of health care as well as the advancement of the nursing profession. These efforts can exert a major impact on the morbidity and mortality of colorectal cancer, as evidenced by savings in health care dollars, lost incomes, and the prevention of incalculable human suffering.

REFERENCES

American Cancer Society. (1986). *1986 Cancer Facts and Figures. New York: Author.*

American Cancer Society. (1985). *Professional Education Newsletter, 1* (1), 1-3.

American Cancer Society. (1983). Cancer of the colon and rectum: Summary of a public attitude survey. *In Detecting colon and rectum cancer.* New York: Author. Professional Educational Publication.

Cancer nursing news. (1984, January/February). *American Cancer Society Newsletter for Nurses*, pp.1-4.

DeVita, V. T., Hellman, S., & Rosenberg, S. A. (1982). *Cancer: Principles and practices of oncology.* Philadelphia: J. B. Lippincott.

Eddy, D. M. (1983). Early detection: How beneficial is it? *Your Patient and Cancer, 3*(2), 3-8.

Fink, D. J. (1983). Facts about colorectal cancer detection. *In Detecting colon and rectum cancer.* New York: American Cancer Society, (Professional Education Publication).

Fleisher, M., Schwartz, M. K., & Winawer, S. J. (1980). Laboratory studies on the Hemoccult slide for fecal occult blood testing. In S. J. Winawer, D. Shottenfield, & P. Sherlock (Eds.), *Progress in cancer research and therapy: Vol. 13. Colorectal cancer: Prevention, epidemiology and screening.* New York: Raven Press.

Frame, P. S., & Kowulich, B. A. (1982). Stool occult blood screening for colorectal cancer. *Journal of Family Practice, 15*(6), 1071-1075.

Frommer, D., & Logue, T. (1981). Comparison of five guaiac resin paper tests for demonstrating the presence of blood in feces. *Australian and New Zealand Journal of Medicine, 11*, 494-496.

Gardner, S. S., Messner, R. L., & Webb, D. D. (1985). Serial Hemoccult stool screening for colorectal cancer. *The West Virginia Medical Journal, 81*(1), 5-10.

Greegor, D. H. (1967). Diagnosis of large-bowel cancer in the asymptomatic patient. *Journal of the American Medical Association, 201*, 943-945.

Greegor, D. H. (1971). Occult blood testing for detection of asymptomatic colon cancer. *Cancer, 28*, 131-134.

Hoffman, A., Young, Q., Bright-Asare, P., et al. (1983). Early detection of bowel cancer at an urban public hospital: Demonstration project. *In Detecting Colon and Rectum Cancer* (pp. 16-30). New York: American Cancer Society. (Professional Education Publications).

Hoffman, W. H. (1984). How worthwhile is screening for occult blood? *Diagnostic Medicine, 7*(5), 35-40.

Johnson, B. L. (1985). Prevention and early detection. In B. L. Johnson & J. Gross (Eds.), *Handbook of oncology nursing.* New York: John Wiley.

Larson, E. (1986). Evaluating validity of screening tests. *Nursing Research, 35*(3), 186-188.

Memorial Sloan-Kettering Cancer Center Office of Continuing Medical Education. (1982). Colorectal cancer: Essentials for primary care physicians. *Clinical Round Tables, 1*(4), 1-8.

Messner, R. L., & Gardner, S. S. (1985). Stop a killer with early detection. *Journal of Gerontological Nursing, 11*(11), 8-14.

Messner, R. L., Gardner, S. S., & Webb, D. D. (1986). Early detection – the priority in colorectal cancer. *Cancer Nursing, 9*(1), 8-14.

Mitchell, P., & Silman, A. (1983). Screening for colorectal cancer. *Nursing Times, 79*(9), 58-60-1.

Morris, D., Hansell, J. R., Ostrow, J. D., & Lee, C. S. (1976). Reliability of chemical tets for fecal occult blood in hospitalized patients. *American Journal of Digestive Diseases, 21*(10), 845-852.

Orem, D. (1980). *Nursing: Concepts of practice* (2nd ed.). New York: McGraw Hill.

Ostrow, J. D., Mulvaney, C. A., & Hansell, J. R. (1972). *Annals of Internal Medicine, 76,* 860.

Ostrow, J. D., Mulvaney, C. A., Hansell, J. R., & Rhodes, R. S., (1973). Sensitivity and reproducibility of chemical tests for fecal occult blood with an emphasis of false-positive reactions. *The American Journal of Digestive Diseases, 18*(11), 930-940.

Polit, D. F., & Hungler, B. P. (1983). *Nursing research: Principles and methods.* Philadelphia: J. B. Lippincott.

Shapiro, L. J. (1982). Cancer of the colon and rectum: The public perspective. New York: American Cancer Society.

Sherlock, P., & Winawer, S. J. (1984). *Colorectal cancer.* [Slide set with background information script for professional education]. New York: American Cancer Society.

Smith-Kline Diagnostics. (1980a). *Competitive product update:* Comparisons between Hemoccult, Quick-Cult™ and "Fe-Cult". Data on file at Smith-Kline Diagnostics, Sunnyvale, CA.

Smith-Kline Diagnostics. (1980b). *Product instructions: Hemoccult. [Slides and tape].* Sunnyvale, CA: Author.

Walz, C. F., Strickland, O. L., & Lenz, E. R. (1984). *Measurement in nursing research.* Philadelphia: F. A. Davis.

Whitehead, A. N. (1929). The organization of thought. In A. N. Whitehead (Ed.), *The aims of education.* New York: Macmillan.

Williams, R. B. (1983). Fecal occult blood testing: The basics. Professional Horizons for Gastrointestinal Assistants Address, Washington, DC.

Winawer, S. J., Fleisher, M., Baldwin, M., & Sherlock, P. (1982). Current status of fecal occult blood teting in screening for colorectal cancer. *CA: A Cancer Journal for Clinicians, 32*(2), 110-112.

Winawer, S. J., Miller, D. G., Schottenfeld, D. (1977). Feasibility of fecal occult-blood testing for detection of colorectal neoplasia. *Cancer, 40*(5), 2616-2619.

Winawer, S. J., Miller, D. G., & Sherlock, P. (1984). Risk and screening for colorectal cancer. In G. H. Stollerman (Ed.), *Advances in internal medicine* (Vol. 30, pp. 471-496). Chicago: Year Book Medical Publishers.

Winchester, D. P. (1983). Colon and rectal cancer. *CA: A Cancer Journal for Clinicians, 33*(6), 359-365.

Winchester, D.P., Sylvester, J. A., & Maher, M. L. (1983). Risks and benefits of mass screening for colorectal neoplasia with the stool guaiac test. *Detecting Colon and Rectum Cancer* (pp. 5-15). New York: American Cancer Society, Professional Education Publication.

Young, J. L., Percy, C. L., Asire, A. J., Berg, J. W., Cusano, M. M., Gloeker, L. A., Horm, J. W., Laurie, W. I., Pollack, E. S., & Shambough, E. M. (1981). Cancer incidence and mortality in the United States, 1973-77. *National Cancer Institute Monograph, 57,* 1-49.

21

The Measurement of Client Outcomes in Home Health Care Agencies

Sarah B. Keating

This chapter discusses development of a list of nursing diagnoses relevant to home care, and an evaluation tool that measures client outcomes in home care (utilizing the relevant nursing diagnoses).

PURPOSE

The purpose of the project was to develop a reliable and valid tool for measuring the health status of patients receiving community health nursing through certified home health agencies. It was proposed that such a tool would increase knowledge concerning the nature and quality of nursing care received by clients within the health care system.

REVIEW OF THE LITERATURE

Overview of an Evaluation Theory Applied to Nursing

Stufflebeam's (1974) evaluation model of context, input, process, and product (CIPP) was selected to refine the study's purpose and identify objectives and methods for the development of an evaluation tool. The advantage of the CIPP model was its usefulness in studying the total problem area and the many dimensions within it. Although the CIPP model attempted to identify all aspects of home health care, it was recognized that measurement of quality nursing care is a multivariate construct, and some variables were inadvertently omitted. The model's four components were analyzed as follows:

1. *Context* – the objectives of the evaluation procedure are listed. Overall evaluation of a home health care agency includes the agency's

structure, its process for delivering services, and its end product or expected patient/client outcomes. Objectives for evaluating the three items are developed from (1) agency standards, (2) means standards, or the criteria for measuring the process toward meeting the goals, and (3) ends standards, or criteria to measure the outcome in terms of the client's improved health status.

2. *Input* – the component of the CIPP model that specifies what is to be evaluated. Table 21.1 lists samples of the content of what is to be evaluated and its form for (1) agency (structure), (2) process of the delivery of care, and (3) final client outcomes.

3. *Process* – for each component of what is to be evaluated, a tool for measuring its effectiveness is listed. For example, under structure, or agency standards, a certain staff-client ratio is recommended. Actual numbers of qualified staff on the payroll become a measure for meeting this standard. Each objective in the context component and the content listed in the input component serve as guides for collecting data to measure progress toward meeting the goals and objectives of evaluation. See Table 21.1 for further examples.

4. *Product* – the analyses of the data collected in the process component of the model serve to measure the progress or outcome of the agency's services in meeting the needs of the client. Thus, each previous component of evaluation (context, input, and process) is analyzed and measured against the objectives of evaluation. Decisions are then made for continuing, modifying, or terminating the evaluation process and, ultimately, the services delivered by the agency.

The CIPP model provided an analysis of the many components of home health care services and a framework from which to choose which best met the purpose of the evaluation. It helped to identify the product of

TABLE 21.1 Adaptation of the Context, Input, Process, and Product (CIPP) Model

Context	Input	Process	Product
Develop criteria for patient outcomes (improve health status following and during care)	Client health status as measured by nursing diagnoses classification system and their related outcome criteria (patient-centered)	Documentation of nursing diagnoses and outcome criteria for each; records of improved, same, or not improved status of client	Improve documentation of client outcomes according to health status; improve nursing care process in order to achieve improved client health status (see criteria for process outcomes)

From Stufflebeam 1979.

home health care nursing services: client outcomes. According to the literature review, reliable and valid tools for measuring patient-centered outcomes and nursing's accountability to the consumer are needed (Atwood, 1980; Gordon, 1980; Horn, 1980; Kreuger, 1980). This project focused on one aspect of quality assurance, that of patient health status and its relationship to outcome of nursing care.

Instruments Utilized for Measuring Quality of Nursing Care

The review of the literature identified several tools that were developed specifically for evaluating the quality of nursing care in community health nursing. One of the earliest quality assurance tools developed for home health care is the Phaneuf tool (1973). The major focus for the tool was on process evaluation rather than outcome.

Other tools for measuring quality assurance were reviewed in Ward and Lindeman (1978) and found to partially address client outcomes. Many health care agencies throughout the country have developed evaluation tools specific to their own agency's recordkeeping formats (Albany Visiting Nurse Association, 1982; Florida Association of Home Health Agencies, 1980, Minnesota Department of Health, 1983; Pennsylvania Assembly of Home Health Agencies, 1975). A tool for measuring the final nursing care outcome according to client health status in home health care agencies was not found in the review of the literature.

CONCEPTUAL FRAMEWORK

Nursing, in its quest as a professional health discipline, has been in the process of identifying the part of the health care delivery system that is unique to nursing. Part of the uniqueness lies in the classification of client health problems labeled as nursing diagnosis. Since the 1950s, this term has been found in the nursing literature, and after the first meeting of the National Group for the Classification of Nursing Diagnoses became a model for defining nursing practice (Carpenito, 1983).

Several classification systems have emerged over the years that utilize nursing diagnosis categories. Examples include *Accepted Diagnoses from the Fifth National Conference* (Kim & Moritz, 1982); *Gordon's (1982) Manual of Nursing Diagnosis,* (1982); and *A Classification Scheme for Client Problems in Community Health Nursing* (Visiting Nurse Association of Omaha, 1980). Carpenito's (1984b) definition for a nursing diagnosis was utilized for this study:

> Nursing Diagnosis is a statement that describes a health state or an actual or potential altered interaction pattern of an individual, family, group, to life processes (psychological, physiological, socio-cultural, developmental, and spiritual) which legally, the nurse can identify and order the primary interventions to maintain the health state or to reduce, eliminate, or prevent client alterations. (pp. 1418-1419).

The early classification systems did not include specific goals related to the diagnoses for providing standards of care. Carpenito (1983) and the contributors to her text were among the first to add other components to the nursing diagnosis categories. They included definition, etiological and contributing factors, defining characteristics, focus assessment criteria, nursing goals and principles, and rationale for nursing care. Within this framework, Carpenito defined outcome criteria or client goals as "the expected changes in the status of the client after he has received nursing care" (p. 41).

The evaluation tool that was developed and tested for this study was based on Carpenito's (1983) framework for measuring client-centered outcomes. Outcome criteria include positive criteria: improvement in the client health status by increasing client comfort and coping abilities, maintenance of present optimal level of health, optimal levels of coping with significant others, optimal adaptation to deterioration of health status, optimal adaptation to terminal illness, and collaboration and satisfaction with health care providers. Negative outcome criteria were complications, disabilities, and unwarranted death. According to Carpenito, outcome criteria should include in their format measurable verbs, specific content, and time parameters, and they should be attainable.

The advantage of the nursing diagnosis model for the development of a tool to measure patient outcomes was its wide applicability to nursing practice and its increasing acceptance by the profession as one parameter of practice. The nursing diagnosis model could be part of the data base that fits into the prospective payment method for financing health care applied to hospital care and eventually to home health agencies.

Problem Statement Based on the Conceptual Framework

Based on the review of the literature and the decision to develop an evaluation tool to measure nursing care outcomes, the following research question was formulated: To what extent can quality of nursing care be measured by an instrument that is derived from specific patient outcomes or goals related to the nursing diagnosis classification of client health problems? To develop an instrument to measure quality of nursing care, specific questions relating to the problem statement were developed. They were as follows:

1. To what extent do nursing diagnoses apply to home health clientele?
2. To what extent are the diagnoses and their outcomes found in agency records?
3. To what extent do the nursing diagnoses relate to medical diagnoses?

Design of the Study

Throughout the study the Institutional Review Board (IRB) of the author's place of employment was apprised of the research activities, and it granted approval for conducting the study. The study was conducted in several stages. The first stage addressed the first two specific research questions concerning the relevance of the nursing diagnosis classification system to home health care clientele and documentation in records. The second phase focused on the major question related to the development of an evaluation tool to measure client outcomes.

TABLE 21.2 Blueprint for Measuring the Reliability and Validity of the Relevance of the Nursing Diagnosis Classification System to Home Health Care Agencies

Objectives	Scale			
Diagnosis applies to home health agency clients	Applies Frequently 3 —	Sometimes Applies 2 —	Seldom Applies 1 —	Does Not Apply 0 —
Rate nursing diagnosis 1 through 42				
Diagnosis can be found in current client records	Recorded Frequently 3 —	Sometimes Recorded 2 —	Seldom Recorded 1 —	Never Recorded 0 —
Rate 1 through 42 nursing diagnoses and their definitions				
Outcome criteria relate to actual nursing care delivered to cleints	Relates Frequently 3 —	Sometimes Relates 2 —	Seldom Relates 1 —	Never Relates 0 —
Rate 1 through 42 nursing diagnoses and their outcome criteria				
Outcome criteria are documented in current client records	Frequently Documented 3 —	Sometimes Documented 2 —	Seldom Documented 1 —	Never Documented 0 —
Rate 1 through 42 diagnoses and their outcome criteria				
Outcome criteria have an effect on the improvement of the client's health status	Always have effect 3 —	Sometimes have effect 2 —	Seldom have effect 1 —	No Effect have effect 0 —
Rate 1 through 42 nursing diagnoses and their outcome criteria				
Open-ended comments: List client health problems omitted in this classification system. List the diagnoses and their related outcome criteria that are the 10 most critical when considering (1) improved client health status, (2) quality of nursing care. General comments				

The last phase reexamined the fit of the nursing diagnosis classification system to recorded client health problems, as well as the documentation of medical diagnoses and their relationship to nursing problems. Major statistical procedures included content and descriptive analyses; and for reliability and validity, coefficient alpha and rates of agreement between experts.

TABLE 21.3 Major Nursing Diagnostic Categories

1. Activity intolerance
2. Anxiety
3. Alterations in bowel elimination
4. Alterations in cardiac output (decreased)
5. Alterations in comfort
6. Impaired verbal communication
7. Coping, ineffective individual
8. Ineffective family coping related to domestic violence
9. Diversional activity deficit
10. Alterations in family processes related to an ill family member
11. Fear
12. Fluid volume deficit
13. Fluid volume excess: edema
14. Grieving
15. Alterations in health maintenance
16. Impaired home maintenance management
17. Potential for injury
18. Knowledge deficit
19. Impaired physical mobility
20. Noncompliance
21. Alterations in nutrition: Less than body requirements
22. Alterations in nutrition: More than body requirements
23. Oral mucous membrane, alterations in
24. Alterations in parenting
25. Powerlessness
26. Rape trauma syndrome
27. Respiratory function, alterations in
28. Ineffective airway clearance
29. Ineffective breathing patterns
30. Impaired gas exchange
31. Self-care deficit
32. Disturbance in self-concept
33. Sensory-perceptual alterations
34. Sexual dysfunction
35. Impairment of skin integrity
36. Sleep pattern disturbance
37. Social isolation
38. Spiritual distress
39. Alterations in thought processes
40. Alteration in tissue perfusion
41. Alterations in patterns of urinary elimination
42. Potential for violence

METHODOLOGY

Methodology for Measuring Relevance of Nursing Diagnosis Classification System to Home Health Care

Nursing administrators and staff nurses were asked to rate the relevance of the model to their practice. A detailed blueprint with five objectives to measure the reliability and validity of the nursing diagnoses' relevance to home health care was developed. Table 21.2 presents the blueprint with its five objectives and rating scale. Table 21.3 lists the 42 major diagnostic categories, which were rated by the nurses. In addition to the diagnoses, the staff nurses were asked to rate the relevance of each diagnosis and specific client outcomes to their practice, and to what extent the diagnoses and outcomes are documented in records.

Methodology for Developing a Tool for Measuring Patient Outcomes

After the review of the diagnostic classification system, a preliminary tool for measuring client outcomes was developed, and the nurses were asked to review it (Table 21.4). This tool was pilot-tested in January 1985 through a review (audit) of clients' records. Three community health nursing faculty with experience in home health care conducted the audit. Only the nursing diagnoses and related goals, medical diagnoses, positive and negative outcomes, and time factors were recorded. Interrater reliability was calculated by recording the frequency of observations on the tool by the experts according to the major categories of diagnoses, goals, and time factors. It was found that the range of interrater percent of agreement for the major categories was 60% for time factor observations, 78% for nursing diagnosis, 80% for medical diagnoses, and 81% for expected client outcomes. The percentages demonstrated an acceptable rate of agreement among the experts in their review of client records.

The reviews of these three faculty members were then subjected to analysis by the researcher and two additional community health nursing faculty members. The purpose of the next review was to fit the recorded nursing diagnoses and related outcomes into Carpenito's (1983, 1984a) diagnostic categories. The interrater reliability was at a 60% rate of agreement among the three judges. A content analysis of the raters' comments revealed that there were diagnoses in the records that did not fit into the specific diagnostic statements from Carpenito's classification but could fit into the major categories. Table 21.5 is a sample of one of the rater's responses for interfacing the client record's diagnoses to those of Carpenito.

The client outcomes listed by the staff nurses in records were also subjected to review by the faculty members and compared to those of Carpenito (1983). The percentage of interrater agreement for identifying client outcomes was calculated by counting the number of outcomes

TABLE 21.4 Tool for Measuring Client Outcomes

| Client Identification Number | DRG category | | Nursing diagnosis | | Expected Outcome (S) | | Expected outcome deadline | | Positive outcomes | | | | | Negative outcomes | | | Time Lapse* (Days) |
	Code	Title	Code	Title	Code	Title	Date	Time in Months	Exceeded expectations (5)	Met expectations (4)	Did not meet expectations (3)	Apply to diagnosis (2)	Diagnosis did not apply (1)	Complications (3)	Disabilities (2)	Unwarranted death (1)	

* Time lapse between expected outcomes and evaluation of outcome.

TABLE 21.5 Sample of Review of Client's Records for Documentation of Nursing Diagnoses and Their Relationship to Carpenito's Classification

Client record nursing diagnosis		Carpenito's nursing diagnosis classification and related outcomes	
No. of diagnosis and goal	Title of diagnosis and goal	No. of diagnosis and	Title of diagnosis and outcome
1	Diagnosis ADL deficit: weakness post-operatively	01	Diagnosis Activity intolerance
1.1	Goals Improve strength gradually, and VNSA will provide assistance until patient cares for self	01.2	Outcome Progress to the highest level of mobility possible
2	Diagnosis Potential alteration in skin integrity, incontinence, emaciation	65	Diagnosis Skin integrity, impairment of, related to immobility
2.1	Goal Patient will stay clean and dry and gain 2#/week		Outcome No specific outcome listed that relates to dry and clean skin
3	Diagnosis Alteration in bowel and bladder status, poor muscle control	00	Diagnosis Elimination, alteration in, related to poor sphincter control
3.1	Goal Develop regular schedule for elimination, become fully continent	04.2	Outcomes (adapted from 04) Relate or demonstrate improved bowel elimination
		04.3	Modify elimination routine to cope with interferences
		77	Diagnosis Urinary elimination, alteration in; patterns of; related to incontinence
		77.1	Outcome Eliminate or reduce incontinence episodes
4	Diagnosis Alteration in nutritional status 2: decreased appetite, no meal preparer	37	Diagnosis Nutrition, alterations in: less than body requirements; difficulty/inability to procure food
4.1	Goals Patient will gain 2lb/week and have daily meals on wheels (MOW)	37.2	Outcome Be assisted to acquire food on a regular schedule

recorded by all three raters and dividing them by those outcomes not agreed on by the experts. Although the percentage of agreement among the raters was 81%, the majority of the outcomes in the records did not have a parallel in Carpenito's nursing diagnosis and outcomes taxonomy.

Based on the results, it was decided to conduct one additional pilot study utilizing only the major categories of nursing diagnoses. Twenty-five client records were randomly selected for audit to identify medical diagnoses and major categories of nursing diagnoses. Table 21.6 outlines the tool for collecting medical and nursing diagnoses in relationship to the Carpenito categories.

DATA ANALYSIS

Relevance of the Nursing Diagnosis Categories to Home Health Care

Seventeen directors of home health agencies in the northeastern part of New York state participated in the first pilot study in the summer of 1984. Since this was an initial inquiry into the application of the nursing diagnosis model and related outcomes, the reliability and validity studies were norm-referenced rather than criterion-referenced (Waltz et al., 1984).

The directors were asked to rate all of the nursing diagnoses and subcategories listed by Carpenito (1983) according to their relevance to home health care. They rated the diagnoses on a scale from never (0), seldom (1), and sometimes (2) to frequently (3). Participants were also asked to list the 10 most critical diagnoses to home health care. Comments and suggestions were also solicited.

TABLE 21.6 Tool for Collecting Medical and Nursing Diagnosis Relating to Carpenito Diagnoses from Client Records

Carpenito Diagnoses	VNA diagnosis	Medical diagnosis
01. Activity intolerance		
02. Anxiety		
03. Bowel elimination, alterations in		
04. Cardiac output alterations in		
05. Comfort, alterations in		
06. Communication, impaired		
07. Coping, ineffective		
08. Diversional activity deficit		
↓	↓	↓
42. Violence, potential for		

TABLE 21.7. List of Nursing Diagnoses Rated by Experts as Having Relevance to Home Health Care Clientele[a]

 1. Activity intolerance
 2. Anxiety
 3. Alterations in bowel elimination
 4. Alterations in cardiac output
 5. Alterations in comfort
 6. Impaired verbal communication
 7. Coping, ineffective individual
 8. Coping, ineffective family
 9. Alterations in family processes related to an ill family member
10. Decreased fluid intake
11. Fluid volume excess: edema
12. Grieving
13. Alterations in health maintenance
14. Impaired home maintenance
15. Impaired physical mobility
16. Noncompliance
17. Alterations in nutrition: Less than body requirements
18. Alterations in nutrition: More than body requirements
19. Respiratory function, alterations in
20. Self-care deficit
21. Sensory-perceptual alterations
22. Impairment of skin integrity
23. Sleep pattern disturbance
24. Social isolation
25. Alterations in thought process
26. Alterations in tissue perfusion
27. Alterations in pattern of urinary elimination

[a]Indicated by listing the 10 most critical diagnoses to home health care and by rating each diagnosis on a scale of 1 to 4 according to frequency of encounter in practice.

The data collected from the rating scale were coded and analyzed utilizing the *Statistical Package for the Social Science* (SPSS) (Nie, Hull, Jenkins, Steinbrenner, & Bent; (1975), subprogram: Frequencies. Table 21.7 lists those diagnoses with mean rating scores of greater or equal to 2.0 ("sometimes" to "frequently encountered") and items that were rated by the participants as the 10 most critical to home health practice.

Several reliability and validity procedures were conducted. Reliability measures included the following:

Internal consistency – to measure the consistency of the items (diagnoses) across the instrument. An alpha coefficient of .364 was the index of reliability. While this latter coefficient is low, it would be anticipated if the diagnoses were discriminant classifications of client health problems; that is, each diagnostic category is indeed a separate client or nursing problem. For example, although related, anxiety, fear, and grieving are unique diagnoses.

Interrater reliability – to measure the consistency of performance across the experts, coefficient alpha was utilized and measured .999.

Content validity was determined by having the nurses judge the nursing diagnoses for their relevance to practice. They were also asked to list any client problems that were omitted (none were elicited) and to contribute any general comments concerning the purpose of the research. All statistical procedures were based on the recommendations of Waltz et al. (1984) for reliability and validity studies.

The second phase of the study was conducted in October 1984. Seventeen staff nurses who had direct contact with home health care clients reviewed the nursing diagnosis model's relevance to their practice. Because there were almost 80 diagnoses and related diagnoses, they were divided into four packets containing 20 diagnoses and related outcomes. Thus, each diagnosis and related outcomes were rated by 3 to 5 nurses rather than by the total sample of 17. The nurses reported that the majority of the diagnoses related to practice and were documented in client records.

Overall Interrater Reliability Concerning Content Validity: Relevance of the Nursing Diagnosis Categories to Home Health Care

Each of the staff nurses was asked to indicate whether she agreed or disagreed with the concept that the nursing diagnoses and their related outcomes classification system were relevant to her nursing practice in home health care. The resulting Content Validity Index (CVI) weas .86 (Waltz et al., 1984).

Evaluation Tool for Measuring Patient Outcomes

In addition to asking the nurses to rate the diagnoses and their outcomes, a preliminary tool for evaluating outcomes through record audit was subjected to their review. Each nurse rated the items in the tool according to the following scale: The item applies to present practice and data in client records to the extent that it applies (3), sometimes applies, (2) and does not apply (1). Table 21.8 presents the overall means for each item on the tool. The majority of the items received a mean of over 2.0, which was the criterion set for acceptance.

Pilot Study of Evaluation Tool Through Record Audit

Three community health nursing faculty members reviewed five home health care client records utilizing the evaluation tool. Table 21.9 presents the reliability findings by the percentage of agreement between the three reviewers for each item of the tool. The rates were acceptable; however, due to time constraints and the nature of the client records, the relationship of the recorded diagnoses and outcomes to the Carpenito (1983) model was not accomplished.

TABLE 21.8 Evaluation Tool for Record Review; Results of Staff Nurses' Ratings[a] of the Items' Application to Practice

Item	Mean
Client ID number	No data
DRG code number (or medical diagnosis)	2.94
Nursing diagnosis, title and number	2.94
Expected outcomes, title and number	2.58
Positive Outcomes	
Exceeded expectations	2.44
Met expectations	2.82
Did not meet expectations	2.65
Negative outcomes	
Complications	2.76
Disabilities	2.73
Unwarranted death	2.00
Outcomes applied to diagnosis	No data
Diagnosis did not apply	No data
Expected outcome deadline	No data
Time lapse	No data

[a]Rating: Applies (3) to Does Not Apply (1).

TABLE 21.9 Percentage of Agreement Between Experts' Recordings from Audit of Five Client Records Utilizing Evaluation Tool

Evaluation tool item	% Agreement
Client identification number	100
Medical diagnosis	80
Nursing diagnosis	78
Expected outcome	81
Positive outcome expectations	
Exceeded	No entries
Met	7
Not Met	50
Negative Outcomes	
Complications	1
Disability	100
Unwarranted death	100
Diagnosis did not apply	No entries
Date of admission	100
Time in days and time lapse in number of days	60

Relationship of Diagnoses Collected from the Evaluation Tool to Those of Carpenito

The list of nursing diagnoses from the five client records was reviewed by three additional faculty members with expertise in community health nursing. They were asked to compare the clients' diagnoses to the categories of diagnoses listed by Carpenito (1983). Each client's diagnoses and the experts' comparisons to Carpenito's category were analyzed. An overall rate of agreement for classifying the diagnoses among the three raters was 66%.

Pilot Study of Nursing Diagnosis Documentation in Client Records

While the directors of nursing and staff nurses reported that nursing diagnoses and their related patient outcomes could be found in client records, the audit using the evaluation tool had mixed results. Nursing diagnoses were located, but outcomes were more difficult to find. In addition, the tool did not yield all of the data anticipated. It was decided to return to two of the specific questions of the study: (1) To what extent are the diagnoses and their outcomes found in agency records? (2) To what extent do the nursing diagnoses relate to medical diagnoses? Only medical and nursing diagnoses were sought.

Twenty-five client records were randomly selected and reviewed by two expert community health nurses. Tables 21.10 and 21.11 list the nursing diagnoses with high and low rates of agreement between the experts. Table 21.12 lists those nursing diagnoses not found in client records.

Of the 95 nursing diagnoses identified by the experts, 26 were not related to a medical diagnosis. Additionally, there were 27 medical diagnoses listed that were not nursing diagnoses. The overall rate of agreement between the judges in locating client health problems was 73%. Some of the variance could be accounted for by each judge placing a client health problem in a different nursing diagnostic category. Three client records were randomly selected and subjected to intrarater reliability, with an overall rate of .92.

TABLE 21.10 Identified Nursing Diagnoses with High Percentage of Agreement for Major Categories (N = 25)

Diagnoses	%	No. of Cases
Anxiety	75	4
Bowel elimination, alerations in	100	5
Cardiac output, alterations in	92	13
Comfort, alteration in	88	8
Communications, impaired	100	2
Family processes, alterations in	100	1
Mobility, impaired physical	77	9
Nutrition, alterations in	73	11
Respiratory function, alterations	100	4
Self-care deficit	100	13
Skin integrity, impairment of	83	12
Urinary elimination, alteration in patterns of	100	7

TABLE 21.11 Identified Nursing Diagnoses with Low Percentage of Agreement for Major Categories (N=25)

Diagnosis	%	No. of Cases
Activity intolerance	0	4
Coping, ineffective	33	3
Fluid volume deficit	1	1
Grieving	0	1
Health maintenance, altteration in	25	4
Injury, potential for	0	2
Ineffective breathing patterns	0	1
Self-concept, disturbance in	0	1
Thought processes, alteration in	0	1
Total		9

TABLE 21.12. Nursing Diagnoses Not Listed in Client Records Reviewed by Two Experts in Community Health Nursing (N = 25)

Diversional activity deficit
Fear
Home maintenance management, impaired
Impaired gas exchange
Ineffective airway clearance
Knowledge deficit
Noncompliance
Oral mucous membranes, alterations in
Parenting, alterations in
Powerlessness
Rape trauma syndrome
Sensory-perceptual alterations
Sexual dysfunction
Sleep pattern disturbance
Alterations in tissue perfusion
Social isolation
Spiritual distress
Violence, potential for

SUMMARY OF FINDINGS

Although the sample size was small and applied to one agency, the great majority of the diagnoses were rated by staff nurses, directors, and faculty as (1) relevant to home health clientele and (2) recorded in agency records. There appeared to be three categories of client problems amenable to services by health care providers and documented in client records: nursing diagnoses, collaborative diagnoses (nursing and other health care provides), and medical diagnoses.

Based on the preliminary screening of the data, the conceptual model for applying the nursing diagnosis classification system to home health care appeared to fit. These findings spoke to two of the related specific questions in the inquiry.

The major research question – "To what extent can quality of nursing care be measured by an instrument that is derived from specific patient outcomes or goals related to the nursing diagnosis classification system of client health problems?" – was rated by staff nurses as appropriate to their practice. An audit of client records found that goals for clients were recorded initially, but they were not always related to specific nursing diagnoses. Flow sheets recording each visit and the client's progress did not document the client's progress toward the goal but rather recorded the implementation of the nursing care plan. Thus, the flow sheets reflected mean standards rather than end standards.

It is likely that the selection of client records currently receiving care rather than discharged-from-service records was in error. However, it would be hoped that a few of the initial client short-term goals would be met during the delivery of services. The current-client records reflected process evaluation. Discharged records might have provided the product evaluation data measuring the positive or negative outcomes of care.

INTERPRETATIONS AND IMPLICATIONS

For this study, the nursing diagnosis classification system applied to clients receiving home health care. There were three types of health care problems: collaborative (with other care providers), medical, or uniquely nursing diagnoses (Carpenito, 1984).

Nursing directors and staff indicated that some of the diagnostic categories were not applicable. The audit verified their statement. Further study is indicated, since many categories logically apply to client health situations, such as "sexual dysfunction related to loss of a body part" or "spiritual distress related to the loss of a loved one." Other diagnoses probably do not apply as often in home health care agencies such as "rape trauma syndrome" or "parenting, alteration in." Additional study is indicated to identify the more common categories and from them studies should be conducted to identify standards of care. Each nursing diagnosis could be subjected to analysis for its underlying dimensions relative to client, nurse, and health care system characteristics.

These types of studies cannot take place until the great majority of health care agencies adopt the nursing diagnosis classification system. A review of the literature and contact with administrators of agencies indicate that this is happening with greater frequency. Agencies are beginning to computerize the classification system, which includes assessment criteria, nursing care plans, standards of care, and client outcomes (e.g., Crosley et al., 1985).

If agencies were to adopt the system, this study's tool to measure client outcomes could be utilized for audit of clients' records. According to the participants in this study, all of the categories listed in the tool applied except "Outcome Applied to Diagnosis," "Diagnosis Did Not Apply," "Expected Outcome Deadline," and "Time Lapse." It is advised that these categories be eliminated from the tool except for the last item, "Time Lapse." It is possible to collect the length of time from initial diagnosis to resolution of the problem from records. Future use of the tool should include a larger sample and further reliability and validity studies. One of its advantages is the short length of time for collecting data. In this preliminary study, it took two researchers $1 \frac{1}{2}$ hrs to review 25 client records. A guidebook that further describes and explains the tools categories also should be developed.

REFERENCES

Albany Visiting Nurse Association. (1982). *Patient classification / objectives system – what is it?* (Unpublished Orientation Material: #490, #492, #493, #494, #495)

Atwood, J. R. (1980). A research perspective. *Nursing Research, 29*(2), 105-108.

Carpenito, L. J. (1983). *Nursing diagnosis application to clinical practice.* Philadelphia: J. B. Lippincott.

Carpenito, L. J. (1984a). *Handbook of nursing diagnosis.* Philadelphia. J. B. Lippincott.

Carpenito, L. J. (1984b). Is the problem a nursing diagnosis? *American Journal of Nursing, 11,* 1418-1419.

Crosley, J. M., Bizzaro, C. A., Brooks, C. A., Fink, L. F., Foger, R. S., Graison-Smith, B. A., Molloy, D. E., & O'Brien, J. M. (1985). *Computerized nursing care planning. Utilizing nursing diagnosis: A handbook.* Washington, DC: Oryn.

Florida Association of Home Health Care Agencies. (1980). *Quality assurance program* (2nd ed.) Author.

Gordon, M. (1980). Determining study topics. *Nursing Research, 29*(2), 83-87.

Gordon, M. (1982). *Manual of nursing diagnosis.* New York: McGraw Hill.

Horn, B. J. (1980). Establishing valid and reliable criteria: A researcher's perspective. *Nursing Research, 29*(2), 88-90.

Kim, J. M., & Moritz, S. (1982). *Classification of nursing diagnoses: Proceedings of the third and fourth national conferences.* New York: McGraw-Hill.

Krueger, J. C. (1980). Establishing priorities for evaluation and evaluation research: A nursing perspective. *Nursing Research, 29*(2), 115-118.

Section of the Public Health Nursing Minnesota Department of Health. (1983). *Outcome criteria: public health nursing services and home health care services.*

Nie, N. H., Hull, H. C., Jenkins, T. G., Steinbrenner, K., & Brent, D. H., (1975). *Statistical package for the social sciences* (2nd ed.). New York: McGraw-Hill.

Pennsylvania Assembly of Home Health Agencies. (1975). *Quality assurance in home health care.* Camp Hill, PA: Author.

Phaneuf, M. C., (1973). Quality assurance: A nursing view. *Hospitals, 47,* 62-68.

Stufflebeam, D. L. (1974). In W. J. Popham (Ed.), *Evaluation in education.* (pp. 116-123) Los Angeles: McCutchen.

Visiting Nurse Association of Omaha. (1980). *A Classification scheme for client problems in community health nursing* (DHHS Publication No. HRA 80-16). Washington DC: U.S. Department of Commerce, National Technical Information Service.

Waltz, C. F., Strickland, O. L., & Lenz, E. R. (1984). *Measurement in nursing research.* Philadelphia: F. A. Davis.

Ward, M. J., & Lindeman, C. A. (Eds.). (1978). *Instruments for measuring nurse practice and other health care variables* (Vols. 1-2). Washington, DC: U.S. Department of Health, Education and Welfare.

22

A Measure of Nursing Outcomes for Home Health Care

Janet I. Feldman and Robert J. Richard

This chapter discusses an Episode Coding Form for evaluating nursing outcomes in home health care agencies.

PURPOSE AND BACKGROUND

Although the discipline of nursing has at least a 30-year history of research devoted to problems, issues, and concern with the allocation of nursing services, there are still questions of quality, productivity, and care outcomes. The goal of this work, part of a larger study of home health care, was to develop quantitative measures of the nursing care status of elderly patients at the beginning and again at the end of episodes of home care. The result is a patient classification method based on nursing diagnosis-like statements. An overall classification score reflects both the number of nursing problems/diagnoses unresolved at the end of an episode of care and the difficulty of remaining at home with such problems. It summarizes scores in four major problem areas, which in turn includes a total of 22 subscale scores.

A definition of patient/nursing care outcomes may be found in *Health Care at Home: An Essential Component of National Health Policy* (American Nurses Association, 1978): "Outcomes are measures of alteration in health status. For the patient, an outcome criterion would be a measurable change in the state of his/her health. Outcomes may be positive or negative and are the ultimate indicators of quality care" (p. 13). According to Rowland and Rowland (1980) such criteria for health care outcomes have been fairly well agreed on and thus are attractive because of face validity. The first step in the development of the classification score for an outcome measure was a computerized literature search. The review revealed that studies concerned with nursing outcomes were infrequent. However, there were a number of studies from disciplines other than nursing concerned with care outcomes (Appelbaum, Seidl, & Austin,

1980; Blenkner, Bloom, & Neilsen, 1971; Eggert, Bowlyow, & Nichols, 1980; Groth-Junker, Zimmer, McKuskey, & Williams, 1983; Hughes, 1982; Hunt & Crichton, 1977; Katz, Ford, Downs, Adams, & Rusby, 1972; Kraus & Armstrong, 1977; Malcom & Higgins, 1983; Nielsen, Blenkner, Bloom, Downs, & Begg, 1972; Wan, Weissert, & Livieratos, 1980).

In addition, 28 community health evaluation research studies were identified by Highriter (1977). Twenty-one of these studies used patient outcomes as evaluation indicators, but only a few nursing outcome studies were related to home health care (Daubert, 1979; Decker, Stevens, Vancini, & Wedcking, 1979; Flett, Last, & Lynch, 1980; Gibbon & Stevens, 1978; Kodadek, 1976; Stone, Patterson, & Felson, 1968; Waller & Davis, 1972).

The care outcome studies done by disciplines other than nursing indicates positive changes overall when social/health care interventions were attempted with elderly patients, but these interventions were reported as expensive. In the final analysis, the causes for patient improvement were not clearly related to specific interventions. Nursing outcome studies reported substantially the same conclusions. The findings were mixed or inconclusive as to the direct relationship of the nursing care and its influence on the outcome of the patient's status. This literature did support the premise that nursing care has positive influence on patient care outcomes.

Only two reports of classification systems were found that assessed patients for home health care. The first was a method used by Daubert (1979) in a nursing outcome study. The second classified the patient's functional status for the purpose of determining the need for nursing resources (Fortinsky, Granger, & Seltzer, 1981).

Giovannetti (1978) stated that there were no patient calssification systems in general use in community health nursing as late as 1978. Simmons (1980) developed a classification scheme that provided a uniform nomenclature for identifying client problems in community nursing. The statements used by Simmons closely resembled those used by Daubert (1979). They were obvious precursors for what since has become nursing diagnostic statements (Gordon, 1982). Indeed, Simmons (1980) stated that her problem statements resembled nursing diagnoses and that work was ongoing to transform this scheme into a method for assessing nursing outcomes. The Simmons format and conceptual framework were chosen for this study to measure nursing care outcomes. Simmons describes this classification scheme as

> ...an orderly arrangement of a nonexhaustive list of patient problems diagnosed by nurses in a community health setting ... subdivided into four major domains each including the names of problems identified in each domain ... modifiers of the problems and signs and symptoms of the problems ... The four major domains of classification scheme represent broad areas of patient problems which are addressed by the community health nurse. The four domains are environmental, psycho-social, physiological and health behav-

iors. The patient problems are grouped within these four major domains. Problems are described by a cluster of signs and symptoms which are listed beneath each problem in the scheme. The signs or symptoms are general statements which condense more specific information about the patient. (p. 6)

This description of the classification scheme indicated several factors that made it attractive as a basis for data collection and coding for this study. These factors were as follows:

1. It was the only scheme developed specifically for community/home health nursing by 1980.
2. The materials describing the development of the scheme indicated that it had been developed with the idea that it might be useful for identifying nursing care outcomes (Simmons, 1980).
3. The language used to state the patient problems/needs was that which has since been adapted with few changes to standardized statements for nursing diagnoses (Gordon, 1982; Simmons, 1980). This meant that the scheme was more than a patient problem/need list but an organization of common nursing diagnoses found in community health nursing practice. This made it, in the opinion of the researchers, all the more suitable as a base for a patient classification method as well as adaptable for future work.
4. This scheme easily adapted to use with computer information systems (Simmons, 1980).
5. The scheme had been derived empirically from the actual practices of community health nursing and field-tested numerous times.
6. This scheme conceptualized classification in a multidimensional hierarchical manner that captured relationships among domains and subdomains of the patient's nursing care status.

These considerations provided a specific rationale for using this particular scheme. It (with several modifications) was used to develop a rudimentary patient classification method for home health patients aged 65 and older.

METHOD AND RESULTS

Data were obtained from closed patient care records of 12 home care agencies in one midwestern state. The agencies represented one each of four ownership groups (not for profit, proprietary, hospital-based, and health department) in three locations (rural, suburban, and small city). The 436 cases reviewed were a 10% random sample of the unduplicated censuses of the 12 agencies. Patients under age 65 were excluded. The data included the standard demographic information for the patients as well as items describing the independency level and problems, and needs at the beginning and end of each episode of care during the study year. There was a total of 528 care episodes for the 436 patients.

An edited version of the Simmons (1980) problem list was used to abstract and then code each patient's status and situation at the beginning and end of each episode of care. Three adjustments were made to adapt and edit the problem list for the coding. First, those items that did not pertain to patients over age 65 were deleted. This reduced the problem/ nursing diagnoses list to 199 items. Second, this list was given to a panel of three experts who weighted them by making a judgment on each individual item in relation to the question; How serious is this problem for an older individual in relation to his/her ability to function at home? The weights that the panel was asked to use were: 1 equals not very serious; 2 equals moderately serious; and 3 equals very serious.

The three nursing experts who assisted in this included two Ph.D.-prepared nurses and a master's-prepared nurse clinical specialist in gerontological nursing. One of the doctorally prepared nurses had extensive background in anatomy and has done clinical work and teaching in gerontological nursing and research in gerontological microanatomy. The master's-prepared nurse has worked with gerontological patients for the past 5 years and was currently an instructor of gerontological nursing in a university setting.

An analysis was done to ascertain how often the three panel members agreed or disagreed on the weights for individual items. The results were that the three nurses assigned the same weight to 58 items (29%). For 126 items (63%), two of three nurses assigned the same weight; and 15 items (8%) were weighted differently by the three nurses. Overall for 184 of the 199 items (92%), two out of the three nurses or all three nurses agreed as to the weight to be assigned to the items. This high level of agreement as to the weight, or seriousness, of the particular problem/ nursing diagnosis of an elderly individual's functional status at home provided some additional assurance that the items did in fact reflect the problems and/or needs of a home health patient and that the problem classification scheme could be used with the weights as a patient classification method suitable for the purposes of the larger study. These assigned weights were averaged for each of the items.

Unfortunately, 199 statements were still too many for data analysis. The weighted statements were reviewed two more times with additional criteria in mind: (1) how frequently, in the opinion of the researchers, had this statement appeared during data collection; (2) what subtlety of information would be lost if a statement were combined or subsumed into a higher level descriptor; (3) would it really matter if the more detailed descriptor was subsumed; and (4) was it urgent that this particular level of detail be represented in this study or that this particular need/problem be at a fine level of detail. The result was a final total of 111 items. These items were assigned either the original weights or, when the statements were subsumed or adapted into more general descriptors, the average weights. A single data collector was used.

These adaptations of the original Simmons problem list were pilot tested. The total average time to abstract a single home care record was less than 20 min, while the time to abstract a single episode of care (start and end) averaged about 10 min. The admission visit and two subsequent visits were abstracted for the start classification data, and the last or discharge visit and two prior visits were used for the end classification data. Each episode of care was coded separately. If a patient had had one episode of care during the fiscal year, then one such coding form was completed. If the patient had had five episodes of care during the fiscal year, then five episode forms were completed. The 111 need/problem statements were answered either yes (1) or no (0).

The category of "unknown" was subsumed into the no answer, or 0. This coding decision masked an important issue for this retrospective record review: whether or not the original records might be a reliable and valid picture of the patient and the health care provided. Usually, the category "unknown" has meant that there was no possible way to find this particular information at the agency. In this instance, due to the coding decision, it was categorized as no. In other words, a presumption was made that if the problem was not noted, charted, or indicated in some way on the chart, it in fact did not exist. As there was no way to check such an existence, it was perceived as the only reasonable position. In contrast to "unknown," missing data (code 8) represented the data collector's own field coding and data collection errors. Thus, where 8 had to be coded, it was in no way a reflection on the agency's records.

In addition, a format to assess the agency records was devised as a method to alleviate a concern in regard to the adequacy of the records used as a data source. The form was filled out at the completion of the data collection period in the agency. In essence, the form listed those factors, components, and issues that a basic nursing text (Wolff et al., 1979) indicated as fundamental to adequate, appropriate, and legally correct charting in any health care agency. A general ranking of the agencies in relation to the adequacy, convenience, and correctness of their records, as assessed by a nonemployee health professional, indicated that three could be categorized as superior, six very good, and three fair. None of the original sample agencies had to be replaced because of poor records.

The next step was the formation of a linear scale by summing the weighted responses. First, each item as coded (0 = no; 1 = yes) was multiplied by the assigned weight to obtain the item value. Second, all of the item values for each of the subscales were summed to obtain the subscale values. Third, all subscale totals were summed for each major scale value. Finally, the major scale values were summed to produce the classification score for either the beginning or the end of a case episode.

The goal was the development of an overall patient classification index that would be applicable at both the beginning and the end of a care episode. The 111 items were organized into a hierarchy of subscales using the framework from the Simmons (1980) study. The resulting four scales for the classification index reflected the original conceptual framework: environment, psychosocial, physiological, and health behaviors. Table 22.1 includes the item assignments and weights for the index.

This overall index (PTCLASS) required several steps as intermediate subscales were formed due to the large number of items involved. The final PTCLASS index was made up of the four scales. These were devised by combining 22 subscales based on the original 111 items. One of the major scales, Environment, did not require the formation of subscales as there were only a few items. Using the *Statistical Package for the Social Science* (SPSS) (Nie, Hull, Jenkins, Steinbrenner, & Bent, 1970) programs, Pearson's correlations were obtained for each of the initial 22 subscales and the four major scales. The correlations were reviewed, and where the researchers felt that some improvement in the *r* could be obtained, items were reassigned. No items were dropped from the subscales.

Lower correlations were found when there were scales that included items that were conceptually related from a nursing point of view but the origin of which reflected different disciplines. This was not unanticipated, as a number of authors and researchers reporting on the development of patient classification systems described this and similar problems (Chagon, Audette, Lebrun, & Tiliquin, 1978; Connor, 1964; Des Orneaux, 1977; Leatt, Kyuns, & Stinson, 1981; McPhail, 1975; Overton, Harrison, & Stinson, 1977; Parker & Boyd, 1974; Plumner, 1976; Roehrl, 1979; Tilquin, 1976; Trivedi, 1979). In general, the subscales with a strong biophysical orientation had higher interitem correlations than those concerned with psychosocial factors.

Then the PTCLASS index was tested for reliability. For this correlational analysis, the data of 528 episodes of care from all 12 agencies were used. This was done because the original frequency distributions for each of the 111 items indicated that with a few exceptions, the yes responses were under 25% per item. Thus, it seemed unlikely that any one or even two of the agencies would provide enough responses for analysis. The goals were to build a single scale with internal consistency appropriate to the hierarchial framework used and to identify, insofar as time and money permitted, multiple item indicators for each subscale of each subdomain. Since neither stability nor equivalence were design issues, the coefficient alpha (Cronbach's alpha) was the method used to determine reliability. An SPSS program was used. To accomplish this, the various subscale totals were used as the variables to test the reliability of the major scales. Table 22.2 presents these reliability coefficients. It is to be noted that the reliability coefficients reported represent major scales created from subscales used as items versus the alternative of major scales made from the individual 111 items.

TABLE 22.1 Subscale Item Assignment and Weights for Patient Classification Scale

Scale	Weight
Environment	
Income deficit	2.33
Sanitation deficit	2.25
Residence safety hazard	2.06
Psychosocial	
Subscale: Maladaptive Behaviors, Grief	
Language barrier/dissatisfied with services	1.33
Social isolation	1.58
Suspicious behavior pattern	1.66
Compulsive behavior pattern	1.33
Role change	1.11
Interpersonal conflict	1.83
Grief	1.40
Subscale: Confusion	
Confusion: attention span	1.60
Confusion: time, place, person	2.33
Confusion: forgetfulness	1.33
Subscale: Depression	
Feeling of hopelessness/worthlessness	2.00
Excessive inward focus	2.00
Expresses wish to die	1.66
Fails to meet personal needs	2.00
Subscale: Anxiety, Caretaking	
Feeling of apprehension	1.66
Irritable	1.33
Much purposeless activity	1.33
Lacks caretaking skills	2.66
Lacks consistent routine for caretaking	2.00
Neglect	1.90
Abuse	2.05
Behavior inappropriate for age	1.33
Physiological	
Subscale: Sensory, Communication	
Hearing impairment	1.41
Vision impairment	1.52
Lacks ability to speak	2.00
Inability to understand	2.66
Relies on nonverbal communication	2.00
Dentition impairment	2.00
Subscale: Respiratory	
Abnormal breath patterns (SOB/dyspnea)	1.66
Cough	1.00
Cyanosis	2.33
Noisy respiration	2.00
Rhinorrhea	1.00
Abnormal breath sounds	2.00

cont.

TABLE 22.1 *(continued)*

Subscale: Circulatory	
Edema	2.00
Cramping/pain in extremities	2.00
Decreases pulses	2.66
Discoloration of skin/cyanosis	2.33
Temperature change in affected areas	2.00
Varicosities	1.00
Fainting/syncopal episodes	3.00
Abnormal blood pressure	1.66
Pulse deficit	2.00
Irregular heart rate	1.66
Excessive rapid/slow heart rate	2.00
Reports anginal pain	3.00
Abnormal heart sounds	1.66
Subscale: Mobility, Muscoloskeletal	
Limited ROM/contractures	1.33
Poor coordination	2.00
Gait/ambulation disturbance	2.00
Decreased muscle strength/muscle tightness	1.66
Inability to manage ADL	3.00
Tremors	2.00
Subscale: Gastrointestinal	
Nausea/vomiting	3.00
Difficulty chewing/swallowing	2.33
Indigestion/heartburn	1.66
Anorexia	2.33
Anemia	2.00
Abnormal weight loss	2.66
Subscale: Life-style	
Inability to cope with body changes	1.83
Life-style incongruent with physiological changes	1.83
Subscale: Bowel	
Diarrhea	2.66
Constipation	1.66
Pain with defecation	1.66
Minimal bowel sounds	1.66
Blood in stool	2.66
Abnormal colon	2.33
Cramping/abdominal discomfort	2.00
Increased frequency of stools	1.66
Incontinent of stools	2.66
Subscale: Bladder	
Incontinent of urine	2.66
Urgency/frequency	2.00
Burning/painful urination	1.66
Inability to empty bladder	2.33
Nocturia	1.66
Polyuria	2.00
Oliguria	2.00
Hematuria	2.66
Subscale: Skin	
Lesion (wound/burn/incision)	2.00
Rash	1.66

cont.

TABLE 22.1 *(continued)*

Inflammation	2.00
Drainage	2.33
Subscale: Pain	
Pain: client statement	2.33
Pain: elevated pulse, respiration, BP	2.33
Pain: compensatory movement	2.33
Pain: pallor, sweating	2.66
Lacks response to normal stimuli	3.00
Health Behaviors	
Subscale: Nutrition	
Abnormal intake of essential food/fluids	2.00
Emaciated/obese	2.33
Subscale: Sleep	
Awakens frequently	1.00
Insufficient rest/sleep	2.33
Subscale: Lifestyle/Personal Hygiene	
Sedentary life-style	1.33
Inappropriate exercise	2.00
Personal hygiene deficit	1.44
Substance misuses	2.83
Subscale: Compliance, Knowledge, Weight Skill	
Noncompliance with medical visits	1.58
Noncompliance with Rx	1.66
Fails to obtain necessary equipment	1.66
Deviates from prescribed dosage	2.33
Lacks system for taking medication	2.00
Medications improperly stored	3.00
Does not obtain med refills	2.00
Unable to integrate diet into balanced nutrition	2.00
Does not adhere to diet Rx	1.66
Unable to demonstrate/relate procedure accurately	2.00
Requires nursing skill	2.33
Unable to perform procedure without assistance	2.66
Unable to operate special equipment properly	2.66

The reliability coefficient of the PTCLASS index was a Cronbach's alpha of .48. Again, this index was created from the four major scale totals rather than the individual items. The interpretation was that the index was moderately reliable, as alpha values of .70 to .89 or higher are indicative of reliable scales. Face validity of the index was assumed, as it was conceptually based on previous works where this issue had been addressed and tested (Simmons, 1980).

Next, separate PTCLASS scales were defined for each episode of care at two points in time. The Start Patient Classification, SPTCLASS, used the data that described patient care/nursing needs at the beginning of an episode of care, and the End Patient Classification, EPTCLASS, used identically weighted items to describe the patient care nursing needs and problems unresolved and or identifiable at the end of each episode of home care. These two scales were also tested for reliability: EPTCLASS obtained a Cronbach's alpha of .55; SPTCLASS an alpha of .48. The two linear scales, SPTCLASS and EPTCLASS, were then used to assess the aggregated episode data of each of the 12 home health agencies.

Mean SPTCLASS and EPTCLASS scores were defined for each home health agency. These mean scores represented the average nursing care problems and/or nursing diagnoses and needs at the beginning and end of an episode of care for the subject-patients of each agency. A high numerical score indicated many nursing problems and therefore a high need for nursing care. Paired *t*-tests were used to compare the start and the classification mean scores for each agency.

The null hypothesis was that no difference between the start classification score and the end classification score for each of the 12 agencies would be found. The results of the paired *t*-tests were that the null hypothesis had to be rejected 11 out of 12 times (*p* = .05). These results indicated there were statistically significant differences between start and end classification scores for all but one agency. This agency had an end classification mean score that was higher than the start classification mean score. This was an agency that had a high recidivism rate to the hospital. Table 22.3 presents the sample size, mean, and standard deviation for the two classification mean scores and *t*-value of the 12 agencies.

TABLE 22.2 Reliability Coefficients (Cronbach's alpha) for Start and End Major Scales

Major scale	alpha (start)	alpha (end)
Environment	.56	.70
Psychosocial	.46	.63
Physiological	.39	.65
Health Behaviors	.24	.40

TABLE 22.3 Paired *t*-tests for Agency Start and End Classification Mean Scores

Agency	N	M (start)	SD (start)	M (end)	SD (end)	t
1	61	25.858	13.027	17.232	16.968	4.56*
2	22	7.196	4.157	4.385	5.885	3.16*
3	37	15.042	11.421	15.461	14.968	−.30
4	77	19.427	12.621	12.029	13.487	4.42*
5	115	16.218	9.522	9.714	13.931	6.39*
6	40	16.786	6.672	8.032	7.916	5.71*
7	16	22.099	12.279	3.788	6.889	5.30*
8	61	14.829	6.830	5.647	8.784	7.84*
9	64	22.522	12.793	11.792	14.778	7.21*
10	10	20.292	5.147	5.805	5.466	6.70*
11	10	20.357	7.267	7.111	6.825	4.35*
12	15	23.101	11.389	7.088	10.206	4.39*

*p = .05

CONCLUSION

The conclusions reached regarding this method for measuring nursing care outcomes were the following:

1. The patient classification methods themselves were moderately reliable. The end classification score was more reliable than the start classification score.
2. The reliability for the subscales was not as high as it might have been. The psychosocial items included in several of the subscales caused problems and difficulties in achieving good internal consistency. The psychosocial items fit the scales in terms of nursing concepts but did not foster statistical reliability. The problem with psychosocial items was not unusual, as it had been noted by Connor (1964) when the first patient classification systems were developed.
3. The trend for 11 of the 12 agencies was that the end classification mean scores were lower than the start classification mean scores for this sample. (This was interpreted to mean that the subjects had on average fewer nursing care problems at the end of an episode of home care than at the beginning.)
4. Using these measures, a statistical difference was demonstrable between the beginning and end of an episode of home care for elderly patients.
5. The end classification mean scores could be considered as an indicator of care outcomes for home care at an agency level.
6. Additional refinements were needed for the subscales and for the start and end indices, including additional revisions and field testing.

These refinements should include using fewer items to achieve the same or improved reliability coefficients, or at minimum, another review of the present correlation coefficients.

Revision of the subscales might include the reassignment of items, the addition and/or deletion of items to update the indices to reflect the current changes in home health care practice, the prospective testing of the patient classification at one or more of the other home care classification systems now emerging. A future field test could also include using the scales on an individual patient basis to assess care outcomes rather than in the aggregate, as was done in this study.

Implications for Nursing

Using statements similar to nursing diagnoses to classify patient care outcomes has not often been attempted. Although considerable refinement would be necessary, this approach affords both a method for interagency comparisons and for addressing workload and staffing issues for home care. Indeed, the PTCLASS index has been used to study the effects of agency ownership, location, and nurse staffing patterns of care outcomes (Feldman & Richard, 1985). Different nursing approaches to meeting the care needs resulting from the various nursing diagnoses might also be evaluated across agencies. An example would be to obtain mean end classification scores for groups of patients with various nursing diagnoses, medical diagnoses, or functional status levels, which could be compared and contrasted across home care agencies. Ultimately, a standardized formative evaluation based on nursing diagnostic problem statements might emerge. Also, the outcome measures could be combined with data about home care visits and episodes of care patterns to determine workload and staffing for home care. The related management issues of providing safe and effective care and for controlling productivity might also be addressed through the use of this method. Finally, this approach would encourage the professional practice of nursing through the application of nursing diagnoses in home care documentation.

REFERENCES

American Nurses' Association. (1978). *Health care at home: An essential component of a national health policy.* Kansas City, MO: Author.

Appelbaum, R., Seidi, F. W., & Austin, C. D. (1980). The Wisconsin community care organization: Preliminary findings from the Milwaukee experiment. *The Gerontologist, 20,* 350-355.

Blenkner, M., Bloom, M., & Nielsen, M. (1971). A research and demonstration project of protective services. *Social Caseworker, 52,* 483-499.

Chagon, M., Audette, L. M., Lebrun, L., & Tilquin, C. (1978). A patient classification system by level of nursing care required. *Nursing Research, 27,* 103-113.

Connor, R. H. (1964). Hospital inpatient classification system. *Dissertation Abstracts International,* 183364. (University Microfilms No. 60-3319).

Daubert, E. A. (1979). Patient classification system and outcome criteria. *Nursing Outlook, 27,* 450-454.

Decker, F., Stevens, L., Vancini, M., & Wedeking, L. (1979). Using patient outcomes to evaluate community health nursing. *Nursing Outlook, 27,* 278-282.

Des Ormeaux, S. P. (1977). Implementation of the C.A.S.H. patient classification system for staffing determination. *Supervisor Nurse, 8*(4), 29-35.

Eggert, G. M., Bowlyow, E. J., & Nichols, C. W. (1980). Gaining control of the long-term care system: First returns from the ACCESS experiment. *The Gerontologist, 20,* 356-363.

Feldman, J., & Richard, R. J. (1985, May). *The relationship between home health nurse staffing patterns and care outcomes.* Poster presented at the Fourteenth Annual Center for Nursing Research Spring Research Symposium, Ohio State University, Columbus, OH.

Flett, D. E., Last, J. M., & Lynch, G. W. (1980). Evaluation of the public health nurse as a primary health-care provider for elderly people. In V. W. Marshall (Ed.), *Aging in Canada: Social perspectives* (pp. 177-188). Toronto: Fitzhenny & Whiteside.

Fortinksy, R. H., Granger, C. V., & Seltzer, G. B. (1981). The use of functional assessment in understanding home care needs. *Medical Care, 19,* 489-497.

Gibbon, M., & Stevens, E. (1978). Nurse influence on the quality of life of elderly patients with chronic illness. In *Proceedings of the Fifth Annual Ontario Psychogeriatric Association* (pp. 15-20).

Giovannetti, P. (1978). *Patient classification systems in nursing: A description and analysis* (DHEW Publication No. HRA 78022). Washington DC: U.S. Government Printing Office.

Gordon, M. (1982). *Manual of nursing diagnosis*. New York: McGraw-Hill.

Groth-Junker, A., Zimmer, J., McKuskey, J., & Williams, T. F. (1983, April). Home health care team, randomized trial of new team approach to home care. *Research Activities No. 51*. (Available from National Center for Health Services Research, 5600 Fischers Lane, Rockville, MD 20857).

Highriter, M. E. (1977). The status of community health nursing research. *Nursing Research, 26*, 183-192.

Hughes, S. L. (1982). Home health monitoring, ensuring quality in home care services. *Hospitals, Journal of the American Hospital Association, 52*, 74-80.

Hunt, T. E., & Crichton, R. D. (1977). One third of a million days of care at home, 1959 to 1975. *Canadian Medical Association Journal, 116*, 1351-1355.

Katz, S., Ford, A. B., Downs, T. D., Adams, M., & Rusby, D. (1972). *Effects of continued care: A study of chronic illness in the home* (DHEW Publication No. HSM 73-3010). Washington, DC: U.S. Government Printing Office.

Kodadek, S. (Ed.). (1976). *Inventory of innovations in nursing*. Boulder, CO: Western Interstate Commission for Higher Education.

Kraus, A. S., & Armstrong, M. I. (1977). Effect of chronic home care on admission to institutions providing long-term care. *Canadian Medical Association Journal, 117*, 747-749.

Leatt, P., Kyung, S. B., & Stinson, S. M. (1981). An instrument for assessing and classifying patients by types of care. *Nursing Research, 30*, 145-150.

Malcom, L. A., & Higgins, C. S. (1983). A study of recipients of district nursing services in Christchurch. *New Zealand Medical Journal, 96*, 763-765.

McPhail, A. (1975). The meaning of patient classification. *Dimensions in Health Services, 52*(6), 30-39.

Nie, N. H., Hull, C. H., Jenkins, J. G., Steinbrenner, K., & Bent, D. H. (1970). *Statistical package for the social sciences* (2nd ed.). New York: McGraw-Hill.

Nielsen, M., Blenkner, M., Bloom, M., Downs, T., & Beggs, H. (1972). Older persons after hospitalization: A controlled study of home aids services. *American Journal of Public Health, 62*, 1094-1101.

Overton, P., Harrison, F., & Stinson, S. (1977). Patient classification by types of care. *Dimensions in Health Services, 54*(8), 27-30.

Parker, R., & Boyd, J. (1974). A comparison of a discriminant versus a clustering analysis of patient classification for chronic disease care. *Medical Care, 12*, 944-957.

Plummer, J. (1976). Patient classification proves staffing needs. *Dimensions in Health Services, 53*(5), 36-38.

Roehrl, P. K. (1979). Patient classification, a pilot test. *Supervisor Nurse, 10*(2), 21-27.

Rowland, H. S., & Rowland, B. L. (1980). *Nursing Administration Handbook*. Germantown, MD: Aspen Systems.

Simmons, D. A. (1980). *A classification scheme for client problems in community health nursing* (DHHS Publication No. HRA 8016). Washington DC: U.S. Government Printing Office.

Stone, J. R., Patterson, E., & Felson, L. (1968). The effectiveness of home care for general hospital patients. *Journal of the American Medical Association, 205*, 716-719.

Tilquin, C. (1976). Patient classification does work. *Dimensions in Health Services, 53*(1), 12-16.

Trivedi, V. M. (1979). Nursing judgement in selection of patient classification variables. *Research in Nursing and Health, 2*(3), 109-118.

Waller, M. V., & Davis, D. J. (1972). Performance profiles based on nursing activity records. *Journal of Nursing Administration, 2*(4), 26-30.

Wan. T. H., Weissert, W. G., & Livieratos, B. B. (1980). Geriatric day care and homemaker services: An experimental study. *Journal of Gerontology, 35,* 256-274.

Wolff, L., Weitzel, M. H., & Fuerst, E. (1979). *Fundamentals of nursing* (6th ed.). J. B. Lippincott.

EPISODE CODING FORM

Begin
Card 1
Agency _____ ID code __ __ 2   /01-03
Patient _____ ID code __ __   /04-05
Episode number __ Card 1   /06-07
(column 08 is left blank)   /08

START OF EPISODE

	Response category					Don't know	Missing data	
Overall dependency	1	2	3	4		7	8	/09
Vision	1	2	3	4		7	8	/10
Hearing (w/aid if used)	1	2	3	4		7	8	/11
Expressive communication	1	2	3	4	5	7	8	/12
Receptive communication	1	2	3	4	5	7	8	/13
Bathing/showering	1	2	3			7	8	/14
Dressing	1	2	3			7	8	/15
Toileting	1	2	3			7	8	/16
Transferring (bed/chair)	1	2	3			7	8	/17
Continence	1	2	3	4		7	8	/18
Eating	1	2	3			7	8	/19
Walking	1	2	3			7	8	/20
Mobility	1	2	3	4		7	8	/21
Adaptive tasks	1	2				7	8	/22
Behavior problems	1	2				7	8	/23
Disorientation/memory impairment	1	2				7	8	/24
Mood disturbance	1	2				7	8	/25

	No	Yes	Missing data	
Income deficit	0	1	8	/26
Sanitation deficit	0	1	8	/27
Residence safety hazard	0	1	8	/28
Language barrier/dissatisfied with services	0	1	8	/29
Social isolation	0	1	8	/30
Suspicious behavior pattern	0	1	8	/31
Compulsive behavior pattern	0	1	8	/32
Role change	0	1	8	/33
Interpersonal conflict	0	1	8	/34
Grief	0	1	8	/35
Confusion: attention span	0	1	8	/36

	No	Yes	MD	
Confusion: time, place, person	0	1	8	/37
Confusion: forgetfulness	0	1	8	/38
Feeling of hopelessness/worthlessness	0	1	8	/39
Excessive inward focus	0	1	8	/40
Expresses wish to die	0	1	8	/41
Fails to meet personal needs	0	1	8	/42
Feeling of apprehension	0	1	8	/43
Irritable	0	1	8	/44
Much purposeless activity	0	1	8	/45
Lacks caretaking skills	0	1	8	/46
Lacks consistent routine for caretaking	0	1	8	/47
Neglect	0	1	8	/48
Abuse	0	1	8	/49
Behavior inappropriate for age	0	1	8	/50
Hearing impairment	0	1	8	/51
Vision impairment	0	1	8	/52
Lacks ability to speak	0	1	8	/53
Inability to understand	0	1	8	/54
Relies on nonverbal communication	0	1	8	/55
Dentition impairment	0	1	8	/56
Abnormal breath patterns (SOB/dyspnea)	0	1	8	/57
Cough	0	1	8	/58
Cyanosis	0	1	8	/59
Noisy respiration	0	1	8	/60
Rhinorrhea	0	1	8	/61
Abnormal breath sounds	0	1	8	/62
Edema	0	1	8	/63
Cramping/pain in extremities	0	1	8	/64
Decreased pulses	0	1	8	/65
Discoloration of skin/cyanosis	0	1	8	/66
Temp. change affected area	0	1	8	/67
Varicosities	0	1	8	/68
Fainting/syncopal episodes	0	1	8	/69
Abnormal blood pressure	0	1	8	/70
Pulse deficit	0	1	8	/71
Irregular heart rate	0	1	8	/72
Excessive rapid/slow heart rate	0	1	8	/73
Reports anginal pain	0	1	8	/74
Abnormal heart sounds	0	1	8	/75
Limited ROM/contractures	0	1	8	/76
Poor coordination	0	1	8	/77
Gait/ambulation disturbance	0	1	8	/78

(column 79 is left blank)   /79
Episode data code E   /80

Begin
Card 2

Agency ID __ __ 2   Patient ID __ __   Episode __ __ 2   /01-07
(column 08 is left blank)   /08

	No	Yes	MD	
Decreased muscle strength/muscle tightness	0	1	8	/09
Inability to manage ADL	0	1	8	/10
Tremors	0	1	8	/11
Nausea/vomiting	0	1	8	/12
Difficulty chewing/swallowing	0	1	8	/13
Indigestion/heartburn	0	1	8	/14
Anorexia	0	1	8	/15
Anemia	0	1	8	/16
Abnormal weight loss	0	1	8	/17
Inability to cope with body changes	0	1	8	/18
Lifestyle incongruent with physiological changes	0	1	8	/19
Diarrhea	0	1	8	/20
Constipation	0	1	8	/21
Pain with defecation	0	1	8	/22
Minimal bowel sounds	0	1	8	/23
Blood in stool	0	1	8	/24
Abnormal colon	0	1	8	/25
Cramping/abdominal discomfort	0	1	8	/26
Increased frequency of stools	0	1	8	/27
Incontinent of stools	0	1	8	/28
Incontinent of urine	0	1	8	/29
Urgency/frequency	0	1	8	/30
Burning/painful urination	0	1	8	/31
Inability to empty bladder	0	1	8	/32
Nocturia	0	1	8	/33
Polyuria	0	1	8	/34
Oliguria	0	1	8	/35
Hematuria	0	1	8	/36
Lesion (wound/burn/incision)	0	1	8	/37
Rash	0	1	8	/38
Inflammation	0	1	8	/39
Drainage	0	1	8	/40
Pain: client statement	0	1	8	/41
Pain: elevated pulse, respiration, BP	0	1	8	/42
Pain: compensatory movement	0	1	8	/43
Pain: pallor, sweating	0	1	8	/44
Lacks response to normal stimuli	0	1	8	/45
Abnormal intake of essential food/fluids	0	1	8	/46
Emaciated/obese	0	1	8	/47
Awakens frequently	0	1	8	/48
Insufficient rest/sleep	0	1	8	/49
Sedentary lifestyle	0	1	8	/50
Inappropriate exercise	0	1	8	/51
Personal hygiene deficit	0	1	8	/52
Substance misuse	0	1	8	/53
Noncompliance with medical visits	0	1	8	/54
Noncompliance with Rx	0	1	8	/55
Fails to obtain necessary equipment	0	1	8	/56
Deviates from prescribed dosage	0	1	8	/57
Lacks system for taking medications	0	1	8	/58

		No	Yes	MD	
Medications improperly stored		0	1	8	/59
Does not obtain med refills		0	1	8	/60
Unable to integrate diet into balanced nutrition		0	1	8	/61
Does not adhere to diet Rx		0	1	8	/62
Unable to demonstrate/relate procedure accurately		0	1	8	/63
Requires nursing skill		0	1	8	/64
Unable to perform procedure without assistance		0	1	8	/65
Unable to operate special equipment correctly		0	1	8	/66

(columns 67-79 are left blank) /67-79

episode data code _E_ /80

Begin
Card 3

Agency ID _ _ 2   Patient ID _ _   Episode _ _ 3   /01-07

(column 08 is left blank) /08

END OF EPISODE

	Response category				DK	MD	
Overall dependency	1	2	3	4	7	8	/09

Length of episode (days) _ _ _ /10-12

Reason for discharge

recovered .... 1 /13
stable condition 2
financial problems 3
acutely ill 4
deceased 5
moved out of area 6
other 7
missing data 8

Disposition at D/C

own care .... 1 /14
family care 2
residential care 3
nursing home 4
hospital 5
moved out of area 6
other services 7
missing data 8

Primary diagnosis _ _ _ /15-17

Second diagnosis _ _ _   Third diagnosis _ _ _ /18-23

(columns 24-25 are left blank) /24-25

	No	Yes	MD	
Income deficit	0	1	8	/26
Sanitation deficit	0	1	8	/27
Residence safety hazard	0	1	8	/28
Language barrier/dissatisfied with services	0	1	8	/29
Social isolation	0	1	8	/30
Suspicious behavior pattern	0	1	8	/31
Compulsive behavior pattern	0	1	8	/32
Role change	0	1	8	/33
Interpersonal conflict	0	1	8	/34
Grief	0	1	8	/35
Confusion/attention span	0	1	8	/36
Confusion/time, place, person	0	1	8	/37
Confusion/forgetfulness	0	1	8	/38
Feeling of hopelessness/worthlessness	0	1	8	/39
Excessive inward focus	0	1	8	/40
Expresses wish to die	0	1	8	/41
Fails to meet personal needs	0	1	8	/42
Feeling of apprehension	0	1	8	/43
Irritable	0	1	8	/44
Much purposeless activity	0	1	8	/45
Lacks caretaking skills	0	1	8	/46
Lacks consistent routine for caretaking	0	1	8	/47
Neglect	0	1	8	/48
Abuse	0	1	8	/49
Behavior inappropriate for age	0	1	8	/50
Hearing impairment	0	1	8	/51
Vision impairment	0	1	8	/52
Lacks ability to speak	0	1	8	/53
Inability to understand	0	1	8	/54
Relies on nonverbal communication	0	1	8	/55
Dentition impairment	0	1	8	/56
Abnormal breath patterns (SOB/dyspnea)	0	1	8	/57
Cough	0	1	8	/58
Cyanosis	0	1	8	/59
Noisy respiration	0	1	8	/60
Rhinorrhea	0	1	8	/61
Abnormal breath sounds	0	1	8	/62
Edema	0	1	8	/63
Cramping/pain in extremities	0	1	8	/64
Decreased pulses	0	1	8	/65
Discoloration of skin/cyanosis	0	1	8	/66
Temp. change affected area	0	1	8	/67
Varicosities	0	1	8	/68
Fainting/syncopal episodes	0	1	8	/69
Abnormal blood pressure	0	1	8	/70
Pulse deficit	0	1	8	/71
Irregular heart rate	0	1	8	/72
Excessive rapid/slow heart rate	0	1	8	/73
Reports anginal pain	0	1	8	/74
Abnormal heart sounds	0	1	8	/75
Limited ROM/contractures	0	1	8	/76

	No	Yes	MD	
Poor coordination	0	1	8	/77
Gait/ambulation disturbance	0	1	8	/78
	(column 79 is left blank)			/79
	Episode data code E			/80

Begin
Card 4

Agency ID _ _ 2   Patient ID _ _   Episode _ _ 4   /01-07
(column 08 is left blank)   /08

	No	Yes	MD	
Decreased muscle strength/muscle tightness	0	1	8	/09
Inability to manage ADL	0	1	8	/10
Tremors	0	1	8	/11
Nausea/vomiting	0	1	8	/12
Difficulty chewing/swallowing	0	1	8	/13
Indigestion/heartburn	0	1	8	/14
Anorexia	0	1	8	/15
Anemia	0	1	8	/16
Abnormal weight loss	0	1	8	/17
Inability to cope with body changes	0	1	8	/18
Lifestyle incongruent whith physiological changes	0	1	8	/19
Diarrhea	0	1	8	/20
Constipation	0	1	8	/21
Pain with defecation	0	1	8	/22
Minimal bowel sounds	0	1	8	/23
Blood in stool	0	1	8	/24
Abnormal colon	0	1	8	/25
Cramping/abdominal discomfort	0	1	8	/26
Increased frequency of stools	0	1	8	/27
Incontinent of stools	0	1	8	/28
Incontinent of urine	0	1	8	/29
Urgency/frequency	0	1	8	/30
Burning/painful urination	0	1	8	/31
Inability to empty bladder	0	1	8	/32
Nocturia	0	1	8	/33
Polyuria	0	1	8	/34
Oliguria	0	1	8	/35
Hematuria	0	1	8	/36
Lesion (wound/burn/incision)	0	1	8	/37
Rash	0	1	8	/38
Inflammation	0	1	8	/39
Drainage	0	1	8	/40
Pain: client statement	0	1	8	/41
Pain: elevated pulse, respiration, BP	0	1	8	/42
Pain: compensatory movement	0	1	8	/43
Pain: pallor, sweating	0	1	8	/44
Lacks response to normal stimuli	0	1	8	/45
Abnormal intake of essential food/fluids	0	1	8	/46
Emaciated/obese	0	1	8	/47

	No	Yes	MD	
Awakens frequently	0	1	8	/48
Insufficient rest/sleep	0	1	8	/49
Sedentary lifestyle	0	1	8	/50
Inappropriate exercise	0	1	8	/51
Personal hygiene deficit	0	1	8	/52
Substance misuse	0	1	8	/53
Noncompliance with medical visits	0	1	8	/54
Noncompliance with Rx	0	1	8	/55
Fails to obtain necessary equipment	0	1	8	/56
Deviates from prescribed dosage	0	1	8	/57
Lacks system for taking medications	0	1	8	/58
Medications improperly stored	0	1	8	/59
Does not obtain med refills	0	1	8	/60
Unable to integrate diet into balanced nutrition	0	1	8	/61
Does not adhere to diet Rx	0	1	8	/62
Unable to demonstrate/relate procedure accurately	0	1	8	/63
Requires nursing skill	0	1	8	/64
Unable to perform procedure without assistance	0	1	8	65
Unable to operate special equipment correctly	0	1	8	/66

(columns 67-79 are left blank) /67-79

episode data code E /80

PART IV
Measuring Quality of Care

23

The Individualized Care Index

Gwen van Servellen

This chapter discusses the Individualized Care Index, a measure of the extent to which nurses individualize their care of patients.

The concept of individualized care is frequently alluded to in professional nursing literature. It is described as both the process by which high levels of quality care and patient satisfaction are achieved and the outcome of primary nursing. Background on the reliability and validity assessments of the Individualized Care Index will be discussed. Further, a specific account of the most recent assessment will be provided. This study was undertaken to establish the discriminate validity of the Individualized Care Index (ICI)-Survey Format. A comparative study of registered nurse responses to the frequency with which they perform individualized care when their units are organized around team, total patient care, or primary nursing modalities was conducted. Finally, implications of the use of the ICI in its present form will be discussed along with indications for future tests of validity and reliability.

CONCEPTUAL BACKGROUND

Individualized nursing care translates all standardized nursing procedures and activities in terms of the unique peculiarity of each patient situation (Marram, Barrett, & Bevis, 1974, 1979). Individualized care can also be said to include patient-centered communicative responses where concern for the patients' thoughts or problems is expressed and a willingness to listen and to stimulate the patients' self-care potential is provided (Chapman, 1977). High levels of individualized nursing care are reported to be both an outcome of a nursing care modality (primary nursing) and the process by which high levels of patient satisfaction and quality care are achieved.

This study was funded in part by an Academic Senate Grant from the University of California, Los Angeles. Recognition is given to Dr. Noel Wheeler, Ph.D., Director of Statistics/Biomathematic Consulting Clinic, and Ms. Sarah Forsythe, M.S., statistician, UCLA, for their assistance in the data analysis.

As early as 1961, individualized approaches to nursing care were advocated (Abdellah, 1961). The essential element of patient-centered nursing care is seen as the individualization of the nursing approach to the patient's needs. "Individualized care" also emerged in descriptions of the nursing process and quality patient care. The purpose of the nursing process is to motivate nurses to think in terms of each individual patient (Yura & Walsh, 1973). Subsequent to these endorsements, it was used in descriptions of patients' bills of rights and was associated with the achievement of quality patient care (Haussmann, Hegyvary, & Newman, 1976; Johnson & Tingey, 1976) and patient satisfaction (Hinshaw, Gerber, Atwood, & Allen, 1983). In addition, the concept is intimately linked with primary nursing, a nursing care modality that has been considered and implemented by large numbers of hospitals both in the United States (Van Servellen, 1980) and overseas (Hegyvary, 1982). In various pilot studies conducted by Marram, Flynn, Abaravich, and Carey (1976) and Van Servellen (1980) it was found that greater numbers of individualized care behaviors (on the part of the nurse) were perceived by patients on primary nursing units compared to those units practicing team and functional nursing. Furthermore, it was suggested that greater levels of individualized care may be a distinguishing facet of this mode of organizing care in a hospital setting.

Instruments to measure individualized care were not to be found in the nursing literature. An extensive review was undertaken to identify measures that related directly or indirectly to the concept. The concepts of personalized care, patient-centered care, and individualized patient care instruction were reviewed, as were the concepts of coordinated care, comprehensive care, and patient-centered assessment. With the exception of the development of the ICI, nothing was found in the way of nurse behavior observational checklists or surveys (interviews or questionnaires) that was a measurement of individualized care. The following is a summation of studies of two related measures that have been used to test the presence of patient-centered individualized care.

The first of these studies is the work of Chapman (1977). Chapman attempted to measure the effects of three different nursing approaches on related postoperative responses of male herniorrhaphy patients. The approaches were categorized as (1) individualized, (2) informative, and (3) routine nursing care approaches to preoperative patients.

Chapman's (1977) "individualized" nursing approach was based on the Type I response in the Social Interaction Inventory (Methuen & Schlotfeldt, 1962) which is reported to denote the most skill in reducing patient stress and promoting patient welfare. Briefly, Methvan and Schlotfeldt (1962) generated a Type I nurse response in differentiating between five prototypical social responses of nurses to patients. A nurse response is judged a Type I reply if it indicates

> ...the nurse's awareness that the person involved is experiencing an unmet
> need or a problem, and conveys a concern to understand the nature of his

difficulty. It encourages verbalization, and conveys a willingness to listen. It seeks to promote reduction of stress experienced by the patient (or family members) and stimulates him to use his own resources in solving his problem. (p. 85)

Methven and Schlotfeldt proposed that Type I responses had the greatest impact in reducing patient anxiety. Chapman indicated that with an individualized approach the nurse "follows the direction of conversation initiated by the patient, indicates cognizance of his interests and expresses a concern to understand the nature of his thoughts or of his problems, conveys a willingness to listen, and stimulates him to use his own resources to their maximal potential" (p. 16).

To evaluate the extent to which the nurse was successful in achieving an individualized care approach, 10 preoperative and 12 postoperative randomly selected tape-recorded investigator-subject interactions were analyzed. Two independent judges, using Chapman's definition of individualized nursing, were reported to indicate a high degree of success by the investigator in administering the prescribed nursing approach. No details are provided as to the specific behaviors or interactions that were used to denote the individualized approach. In addition, no interrater reliability results are reported. It can be presumed that, at best, the results were based on criteria that had face validity. In addition, although the purpose is not explained, Chapman coded the interactions of staff in terms of "instrumental" and/or "expressive" nursing functions. Zelditch (1955) defines instrumental as "task-oriented" and expressive as "person-oriented." Chapman is very vague about the use of these coded interactions but indicates they too were means of judging the interaction introduced by the investigator with the individualized patient group. Rather than continue to fault the investigator for inadequacies in study design, it is important to examine further the adaptability of either the Social Interaction Inventory Type I response or the expressive"/"instrumental" dichotomy in measuring individualized nursing care behaviors.

The University of Minnesota (Anderson & Choi, 1981), in a comparative nursing care study measuring the differences in care delivered under a primary and total patient care modality, utilized the phenomenon of "expressive" nursing functions to depict similarities and differences in nursing interactions with patients on these two types of units. Nurse questionnaires, recorded nurse-patient interactions, medical record audits, and patient questionnaires were evaluated to determine the extent to which certain indicators of expressive nursing functions were present in nurse-patient relationships and documented on the nursing record.

It should be noted that tests for validity and reliability were unspecified in this unpublished report. However, the criteria were deemed sensitive to depicting differences in nursing care with primary and total patient care modalities. The primary nursing units were found to provide higher levels of expressive nursing functions when compared to the total patient care units.

These measures give general directions for the development of an individualized care index that is reliable, valid, and sensitive. Chapman's criteria, although unspecified, provide a global context in which to consider the definition of the concept.

Unfortunately, the criteria are quite general and open to a wide range of interpretation. Although they may be somewhat helpful in evaluating nurse-patient communications, these criteria are not specific enough in their current form to generate reliable measures of individualized care.

Instruments that judge the extent to which nursing care is "expressive" or "nonexpressive" (to use the University of Minnesota researchers' terminology) would seem to be somewhat helpful in measuring individualized care. Expressive nursing care, as was discussed earlier (Anderson & Choi, 1981), is linked with patient-centered care. The study conducted at the University of Minnesota provides some specific criteria on which to judge this phenomenon in nursing practice. Specific behaviors in these instruments parallel those in the ICI. A case in point is the item "Give information to my patients about their illness" (Nurse Questionnaire), which parallels several ICI behaviors, including "Discussing with the patient how his illness will affect him and his family."

These measures have not been adequately tested; a further drawback is the fact that patient-centered care such as that detailed in expressive nursing activities is not synonymous with individualized care. As is detailed later, individualized care, while largely patient-centered, includes specific aspects of coordination and comprehensiveness of care (as well as patient-centered inquiry/communications) not found in descriptions of expressive nursing functions.

The following is an outline of the steps taken over a 2-year period to refine and test the ICI. Included here is a review of the steps that have occurred to date and a detailed discussion of a test of discriminate validity. The issues of validity as well as reliability (measure of internal consistency) are discussed.

DEVELOPMENT OF THE ICI

The first step in designing the measure was to establish a valid definition of the concept. The initial content validity of the ICI was assured by establishing a list of individualized care behaviors by three means: a review of the literature, the input of a panel of judges, and an initial pretest.

An extensive review of the literature dating back to 1960 was conducted. The concept of individualized care, as well as various related phenomena, was explored: patient-centered care, comprehensive care, and coordinated-continuous patient care delivery. It was believed that these concepts may not be independent of one another and may form a cluster of related phenomena.

A panel of judges, which consisted of three graduate faculty and two graduate students, was asked to review a list of nursing care behaviors generated by the researcher and research assistants from the literature. They were asked to complete two tasks: (1) to differentiate those behaviors judged to be individualized care behaviors from irrelevant and bureaucratic care behaviors, and (2) to classify the individualized care items, if they could, according to the following categories: patient-centered care, comprehensive care, coordinated care, and continuity of care. In addition, each member was asked to alter the items to make them clearer and more precise. An analysis of the nursing care behaviors revealed that 64 of 80 individualized care items were judged to be individualized care actions.

This complete list of behaviors was subjected to another validity test, in which a larger group of nurses was asked to judge the items for their representatives. A sample of 41 graduate students who were practicing as part-time staff nurses was asked to rate each item on a 5-point Likert-type scale. They were asked to judge how well each behavior fit their concept of individualized care, with 5 = Strongly agree and 1 = Strongly disagree. Of the initial full 80 nursing care items, 55 were perceived to be individualized care actions with mean scores of 4.0 and above.

INSTRUMENT

The purpose of the ICI-Survey Format is to measure the extent to which nurses individualize their care to their patients. Its subscales allow the researcher to differentiate what categories of individualized care are practiced at greater or lesser frequency.

The ICI-Survey Format consists of two sections; the first section is a set of eleven questions derived from the American Nurses' Association (1981) Inventory of Registered Nurses, aimed at obtaining key demographic information about the respondents. The second section elicits responses about the frequency with which nurses perceive themselves as fulfilling each of 32 nursing actions for their patients. For example, how frequently do you "ask patients what they would like to know about their illness" and "discuss with patients the care that is planned for them while they are in the hospital." Nurses are asked to respond to a 5-Point Likert scale, as follows: "With *none* of my patients" = 1 and "With *all* of my patients" = 5. An additional 13 items were included from the Qualpacs instrument (Wandelt & Ager, 1974) to mask the intent of the questionnaire, which focused heavily on patient-centered interactions of the nurse-patient dyad.

Such items included "Make decisions that reflect knowledge of facts and good judgment" and "Communicate clearly ideas, facts, and concepts about the patient in charting." A social desirability response pattern was expected to influence the respondent's answers. Hinshaw (personal communication, June, 1984) suggests that in relationship to the Measurements of Clinical and Educational Nursing Outcomes Projects, such a subset of quality nursing care items, if included, could mask the intent or essence of the study.

SCORING AND ADMINISTRATION

Procedures for administering the survey include the following steps. The ICI is a survey addressed specifically to registered nurses who deliver direct patient care. The sample of RNs should be identified. The researcher may either survey the behaviors of all RNs on particular nursing units or sample randomly from these units or the hospital as a whole. The ICI can yield an overall estimate of individualized care practices at the unit level or be used to identify weaknesses in the practice of individual nurses. The survey should be administered to staff when on duty, and directions to staff about estimating their practice behaviors should be given. An alternative form of the ICI has been developed that asks the nurse to identify those behaviors performed for a specific patient.

Scoring of the ICI requires the researcher to calculate the mean score and standard deviation for each respondent on each subscale of the ICI as well as on the ICI as a whole. All items are assigned an equal weight. Interpretation of the scores is based on judging scores as "high" or "low" given the average score of the nurse population under study.

RELIABILITY OF THE ICI

Reliability of the ICI was determined by two means: a test-retest measure and a measure of internal consistency.

A test-retest procedure was used with a preliminary pilot test of the instrument. The ICI was administered to 10 students. Reliability of the ICI was established by a test-retest trial in which a correlation coefficient of .86 was found when these students were tested 1 week apart.

A measure of internal consistency of items using Cronbach's alpha was undertaken with a sample of 838 practicing RNs in 18 hospitals. Cronbach's alpha was calculated for each factor in the ICI: patient-centered comprehensive care, patient-centered coordinated care, and patient-centered inquiry/assessment. Cronbach's alpha, calculated from the average interitem correlation, is interpreted as a measure of the reliability of each factor (Carmines & Zeller, 1969, pp. 47-48). The interitem correlations were only moderate: Factor I, .35; Factor II, .56; and Factor III, .49. Each subscale, however, had an acceptable alpha coefficient: Factor I, .85; Factor II, .91; and Factor III, .91. These alpha values indicate good reliability for each factor considered as a sum of ratings for its items.

VALIDITY OF THE ICI

Tests of the validity of the ICI were undertaken with two separate studies: one measuring the construct validity of the ICI; another, its discriminate validity. Particular detailed attention will be given the test of discriminate validity since it represents the latest study utilizing the ICI.

The construct validity of the ICI items was the focus of a study of a large sample of RNs practicing nursing in a hospital setting. The purpose of this study was to employ a factor analytic procedure to identify the specific subdimensions of the ICI. A ratio of 10 respondents for each item set the outer limits for sampling RNs for this phase of the research. The factor analytic procedure was employed to accomplish two things: (1) to reveal the underlying dimensionality of the concept and (2) to provide a valid means of reducing a large set of items to a smaller representative set of indices. The ICI was administered to 838 practicing RNs in 19 randomly selected hospitals.

Because of skew of the distributions of the nursing behavior item ratings, the conventional factor analysis assuming normal distributions is not applicable. Therefore, it was decided to dichotomize the distributions at a value of 4 (> 4 vs. < 4) and to employ Muthen's (1981) two-procedure factor analysis for dichotomous variables. The first procedure is an exploratory factor analysis that enables one to determine the number of factors present and to form hypotheses regarding factor structure. The second procedure is a confirmatory analysis that tests the goodness of fit of a model for which one specifies both the number of factors and the items (nursing behaviors) that have loadings on each of the factors.

Results of the exploratory factor analysis were the following. Of the 80 items (excluding five nonsense items) 44 items were selected most useful to determine subfactors of individualized care. The criterion for selecting these items was that they showed sufficient variability in ratings to provide useful information on subjects' differing perceptions of nursing behavior. Results of the exploratory factory analysis indicated that four factors could be differentiated: a bureaucratic factor and a three-factor individualized care model. The individualized care factors were interpreted and categorized as follows: Factor I: patient-centered comprehensive care; Factor II: patient-centered coordinated care; and Factor III: patient-centered inquiry/assessment.

Table 23.1 presents the factor loadings for those items (behaviors) loading .40 for the confirmed three-factor individualized care model. Two factors loaded >.40 on two factors simultaneously. These items were "Asking the patient if he has any questions about his care" and "Discussing with the patient the care that is planned for him while he is in the hospital."

TABLE 23.1 Individualized Care Index Factor Loadings Within Each Factor (*N* = 838)

Item No.	Item	Patient-centered coordinated care	Patient-centered comprehensive care	Patient-centered inquiry/ assessment
76.	Making sure the patient knows what roles physicians will play in his care	.74	0.0	0.0
79.	Discussing with the dietitian the diet plan for the patient	.73	0.0	−0.12
52.	Asking the patient what his usual daily activities are, including: work, hobbies, and recreation	.59	0.0	0.0
39.	Making sure the patient knows the names of the persons responsible for specific procedures and/or treatements	.56	0.0	0.0
68.	Making sure the patient understands who will be taking care of him	.54	0.11	0.0
44.	Informing the doctor that you are the patient's nurse	.54	0.0	0.0
63.	After completing the nursing assessment, validate with the patient what you have identified as his problem	.50	0.0	0.0
42.	Allowing the patient to set the times for his activities and treatments as much as possible, i.e., bath, medications, bedtime	.48	0.0	0.0
70.	Writing 24-hr nursing orders for the patient on the care plan	.46	0.0	0.0
72.	Asking the patient if he has any questions about his care	.42	.50	0.0
77.	Discussing with the patient the care that is planned for him while he is in the hospital	.41	0.0	0.40
51.	Allowing the patient time to talk about his fears or concerns	0.0	.84	0.16
26.	Meeting with the oncoming shift to discuss the patient's problems	0.0	.76	0.0

cont.

41.	Completing all "hands on" nursing procedures for the patient with skill and sensitivity patient needs	0.0	.65	0.0
34.	Allowing the patient to assume as much responsibility for his own care as he can	0.0	.64	0.0
59.	Supporting the patient in learning about his care	0.34	.55	0.0
35.	Including the patient's family in planning the patient's care upon discharge	0.0	.54	0.18
27.	Through talking with the patient and/or his family, determine what nursing care needs the patient has that are different from the expected or anticipated needs	0.0	.54	0.28
72.	Asking the patient if he has any questions about his care	0.42	.50	0.0
49.	Reviewing the information that you gave the patient to be sure that he understood	0.32	.44	0.0
53.	Making sure the patient understands about his medications, such as reason why he is receiving them and/or possible side effects	0.26	.42	0.0
17.	Discussing with the patient the impact his hospitalization will have on his life and family	0.0	0.0	.86
15.	Sitting down with the patient to discuss his care	0.0	0.0	.81
14.	Discussing with the patient how his illness will affect him and his family	0.0	0.0	.76
11.	Talking with the patient about what he knows about his illness	0.0	0.0	0.74
9.	Asking the patient if he understood all the things that his physician had told him	0.0	0.0	0.70
20.	Asking the patient if he has any preferences about any aspect of his care	0.0	0.0	0.69
13.	Assessing the patient's emotional state frequently	0.0	0.0	0.64
12.	Finding out if the patient	0.0	0.0	0.61

cont.

TABLE 23.1 *(continued)*

	has ever talked with any-one who has the same illness			
1.	Discussing with the family what role they would like to assume in providing care for the patient while he is in the hospital	0.0	0.0	0.49
77.	Discussing with the patient the care that is planned for him while he is in the hospital	0.41	0.0	.40

Finally, a test of discriminate validity was conducted to examine the ability of the ICI to distinguish between different modalities of nursing care that were purported to yield lower or higher levels of individualized care. Some empirical evidence and many anecdotal accounts have shown that higher levels of individualized care can be expected with the primary nursing care delivery system, compared to team and functional modes. Greater numbers of certain patient-centered expressive care behaviors were found in a study of a primary nursing setting compared to a total patient care setting. It was hypothesized that nurses' performance of individualized care behavior (as measured by the ICI) will vary depending on the modality practiced.

The hypotheses of the study were

1. Nurses' performance of individualized care behavior (as measured by the ICI-Survey Format) will be significantly higher for primary nursing staff than for total patient care and team nursing staff.
2. Nurses' performance of individualized care behaviors (as measured by the ICI-Survey Format) will be significantly higher for total patients care than for team nursing staff.

Performance of individualized care was defined as nurses' self-reported frequency with which they performed nursing actions specified in the ICI.

Three nursing care modalities were compared. These were team nursing, total patient care, and primary nursing. Each modality was seen to have a distinct method of nurse-patient assignment. For the purpose of this study these modalities were defined in the following manner.

Team nursing – An RN and aide and/or LVN are assigned to a group of patients, usually 12 to 15. The RN team leader administers medications and treatments, the LVN and/or aide complete other aspects of care for these 12 to 15 patients.

Total patient care – Nurses are assigned to 4 to 7 patients for whom they deliver total patient care. These nurses may be RNs or LVNs; however, their care (on a single shift) is not supplemented by another nurse or aide. There is no expectation that the same nurse(s) when on duty will be reassigned the same patients.

Primary nursing – Nurses are assigned to 4 to 7 patients for whom they deliver total patient care. Nurses are designated as primary nurses or associate nurses. However, only RNs can be primary nurses; associate nurses can be either RNs or LVNs and can care for the patient when the primary nurse is not on duty. There is an expectation that primary nurses be reassigned to the same patients throughout these patients' hospitalization.

By definition these modalities differ in the extent that continuity of the nurse-patient relationship is upheld. A secondary hypothesis was that different levels of continuity will be observed across modalities. Continuity is a measure that can be assigned to a unit as a whole and represents the average rate that nurses are assigned to care for the same patient. For the purpose of this study, average continuity rate represented the proportion of time the nurse on duty has been assigned to the same patient from the day of admission.

METHOD

Sample and Setting

A systematic sampling of nursing units in randomly selected hospitals was used for this study.

Using the criteria of 200 beds and Joint Commission for the Accreditation of Hospitals accreditation, a sample of eight hospitals was randomly drawn from American Hospital Association (1983) hospital listings, using a table of random numbers. The sampling criteria for choosing units from participating hospitals were as follows: (1) the unit should service largely general medical-surgical patients and (2) the unit had to practice one of the following three modalities: team nursing, total patient care, or primary nursing, as previously defined. A double-level screening process was conducted to choose appropriate units. Directors of nursing in these hospitals were asked to select units that met these criteria; then head nurses on these units were asked to verify these judgments by completing a head nurse survey. The survey asked for clarification about staffing patterns, assignments of staff to patients, and the role of the staff RN in caring for patients.

A total of 11 hospital units were chosen to participate. Of these units three were primary nursing units; four, team nursing; and four, total patient care units. The objective of sampling RNs from these units was to enlist all consenting RNs to complete the survey. A minimum of 80% of the total RN staff on each unit was required if the unit was to remain in the study.

A survey was delivered to each RN by the head nurse on the unit. The surveys, enclosed in sealed envelopes, were returned to a large manila envelope on the unit, addressed to the researcher, and subsequently picked up by the researcher two weeks from the day of distribution.

Customary procedures to protect the rights of human subjects were utilized. Nurses were informed of their rights and signed a consent form to participate in the study.

RESULTS

Sample Characteristics

A total of 164 nurses were surveyed in 11 hospital units of eight hospitals. The sample breakdown was the following: Team nursing, 55; total patient care, 53; and primary nursing, 56.

The majority of the nurses surveyed (95.1%) were female; the median age range was 35 to 39 years. Nearly two-thirds (105, or 64%) of the sample were Caucasian; the next most common ethnicity and the only other group represented in significant numbers was Asian (43, or 26.2%). The *basic* RN preparation included 44.5% from AA programs, 27.4% from diploma programs, and 27.4% from BSN programs. When *highest level* of nursing education was considered, nurses graduating from AA programs were still greatest in number: 40.9% had attained an AA degree; 25.6%, a diploma; and 31.1%, a BSN/BS degree. Only two nurses held a MN or MSN degree. The majority worked full-time (79.3%), were career appointments (76.2%), and were considered permanent staff (83.5%). The majority also worked 8-hr shifts; either days (37.8%) or evenings (34.1%). As for their area of specialization, all nurses worked in medical-surgical nursing; 29.3% worked in a combination of medical-surgical services (e.g. medical and oncology or medical-general/surgery). Sixty-four percent of the sample had less than 10 years of nursing experience; the median range was 5 to 10 years. In comparison, 14.4% of the sample had less than 10 years hospital nursing experience, and the median range was 3 to 5 years.

Individualized Care as a Function of Nursing Care Modality

The primary hypothesis of interest is this study was that nurses' performance of individualized care behaviors (as measured by the ICI) would vary across nursing care modalities. Results should indicate a low level for staff practicing team nursing to a high level for staff practicing primary nursing, with staff practicing total patient care (TPC) somewhere in between. Although the data indicated a trend in the expected direction for the average total ICI scores, this result was not statistically significant (see Table 23.2). Examination of Table 23.2 also shows that this lack of a significant difference in the total ICI scores among the 3 nursing modalities held for each of the 3 ICI subdimensions.

It was also of interest to determine if differences in the demographic makeup of the staff had any effect on the relationship between modality and the performance of individualized care. The data failed to indicate

TABLE 23.2 ICI Scores by Nursing Modalities (Mean ± SD)

Scales	Nursing modality			F-ratios	df	p-value [a]
	Team (N = 55)	Total patient care (N = 53)	Primary N = 56			
ICI overall score	107 ±16	108 ±13[b]	111 ±16	1.3	(2,160)	0.29
ICI subscales						
Inquiry/ assessment	37 ±6	37 ±6	39 ±7	2.5	(2,161)	0.09
Comprehensive care	40 ±5	40 ±5	40 ±5	0.4	(2,160)	0.65
Coordinated care	39 ±7	39 ±5	40 ±6	0.2	(2,161)	0.79

[a]Results of a one-way ANOVA F-test of the hypothesis that there are no differences in the average total ICI score for team, total patient care, and primary nursing modalities.
[b]N = 52.

any significant differences in the average total ICI scores between modalities when controlling for education (basic as well as higher), area of nursing (e.g., surgical), and number of years practiced (in general as well as exclusively as an RN in a hospital setting). There was also no evidence that education, area of nursing, or length of experience in themselves had a significant effect on the reported level of individualized care practiced.

As would be expected, night nurses practiced individualized care differently from either day or evening nurses. There was a statistically significant difference in the average total overall ICI scores between nurses on days and evenings ($\overline{X} = 112 \pm 13$ and 112 ± 14, respectively) and nurses on nights ($\overline{X} = 100 \pm 17$). Results of a one-way ANOVA indicated an F-ratio of 9.96 ($df = 2,159$, $p = .0001$).

Due to sample size constraints, only Caucasian and Asians were used in analyzing the effect of ethnicity on reported practice of individualized care behaviors. There was a statistically significant difference in the average total overall ICI score among the three nursing modalities when taking into account differences in ethnicity results of a two-way ANOVA F-ratio of 3-3 ($df = 2,140$, $p = 0.04$). Table 23.3 presents the average total overall ICI scores for the six ethnic-modality combinations as well as the results of a one-tailed, two-group t-test. These results are also presented graphically in Figure 23.1. The trend in individualized care behaviors expected (see statement of primary hypotheses) is most evident in Asian nurses. Specifically, Asian nurses practicing team nursing have a significantly lower average total overall ICI score than Asian nurses practicing TPC ($p = 0.03$) and primary nursing ($p = 0.02$). Caucasian nurses practicing primary nursing appear to perform more individualized care behaviors than Caucasian nurses practicing TPC ($p = 0.04$). Perusal of Figure

23.1 and Table 23.3 also shows that Asian nurses had a lower average ICI score than Caucasian nurses when practicing team nursing but that this relationship was reversed for Asian nurses practicing TPC and primary nursing. Thus, it appears that ethnicity of the nurse is not only an important factor to take into account when assessing individualized care within a given nursing modality but that the pattern of individualized care behavior across nursing modalities varies depending on the ethnic background of the nurse.

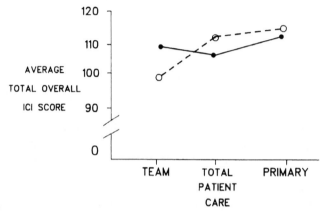

FIGURE 23.1 Total overall ICI score: ethnicity versus nursing modalities. *Solid line* = Caucasian; *dashed line* = Asian.

TABLE 23.3 Overall ICI Score by Ethnicity versus Nursing Modalities (Mean ± SD)

Ethnicity	Team	Nursing modality		Comparison	*t-*values	*df*	*p*-value[a]
		Total patient care	Primary				
Caucasian	109 ± 15	106 ± 14	112 ± 13	Team vs. TPC	−0.8	101	0.21
	N = 43	*N* = 28	*N* = 33	Team vs. primary	1.1	101	0.15
				TPC vs. primary	1.9	101	0.04
Asian	99 ± 22	112 ± 11	115 ± 21	Team vs. TPC	1.9	39	0.03
	N = 10	*N* = 21	*N* = 11	Team vs. primary	2.1	39	0.02
				TPC vs. primary	0.5	39	0.32

[a]Results of a one-sided two-sample *t*-test of the hypothesis that there are no differences in the average total overall ICI score for team, total patient care, and primary nursing modalities; significant at 0.05.

As indicated previously a secondary purpose of the study was to examine the continuity of care on each unit to determine how well these units practiced a single modality. Continuity of care was measured in two ways: average and corrected continuity. Table 23.4 shows the mean continuity ratings for each of the three nursing modalities. Although the expected relationship between average continuity and modality was evident (i.e., lower continuity for team nursing to higher continuity for primary nursing), it is of interest to note that this trend was not apparent when continuity was measured by corrected continuity, which was thought to be a better measure than average continuity.

DISCUSSION

The overall aim of this program of research was to establish the validity and reliability of ICI-Survey Format. The specific purpose of the most recent study was to test the discriminant validity of the ICI with nurses practicing in different nursing care modalities.

The general implications of the reliability and validity assessments indicate that the ICI should undergo further tests of validity and reliability. As was noted, the ICI could not discriminate between nursing care modalities. This fact could be related to more than one phenomenon. First, the nursing care modalities may not have been sufficiently different to reveal differences in performance. One should also consider that the results may be due to the self-report nature of the tool. Observations of nursing behaviors may be the best approach to measuring this variable. Of significance here was that the researcher's communications with head nurses suggested that no modality was practiced in its pure form. Primary nursing units had difficulty preserving the continuity of nurse-patient relationship, and team nursing units sometimes did TPC with selected patients, for example, medical-oncology patients. Also, TPC units were sometimes low on RN staff and employed a mini-team arrangement and in still other instances used a primary nursing mode, when staffing permitted, with selected patients. The fact that these modalities were probably not discreetly different was also evident in the analysis of continuity of assignment and nursing care modality. Continuity of care should be strongly related to modality, and the lack of a strong relationship could explain, in part, why the relationship between modality and individualized care

TABLE 23.4 Continuity versus Nursing Modalities (Mean ± SD)

Continuity	Team (N = 55)	Total patient care (N = 53)	Primary (N = 56)
Average	0.11 ± 0.10	0.15 ± 0.04	0.016 ± 0.04
Corrected	0.22 ± 0.08	0.26 ± 0.05	0.20 ± 0.05

was not strongly evident. That is, it is further evidence that the modalities were not practiced in a pure enough form. This, obviously, would make it difficult for the ICI to discriminate between the modalities.

Future research that further establishes the validity and reliability of the ICI is warranted. Specifically, discriminate validity may be obtained if the researcher is able to locate units that adhere to a specific staffing pattern most of the time. Variability in practices will always be found but may be controlled to a greater extent if the researcher selects purer forms of the modalities and is not confined to geographically accessible hospitals. Second, more attention should be given to a comparison of philosophical components of the nursing care modalities. The philosophy of patient care in the hospital, standards of practice, and job descriptions of RNs are likely to reveal why two units practicing different modalities score similarly on the ICI, a finding in this study.

Future studies to evaluate the difference between nursing care modalities need to develop objective criteria in determining the actual degree of implementation of these modalities on selected hospital units. This study examined an important practice pattern of nurses, continuity of care. Evaluations such as these assist in making finer distinctions between units practicing a modality in its pure form from those that, in reality, are using a combination of nursing care methods (Alexander, Weisman, & Chase, 1981).

Studies of discriminate validity can be repeated; those that utilize an observational format based upon the ICI should make a significant contribution. A sound measure of individualized nursing care practices is needed. Individualized care is not only linked with certain nursing care modalities, it is also associated with patient satisfaction and quality care. Such a measure is important in discriminating among modes of organizing care at the unit level but equally important in predicting the outcomes of nursing care.

REFERENCES

Abdellah, F. (1961). *Patient-centered approaches to nursing*. New York: Macmillan.

Alexander, C. S., Weisman, C. S., & Chase, G. A. (1981). Evaluating primary nursing in hospitals: Examination of effects on nursing staff. *Medical Care, 19,* 80-89.

American Hospital Association. (1983). *American Hospital Association guide to the health care field*. Chicago: Author.

American Nurses' Association. (1981). *Inventory of registered nurses*. Kansas City, MO: Author.

Anderson, M., & Choi, T. (1981). *Study on behavioral outcomes achieved through differing organizational patterns for delivery of nursing care*. Unpublished manuscript, University of Minnesota Hospitals and Clinics, Center for Health Service Research.

Carmines, E., & Zeller, R. (1979). *Reliability and validity assessment*. Beverly Hills, CA: Sage.

Chapman, J. (1977). Effects of different nursing approaches upon selected postoperative responses of male herniorrhaphy patients. In F. Downs & M. Newman (Eds.), *A source book of nursing research* (2nd ed.) (pp. 15-23). Philadelphia: F. A. Davis.

Haussman, R. K. D., Hegyvary, S. T., & Newman, J. F. (1976). *Monitoring quality of nursing care: II. Assessment and study of correlates* (DHEW Publication No. (HRA) 76-7). Bethesda, MD: Department of Health, Education and Welfare.

Hegyvary, S. (1982). *The change to primary nursing - a cross cultural view of professional nursing practice.* St. Louis: C. V. Mosby.

Hinshaw, A. S., Gerber, R. M., Atwood, J. R., & Allen, J. R. (1983). The use of predictive modeling to test nursing practice outcomes. *Nursing Research,* *33*(1), 35-42.

Johnson, G. V., & Tingey, S. (1976). Matrix organization: Blueprint of nursing care organization for the 80's. *Hospital and Health Services Administration, 21,* 27-39.

Marram, G., Barrett, M., & Bevis, E. (1974). *Primary nursing - a model for individualized care.* St. Louis: C. V. Mosby.

Marram, G., Barrett, M., & Bevis, E. (1979). *Primary nursing - a model for individualized care* (2nd ed.). St. Louis: C. V. Mosby.

Marram, G., Flynn, K., Abaravich, W., & Carey, S. (1976). *Cost-effectiveness of primary and team nursing.* Wakefield, MA: Contemporary.

Methuen, D., & Schlotfeldt, R. M. (1962). The Social Interaction Inventory. *Nursing Research, 11,* 84-85.

Muthen, B. (1981). Factor analysis of dichotomous variables. In E. Borgatta & D.J. Jackson (Eds.), *Factor analysis and measurement in sociological research: a multidimensional perspective* (p. 85). San Francisco: Sage.

Van Servellen, G. (1980). Primary nursing - the adoption of a nursing care modality. *Nursing and Health Care, 1*(3), 144-150.

Wandelt, M., & Ager, J. (1974). *The nursing process - assessing, planning, implementing, evaluating* (2nd ed.). New York: Appleton-Century-Crofts.

Yura, H., & Walsh, M. (1973). *The Nursing process – assessing, planning, implementing, evaluating* (2nd ed.). New York: Appleton-Century-Crofts. Inc.

Zelditch, M. (1955). Role differentiation in the nuclear family. In T. Partons, R.F. Bales, J. Olds, & P. E. Slater, (Eds.), *Family, sociation and interaction process* (p. 307). Glencoe, IL: The Free Press.

NURSING CARE SURVEY

Dear Research Participant: In the course of delivering care to their patients, nurses perform many nursing care activities. We are asking you to provide us specific information about the extent to which you perform certain nursing care actions with your patients.

This survey consists of two parts.

Part I asks a number of questions about you and your background. The purpose of these questions is to assist the researcher in developing a profile of the participants in the study.

Part II of the survey asks you to specify the extent to which you practice certain nursing actions. Your task is to judge the frequency you perform these activities and circle the response that best fits your judgment.

Please proceed in completing the enclosed survey. You will be given as much time as you need to complete the questionnaire. Your answers will remain anonymous. When you have completed the questionnaire, please enclose it in the envelope provided, then insert it in the larger envelope entitled "Nursing Activity Survey." A summary of the study will be made available to your Head Nurse at a later date.

Thank you for your important contribution to this effort. Please feel free to contact the researcher if you have any questions or concerns

I. DEMOGRAPHIC DATA

For Office Use Only

Please check the ONE answer that best describes you.

1. Your sex is: ____ male or ____ female.
       (1)   (2)   ____
                                                              (6)

2. Your age is: ____ Under 25
       (1)

____ 25-29   ____ 30-34   ____ 35-39
(2)   (3)   (4)

____ 40-44   ____ 45-49   ____ 50-54   ____
(5)   (6)   (7)   (7)

____ 55-59   ____ 60 and over
(8)   (9)

3. Your racial/ethnic background is (optional):

____ Caucasian/White   ____ Negro/Black
(1)   (2)

____ American Indian/   ____ Oriental/Asian   ____
(3) Native American   (4)   8

____ Spanish origin or   ____ Other (please
(5) descent   (6) specify)

4. What is your basic nursing education?

___ LVN ___ RN/AA ___ DIPLOMA ___ RN/BSN ___
(1)   (2)   (3)   (4)   (9)

5. What is the highest level of nursing education you've attained?

___ LVN ___ AA ___ DIPLOMA ___ BSN/BS ___
(1)   (2)   (3)   (4)   (10)

___ MN/MSN
(5)

6. Do you hold an advanced degree in another field, other than nursing?

___ no ___ yes ___ other (please specify degree
(1)   (2)   (3) and field)

7. What is your current employment status?   (11)
   a. (check one) __ (1) full time (32 hr or more per week)
                 __ (2) part time (less than 32 hr/week)
   b. (check one) __ (1) career employee (permanent   (12)
                          employee, with benefits)
                 __ (2) per diem (at least one
                          shift per week)
   c. (check one) __ (1) permanent floor assignment   (3)
                 __ (2) float assignment

                                              (14)

8. What shift do you work most often? (check one)
   __ (1) Days (8-hr shift)
   __ (2) Evenings (8-hr shift)
   __ (3) Nights (8-hr shift)
   __ (4) Rotate
   __ (5) Days (12-hr shift)
   __ (6) Eves/Nights (12-hr shift)

                                              (15)

9. In what specific area of nursing do you work? If you work in more than one area, please identify *one* as your primary.

__ Medical (01)	__ Surgical (08)
__ Med/Surg Combination (02)	__ Orthopedic (09)
__ Obstetrics/Newborn (03)	__ Urology (10)
__ Intensive Care (ICU, CCU) (04)	__ Oncology (11)
__ Pediatrics (05)	__ Dialysis (12)

                                    (16) (17)

    — Neurology   — Psychiatric
      (06)   (13)
    — Gynecology   — Other, Please
      (07)   specify
                                   (14) _____

10. How many years have you practiced nursing?

	Less than 1 year		1-3 years	
(1)		(2)		
	3-5 years		5-10 years	
(3)		(4)		
	10-15 years		15-20 years	
(5)		(6)		(18)
	over 20 years			
(7)				

11. How many years have you practiced nursing exclusively as an RN in a hospital setting?

	Less than 1 year		1-3 years	
(1)		(2)		
	3-5 years		5-10 years	
(3)		(4)		
	10-15 years		15-20 years	
(5)		(6)		(19)
	over 20 years			
(7)				

PERFORMANCE OF NURSING ACTIONS

Nurses complete many tasks in caring for patients. Some of these tasks may be performed more frequently than others. You are asked to judge how frequently you do these things by indicating the proportion of patients for whom you complete these activities. That is, how frequently do you perform these behaviors in the administration of nursing care to the patients to whom you are assigned?

Choice 1: With none of my patients
Choice 2: With a few of my patients
Choice 3: With some of my patients
Choice 4: With most of my patients
Choice 5: With all of my patients

Circle the answer that best reflects your judgment.

	With none of my patients	With a few of my patients	With some of my patients	With most of my patients	With all of my patients
1. Discuss with the family what role they would like to assume in providing care for patient while he/she is in the hospital.	1	2	3	4	5
2. Give patients an opportunity to explain their feelings.	1	2	3	4	5
3. Meet with the oncoming shift to discuss the patient's problems.	1	2	3	4	5
4. Sit down with patients to discuss their care.	1	2	3	4	5
5. Make sure patients know what roles physicians will play in their care.	1	2	3	4	5
6. Allow the patients time to talk about their fears or concerns.	1	2	3	4	5
7. Meet patient's daily hygiene needs for cleanliness and acceptable appearance.	1	2	3	4	5
8. Discuss with patients the care that is planned for them while they are in the hospital	1	2	3	4	5

9. After completing the nursing assessment, validate with the patient what you have identified as his/her problems.   1   2   3   4   5

10. Discuss with the dietitian the diet plan for the patient.   1   2   3   4   5

11. Allow patients to assume as much responsibility for their own care as they can.   1   2   3   4   5

12. Make sure patients understand who will be taking care of them.   1   2   3   4   5

13. Ask patients what they would like to know about their illness.   1   2   3   4   5

14. Ask patients if they have any preferences about any aspect of their care.   1   2   3   4   5

15. Allow patients to set the times for their activities and treatments as much as possible, e.g., baths, medications, bedtime.   1   2   3   4   5

16. Help patients accept dependence/independence (as appropriate to their condition).   1   2   3   4   5

17. Find out if the patient has ever talked with anyone who has the same illness.   1   2   3   4   5

18. Participate in conferences concerning your patients' care.   1   2   3   4   5

19. Take action to meet the patient's need for adequate hydration and elimination.   1   2   3   4   5

20. Adapt expected patient activities to the physical and mental capabilities of the patient.   1   2   3   4   5

21. Make sure patients know the names of the persons responsible for specific procedures and/or treatments.   1   2   3   4   5

22. Include the patient's family in planning the patient's care upon discharge.   1   2   3   4   5

23. Make sure patients understand about their medications, such as reason why and side effects.   1   2   3   4   5

24. Write 24-hr nursing orders for the patient on the care plan.	1	2	3	4	5
25. Support patients in learning about their care.	1	2	3	4	5
26. Talk with patients about what they know about their illness.	1	2	3	4	5
27. Review the information that you gave the patient to be sure that he understood.	1	2	3	4	5
28. Carry out medical and surgical asepesis during treatments and special procedures.	1	2	3	4	5
29. Approach patients in a kind, gentle, and friendly manner.	1	2	3	4	5
30. Discuss with the patient the impact their hospitalization will have on their lives and families.	1	2	3	4	5
31. Complete all "hands on" nursing procedures for the patient with skill and sensitivity to patient needs.	1	2	3	4	5
32. Keep informed of your patients' condition and whereabouts during your assigned shifts.	1	2	3	4	5
33. Ask patients what their usual daily activities are, such as work, hobbies, and recreation.	1	2	3	4	5
34. Report the pertinent incidents of the patient's behavior during interaction with other staff.	1	2	3	4	5
35. Protect patients sensitivities and rights to privacy.	1	2	3	4	5
36. Through talking with patients and/or their families, determine what nursing care needs the patient has that are different from the expected or anticipated needs.	1	2	3	4	5
37. Inform the doctor that you are the patient's nurse.	1	2	3	4	5
38. Ask patients if they have any questions about their care.	1	2	3	4	5
39. Give patients explanations and verbal reassurances when needed.	1	2	3	4	5

40. Ask patients if they   1   2   3   4   5
    understood all the things that
    their physician has told them.
41. Communicate clearly ideas,   1   2   3   4   5
    facts, and concepts about the
    patient in charting.
42. Make sure that changes   1   2   3   4   5
    in care and the care plans for
    your patients reflect the continu-
    ous evaluation of nursing care
    given.
43. Make decisions that reflect   1   2   3   4   5
    knowledge of facts and good
    judgment.
44. Assess the patient's   1   2   3   4   5
    emotional state frequently.
45. Discuss with patients how   1   2   3   4   5
    their illness will affect them and
    their family.

24

Measuring Patient Satisfaction with Nursing Care: A Magnitude Estimation Approach

Lillian Eriksen

This chapter discusses the satisfaction with Nursing Care Questionnaire, a measure of patient satisfaction with nursing care in the hospital setting.

PURPOSE

The purpose of this instrument is to measure patient satisfaction with nursing care in the hospital setting. The objectives were to create a reliable, valid, and sensitive instrument that can be used by nurse administrators as a tool for evaluating nursing care from the perspective of the patient and by nurse researchers studying the variable of patient satisfaction.

CONCEPTUAL BASE

Donabedian (1980) viewed client satisfaction as an objective or outcome of care representing the patient's judgment on the quality of care. Patient satisfaction, a fundamental measure of quality of care, furnishes the evaluator with information regarding "the provider's success at meeting those client values and expectations which are matters on which the client is the ultimate authority" (Donabedian, 1980, p. 25). Donabedian also noted that the client is limited in some judgments of quality of care due to lack of knowledge concerning the science and technology of care.

Several authors have identified what patients expect from nurses. When constructing the patient satisfaction checklist, Abdellah and Levine

(1957) interviewed patients for the purpose of identifying satisfying and unsatisfying events patients encountered while hospitalized. These patient-identified events formed the base for the entire instrument. The items were placed into seven categories determined by substantive review of the responses given by the patients during the interviews. The seven dimensions included events indicating satisfaction with care, rest and relaxation, dietary needs, elimination, personal hygiene and supportive care, reaction to therapy, and contact with nurses.

Tagliacozzo (1965) reported that patients are sensitive reactors to the personality and attitudes inferred from nurse behavior. When asked to identify what they expected from a nurse, patients included in Tagliacozzo's study sample mentioned a kind and friendly personality, cheerful smiling personality, knowledge of the patient, dedication, spontaneous service, a fast response, some encouragement, patience and tolerance, enough time, interest, kindness, personalized care, some sympathy and efficiency.

When combining the patients' expectations into more general categories, Tagliacozzo (1965) found that 81% of the respondents identified personalized care and personality attributes of the nurse as important dimensions of patient expectation of nursing care. Forty-five percent of the respondents indicated that prompt and efficient service was an important expectation. In addition, knowledge and technical skill were mentioned by 29% of the respondents as important. The most criticized behavior was slow response to patient requests and needs.

On a questionnaire given to patients before discharge, for the purpose of evaluating hospital services, patients commented on the human interpersonal qualities of nurses (Doll, 1979). Positive comments included kindness, friendliness, courtesy, good communications, concern, personal touch, and cheerfulness. Negative comments referred to nurses as rude, hateful, or slow. None of the respondents commented on the skill or expertise of the nurses.

Occasionally patients write about their expectations of nurses. Fellows (1983) enumerated a number of qualities and behaviors he expected of nurses. The most important was for the nurse to treat the patient as an individual. The nurse should be bright, intelligent, capable, calm, attentive, attractive and personable, should display empathy and be able to establish a mutual relationship of trust. In addition, the nurse needs to be a good listener and at the same time be able to communicate intelligently with doctors and supervisors, must be able to recognize early signs of deterioration or change in the patient, and must be able to cope well with emotional interaction. Most of the items in this list deal primarily with the interpersonal skill of the nurse. Observational skills were also identified by Fellows as being an expectation of a patient.

Another patient, Perkins (1983), expressed his thoughts regarding satisfying nurse behaviors. The first behavior focused on explanation of procedures and equipment, including their purpose. Displaying personal interest in the patient's welfare and recovery was another significant nurse behavior identified by Perkins. Other attributes cited by Perkins include promptness, efficiency, poise, calm manner, ability to alleviate fear, being technically informed and trained in skills and encouraging.

Care providers have also studied patient satisfaction with care. Ware and associates have published a number of articles related to patient satisfaction with health care (Ware & Snyder, 1975; Ware, Snyder, & Chu, 1975; Ware, Snyder, & Wright, 1976; Ware, Davies-Avery, & Snyder, 1978). Ware and associates (1978) identified eight dimensions of satisfaction that were defined and supported by factor analytic studies conducted and published by these investigators. The eight dimensions were labeled art of care, accessibility/convenience, finances, physical environment, availability, continuity of care, and efficacy/outcomes of care.

These eight dimensions were further defined by Ware and associates (1978). Art of care focuses on the amount of "caring" demonstrated by the health care provider. Satisfying characteristics included concern, consideration, friendliness, patience, and sincerity. On the negative side, health care provider behaviors were abruptness, disrespect, and causing embarrassment, hurt, insult, or unnecessary worry.

Technical quality of care refers to the technical skills and abilities of providers as well as the quality and modernness of facilities and equipment. At the positive end are provider ability, accuracy, experience, thoroughness, training, paying attention to details, avoiding mistakes, giving good examinations, and providing clear explanations to patients. The negative behaviors included defective equipment and facilities, outdated methods, taking of unnecessary risks, and overprescribing.

Accessibility/convenience pertains to those factors associated with arranging to get health care. Variables included in this dimension were time and effort required to obtain an appointment, distance from the site to receive care, time and effort required to travel to the site, service hours, waiting time at the site, availability of assistance over the phone, and whether care is provided in the home.

Finances refers to the ability of the recipient to arrange for payment of services. Included were costs of care or insurance, flexibility of payment, and comprehensiveness of insurance.

Physical environment pertains to the environment in which the care is delivered. Satisfactions with the environment included pleasant atmosphere, comfortable seats, attractive waiting rooms, clear signs and directions, good lighting, cleanliness, and neatness.

Availability focuses on both services and personnel. Measures of this dimension include quantities of health care personnel and facilities. Continuity of care is defined in terms of delivery of care from the same facility or provider.

Efficacy/outcomes of care regard the efficacy of treatment in improving or maintaining health status. This dimension was found to be infrequently measured in studies of patient satisfaction.

While these eight dimensions were identified for patient satisfaction with health care services in ambulatory settings, most seemed also to be appropriate for consideration as dimensions of satisfaction in the hospital setting. After review, the dimensions of finance and accessibility/ convenience were deleted, as they dealt with the need for patients to make arrangements regarding the provision of nursing care.

Finances referred to the arranging for payment of services, which is not a function currently involved with nursing care. Nursing care costs are most typically included as a part of hospital costs, not arranged for as a separate bill. Also, the issue of accessibility or convenience pertained to arranging for care. Again, patients are not usually involved in arranging for their nursing care, as it is associated with hospitalization.

With the deletion of finances and accessibility, six dimensions remained for the framework of the instrument. (Ware & Associates, 1978). The six proposed dimensions included (a) art of care, (b) technical quality of care, (c) physical environment, (d) availability, (e) continuity of care, and of efficacy/outcomes.

METHODS

Instrument

The instrument used a norm-referenced measurement framework. A magnitude estimations scaling approach was selected in an attempt to develop an instrument that is more sensitive than those currently in the literature.

Thirty-five items for the instrument were identified from the literature and previous patient satisfaction tools. Items were formulated in terms of nurse characteristics or behaviors and events likely to be encountered in the hospital setting. As seemed appropriate, the 35 items were grouped into the six dimensions identified above. An additional global patient satisfaction item was not assigned to a dimension.

For purposes of testing reliability and validity of the instrument all items were randomly ordered for each respondent, with each presented sideways on a single sheet of legal-size paper. This was necessary to avoid fatigue factors in responses to items, prevent comparison of responses to previous responses, and provide adequate room for line production responses of the subsample used for psychophysical validation of respondent performance in making ratio judgments.

Scoring and Administration

The instrument is in the form of a self-administered questionnaire. Scores for each of the six dimensions are calculated by averaging log transformations of the responses to the items in each dimension. Thus, there are six scores.

Setting

A small general community hospital in a small western city was used as the setting for this initial testing of the instrument for patient satisfaction with nursing care. Two 30-bed general medical-surgical patient care units were used to select respondents.

Respondents

Respondents included in the study were patients on their patient care unit of discharge a minimum of three days, oriented to person, place,and time, at least 21 years of age, and capable of responding to a questionnaire in English. Demographic variables collected regarding the respondents included age, sex, length of hospital stay,length of stay on unit of discharge, number of times previously hospitalized in current hospital, and number of times hospitalized in other hospitals.

Procedures

After obtaining a list of patients being discharged, eligible respondents were identified. Each eligible respondent on each of the two patient care units was approached for willingness to participate in the study. At that time the purposes of the study and an estimate of the time required to complete the questionnaire were read to the respondent by the investigator. Confidentiality of responses was assured. If the respondent was willing to participate, the investigator reviewed the written directions with the patient and answered any questions the respondent initiated. After answering the respondent's concerns or questions, the instrument was left with the respondent. An envelope that could be sealed was provided to maintain confidentiality of responses. The investigator returned to each respondent to retrieve the questionnaires.

Prior to responding to the instrument for assessing patient satisfaction with nursing care, respondents completed a calibration procedure. The purposes of the calibration procedure were to provide instruction and practice in making magnitude judgments, to determine whether respondents were making proportional judgments accurately, and to estimate response bias (Lodge, 1981). The calibration procedure used numeric estimation (NE) of predetermined line lengths and line production (LP) of predetermined numbers.

The format for NE included the following:
1. Use of legal-size paper with print lengthwise.
2. Directions for completion.
3. Reference line with number 100 was presented on first page following directions.
4. One stimulus per page with pages randomly ordered.
5. Nine lines: 5 mm, 7 mm, 20 mm, 35 mm, 50 mm, 70 mm, 150 mm, 225 mm, 300 mm.

The format for LP included the following:
1. Use of legal-size paper with print lengthwise.
2. Directions for completion.
3. Reference number 100 with a 100-mm line will be on the first page following directions.
4. One stimulus per page with pages randomly ordered.
5. Nine numbers: 3, 6, 20, 35, 50, 75, 150, 225, 300.

A cross-modality matching paradigm was also incorporated into the study for the purposes of psychophysical validation of the instrument. A randomly selected subsample of 18 respondents used both NE and LP for responses to each of the stimuli in the Satisfaction with Nursing Care Questionnaire.

Reliability and Validity Testing

Prior to testing instrument reliability and validity it was necessary to examine the ability of hospitalized patients to use a magnitude estimation scaling model for expressing their satisfaction with nursing care. The calibration and cross-modality matching paradigm procedures suggested by Lodge (1981) were used to assess the ability of hospitalized patients to make proportional judgments. The psychophysical validation of respondent performance was obtained by regressing both the geometric means of the numeric responses (NE) against the actual predetermined line lengths and the geometric means of the lien productions (LP) against the predetermined numbers.

The analysis of the cross-modality matching paradigm was compared to the empirical exponents obtained from the estimates of the responses on the patient Satisfaction with Nursing Care Questionnaire to the empirical exponents obtained from the same subjects when they matched the same two response modalities to metric stimuli. The assumption was that any biases affecting the response to the metric stimuli are similarly affecting the responses on the Patient Satisfaction with Nursing Care Questionnaire.

An estimate of internal consistency for each of the six potential subscales was planned for, using coefficient theta, a maximized alpha coefficient. Coefficient theta is dependent on the principal components of factor analytic techniques. Also, an item analysis using item-item and item-total score correlations for each of the subscales was planned.

Validity testing was planned to include predictive validity and construct validity. Predictive validity was tested as evidenced by the prediction of nurse managers in the setting of which of the two units would have the highest patient satisfaction scores. Construct validity was examined using factor analytic approaches to substantiate the existence of the six subscales.

MAJOR FINDINGS AND RESULTS

Findings and results will be discussed first in relation to the respondent sample. Second, initial findings concerning instrument reliability and validity will be addressed.

A total of 90 patients from two patient care units responded to the Patient Satisfaction with Nursing Care Questionnaire, 47 males and 43 females. Thus, slightly more than half of the respondents were males. The ages ranged from 20 to 89, with a mean age of 44. There were a larger number of younger respondents than might be expected, with 24 in the 20 to 29 age range and 25 ages 30 to 39.

This finding is most likely related to the number of orthopedic patients hospitalized on one of the units from which the sample was selected. In addition there were 4 respondents between 40 and 49, 12 between 50 and 59, 15 between 60 and 69, 7 between 70 and 79, and 3 between 80 and 89 years of age.

Approximately 73% of the respondents were hospitalized for 3 to 5 days, and 90% stayed less than 10 days. This was the first contact with nursing care in this hospital for almost half of the sample ($N = 42$). On the other hand, more than half had had previous hospitalizations in the facility in which the study was conducted, 38 had 2 to 4 previous hospitalizations, 8 had 5 to 10, and 2 had 20 or more. Approximately 75% of the respondents ($N = 57$) had had prior hospitalization experience in institutions other than the study hospital, 43 having 1 to 3 prior hospitalizations, 21 having 4 to 10 and 3 having 20 or more.

Testing of instrument reliability and validity necessitated the examination of the ability of hospitalized patients to use a magnitude estimation scaling model for expressing their satisfaction with nursing care. The calibration and cross-modality paradigm procedures suggested by Lodge (1981) were used to assess the ability of hospitalized patients to make proportional judgments. The psycho-validation of respondent performance was obtained by regressing both the geometric means of the numeric responses (NE) against the actual predetermined line lengths and the geometric means of line production (LP) against the predetermined numbers. The closer the regression is to one and the closer the data points are to the 45° line on logarithmically ruled graph paper, the more the data can be treated as psychophysically valid ratio measures (Lodge, 1981).

In Figure 24.1, it can be seen that hospitalized patients did extremely well in estimating line lengths in response to the drawn predetermined line stimuli. The regression analysis yielded an R^2 of 0.99. The same results ($R^2 = 0.99$) were obtained for the line productions that the respondents drew in response to the number stimuli (see Figure 24.2).

When respondents were making numeric estimations of the line stimuli they tended to overestimate the lengths of the line stimuli (see Figure 24.1). When drawing lines in response to number stimuli, the respondents tended to draw lines that were too long for smaller numbers and too short

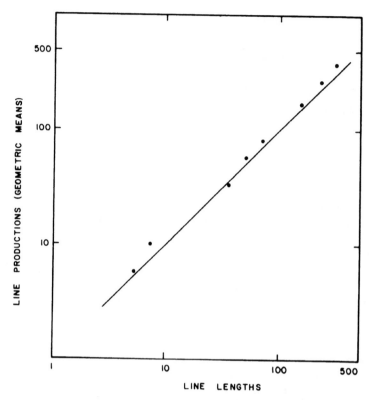

FIGURE 24.1 Numeric estimations plotted as a function of nine lines of varying lengths on logarithmic coordinates. Each point represents the geometric mean of the numeric estimates averaged over 90 respondents. The solid line represents the theoretical exponent of 1.0. The empirically obtained R^2 was .99.

for larger numbers (Figure 24.2). These findings are consistent with those reported by Lodge (1981). A plot of the line production responses against the numeric estimates to a common set of six stimuli (Figure 24.3) again showed a very strong relationship, indicating that the respondents were indeed using the two response modalities to make ratio judgments. These findings, illustrated in Figures 24.1, 24.2, and 24.3 indicate that hospitalized patients, ready for discharge, can indeed make magnitude judgments concerning metric stimuli.

The analysis of the cross-modality matching paradigm compared the empirical exponents obtained from the estimates of the responses on the Patient Satisfaction with Nursing Care Questionnaire to the empirical exponents obtained from the same subjects when they matched the same two response modalities to metric stimuli. The assumption is that any biases affecting the responses to the metric stimuli are similarly affecting the responses on the Patient Satisfaction with Nursing Care Questionnaire.

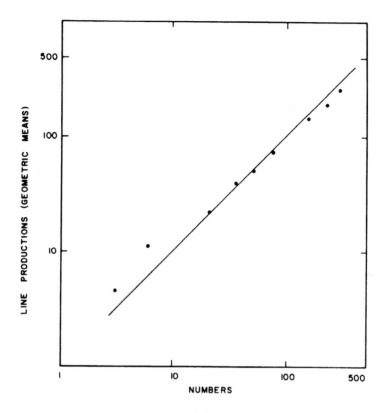

FIGURE 24.2 Line production responses plotted as a function of nine numeric stimuli on logarithmic coordinates. Each point represents the geometric mean of the length of the line production responses averaged over 90 respondents. The solid line represents the theoretical exponent of 1.0. The empirically obtained R^2 was .99.

The results of the analysis of the cross-modality paradigm, illustrated in Figure 24.4 indicate a strong relationship (.93) between the predicted and obtained exponents. The empirically obtained exponents from the matches to both the metric stimuli and the responses to the Patient Satisfaction with Nursing Care Questionnaire are not expected to be statistically significant from one another at the .05 level. In this sample, the empirical exponent in the metric stimuli was .99; in the responses to the Patient Satisfaction with Nursing Care Questionnaire, .93. There was no statistically significant difference in these two exponents; therefore, the scale is psychophysically valid.

Internal consistency reliability was planned to be estimated using coefficient theta. The use of coefficient theta is predicated on the existence of the six subscales in the instrument. Since the exploratory factor analysis, using this initial sample did not substantiate the subscale structure of the instrument, coefficient theta was not calculated. The evidence of predic-

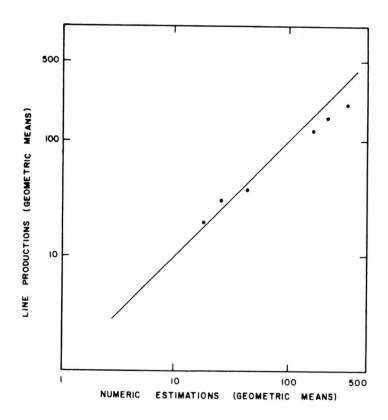

FIGURE 24.3 Line production responses are plotted on logarithmic coordinates as a function of numeric estimates to a common set of six metric stimuli. Each point represents the geometric mean averaged over 90 respondents. The solid line is the predicted exponent of 1.0. The empirically obtained R^2 was .99.

tive validity does, however, substantiate reliability of measurement because an instrument cannot have validity without having reliability.

An initial exploratory factor analysis, using the SPSS program for Varimax rotation, identified five factors with eigenvalues greater than one. The first factor had an eigenvalue of 23.258 and accounted for 81.4% of the variance. A substantive review of the variables loading on this factor revealed a preponderance of interpersonal skills (art of care) and technical nursing skills. Also many of the variables associated with factors 2 and 3 appear to be of an interpersonal or art of care nature. Ware and associates (1976) and Hinshaw and Atwood (1982) reported the tendency for variables associated with art of care and technical skill to load as a single factor rather than as two distinct factors underlying patient satisfaction with care.

The variables that loaded on factors 4 and 5 can best be described as environmental factors. Thus, it would appear that this initial instrument

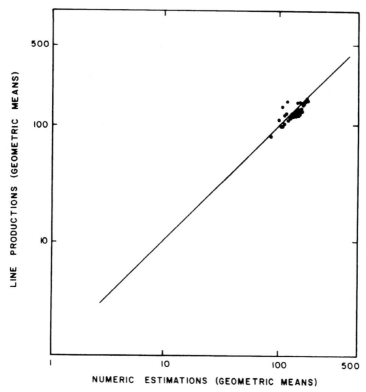

FIGURE 24.4 Line production responses are plotted as a function of numeric estimates to 36 items on the Patient Satisfaction with Nursing Care Questionnaire. Each point represents the geometric mean averaged over 18 respondents. The solid line is the predicted exponent of 1.0. The empirically obtained R^2 was .93.

may be sampling two factors, one concerned with art and technique of care and the other related to the patient's environment.

Evidence for predictive validity was obtained from the director of nursing and two nursing supervisors. Each predicted the same unit would score highest on the Patient Satisfaction with Nursing Care Questionnaire. The results indicated that there were statistically significant differences ($<.05$) between the units, thus corroborating the predictions of the nursing director and the nursing supervisors.

The initial testing of the Patient Satisfaction with Nursing Care Questionnaire revealed that it is a psychophysically valid instrument. There is also evidence for predictive validity and inferred reliability based on the results of this initial testing.

MAJOR IMPLICATIONS FOR NURSING

The findings from this one sample imply that patients ready for discharge from the hospital are able to make valid magnitude judgments in expressing their level of satisfaction with nursing care. Thus, it would seem that magnitude scaling is a viable scaling model for use by nurse researchers with similar patient samples. Since the mean age of the sample was relatively young, it would be appropriate to examine further the variable of age in using this scaling model with patients.

The major implications for nursing at this early stage of development and testing of this instrument and scaling model are for instrument revision and additional reliability and validity research. Plans for the continued development and testing of the Patient Satisfaction with Nursing Care Questionnaire include further item analysis and revision of items with the addition and deletion of items as indicated. Sampling from other populations and settings is planned for the near future. Subscale reliability will be estimated, using coefficient theta once the existence of the subscales is substantiated during further development and testing. Construct validity will be examined using factor analytic techniques as well as the multitrait, multimethod approach.

REFERENCES

Abdellah, F., & Levine, E. (1957). Developing a measure of patient and personal satisfaction with nursing care. *Nursing Research, 5*, 100-108.

Donabedian, A. (1980). *The definition of quality and approaches to its measurement.* Ann Arbor, MI: Health Administration Press.

Doll, A. (1979). The things patients say about their nurses. *Nursing 79, 7* (5), 113-120.

Fellows, K. (1983, May/June). What I expect from the nurse. *Geriatric Nursing,* pp. 154-155.

Hinshaw, A., & Atwood, J. (1982). A patient satisfaction instrument: Precision by replication. *Nursing Research, 31,* 170-175.

Lodge, M. (1981). *Magnitude scaling: Quantitative measurement of opinions.* Beverly Hills, CA: Sage.

Perkins, R. (1983, May/June). What I expect from the nurse. *Geriatric Nursing,* pp. 155-157.

Tagliacozzo, D. (1965). The nurse from the patient's point of view. In J. K. Skipper & R. C. Leonard (Eds.), *Social interaction and patient care,* 219-227. Philadelphia: J. B. Lippincott.

Ware, J., Jr., & Snyder, M. (1975). Dimensions of patient attitudes regarding doctors and medical care services. *Medical Care, 13* (18), 669-682.

Ware, J., Jr., Snyder, M., & Chu, G. (1975). Consumer perceptions of health care services: Implications for the academic medical community. *Journal of Medical Education, 50,* 839-848.

Ware, J., Jr., Snyder, M., & Wright, W. (1976). *Development and validation of scales to measure patient satisfaction with health care services: Volume 1 of a final report.* Southern Illinois University, Carbondale, IL: School of Medicine.

Ware, J., Jr., Davies-Avery, P., & Snyder, M. (1978). A taxonomy of patient satisfaction. *Health & Medical Care Services Review, 1* (1), 1-15.

Satisfaction with Nursing Care Questionnaire

DIRECTIONS FOR COMPLETING THE QUESTIONNAIRE

Listed below are some characteristics or behaviors of nurses that patients have identified as having an influence on their satisfaction with nursing care.

Think about YOUR expectations of nursing care. Assign your expectations the number 100.

Now read each item and determine to what DEGREE *your* experience with nursing care on *this* floor:

did not meet your expectations

did meet your expectations

exceeded your expectations

With the number 100 as a reference point for your expectations, assign ANY NUMBER (2, 10, 75, 120, 465, etc.) which reflects what YOU THINK about each item. For example, if you think your nursing care in relation to an item was twice as good as you expected, then assign the number 200 to that item. If on the other hand you think your nursing care in relation to an item was only one-tenth as good as you expected, then assign the number 10.

You are free to assign any number you think appropriate, keeping in mind how you would rate the item in relation to your expectations which are assigned 100.

In order to understand how different people with difference experience respond to the questionnaire, would you please provide the following information about yourself.

1. Your age
2. Your sex
3. Number of days in the hospital this time
4. Number of times a patient in this hospital
5. Number of times a patient in other hospitals

Art of Care

1. Courtesy of my nurses. _____
2. Nurse's understanding of how I feel. _____
3. Patience of my nurses. _____
4. Attention of my nurses to me. _____
5. Nurses use terminology I clearly understand. _____
6. Kindness of my nurses. _____
7. Listening to what I have to say. _____
8. Friendliness of my nurses. _____
9. Privacy provided by my nurses. _____

Technical Quality of Care

1. Skill of my nurses in doing procedures such as starting
    intravenous fluids, giving injections, enemas, or irrigations,
    and changing dressings.   _____
2. Knowledge of my nurses in taking care of patients with my
    condition.   _____
3. Explanations given to me by nurses regarding treatments,
    procedures, or medications.   _____
4. Teaching me how to do things for myself.   _____
5. Assisting me as needed with bathing.   _____
6. Assisting me with eating as needed   _____
7. Assisting me with toileting as needed.   _____
8. Organization of the nurse when caring for me.   _____

Physical Environment

1. Nurses kept supplies and things I needed in reach.   _____
2. Nurses straightened my tables and bed as needed.   _____
3. Nurses adjusted light in my room as needed.   _____
4. Nurses adjusted the temperature in my room as I needed.   _____
5. Nurses controlled the noise in my room.   _____

Availability

1. Getting a nurse when I needed one.   _____
2. Nurses checking on me and my condition.   _____
3. Nurses getting me what I need.   _____

Continuity of Care

1. Nurses follow through on things I need from one shift to another. _____
2. Different nurses from day to day or shift to shift know what I
    need without me telling them.   _____
3. The same nurses take care of me each day.   _____

Efficacy/Outcomes of Care

1. Nurses made me comfortable or relieved pain.   _____
2. Nurses made me feel calm and relaxed.   _____
3. Nurses made me feel secure.   _____
4. I felt prepared by the nurses for things that happened to me.   _____
5. Know what to do for myself during hospital stay.   _____
6. Know what to do for myself when I go home.   _____
7. Nurses made me feel clean and refreshed.   _____

DIRECTIONS FOR NUMERIC ESTIMATION (NE)

This booklet contains a series of lines of varying lengths. Please take a brief look through the booklet and note that some lines are longer than the first while others are shorter.

You will be asked to compare each of the lines to the first. The first line is your reference. We have given it the number 100. The number 100 is your reference or standard. All you need to do is write a number in the box for each line.

If a line seems longer than the reference line, you would write the number 200 in the box. If it is 10 times longer you would write the number 1000 in the box.

On the other hand, some of the lines are shorter than the reference. If the line is one-half as long, you would write the number 50, which is one-half of 100. Another line about one-tenth as long would be given the number one-tenth of 100, that is, 10.

Give each line a number, whatever number seems appropriate to express how the line compares to your reference line: The longer the line, the bigger your number compared to 100. The shorter the line, the smaller your number compared to 100. You may use whatever number you think is right.

ONCE YOU BEGIN, PLEASE DO NOT LOOK BACK TO CHECK OTHER NUMBERS OR LOOK AT THE REFERENCE LINE. WE ARE ONLY INTERESTED IN YOUR GENERAL IMPRESSIONS.

(Patients were presented with nine lines, one per page, of varying lengths for which they will make a numeric estimation).

DIRECTIONS FOR LINE PRODUCTION (LP)

This section contains a series of numbers of varying sizes. Please take a brief look through and note that some of the numbers are larger than the first, while others are smaller.

Your task is to draw a line representing each of the numbers. Each line you draw should be in comparison to the reference number and line on the first page. The first number is 100. We have drawn a line to represent 100. All you need to do is draw a line under the number of each page that you think represents that number.

If the number is larger than 100, you will draw a line larger than the reference line. For instance, if one of the numbers is 200, you would draw your line twice as long as the reference line. If the number is 150, you would draw your line 1 $^1/_2$ times as long as the reference line.

On the other hand, some of the numbers are smaller than the reference number of 100. If the number is 50, you would draw a line half the length of the reference line, which represents 100. The number 10 would be represented by a line of one-tenth the length of the reference line.

Draw a line for each number of whatever length seems appropriate to express how the number compares to the reference number line: The higher the number compared to 100, the longer the line you will draw. The smaller the number compared to 100, the shorter the line you will draw.

ONCE YOU BEGIN, PLEASE DO NOT LOOK BACK TO CHECK OTHER NUMBERS OR LOOK AT THE REFERENCE LINE. WE ARE ONLY INTERESTED IN YOUR GENERAL IMPRESSIONS.

(Patients were presented with nine numbers, one on each page, for which they will make line productions.)

PART V
Future Directions

25

Measurement of Clinical Outcomes for the Improvement of Nursing Care: Issues, Dilemmas, and Future Directions

Marianne K. Zalar

Nurse administrators, managers, and staff are very concerned about the realities of reduced budgets, decreasing hours of care, increased patient acuity, and decreased lengths of hospital stay. There is no question that this is a critical period for nurses, patients, and hospitals. The potential impact of the evolving methods of payment for health care services is great. Payment of health care services will be based on financial incentives intended to encourage cost control and to foster price competition. The first step toward this end was the passage of the prospective payment system for Medicare in 1983. Other third-party payors are rapidly moving to implement similar payment programs.

Before discussing the improvement of nursing care through measurement of clinical outcomes, it is necessary first to discuss some of the national issues relative to the future of health care services and then some of the issues affecting the conduct and measurement of clinical nursing research.

CHANGING HEALTH CARE DELIVERY SYSTEM

The future impact of this changing health care delivery system is dramatically reported in a study titled "Health Care in the 1990s: Trends and Strategies." The study was sponsored by the American College of Hospital Administrators and conducted by Arthur Anderson & Co. 1984, an international accounting and consulting firm. The purpose of the study was to determine the consensus of health care experts concerning the future direction of the health care system.

A survey sample of 1,000 experts was assigned to one of six panels. There was one panel for each of the following groups: hospital leaders, physicians, other providers (defined as nursing homes, extended care facilities, specialty care institutions, ambulatory care facilities, legislators/regulators, suppliers, and payors. At no place in the document is there any mention of nursing input. Quite possibly nurse administrators were included among the hospital leaders.

Time does not permit discussion of all of the findings from the study, but a few of the findings that are most germane to the discussion of clinical outcome measurement will be shared.

1. *Quality of care will be a concern:* There was 87% agreement that uninsured persons without the ability to pay will experience the most significant decline in the quality of health care services by 1995. Medicare and Medicaid beneficiaries will also experience a decline in services.

2. *More emphasis on wellness:* Wellness and preventive medicine programs are perceived to be making some contribution to lowering the cost of care. There is no coordinated effort, however, to educate the public about the necessity of preventive measures.

3. *Congress will define life and death:* Eight of 10 participants predict that by 1990 the Medicare program will limit the dollar expenditure for the extension of life for the chronically ill aged. Ninety-five percent of the panelists believe that by 1990 life and death will be defined legislatively to allow the withdrawal or nonuse of life support systems in cases of terminal illness.

4. *Patients will become prudent buyers:* According to 99% of the respondents, as patients become responsible for the greater share of their health care expenditures, their price awareness will increase. Almost all think that this development will increase competition among providers.

5. *No shortage of physicians or other health professionals:* Shortages are expected in relatively few health care professions. The panels were divided on the projected surplus or deficit of physician assistants, registered nurses, vocational nurses, nurse aides, and allied health personnel.

6. *Investor-owned hospitals will increase 60% by 1995:* Investor-owned hospitals will constitute 10% of the nation's hospitals by 1990 and 23% by 1995.

7. *Multihospital systems will grow significantly:* The respondents predict that over 40% of nongovernmental hospitals will be owned, leased, or controlled by multihospital systems by 1995.

8. *Productivity is a key to hospital financial success:* Attention to cost will be imperative. Because well over one-half of a typical hospital's costs are related to personnel, productivity improvements hold the most potential for substantially affecting operating expenses.

Panelists were asked to provide the three most innovative steps their organizations have taken in response to the introduction of prospective payment. For nursing, improved productivity measurement and monitoring was ranked first, reassignment of work tasks was ranked second, and improved employee training was ranked third.

These findings certainly make very clear to professional nurses the direction research efforts must take if nursing is to survive as a profession. There is no question, in light of these findings, that cost variables must be measured along with quality care measures. Donabedian (1985) has said that health care professions today are caught between the opposite pulls of two implacable imperatives: to maintain quality and to contain cost. Ideally, health professionals owe their allegiance to quality, but the demands for cutting costs have become increasingly more insistent and more skillfully orchestrated. Nurses are obliged to demonstrate that nursing care makes a difference. Research utilization must continue to be a top priority for the professional nurse.

Nursing research is one of the most valuable tools available for answering nursing administrative, educational, and clinical practice questions. Only through research can objective facts be obtained to support or refute cost-containment measures. Only through research, together with the systematic use of findings, can nursing improve its practice, demonstrate its value, and acquire the evidence that is necessary to influence its future.

Claire Fagin (1982) reviewed nursing research studies done over a 10-year period that reported cost-effective findings. Studies reviewed dealt with direct patient care, patient education, adding to patient-care knowledge, and alternatives to hospitalization. The cost-savings from all of the reported studies were very impressive. Nine of these studies documented a savings of $696,100 for their respective hospitals.

Two studies, one study cited by Dr. Fagin in her article and another study done at Stanford, show how two investigators dealt with cost/quality issues. Measel and Anderson (1979) studied restless premature infants who were developing intestinal distention. The researchers hypothesized that infants would become relaxed and could be tube-fed successfully if allowed to suck on a pacifier during and following each feeding. Measel and Anderson found that treated infants showed readiness for bottle feeding 3.4 days earlier and were discharged 4 days sooner than the control group.

The study was replicated. Findings were identical with regard to weight gain and readiness for bottle feeding. The 30 treated infants were discharged 8 days sooner. The actual cost savings reported was $104,000. The potential savings from this nursing intervention alone could yield $52 million a year nationally. The research funding for the first study was $4,000. This study is a very dramatic example of the contribution of nursing research to both quality of nursing care and cost-effective care for a very small expenditure of funds.

Joan Mersch, clinical nurse coordinator of the coronary care unit at

Stanford University Hospital, recently completed a study of 29 patients who underwent routinely scheduled cardiac cathetization (Dailey & Mersch, 1987). She wanted to determine whether room-temperature injectate or iced-temperature injectate correlated more closely with the Fick method for determining cardiac output. It was hypothesized that if room-temperature injectate provides equally accurate and reproducible cardiac output values, nursing time, patient cost, and contamination potential could be reduced.

Findings from her study showed that there was a higher correlation between the Fick method and the thermodilution method using room-temperature injectate ($r = 0.84$) than the thermodilution method using iced-temperature injectate ($r = 0.72$). There was also a high correlation ($r = 0.90$) between cardiac output values determined by the two thermal indicators, room injectate and iced injectate.

This study indicates that room-temperature injectate and iced-temperature injectate closely correlate with the Fick method for determining cardiac output and closely correlate with one another. Therefore, room-temperature injectate can accurately be used to determine cardiac output, thereby reducing nursing time, cost, and potential contamination.

Ms. Mersch's study (Dailey & Mersch, 1987) has quality care implications related to decreasing the potential of contamination, since contamination is an issue when iced-injectate syringes are stored in a water bath that has been identified as a source of contamination if syringes are not watertight. The use of room-temperature injectate removes that additional step. Nursing time required to prepare the iced injectate using sterile procedures will not be necessary if room-temperature injectate is used. Finally, patient cost will be reduced because it is not necessary to maintain injectate equipment and the increased supplies.

The two studies cited above are excellent examples of the quality of nursing clinical research that deals with both quality care and cost-containment issues.

Dr. Fagin (1982) suggests that nursing research, from an investment viewpoint, needs only to return $1.5 million per year on a $5-million investment. Hospital costs have reached over $100 billion per year. Therefore, if production costs are reduced by only 1.5 parts in 100,000 as a result of nursing research, that research is a good return on investment.

THE RESEARCH TEAM

Nurses obviously have considerable work to do in a short period of time 1990 is only 5 years away. All of the nursing talents available must be employed to take on the challenge of conducting research and utilizing research findings to provide cost-effective/quality care in a radically changing health care system.

The major responsibility for conducting research can no longer be the responsibility of the research academician alone. While the need for tested answers to vital questions in all areas of practice is immense, the lack of qualified investigators to meet the need is equally great. Of the 112 million employed nurses in the U.S. in 1980, only about 3,000 (0.0025%) had a doctorate and fewer than 6% of those were primarily engaged in research. It is obvious that 3,000 doctorally prepared nurse researchers cannot meet the current demand for nursing research.

The nursing administrator plays a very important role in facilitating clinical research. She legitimates research activity by nurses and formally recognizes nursing research through the institution's formal reward system (Davis,1981). For example, Duane Walker, director of nursing at Stanford University Hospital, established a department of nursing research within the administrative structure. Nursing research activities by staff nurses are included in the criteria for advancement in the clinical ladder for staff nurses.

The nurse manager also plays a key role in both the conduct of research and the utilization of research findings. A manager who is committed to research as an integral component of practice encourages staff nurse research on the unit, arranges scheduling so that staff nurses can attend research courses, is actively involved in the identification of practice-relevant research problems, and facilitates policy and procedure changes when indicated by the research findings.

Finally, clinicians who work in a research-supportive environment are anxious to participate actively in research activities. Carol Lindeman (1979) identified five factors that staff nurses have identified as important for an effective research program: (1) conducting the research in a manner that allows the staff to feel a part of the study, (2) adequate staff development either on "duty time" or as "time back", (3) integrating the research as part of the daily assignment, (4) adequate released time from patient care to participate in the planning phase, and (5) ready access to a prepared nurse researcher, preferably someone employed by the institution in a staff position.

Through the combined efforts of the clinician, researcher, administrator, and manager, an environment or the conduct of research and utilization of findings is made possible. The clinician is best able to identify clinically relevant research problems; the researcher assists the clinician to translate the clinical problem to a research problem and assists in proposal development. The administrator legitimizes and rewards research activities in the organization and the managers facilitate clinical research activities and implementation of findings.

ISSUES AFFECTING CLINICAL DECISION MAKING

Problems related to generalization of research findings, replication of studies, standardization of instruments, dissemination and utilization of clinical research findings, and evaluation of clinical outcomes are not new to nurse researchers and psychometricians. The nursing literature is replete with discussions of how these problems affect the state of the art of nursing research.

There is no question that these issues have an impact on clinical decision making. Therefore, some time will be spent discussing how these issues affect practice-relevant decisions from the perspective of clinicians, nursing administrators, and managers.

Impact on Clinicians

Through the use of research findings, nurses can improve patient care, promote higher standards of nursing, upgrade education programs, strengthen nursing services and organization, and advance the profession of nursing (Rettig,1981). For this to occur, the practicing nurse must be able to evaluate the quality of research before findings can be incorporated into practice. Unfortunately, many nurses are not prepared to critique research reports or make judgment calls regarding the clinical significance of research findings. This problem is confounded by the way research reports are written. The nurse who has had an introductory course in research as part of a baccalaureate nursing program or who has graduated from a two-year or three-year nursing program is not prepared to read reports of studies in journals such as *Nursing Research*. In addition, staff nurses seldom attend research conferences. When they do attend, they report feelings of inadequacy because they do not understand the language of the nurse scientist.

Even when a nurse is able to review published research findings critically, frustration often occurs. Frequently, there are no nursing studies in the topic area. Sometimes reports of excellent clinical studies are found, and the findings cannot be utilized in practice because they cannot be generalized to the patient population or to the work setting. Therefore, a replication of the study would be required before research utilization could occur.

There are times, however, when the clinician finds a report of a study that answers the clinical practice question, is generalizable to the patient population and setting, and would predictably improve patient care. The nurse must work in an environment where management and administration is receptive to change. In a receptive environment the nurse is able to develop a plan and evaluate the projected change from a quality/cost perspective to answer questions of interventive effectiveness. Once this has been done, policies and procedures must be written and in-service education conducted. Obviously, this process is very time-consuming and requires a great deal of commitment on the part of the clinician.

Dr. Elaine Larson (1983) has combined nursing quality assurance with the research program at the University Hospital in Seattle, Washington, in an attempt to facilitate the process of research utilization. She recognizes that there are certain disadvantages, but she believes that the advantages far outweigh the disadvantages because nursing research can be introduced into the clinical setting via quality assurance. When incorporated as part of quality assurance, studies are more likely to have clinical relevance. Results are more likely to be integrated into practice when programs are combined rather than separate. Finally, combined programs are more cost-effective.

Impact on Managers and Administrators

At no time in the recent history of nursing has there been a greater need to demonstrate that nursing care makes a difference in patient outcomes than now exists. Nurse managers and administrators are obliged to prove that safe (not quality) care is provided. There is no better ammunition than facts that can be given to administrators and hospital boards. Research can provide those facts.

Fawcett (1980) suggests that administrators must demonstrate their commitment to nursing research as the basis for practice in the following ways: (1) seeking personal self-development with respect to learning about the research process, change theory, and the practical application of research findings; (2) facilitating staff development toward familiarity with research methods and appreciation of research-based practice; and (3) hiring staff members who can demonstrate both the commitment and the ability to apply research-based knowledge to practice.

DEVELOPMENT OF RESEARCH SPECIALITY CENTERS

Collaborative efforts of nurse clinicians, researchers, administrators, and managers can make significant contributions to scientifically based nursing practice. Research speciality centers should be instituted in selected hospital-based departments of nursing research to do in-depth research on clinical topics like pain control, stress management, wound care, and nursing needs of the elderly hospitalized patient. A national body such as the ANA Council of Nurse Researchers might serve as the unifying group to facilitate judicious identification of problem areas, centralized recruitment of research centers, publication of center activities, and direction for funding.

The centers would assume responsibility for developing research protocols. When the pilot testing was completed, the center would issue a "call for collaborative research" to recruit research sites. (The calls would be patterned after the successful mechanism for soliciting papers for research conferences).

Staff from the center would supervise data collection from the research sites, process and analyze data, and disseminate findings through publications and presentations. The centers would also provide direction for utilization of clinically significant findings and evaluation of patient outcomes.

The advantages for this type of center are many:

1. The lag time between completion of research studies and dissemination of findings would be greatly reduced.
2. Large studies could be conducted, thus facilitating generalizability of findings to larger patient populations and settings.
3. It would conserve nurse researcher resources because studies would be centrally designed.
4. Smaller hospitals that do not have access to researchers, statisticians, psychometricians, and mainframe computers could actively participate in nursing research studies.
5. The center could serve as a central data bank.
6. It would be more cost-effective.

CONCLUSION

In conclusion, nurses are experiencing a crisis in the health care system. As a profession, nurses must collectively accept the challenge to offer quality nursing care to all patients regardless of their age, level of disability, or socioeconomic status. The development of speciality research centers is one example of how nurses might meet the challenge.

REFERENCES

Arthur Anderson & Co. (1987). *Health care in the 1990s: Trends and strategies* (Report prepared for the American College of Hospital Administrators). Chicago: Author. (Available from author, 33 West Monroe St., Chicago, IL 60603).

Dailey, E. K. & Mersch, J. D. (1987). Thermodilution cardiac output using room and ice temperature injectate: Comparison to the Fick method. *Heart and Lung, 16* (3), 294-300.

Davis, M. Z. (1981). Promoting nursing research in the clinical setting. *Journal of Nursing Administration, 11*, 22-27.

Donabedian, A. (1985). Quality, cost and cost containment. *Nursing Outlook, 32*, 142-145.

Fagin, C. (1982). The economic value of nursing research. *American Journal of Nursing, 12*, 1844-1849.

Fawcett, J. (1980). A declaration of nursing independence: The relation of theory and research to nursing practice. *Journal of Nursing Administration, 10*, 36-39.

Larson, E. (1983). Combining nursing quality assurance and research programs. *The Journal of Nursing Administration, 13*, 32-38.

Lindeman, C. A. (1979). Nursing research: A visible, viable component of nursing process. *Nursing Digest, 6*, 45-95.

Measel, C. P., & Anderson, G. C. (1979). Nonnutritive sucking during tube feedings: Effect on clinical course in premature infants. *Journal of Obstetrics and Gynecology, 8*, 265-272.

Rettig, F. C. (1981). Assessing research for clinical use. *American Operating Room Nurse's Journal, 33*, 873-880.

APPENDIX: Measurement of Clinical and Educational Nursing Outcomes Project: Project Participants and Topic Areas

Participant	Topic area
Lois Ryan Allen, R.N., M.A. Widener University Chester, Pennsylvania	Attitude Toward Computer-Assisted Instruction
Jean M. Arnold, R.N., Ed.D. Rutgers University Newark, New Jersey	Diagnostic Reasoning Protocols for Nursing Clinical Simulations
Patricia M. Bailey, R.N., Ph.D. University of Kentucky Lexington, Kentucky	Comparison of Ideal Values of Nurse Faculty and Values Taught
Betsy M. Barnes, R.N., M.S.N., C.C.R.N. Lander College Greenwood, South Carolina	Student Performance Evaluation Form – The Nurse as Teacher with Basic Knowledge
Elizabeth A. Barrett, R.N., Ph.D. The Mount Sinai Medical Center New York, New York	Measuring Quality of Nursing Care for DRGs Using the HEW-Medicus Nursing Process Methodology – A Pilot Study
Clarissa Beardslee, R.N., Ph.D. University of Pittsburgh Pittsburgh, Pennsylvania	Evaluation of the Advanced Clinical Nursing Component of a Graduate Program in Nursing in Preparing Students For "On-the-Job" Functioning
Doris R. Blaney, R.N., Ed.D., F.A.A.N. Indiana University Gary, Indiana	Development and Psychometric Analysis of a Scale to Measure Attitude Toward Cost-Effectiveness in Nursing
Patricia Bohachick, R.N., Ph.D. University of Pittsburgh Pittsburgh, Pennsylvania	Level of Physical Activity Questionnaire

Participant	Topic area
Marion E. Broome, R.N., Ph.D. Medical College of Georgia Augusta, Georgia	Development and Testing of an Instrument to Measure Children's Fears of Medical Experiences
Linda Brown, R.N., Ph.D. University of Chicago Chicago, Illinois	Information Processing and Actions Taken by Nurses in Response to Advanced Information Technology
Kathleen Buckwalter, R.N., Ph.D. Iowa University Iowa City, Iowa	Development and Testing of the Iowa Self-Assessment Inventory
Shirley Metz Caldwell, R.N., Ed.D. Vanderbilt University Nashville, Tennessee	Family Well-Being Assessment: Conceptual Model, Reliability, Validity, and Use
Shirley A. Carter, R.N., Ed.D. University of Delaware Newark, Delaware	Quantification and Analysis of Selected Intervening Variables Affecting Course Outcomes
JoAnn H. Collier, R.N., M.S. University of Akron Akron, Ohio	Impact of Computer-Assisted Decision Making in an Existing Diabetes Patient Education Program
Carol Collison, R.N., Ph.D. University of South Carolina Columbus, South Carolina	Family Functioning as Conceptualized from a Systems Perspective
Nancy S. Creason, R.N., Ph.D. University of Illinois Urbana, Illinois	Operational Definitions of Statements of Nursing in the PES (Problem, Etiology, Signs, and Symptoms) Format
Linda Cronewett, R.N., Ph.D. University of Michigan Chelsea, Michigan	Child Care Activities Scale
Ann D. Crutchfield, R.N., M.S.N. Kennesaw College Marietta, Georgia	Nursing Competencies Related to Assessment
Gail C. Davis, R.N., Ed.D. Texas Christian University Fort Worth, Texas	Measurement of the Clinical Outcomes of the Patient with Chronic Pain
Mary E. Duffy, R.N., Ph.D. University of Texas Austin, Texas	The Research Appraisal Checklist: Development and Validation of an Instrument to Appraise Nursing Research Reports

Participant	Topic area
Sandra R. Edwardson, R.N., Ph.D. University of Minnesota Minneapolis, Minnesota	Revision and Testing of the Haussman and Hegyrary Outcome Measure for Myocardial Infarction
Lillian Eriksen, R.N., D.S.N. University of Wyoming Laramie, Wyoming	Patient Satisfaction with Nursing Care: A Magnitude Estimation Approach
Sr. Mary Jean Flaherty, R.N., Ph.D. The Catholic University of America Washington, D.C.	Grandmother Functioning Scale
Martha J. Foxall, R.N., Ph.D. University of Nebraska Omaha, Nebraska	Evaluation of Measurements to Assess Family Response to Chronic Illness
Linda Holbrook Freeman, R.N., M.S.N. University of Louisville Louisville, Kentucky	Evaluation of Assertive Behavior in Registered Nurses Following a Continuing Education Program
Lorraine Gentner, R.N., Ph.D. Baylor University Dallas, Texas	A Proposal for the Development of a Tool to Measure Loneliness
Valerie D. George, R.N., Ph.D. Cleveland State University Cleveland, Ohio	Measuring the Sense of Coherence
Louise M. Givens, R.N., M.S.N. Children's Hospital National Medical Center Washington, D.C.	Clinical Competencies and Adjustment Levels of Nurse Orientees
Davina Gosnell, R.N., Ph.D. Kent State University Kent, Ohio	Development of a Reliable and Valid Instrument to Assess Persons' Potential Risk for Pressure Sores
Carol Gramse, R.N., Ph.D. State University of New York Stony Brook, New York	Assessment of Validity and Reliability of a Measure of Women's Health Beliefs Using the Multitrait, Multimethod approach
Elsie Gulick, R.N., Ph.D. Rutgers College of Nursing Newark, New Jersey	Development of the Self-Administered ADL Scale for Persons with Multiple Sclerosis
Blossom Gullickson, R.N., M.S. St. Olaf College Northfield, Minnesota	Development of a Simulated Clinical Performance Examination

Participant	Topic area
Ann Gunnett, C-N.P., M.S.N. University of Maryland Baltimore, Maryland	Improving Measurement of Student Clinical Performance
Cathie Guzzetta, R.N., Ph.D. The Catholic University of America Washington, D.C.	Development of a Protocol for Validating Nursing Diagnosis
Winifred B. Hagan, R.N., M.S.N. The Hospital of the Albert Einstein College of Medicine Bronx, New York	Nursing Staff Behaviors and Acutely Ill Older Adult Outcomes in a Twenty-Four Hour Reality Orientation Program
Donna Hawley, R.N., Ed.D. Wichita State University Wichita, Kansas	Development of a Questionnaire That Identifies Persons Who Have Symptoms Consistent with Fibrositis
Kathryn Hegedus, R.N., D.N.Sc. The Children's Hospital Boston, Massachusetts	Examination of Clinical Performance
Sharron Humenick, R.N., Ph.D. University of Wyoming Laramie, Wyoming	The MICAM: The Maturation Index for Colostrum and Mature Milk
Helen M. Jenkins, R.N., Ph.D. George Mason University Fairfax, Virginia	Clinical Decision Making Measured by the Clinical Decision Making in Nursing Scale
Joan M. Johnson, R.N., Ph.D. University of Wisconsin Oshkosh, Wisconsin	Assessment of Students in Relation to Curriculum Objectives and Correlated with Other Data
Colette Jones, R.N., Ph.D. University of Maryland Baltimore, Maryland	An Instrument to Measure the Perceptions of Both Fathers and Mothers Regarding Their Infants' Characteristics
Sarah Keating, R.N., C-P.N.P., Ed.D. Russell Sage College New York, New York	The Measurement of Client Outcomes In Home Agencies
Marguerite Kinney, R.N., D.N.Sc. University of Alabama Birmingham, Alabama	Development of a Protocol for Validating Nursing Diagnosis
Imogene King, R.N., Ed.D. University of South Florida Tampa, Florida	A Criterion-Referenced Measure of Goal Attainment

Participant	Topic area
Lark Kirk, R.N., M.S.N. Washington Hospital Center Washington, D.C.	Models in Nursing Care: Clinical Comparisons
Margaret Kostopoulos, R.N., M.S.N., C.N.A. Doctor's Hospital of Prince Georges County Lanham, Maryland	Reliability and Validity of the Registered Nurse Performance Evaluation
Janet W. Krejci, R.N., M.S., C.N.S. St. Michael Hospital Milwaukee, Wisconsin	Attributions of Chronic Pain Patients
Ursel Krumme, R.N., Ph.D. Seattle University Seattle, Washington	Measurement of Baccalaureate Students' Nursing Process Competencies: A Nursing Diagnosis Framework
Therese G. Lawler, R.N., Ed.D. East Carolina University Greenville, North Carolina	Measuring Socialization to the Professional Role
Helen Lerner, R.N., Ph.D. Lehman College Bronx, New York	Questionnaire Identification of Social and Intellectual Stimulation Available to Young Children in Their Home
Dona J. Lethbridge, R.N., Ph.D. University of New Hampshire Durham, New Hampshire	The Childbirthing Decision Aid
Margaret Louis, R.N., Ph.D. University of Nevada Las Vegas, Nevada	Nursing Instrument to Test Neuman's Conceptual Framework
Margaret Lunney, R.N., M.S.N. Hunter College-Bellevue New York, New York	The Concept of Nursing Diagnosis: Dimensions and Issues
Francine R. Margolius, R.N., M.S.N. Medical College of South Carolina Charleston, South Carolina	Coping of a Child and Family During Hospitalization
Beverly J. McElmurray, R.N., Ed.D. University of Illinois Chicago, Illinois	A Multidimensional Measure of Health in Older Women
Elizabeth McFarlane R.N., D.N.Sc. The Catholic University of America, Washington, D.C.	Determinants of Cardiovascular Patients' Compliance with Prescribed Health Regimens

Participant	Topic area
M. Denise McHugh, R.N., M.S. University of Wisconsin Oshkosh, Wisconsin	Nursing Assessment: Data Specified on Nursing Assessment Formats
Elaine McIntosh, R.N.C., M.S.N. Tennessee Department of Health and Environment Nashville, Tennessee	Women's Learning Needs Assessment Tool
Susan C. McMillan, R.N., Ph.D. University of South Florida Tampa, Florida	Reliability and Validity of Selected Measures of Chemotherapy-Induced Nausea and Vomiting
Michelle Miller, R.N., M.S. St. Michael Hospital Milwaukee, Wisconsin	Professional Practice Climate in Nursing
Barbara Mims, R.N., M.S.N., C.C.R.N. Parkland Memorial Hospital Lewisville, Texas	Development of a Clinical Performance Examination for Critical Care Nurses
Linda Moody, R.N., Ph.D. University of Florida Gainesville, Florida	Nursing/Health Policy Survey
Ann Morgan, R.N., M.S.N. University of Maryland Baltimore, Maryland	Measurement of the Impact of a Continuing Education Physical Assessment Course on Nursing Practice in a Selected Community Hospital
Doris E. Nicholas, R.N., Ph.D. Howard University Washington, D.C.	Measurement of Helping Outcomes in Nursing
L. Claire Parsons, R.N., Ph.D. University of Virginia Charlottesville, Virgina	Development of a Nurse Neurologic Assessment Tool
Mary Lou Peck, R.N., Ph.D. Russel Sage College New York, New York	Application of the Bondy Scale and Videotapes to Measure Short-Term Skill Development of Student Nurses
Shirley Pisarek, R.N., M.S.N. Veterans Administration Medical Center Hampton, Virginia	Perceptual Adaptation Differences in Medication Teaching

Participant	Topic area
Marjorie Ramphal, R.N., Ed.D. Columbia University New York, New York	Urinary Incontinence
Olive J. Rich, R.N., Ph.D. Temple University Philadelphia, Pennsylvania	Maternal Tasks in Taking on a Second Child
Judy Richter, R.N., Ph.D. University of Northern Colorado Greeley, Colorado	Reliability and Validity of the Lifestyle Assessment Questionnaire
Karen Robinson, R.N., M.S. Veterans Administration Medical Center Fargo, North Dakota	Denial and Anxiety in Second- Day Myocardial Infarction Patients
Joanne Scungio, R.N., Ph.D. University of Alabama Birmingham, Alabama	Parental Coping of Childhood Cancer
Ann Sheridan, R.N., Ed.D. Massachusetts General Hospital Boston, Massachusetts	Development of a Criterion- Referenced Tool to Measure Knowledge of Research Consum- erism: Phase I
Judith Shockley, R.N., M.S.N. University of Texas San Antonio, Texas	Advanced Placement Examination in BSN Programs: Development of Domain-Referenced Instruments
Bonnie Ketchum Smola, R.N., Ph.D. University of Dubuque Dubuque, Iowa	Refinement and Validation of a Research Tool to Measure Lead- ership Characteristics Of Bacca- laureate Nursing Students
Janet R. Southby, R.N., D.N.Sc. U.S. Army Nurse Corps Washington, D.C.	Attitudes About and Expectations of Graduate Nursing Education
Jacqueline Stemple, R.N., Ed.D. West Virginia University Morgantown, West Virginia	Self-Care Professional Role Ori- entation: Instrument Development
Nancy A. Stotts, R.N., Ed.D. University of California San Francisco, California	Testing a Wound Assessment Instrument
Cheryl B. Stetler, R.N., Ph.D. Massachusetts General Hospital Boston, Massachusetts	Development of a Criterion- Referenced Tool to Measure Knowledge of Research Consum- erism: Phase I

Participant	Topic area	*Appendix*

Sarah S. Strauss, R.N., Ph.D.
Medical College of Virginia
Hospitals, Richmond, Virginia

Information References and
Information-Seeking in Hospitalized Surgery Patients

N. Jean Stremmel, R.N., M.S.
University of Maryland
College Park, Maryland

Measurement of the Impact of a
Continuing Education Physical
Assessment Course on Nursing
Practice in a Selected Community
Hospital

Jane P. Taylor, R.N., M.S.
University of Delaware
Newark, Delaware

Clinical Testing to Measure Cognitive Behavioral Changes in
Nursing Students

Gladys Torres, R.N., Ed.D.
Brooklyn Veterans Administra-
tion Center
Brooklyn, New York

Multivariate Evaluation of a Collaborative Practice Project: Preliminary Impressions

James P. Turley
University of South Florida
Tampa, Florida

Measurement of Time as Tempo

Sandra Underwood, R.N., M.S.N.
Chicago State University
Chicago, Illinois

Measuring the Instructional
Validity of Computer-Based
Instruction in the Development of
Higher Level Cognitive Skills in
Nursing

Gwen van Servellen, R.N., Ph.D.
University of California
Los Angeles, California

The Individualized Care Index –
a Test of Discriminate Validity

Peggy L. Wagner, R.N., M.S.N.
St. Michael Hospital
Milwaukee, Wisconsin

Exhaustion of Adaptive Potential:
Measurement in the Clinical
Setting

Clarann Weinert, S.C., R.N.,
Ph.D.
Montana State University
Bozeman, Montana

Revision and Further Development of a Social Support Measure: The Personal Resource
Questionnaire

Mary Wierenga, R.N., Ph.D.
University of Wisconsin
Milwaukee, Wisconsin

Measurement of Diabetes
Well-Being

Janie Wilson, R.N., Ph.D.
San Antonio College
San Antonio, Texas

Clinical Evaluation of Students in
a Management Course

Constance Ziegfield, R.N., M.S.
Johns Hopkins
Baltimore, Maryland

Nursing Knowledge of Principles
of Chemotherapy Management: A
Criterion-Referenced Evaluation

Kenneth Zwolski, R.N., M.S., M.A.
Columbia University
New York, New York

Development of a Tool for the
Measurement of Ability to For-
mulate Nursing Diagnoses.

Index

A

Abaravich, W., 500
Abdellah, F., 523-524
Acceptance, 73, 300
   emotional, 365-366
   of illness, 231, 237, 240
Acceptance of Illness Scale, 231, 237,
   241-243, 244, 274-275
   scoring, 244
   validation, 247-252, 254-258
Accepted Diagnoses from the Fifth
   National Conference (Kim &
   Moritz), 459
Accessibility, of health care, 525, 526
Activities of Daily living (ADL), 29,
   30, 31, 40-41, 130
   assessment of ability to perform,
     111-112, 114, 119-128
   behavior response to, 113, 119-128
   and the elderly, 331
   and goal attainment, 111, 112, 113
   in multiple sclerosis, 129-130; *see*
     also ADL Self-Care Scale for
     Persons with Multiple Sclerosis
   physical ability to perform, 113,
     119-128
Adams, J.E., 234
Adams, T., 189
Adaptation, 8, 48, 49, 67, 400-401
Adherence, 82, 267
Adjustment, to chronic illness,
   236-238, 240
   vs. coping, 240, 241, 255
   definition of, 240
   family, 237, 241, 256
   measurement of, 241, 257, 258
ADL Self-Care Scale for Persons with
   Multiple Sclerosis, 129, 131,
   149-160
   Assistive Devices Checklist, 131,
     134, 135, 138-139, 140-144,
     157-158
   content, 132-133, 137-138, 139,
     141, 142-144
   development of, 131-133
   difference scores in, 142-143, 144
   MS-Related Symptoms Checklist,

     131, 134, 135, 139, 140-144,
     158-159
   pilot testing of, 134
   scale requirements, 132
   scoring, 133
   validation, 136-146
Administration on Aging, 328
Adriamycin, 222-223
Affect Balance Scale (ABS), 231, 237,
   241, 245, 247, 275
   Negative Affect Scale, 241-243,
     245
   Positive Affect Scale, 241-243, 245
   scoring, 245
   validation, 247, 248-252, 254-258
Affective behavior, changes in, 8-9
Age
   and denial, 57-58
   and pressure sores, 190
   and risk for colorectal cancer, 445
Alarm reaction, 8-9
Alcohol use
   and compliance, 85, 86, 88, 89,
     97-98, 106
   as coping behavior, 301
   in life-style assessment, 371
Alteration in Comfort: Pain
   (acute), 164
   (chronic), 162, 163, 164
Altmaier, E.M., 220-221
American Cancer Society, 445, 451,
   453
American College of Hospital Administrators, 541
American Nurses' Association, 25, 26
Amyotrophic lateral sclerosis, 191
ANA Council of Nurse Researchers,
   547
Anderson, G.C., 543
Anxiety, 204
   in acute myocardial infarction, 4, 8,
     12, 25, 28, 49, 57
   in chronic obstructive pulmonary
     disease, 236
   in chronic pain, 172
   and denial, 49-50, 51, 57, 58
   measurement of 28-31, 32-33,
     46-47, 51, 67

Anxiety, *(continued)*
    and nausea and vomiting, 220–221,
        224
    reduction of, 501
    situational, 51–57
    state vs. trait, 51, 54, 55–57, 224
    in surgical procedures, 65, 66
Anxiety–Depression (A–D) Scale for
    Medically Ill Patients, 12
Appel, A.A., 24
Appetite, and pain, 174, 183
Appraisal, of health care situation, 64,
    68
Art of care, nursing, 525, 526, 535
Arthritis Foundation, 169
Arthritis pain, 175
Arthur Anderson & Co., 541
Assistive devices, for multiple sclerosis
    patients, 134–135
Association for the Study of Pain, 162
Atkinson, J.H., 167
Attitude Toward Information Index
    (ATI), 62, 63, 67, 68, 69, 78
    scoring, 69, 74
    validation, 68, 75, 76, 78
Attitudes Toward Disabled Scale, 244
Atwood, J., 532
Auerbach, S.M., 62, 63, 66
Availability of nursing care, 525, 526,
    536

B

Backman, J.G., 403
Barbanel, J.C., 186
Bard, M., 399
Barthel Index, 110
Barton, A.A., 189
Baum, A., 63
Bayley Scales of Infant Development,
    426, 431–437
    administration of, 435–436
Beavers, W.R., 401
Beavin, J., 396
Beck Depression Inventory (BDI), 33,
    237
Bee, H., 425
Behavior Morale Scale, 238
Bell, J.M., 235
Berecek, K.H., 189
Bibring, G.L., 57
Bigelow, D.A., 74
Bigos, K.M., 57

Bille, D.A., 84
Billings, A.G., 299
Biofeedback, 301
Bittman, S., 190
Bloch, D., 25
Body map, 179
Bogdonoff, M.D., 237
Bothwell, S., 238
Bradley, R., 426, 428, 434, 438
Brandt, P., 310, 312
Breast cancer, 377, 443
    statistics, 377
    women's beliefs about, 377–378,
        379, 380, 390
Breast self-examination, 371, 377,
    378, 379, 390
Brief Sympton Inventory (BSI), 167
Bromm, B., 162
Brook, R.H., 24
Brown, B.W., 397
Brown, O.H., 237
Buros, O.K., 397
Bush, C.T., 90

C

Cady, P.,235
Caffeine intake, 85, 86, 88, 89,
    98–99, 107
Caldwell, Bettye, 423, 425, 426, 428,
    437, 438
Campbell, S., 388
Cantor, M.M., 25
Cantril Ladder, 237
Caplan, G., 309
Cardiac catheterization, 544
Cardiovascular disease; *see* Myocardial
    infarction
Carey, S., 500
Carmines, E.G., 258, 297
Carpenito, L.J.
    and acute vs. chronic pain, 161
    and nursing diagnoses, 459–460,
        463, 465, 466, 469–470
Carrieri, V., 309
Cassem, N.H., 48, 49, 50, 52
Catecholamines, 9
Cattell, R.B., 297
Chandler, D.I., 412
Chapion, V., 378
Chapman, C.R.,172
Chapman, J., 233, 500, 501
Chemoreceptor trigger zone (CTZ),

218
Chemotherapy
  administration, 224–225
  and nausea/vomiting, 216, 218,
    219–220
  as toxin, 220
  see also Adriamycin, Cytoxan,
    5-Flouracil
Cheung, B.S., 220
Chiarello, R.J., 238
Child, D., 297
Child Medical Fear Scale, 202
  development of, 207–209
  Fear Survey Schedule, 209
  psychometric testing or, 210
  scoring and administration, 209
  subscales, 209, 211
  validation, 210
Children
  defense mechanisms in, 15
  developmental delay in, 423–424,
    438
  and environmental stimulation,
    424–427
  and Family Response to Chronic Ill-
    ness Questionnaire, 281–282
  fear in, 203–204, 206–207: *see also*
    Children's medical fears
  interviews with, 213
  perceptions of stress, 412
Children's medical fears, 202–213
  testing for, 204–208
Chronic illness
  adjustment to, 236–238
  conceptual model, 239
  coping in, 234, 236–241
  family response to, 232, 241
  self-assessment in, 131
Chronic Impact and coping Instru-
    ment (CICI), 231, 241–242, 243,
    268–271
  scoring, 243
  validation, 247–258
Chronic obstructive pulmonary disease
    (COPD), 231, 232
  response of spouse in, 232, 241
  social behavior changes in, 236
  statistics on, 232
Chua-lin, C., 432
CIPP (context, input, process, prod-
    uct), 457–458
Clark, M.O., 186, 190
Clarke-Steward, K.A., 425
Classification Scheme for Client Problems

in Community Health Nursing, 459
Clay, E., 188
Coelho, G.V., 234
Cognitive appraisal, as coping, 240
Cohesiveness, family, 400
Colonoscopy, 450, 452
Colorectal cancer, 443–444
  case finding, 444, 445, 447, 452
  costs, 453–454
  detection, 444, 445, 453
  public attitude toward, 445–446
  risk factors, 445
  screening tests for, 444,445, 448,
    452–453; *see also* Fecal occult
    blood screening, Hemoccult test
  statistics, 443
Communication
  family, 403
  measuring, 126–127
  in multiple sclerosis, 156
  nonverbal, 127
  nurse–patient, 110
Community Adjustment Profile Sys-
    tem Questionnaire, 245
Community health nursing; *see* Home
    health care
Compliance, 82–84, 90–91
  change involved in, 86–87
  in colorectal cancer screening, 451
  determining, 87
  difficulty involved in, 87
  vs. noncomplicance, 83, 85
  studies on, 84
Compliance Questionnaire, 81, 84–89,
    93–108
  development of,81–82
  interview format of, 89
  judged compliance in, 88
  scoring, 85–87
  wife's judgment in, 88, 101–108
Compromise, as coping behavior, 300
Confidentiality
  in compliance interviews, 90
  in Wellness Inventory, 356, 362
Confrontive coping behavior,
    297–299, 303
Congestive heart failure, 9, 25
Connor, R.H., 485
Consciousness, 123–124
Control, 236, 300
  patient's perception of, 66, 67
Conway-Ratkowski, B., 83
Coons, C., 423, 428, 429, 434
Corsini, D.A., 425

Coping, 49, 233–236
  and adjustment, 240, 241, 255
  with chronic illness, 234, 236–241,
    253, 255
  and cognitive appraisl, 240
  information seeking as, 64, 65, 67
  measurement of, 241, 257,
    287–303, 306–308
  with pain, 174
  research on, 234
  strategies, 62, 66, 234,236, 238,
    257, 297–301
Coping Scale, 231, 241–242, 244,
  271–274
  scoring, 244
  validation, 247–250, 253, 256–258
  see also Jalowiec Coping Scale
Coronary Heart Disease Teaching
  Evaluation Form, 26
Countershock, 8
Cox, D.F., 65, 72
CPK-MB values, 5, 6, 15
Criterion-Referenced Measure of
  Goal Attainment Tool, 109,
  119–128
  scoring, 114
  subscales, 112
  validation, 15–116
Criterion-referenced tools, 110, 111,
  117, 193
  validity in, 115
Cronewett, Linda, 409
Croog, S.H., 233
Cytoxan, 222

D

Daubert, E.A., 476
Dean, A., 237
Decubitus ulcers; *see* Pressure sores
Devense mechanisms, 48, 50; *see also*
  Denial
Demographic Information Form, 243,
  246
Denial
  in chronic illnss, 240
  measurement of, 50; *see also,* Self-
    Appraisal Inventory
  in myocardial infarctaion,8–9,
    48–50, 51
Depression, 8, 25
  in chronic obstructive pulmonary
    disease, 236

  and chroic pain, 172
Derogatis, L.R., 238
Dickoff, J., 196
Diet
  in colorectal cancer screening, 445,
    448, 449
  in Compliance Questionnaire, 85,
    86, 88, 89, 93–94, 101–102
  and pressure sores, 193,. 201
Dimond, M., 238
Dinsdale, S.M., 189
Dirken, J.M., 233
Disability Status Scale, 130, 146
Doerr, B.J., 352, 356
Donabedian, A., 523, 543
Donner, F.J., 300
Dracup, K.A., 83
Drug abuse
  as coping behavior, 301
  in Wellness Inventory, 353,
    363–364
Dunn, M.A., 237, 244
Dyk, R.B., 232

E

Edwards, D.W., 245, 255
Efficacy, of nursng care, 525, 526,
  536
Egbuonu, L., 427
Elardo, R., 426
Elderly
  assessment of, 328–257
  community surveys of, 344–345
  and long-term care, 344
  pressure sores in, 190, 191, 193
Elkins, P.D., 206
Emesis; *see* Vomiting
Emotional management, 365–366
Emotive coping behavior, 298,
  299–300, 303
Endress, M.P., 66
Environmental stimulation, for children, 424
  measurement of, 427–428
  parents; role in, 424, 425
  research on 425
  and socioeconomic status, 425–427
Episode Coding Form, 475, 489–496
  methodology, 477–480
  subscales, 480, 481–483, 485
  validation, 480, 483–484
Exercise

in Compliance Questionnaire, 85, 86, 88, 89, 96, 104
as coping behavior, 297
measuring goal attainment in, 122–123
in Wellness Inventory, 353, 363
Exhaustion, 8
Expressive nursing care, 502
Exton-Smith, A.N., 187, 188

F

Fagin, Claire, 543, 544
Family
  adaptation, 400–401, 406
  cohesion, 400, 406
  illness in, 232, 241, 255–257, 258, 280–281, 402
  as interactional system, 396
  literature on, 397
  role processes, 401, 405
  satisfaction, 399, 406
  stress, 396, 397, 398–399
  structure, 398, 401, 405
  support, 399, 406
  vulnerability, 403, 405, 406
  well-being, 399, 400, 401, 405–407, 424; *see also* Family Well-Being Assessment
Family Environment Scale (FES), 397
Family Functioning Index, 397
Family Measurement Techniques (Straus & Brown), 397
Family Response to Chronic Illness Questionnaire, 231
  data collection and analysis, 246–247
  Ill Partner Version, 246
  Spouse Version, 246, 266–284
  subjects, 246
Family Stress Assessment (FSA), 396, 397
Family Structure and Effective Health Behavior (Pratt), 397
Family Well-Being Assessment (FWA) tool, 396, 398, 412, 417–422
  development, 407
  scoring and administration, 407–408
  subscales, 407, 408, 410, 411
  validation, 409–413
Fandal, A.W., 423, 428, 429, 433
Fawcett, J., 547

Fear, 240–207
  in children, 203–204, 206–207; *see also* Children's medical fears
  preoperative, 67
Fear Survey Schedule for Children (FSS-FC), 204–205, 206, 212
Fecal occult blood screening, 444, 445, 447, 448; *see also* Hemoccult test
Fellows, K., 524
Felton, G.J., 235, 237, 244, 245, 246, 253, 256
Fillenbaum, G.G., 329, 337, 339
Finances, and health care, 525, 526
Fink, D.K., 83
Fiske, S., 388
Fitzgerald, F.F., 233
5-Fluorouracil, 222, 223
Fleiss, J.L., 335
Flynn, K., 500
Folkman, S., 244, 245, 297, 299
Forrester, J.M., 191
Frankenburg, W.K., 243, 428, 429, 433
Freud, Anna, 48, 50
Frommer D., 447
Frytak, S., 217
Fuller, S., 66
Functional abilities, assessment of, 117

G

Gay, E., 423, 428, 429, 433
Giovanetti, P., 476
Gearson, L.W., 190
General adaptation syndrome (GAS), 7
General Health Questionnaire, 237
General systems theory, 240–241
George, L.K., 339
Goal attainment
  measuring, 109, 111, 119–128
  and nurse–patient goal setting, 110, 111
Gordis, K., 85
Gorsuch, R.L., 287
Gossett, J.T., 401
Guaiac resin, 445, 447, 448
Guilford, J.P., 288
Guzzettz, C.E., 4

H

Hackett, Thomas P., 48, 49, 50
Hackett-Cassem Denial Scale, 50–52
Hamburg, D.A., 234
Hammond, M.A., 428, 429
Hargreaves anxiety scale, 28
Harris, R.B., 237
Haussman, R.K.D., 26; *see also* Outcome measure for Myocardial Infarction
Health behaviors, 359–360; *see also* Wellness Inventory
Health beliefs, 378
  in Family Response to Chronic Illness Questionnaire, 270
  see also Women, health beliefs of
Health Beliefs Instrument, 377, 395
  purpose of, 378
  scoring, 381–382
  validation, 378–381,383–390
Health Care at Home (ANA), 475
"Health Care in the 1990s: Trends and Strategies," 541–541
Health hazard appraisal tool, 356–357
Health Information Form, 243, 246, 266–268
Hegyvary, S.T., 26; *see also* Outcome Measure for Myocardial Infarction
Hemoccult test, 443, 449–451, 454
  kits, 449, 451, 451
  objectivity, 450
  performance monitor, 449–450
  sensitivity of, 447–448, 450
Hemoglobin, 445, 450
Hettler, William, 352
Highriter, M.F., 476
Hilles, N.C., 237
Hinshaw, A.S., 503, 532
Hoffman, W.H., 448, 452
Hollenbech, A.R., 428
Holism, 82
Holmes, R.H., 404
Home health care 457–473, 475–486
  evaluation tool for, 466–473; *see also* Episode Coding Form
  and nursing diagnoses, 466–467, 471–472
  and record audit, 468–472
Home Observation for Measurement of the Environment (HOME), 423–424, 425, 426–428, 437
  administration of, 428

in development of Home Screening Questionnaire, 429–430
Home Screening Questionnaire (HSQ), 423, 424, 427, 430,438
  administration of, 432–433, 434
  definition of terms in, 431
  development of, 428–429
  ethnic breakdown of sample, 424, 427, 430, 431–432
  scoring, 429, 432–433
  validation, 429–430, 433–437
  wording, 434, 437
Hopkin's System Checklist, 237
Hospital discharge
  and patient knowledge, 35
  and stress, 4–5, 12–15
Hospital Fear Questionnaire (HFQ), 205–2206
Hospital Fear Scale, 204–205
Hospitalization
  in acute myocardial infarction, 4
  alternatives to, 543
  and children's fears, 203, 204
  for surgery, 63, 204
  see also Hospital discharge
Hospitals, investor-owned, 542
Hughes, L., 356
Human interaction, assessment of, 112, 117, 123–128
Hungler, B.P., 51
Hunter, K.L., 237
Hunter, M., 169
Hunter, W.S., 189
Husain, T., 187, 188
Hutchins, F.B., 352, 356
Hyman, R.B., 237
Humovich, D.P., 236, 243, 253

I

Index of Nausea and Vomiting (INV), 219, 222, 223, 225–226, 227, 228
Individualized Care Index (ICI), 499
  development of, 502–503
  ethnicity in, 510, 511–512
  modalities compared, 508–509, 510–513
  sample, 509–510
  scoring and administration, 504
  survey format, 499, 503, 508, 513, 516–518
  validation, 504–509, 510–514
Individualized nursing care, 499

studies of, 500–502
Infancy, 425, 543
Information preference, 62, 63, 68
  and dental surgery, 62–63
  and desire for control, 66, 67
  measurement of, 67
Information seeking
  in Family Response to Chronic Illness Questionnaire, 273–274
  and control, 67, 79
  as coping process, 65–66, 67
  see also Information-seeking Questionnaire
Information-seeking Questionnaire, 62, 67, 68
  categories, 73
  coding scheme, 72–73
  data collection for, 73–74
  scoring, 70
  validation, 71–73
International Federation of Multiple Sclerosis Societies, 130
Interpersonal Dependency Inventory, 237
Inventory of Registered Nurses, 503
Iowa Self-Assessment Inventory, 328, 345–346, 347–351
  administration of,336, 340
  applications, 343–344
  components of, 329, 332–333, 335, 336
  participants in, 332, 341
  rating criteria, 333–334
  scoring, 334, 336, 340
  validation, 335–337, 341–343
IQ score, 426, 428

J

Jackson, D., 396
Jacobs, G.A., 51, 53
Jalowiec Coping Scale, (JCS), 287, 306–308
  development of, 289–290
  scoring, 290
  three-factor model, 295–303
  validation, 288–289, 301–302
James, P., 196
Johnson, J.E., 62, 66
Johnson, M.H., 221
Johnson, W.L., 84
Joint Commission on the Accreditation of Hospitals, 25, 509

Jordan, M.M., 186

K

Kaplan, G.D., 381
Katz Index of ADL, 110
Keys, J.F., 412
Kiely, W.F., 299–300
Kim, J.O., 297
Klein, R.F., 237
Kobasa, S.C., 300
Kosiak, M., 188
Krantz, D.S., 63, 67, 68
Krantz Health Opinion Survey (KHOS), 62, 63, 64, 68, 69, 78
  scoring, 69, 74
  subscales, 63, 69, 75
  validation, 67, 68, 71, 75–78
Kremer, E., 167

L

Laborde, J.M., 237
LaDou, J., 356
Landermann, R., 339
Larson, Elaine, 452–453, 546
Launier, R., 64–65, 234, 236, 288
Lauzon, R.R.J., 356
Lawton, M.P., 329, 330, 339
Lazarus, R.S.
  on coping patterns, 65, 234, 235, 236, 297, 299
  on psychological stress, 64
  and Ways of Coping Scale, 244, 287–288
Levine, E., 523–524
Lewis, J.M., 401
Lewis, M., 426
Life satisfaction, 404, 407
Life Satisfaction Index A, 237
Lifestyle Assessment Questionnaire (LAQ), 352, 357–358, 361–375
  Alert section, 372–374
  Risk of Death section, 365–372
  Topics for Personal Growth section, 368–369
  Wellness Inventory; *see* Wellness Inventory
Light, R.J., 335
Lindeman, Carol, 459, 545
Lindsey, A., 309

Line Production (LP), 527–532, 537
Linkowski, D.C., 237, 244
Linn, B.S., 340
Linn, M.W., 237, 238, 340
Lipowski, Z.J., 299
LISREL, 290–297, 301–302
Lodge, M., 528, 530
Lofland, J., 208
Logue, T., 447
Long, J.S., 296
Long-term care, 344
Longitudinal Observation and Intervention Study, 427
Lushene, R., 51, 53

M

Maddi, S.R., 300
Mager, R.R., 111, 115
Magnitude scaling, 533
Maides, S.A., 381
Mankad, V.N., 431
Manley, M.T., 186, 190, 191
Manual of Nursing Diagnosis (Gordon), 459
Mapping sentence, 406–407
Marcus, T.LL., 425
Marram, G., 500
Marston, M.V., 84, 85
Martelli, M., 62
Mayman, M., 234
McCause, K.L., 196
McCreary, C., 172
McGill Comprehensive Pain Questionnaire (MCPQ, 161, 163, 175, 178–185
 components of, 163, 167–173
 development of, 164
 pain intensity rating scale, 173, 175
 validation, 169–172
McGill Pain Questionnaire (MPQ), 164, 166–167, 168, 169, 173
Masel, C.P., 543
Medicaid, 542
Medication
 compliance in, 85, 86, 87a–88, 89, 90, 93, 101
 and pressure sores, 191, 193, 199, 201
Meditation, 301
Menniner, K., 234, 235
Mental Development Index (MDI), 433, 435, 436, 437

Mental Measurement Yearbooks (Buros), 397
Mental Scale Record Form, 431, 432, 433, 435
 administration of, 435–436
Meir, Richard, 186
Meissner, W.W., 404
Meleis, A.I., 83
Melzack, R., 164, 167
Menke, E., 204
Mercuri, L.B., 62
Merrick, W.LA., 300
Mersch, Joan, 543–544
Method variance, 380
Methvan, D., 500–502
Miller, M.E., 187
Minnesota Multiphasic Personality Inventory, 237
Minuchin, S., 401
Mirabile, C.S., 223, 227
Money, K.E., 220Mood
 and chronic obstructive pulmonary disease, 236
 and pain, 173, 174, 183–184
Mood Adjective Checklist, 66
Moos, R.H., 234, 299, 330, 397
Morell, D., 220
Morrow, G.R., 220, 224, 237
Morrow Assessment of Nausea and Emesis (MANE), 222, 224, 225–226, 227
Motion sickness, 218
 and ingested toxins, 219–220
Motion Sickness Susceptibility Questionnaire (MSS), 222, 223–224, 225, 226
 predictive ability, 227, 228
Moughton, M., 83
Movement
 assessment of, 112, 117, 121–123
 and pressure sores, 188–189
Mueller, D.C., 297
Mueller, D.P., 245, 255
Muhlenkamp, Ann, 314, 315
Mulholland, J., 189
Multidimensional Functional Assessment Questionaire (MFAQ), 328, 332
Multihospital systems, 542
Multilevel Assessment Instrument, 329
Multiple sclerosis
 ADL strengths and deficits in, 129
 characteristics of, 130
 patients tested, 136–137

self-assessment in, 129–130
Multitrait multimethod (MTMM)
    approach, 378, 380–381, 390
    matrix, 382, 388, 389 390
    statistical analysis, 383–386
Murphy, S., 299
Myocardial infarction, 3–15, 25–35,
    37–47
    compliance in, 81
    see also Compliance Questionnaire
    definition of, 5
    see also Denial
    morality/morbidity, 3–4, 25, 49
    and outcome evaluation measures,
      25–26, 34
    and psychosocial adjustment, 25
    responses to, 48–49
    second-day patients, 48–61
    spouse support in, 81–82
    stress in, 4, 8–9, 13–15, 48, 233
    variables influencing, 5–6, 13,
      14–15, 25

N

Nakamura, C.Y., 204, 205
Nasogastric Intubation Checklist, 66
National Conference for Classification
    of Nursing Diagnosis, 161
National Group for the Classification
    of Nursng Diagnosis, 459
National Multiple Sclerosis Society,
    133, 135, 149
Natow, A.B., 190
Nausea, 217–218
    anticipatory, 220, 224
    and anxiety, 221
    causes of, 217
    chemotherapy-induced, 216, 220
    measuring, 218, 221–228
    post-treatment, 224
    and vomiting, 217
Nickerson, F.T., 240
Nicol, S.M., 186
Nitrogen balance, 189
Noncompliance, 83
    ethical issues in, 90, 91
Norbeck, J., 309
Norm-referenced tools, 9, 110,526
Norris, C.M., 217
Norton,D., 187, 192, 193, 194
Norton Scale, 192–193, 194
Nucholls, K.B., 405

Numeric estimation (NE), 527, 528,
    529, 530, 536–537
Nunnally, J.C., 297, 318, 384
Nurse clinician, 545–547
Nurse manager, 545, 547
Nursing, 459, 541–548
    assessment of, 25, 26, 110
    care behaviors, 503
    and chemotherapy-induced nausea/
      vomiting, 216, 228
    and children's home environment,
      426, 438–439
    and children's medical fears,
      202–203, 213
    and chronic pain, 161, 174–175
    and colorectal cancer screening,
      444, 450, 451, 452, 454
    communication in, 110, 502
    and compliance, 82, 83, 90–91
    costs, 526, 543
    and denial behavior, 49–50, 51, 59
    diagnosis categories, 459; *see also*
      Nursing diagnoses
    and familes with chronic illness, 258
    goal attainment in, 109–110, 114,
      116–118
    and health beliefs, 377–378
    and health-related information, 62,
      63
    and home health care, 485–586; *see
      also* Home health care
    and individualized care, 499, 502
    measurement of quality of, 457,
      500, 523–524
    modalities of, 508–509, 510–514
    and myocardial infarction patients,
      4, 9, 14, 24, 28, 59
    and multiple sclerosis, 131
    patient comments on, 523–525
    and pressure sore prevention, 192,
      196
    primary, 500, 509, 513
    research, 543–548
    role in post-discharge incidents, 4, 9
    and self-care, 453
    and stress reduction, 4, 9, 15, 48
    and therapeutic alliance, 83, 91
    and wellness life-style, 352, 354
Nursing administrator, 545, 547
Nursing Care Survey, 516–518
Nursing Child Assessment Program
    (NCAP), 426, 428–429
Nursing diagnoses, 460, 451, 465,
    475, 485–486
    Alteration in Comfort: Pain, 161

Nursing diagnoses, *(continued)*
  categories, 459, 462, 476; *see also*
    Patient classification
  vs. medical diagnoses, 470
  and record audit, 468–469
  validation of, 470–471
Nurturant behavior, 313–314
Nutrition
  assesment, 353, 355, 362–363
  knowledge, 45–46
  and pressure sores, 189–190
Nyman, B.A., 426

O

O'Brien, M.F., 83
Older Americans Resources and Services (OARS)
  components of, 330
  program, 328–331, 332
Orem, D.E., 131, 132, 143, 146, 453
Ott, C.R., 238
Outcome evaluation, 109
  in assessing nursing care, 24–26, 34,
    35, 109, 460, 463–464, 468; *see
    also* Outcome Measure for Myo-
    cardial Infarction, Nursing
    diagnoses
  in home health care, 460, 463, 464,
    468, 475, 485
  as method of determining compli-
    ance, 87
  studies of, 475–477
  see also Efficacy
Outcome Measure for Myocardial
  Infarction, 24, 26–35, 37–47
  administration and scoring, 28
  anxiety subsale, 29, 30, 32, 32–35
  development of, 26
  evaluation of, 35
  knowledge subscales, 29–31, 41–46
  revision of, 27–28
  validation, 29–34

P

Padila, G.V., 62, 66
Pain, 172
  acute vs. chronic, 161, 165, 173
  attitude toward, 171, 174, 184
  definition of, 162
  demographic data on, 166

effects of, 173–174
measurement of; *see* McGill Com-
    prehensive Pain Ques-
    tionnaire
modifiers, 171, 174
retrospective reporting of, 173
Pain Center, Montreal General Hospi-
    tal, 166
Pain language, 172
Pain rating index (PRI), 163, 167
Palliative coping behavior, 298, 300,
    303
Parents, 403–404, 425
  expectations of, 426
  interaction with chidren, 426
Parrish, J., 74
Patient classification, in home health
    care, 475–479, 480–486
  indices, 480, 483, 486
Patient kowledge, 4, 29, 30, 31, 35,
    41–46, 543
Patient satisfaction, with nursing care,
    523–526
Pavlou, M., 238
Payment systems, 541
Pearlin, L.I., 234, 235, 244
Pederson, F.A., 426
Pelvic pain, 172
Performance Evaluation Procedure,
    25
Performance of Nursing Actions,
    519–522
Perkins, R., 524
Perry, P.R., 237
Personal hygiene, measurement of,
    112, 117, 119–121
Personal Resource Questionnaire
    (PRQ), 309, 310 311, 319,
    321–327
  administration and scoring, 311
  development of, 310, 312, 313
  PRQ-85 version, 313, 315, 319,
    321–327
  subscales, 315–318
  validation, 312–313, 315–318
Peterson, N.C., 190
Pettegrew, L., 397, 405
Phaneuf, M., 25, 459
Philadelphia Geriatric Center, 329
Philips, C., 169
Phillips, V.A., 401
Physical environment, in nursing care,
    525, 526, 536
Pless, I.B., 397

Polit, D.V., 51
Polypoid lesions, 444, 452
Popham, W.J., 115
Poouissant, A.F., 427
Powerlessness, 299
Powers, M.J., 233, 235, 236, 237
Pratt, L., 397, 399, 402, 403, 404,
    405
Present pain intensity (PPI), 163, 167,
    170
Pressure, 187, 188
Pressure Sore Risk Assessment
    tool, 186, 198–201
  criteria for selection of subjects, 194
  development of, 192–193
  modification of, 193
  scoring, 194
  validation, 195
Pressure sores, 187–188, 193
  and age, 190
  and blood pressure, 191
  causes, 187–191
  diseases most com-
        monly contributing to, 190–191
  and medications, 191
  and mobility, 188–189
  and moisture, 189
  and nutrition, 189–190
  prevention costs, 186
Prieto, F.G., 167
Profile of Mood States (POMS), 67,
    68, 78
  scoring, 70, 74
  subscales, 71, 76, 78
  validation, 76
Protein metabolism, and pressure
    sores, 189
Pruyser, P., 234
Psychophysiologic Distress Index, 237
Psychophysiological Stress Model, 7
Psychosocial Adjustment to Illness
    Scale, 238
Psychosomatic symptoms, 404, 412

Q

Qualpacs instrument, 503

R

Rachman, S., 169
Rahe, R., 404

Rawlinson, M.F., 237
Reading, A.E., 172
Recent Life Changes (RLC) Question-
    naire, 233
Record audit, 468–469
Reddy, M.P., 189
Reeder, I., 233
Reiber, G.E., 196
Reichel S.M., 189
Research specialty centers, 547–548
Research utilization, 543–544,
    5464–547
Research team, 544–545
Resignation, as coping strategy, 300
Revenson, T.A., 244, 245
Rheumatoid disease, 162, 165
Rhodes, V.A., 219, 221, 223
Rice, V.H., 66
Robbins, P.R., 299
Roberts, M.C., 206
Role processes, 401
  ambiguity, 405, 407
  conflict, 402, 407
  overload, 402, 407
  nonparticipation, 403, 407
  preparedness, 403–404, 407
Role Tension Index, 237
Rosen, J.L., 57
Rosenbaum, M.S., 431
Rosenberg, M.I., 244
Rosenstock, I.M., 376
Rossi, A., 403
Rowland, B.L., 475
Rowland, H.S., 475
Rubin, C.F., 190
Rubinstein, J.L., 425
Rudd, T.N., 187, 188, 189
Ryan, J., 83

S

Sachs, M.L., 187
Sackett, D.L., 82, 83
Satisfaction with Nursing Care
    Questionnaire, 523, 526,
    535–537
  development of 526–528
  respondents, 529, 533–534
  scoring and administration, 526
  validation, 528, 529–533
Satterwhite, B., 397
Scalzi, C., 49
Schar, M., 233

Scherer, M.W., 204, 205
Schlottfeldt, R.M., 500–501
Schnell, V., 189
Schooler, C., 234, 235, 244
Self-Appraisal Inventory, 48, 51, 61
  administration and scoring, 52–53
  development of, 52
  validation, 58–59
Self-assessment, 343, 344
  components of, 131
  in multiple sclerosis, 129–130
Self-blame, 273
Self-care behavior, 130, 131, 135, 453
  assessment of, 353, 355, 352
  requisites, 131
Self-Concept Instrument, 237
Self-discipline, as coping strategy, 234
Self-esteem, 8, 240, 399
Self-Esteem Scale, 231, 237, 241–243, 244–245, 275–276
  scoring, 245
  validation, 247–252, 254–258
Self-Evaluation of Life Function, 340
Self-report, of compliance, 87–88, 91
  discrepancies in, 88
  of vomiting severity, 219, 224
Selye, Hans 7–8
Sensory dysfunction
  measuring, 124–126
  in multiple sclerosis, 130, 156
Shannon, M., 186, 189, 191, 196
Shantin, L., 237
Sharma, K., 219
Sherwin, M.A., 187, 188
Sherwood, J.N., 356
Shock, 8
Sibling rivalry, 399
Sickness Impact Profile (SIP), 34, 238, 244
Sidle, A., 235, 301
Sigmoidoscopy, 450
Silber, F., 234
Sime, A.M., 65
Simmons, D.A., 476–477, 478, 480
Situational Attitude Schedule, 237
Slavonic, M.J., 338–340
Sleep
  as coping behavior, 300
  measuring goal attainment in, 1233
  and pain, 174, 183
Smoking
  and Compliance Questionnaire, 85, 86, 88, 89, 97, 105–106

and Lifestyle Assessment Question-
  naire, 368–369
Smyer, M.A., 329, 337
Snyder, C., 427, 428
Social Adjustment Scale Self-Report
  (SAS-SR), 231, 241–243,
  245–246, 276–283
  scoring, 246
  validation, 247–252, 254–258
Social Dependency Scale, 131
Social Interaction Inventory, 500–501
Social Readjustment Rating Scale
  (SRRS), 233
Social support
  definition of, 310, 315
  dimensions of, 315
  studies of, 309
  see also Spouse support
Spielberger, C.D., 51, 53, 57
Spouse support, 81–82
Stanford-Binet testing, 427–428
Stanitis, M.A., 83
Stafrield, B., 428
State-Trait Anxiety Inventory (STAI),
  53–54, 57, 237
  and chemotherapy, 222, 224,
  225–227
  and Outcome Measure for
  Myocardial Infarction, 32–35
Statistical Package for the Social Services
  (Nie et al.), 467, 480
Sternbach, R.A., 172
Steward, M.I., 162
Stimulation; *see* Environmental
  stimulation
Stillman, M., 378, 383, 386
Straus, M.A., 397
Streissguth, A.P.426
Stress
  and changes in affective behavior,
  8–9
  in chronic illness, 232, 240–241,
  253, 255
  and coping behavior, 238, 240,
  297–301
  definition of, 5
  emotional response to, 65–66
  family, 399, 400, 402, 403, 404,
  406, 412
  and health information, 62
  and hospital discharge, 4–5, 13–15
  of hospitalization, 204, 205
  job-related, 403
  and learning, 4

measurement of, 4–5, 233, 241, 258
and physiologic changes, 9
psychophysiologic model, 7, 9
and spouse of ill partner, 232,
255–256
variables influencing, 13–15
Stress of Discharge Assessment Tool
(SDAT), 3, 5, 9–16, 19–23
development of, 10–11
and implications for nursing, 15
revision of, 13–14
scoring, 10
testing of, 11
validation, 11–12, 14
Stufflebeam, D.L., 457
Sugjective Stress Scale (SSS), 233
Surgery patients, 62–63
Sutherand, A.M., 232

T

Tagliacozzo, D., 524
Tanck, R.H., 299
Taylor, L.L., 288, 299, 300
Taylor Manifest Anxiety Scale, 237
Team nursing, 508
Thematic Apperception Test, 235
Therapeutic alliance, 82–83
Thomas, R.C., 396, 397, 398
Tissue destruction, 189; *see also*
Pressure sores
Tissue Trauma Research Center, 186
Torgerson, W.S., 167
Total patient care (TPC), 508, 510
Trait variance, 380
Treece, E.W., 92
Treece, J.W., 92
Treisman, M., 219–220
Trimble, H.C., 187, 188, 191
Tsu, V.D., 234

V

Vagg, P.ER., 51, 53
Value Survey, 381, 394
Van der Veen, F., 402
Van Ergen, I.F., 426
Vasoconstriction, 9
Vernon, D.T., 74
Vestibular system stimulation, in
emesis, 219–220
Viney, I.L., 234

Visual analog scale (VAS), 167, 169,
381
instructions for, 173
Vomiting, 218–219
anticipatory, 220–221, 224
and anxiety, 221
chemotherapy-induced, 216, 218,
219–220
measuring, 221–228
post-tratment, 224
symptoms associated with, 219
Vulnerability, 404, 405, 406

W

Wagman, W.J., 245, 255
Walcott, I., 189
Walker, Duane, 545
Wallston, B.S., 381
Wallston, K.A., 381
Ward, M.J., 459
Ware, J., Jr., 525, 532
Watson, P.M., 221
Watzlawich, P., 396
Ways of Coping Scale, 235, 287–288
Weight loss, 85–86, 89, 94–95,
102–103
Weisman, A., 299
Weiss, R., 313
Weissman, M.M., 238, 245
Wellness Inventory, (Lifestyle Assess-
ment Questionnaire), 352,
362–368
components of, 353
development of, 354
scoring and administration, 353
validation, 354–357, 358–359
Westbrook, M.T., 234
Westlake, S.K., 288, 299, 300
White, H., 300
White, R.W., 240
Whitehead, A.N., 453
Wideman, M., 63
Wilhite,H., 432
Williams, A., 187
Wilson, C.D., 426
Wishnie, H.A., 49
Women
and colorectal cancer, 451
health beliefs of, 376–378, 379,
380, 390
see also Breast cancer, Breast self-
examination

Woog, P., 237
Workshop/Symposium on Compliance
    with Therapeutic Regimens, 82
Wortman, C., 309

Y

Yarrow, L.J., 425, 437
Yarvis, R.M., 245, 255
Yeagley, S.C., 412

Z

Zang Self-Rating Depression Scale,
    237
Zelditch, M., 501
Zeldow, P.B., 238
Zeller, R.A., 258, 297
Ziemer, M.M., 66
Zimmer, M., 25, 26
Zimmerman, M., 162
Zingale, H.C., 245, 255

Springer publishing company

Identification of the *Nursing Minimum Data Set*

Harriet H. Werley
Norma M. Lang
Editors

In this book a group of the nation's leading nurses, along with health policy spokespersons and information systems experts, develop a Nursing Minimum Data Set (NMDS) — a groundbreaking step in the development of nursing knowledge. The NMDS enables nurses to use the capabilities of computers to assemble comparable nursing data across clinical populations, geographic areas, and time, through use of consensually derived data categories, variables, and uniform definitions. The availability of comparable nursing data would be a boon to nursing research, help identify trends and develop guidelines for nursing practice, provide necessary information for decisions on the cost and allocation of nursing resources, and give health administrators and policy makers a more complete overview of the health manpower scene. Contributors include Faye Abdellah, Phyllis Giovannetti, Lucille A. Joel, and Margaret D. Sovie.

"This book is a rich and timely contribution to nursing and other health fields. . . . The editors have provided nurses with a challenge for the future. Not only is the volume a collection of scholarly chapters of which one can be proud, but it also gives each of us in nursing a framework and proposes a set of data by which we can study nursing and describe it more fully. These data will enable us to portray nursing as it really is — a discipline in its own right. . . ." —from the Foreword by
Myrtle K. Aydelotte, R.N., Ph.D., F.A.A.N.
496pp / 1988 / $44.95

Order from your bookdealer or directly from publisher.

Springer Publishing Co. 536 Broadway, New York, NY 10012